Preoperative Assessment and Management

Second Edition

Edited by

BobbieJean Sweitzer, MD
Associate Professor of Anesthesia and Critical Care
Director, Anesthesia Perioperative Medicine Clinic
University of Chicago
Chicago, Illinois

Wolters Kluwer | Lippincott Williams & Wilkins
Health

Philadelphia · Baltimore · New York · London
Buenos Aires · Hong Kong · Sydney · Tokyo

Acquisitions Editor: Brian Brown
Managing Editor: Nicole Dernowski
Project Manager: Rosanne Hallowell
Manufacturing Manager: Kathleen Brown
Marketing Manager: Angela Panetta
Design Coordinator: Holly McLaughlin
Cover Designer: Becky Baxendell
Production Services: Aptara Inc.

Second Edition
**© 2008 by LIPPINCOTT WILLIAMS & WILKINS, A WOLTERS KLUWER
BUSINESS**
530 Walnut Street
Philadelphia, PA 19106 USA
LWW.com

First edition © 2000 by Lippincott Williams & Wilkins

Printed in the United States

Library of Congress Cataloging-in-Publication Data

Preoperative assessment and management /
[edited by] BobbieJean Sweitzer.—2nd ed.
   p. ; cm.
   Rev. ed. of: Handbook of preoperative assessment and management.
   Includes bibliographical references and index.
   ISBN-13: 978-0-7817-7498-7
   ISBN-10: 0-7817-7498-5
   1. Preoperative care—Handbooks, manuals, etc.   I. Sweitzer, BobbieJean.
II. Handbook of preoperative assessment and management.
   [DNLM: 1. Preoperative Care—methods—Handbooks.   2. Risk
Assessment—methods—Handbooks. WO 39 H2365 2008]
   RD49.H364 2008
   617´.9192—dc22

                                                    2007042806

Care has been taken to confirm the accuracy of the information presented and to
describe generally accepted practices. However, the authors, editors, and publisher
are not responsible for errors or omissions or for any consequences from application
of the information in this book and make no warranty, expressed or implied, with
respect to the currency, completeness, or accuracy of the contents of the publication.
Application of this information in a particular situation remains the professional
responsibility of the practitioner.

The authors, editors, and publisher have exerted every effort to ensure that drug
selection and dosage set forth in this text are in accordance with current
recommendations and practice at the time of publication. However, in view of
ongoing research, changes in government regulations, and the constant flow of
information relating to drug therapy and drug reactions, the reader is urged to
check the package insert for each drug for any change in indications and dosage and
for added warnings and precautions. This is particularly important when the
recommended agent is a new or infrequently employed drug.

Some drugs and medical devices presented in this publication have Food and
Drug Administration (FDA) clearance for limited use in restricted research settings.
It is the responsibility of the health care provider to ascertain the FDA status of
each drug or device planned for use in their clinical practice.

The publishers have made every effort to trace copyright holders for borrowed
material. If they have inadvertently overlooked any, they will be pleased to make
the necessary arrangements at the first opportunity.

To purchase additional copies of this book, call our customer service department
at (800) 639-3030 or fax orders to (301) 223-2320. International customers should
call (301) 223-2300.

Visit Lippincott Williams & Wilkins on the Internet at: lww.com. Lippincott
Williams & Wilkins. Customer service representatives are available from 8:30 am to
6 pm, EST.

                                        10 9 8 7 6 5 4 3

To Stephen, Sydney, Sheridan, Schuler and Gypsy.
The "Ss" have sacrificed time and attention
so I can accomplish, and "G" requires long walks
which allow me to ponder.

Contents

Contributors

Angela M. Bader, MD, MPH *Associate Professor, Department of Anesthesiology, Pain and Perioperative Medicine, Harvard Medical School; Director, Weiner Center for Preoperative Evaluation, Department of Surgical Services, Brigham and Women's Hospital, Boston, Massachusetts*

Jane C. Ballantyne, MD, FRCA *Associate Professor of Anesthesiology, Harvard Medical School; Chief, Division of Pain Medicine, Department of Anesthesia and Critical Care, Massachusetts General Hospital, Boston, Massachusetts*

Darin J. Correll, MD *Instructor, Department of Anesthesia, Harvard Medical School; Director, Postoperative Pain Service, Department of Anesthesiology, Perioperative and Pain Medicine, Brigham and Women's Hospital, Boston, Massachusetts*

Thomas Cutter, MD, MAEd *Associate Professor, Associate Chairman, Department of Anesthesia and Critical Care, Pritzker School of Medicine, University of Chicago; Medical Director for Perioperative Services, University of Chicago Medical Center, Chicago, Illinois*

Evans R. Fernández Pérez, MD *Instructor in Medicine, Department of Pulmonary and Critical Care Medicine, Mayo Clinic College of Medicine; Fellow, Department of Pulmonary and Critical Care Medicine, Mayo Clinic, Rochester, Minnesota*

Lynne R. Ferrari, MD *Associate Professor, Department of Anesthesia, Harvard Medical School; Medical Director, Perioperative Services, Department of Anesthesia, Critical Care, Pain and Perioperative Medicine, Children's Hospital, Boston, Massachusetts*

Lee A. Fleisher, MD *Robert D. Dripps Professor, Department of Anesthesiology and Critical Care, University of Pennsylvania; Robert D. Dripps Professor and Chair, Department of Anesthesiology and Critical Care, Hospital of the University of Pennsylvania, Philadelphia, Pennsylvania*

Robert R. Gaiser, MD *Professor, Department of Anesthesiology and Critical Care, University of Pennsylvania; Vice Chair for Education, Department of Anesthesiology and Critical Care, Hospital of the University of Pennsylvania, Philadelphia, Pennsylvania*

Ognjen Gajic, MD, MSc, FCCP *Assistant Professor of Medicine, Department of Internal Medicine, Division of Pulmonary and Critical Care Medicine, Mayo Clinic College of Medicine, Rochester, Minnesota*

David B. Glick, MD, MBA *Assistant Professor, Department of Anesthesia and Critical Care, University of Chicago; Medical Director, PACU, Department of Anesthesia and Critical Care, University of Chicago Hospitals, Chicago, Illinois*

Susan B. Glick, MD *Associate Professor of Medicine, Department of Internal Medicine, University of Chicago; Associate Professor of Medicine, Department of Medicine, University of Chicago Hospitals, Chicago, Illinois*

David L. Hepner, MD *Assistant Professor, Department of Anesthesia, Harvard Medical School; Associate Director, Weiner Center for Preoperative Evaluation, Staff Anesthesiologist, Department of Anesthesia, Perioperative and Pain Medicine, Brigham and Women's Hospital, Boston, Massachusetts*

Amir K. Jaffer, MD *Associate Professor of Medicine, Department of General Internal Medicine, Cleveland Clinic Lerner College of Medicine; Medical Director, IMPACT Center, Department of General Internal Medicine, Cleveland Clinic, Cleveland, Ohio*

P. Allan Klock, Jr., MD *Associate Professor, Department of Anesthesia and Critical Care, University of Chicago; Vice Chair for Clinical Affairs, Department of Anesthesia and Critical Care, University of Chicago Medical Center, Chicago, Illinois*

Ajay Kumar, MD, MRCP *Clinical Assistant Professor of Medicine, Cleveland Clinic Lerner College of Medicine, Case Western Reserve University; Assistant Medical Director, IMPACT (Internal Medicine Preoperative, Assessment Consultation and Treatment) Center, Department of Hospital Medicine, Cleveland Clinic Foundation, Cleveland, Ohio*

Padraig Mahon, MSc, FCARCSI *Research Registrar, Department of Anesthesia and Intensive Care, Cork University Hospital, Cork, Ireland*

James B. Mayfield, MD *Assistant Professor, Vice Chair of Clinical Affairs, Department of Anesthesiology and Perioperative Medicine, Medical College of Georgia, Augusta, Georgia*

Benjamin E. McCurdy, MD *Pain Fellow, Department of Anesthesiology and Perioperative Medicine, Medical College of Georgia, Augusta, Georgia*

Vivek K. Moitra, MD *Assistant Professor of Anesthesiology, Division of Critical Care, Columbia University College of Physicians and Surgeons, New York, New York*

Parwane S. Parsa, MD *Assistant Professor, Department of Anesthesia and Critical Care, University of Chicago, Chicago, Illinois*

Marc A. Rozner, MD, PhD *Professor of Anesthesiology and Pain Medicine, Professor of Cardiology, University of Texas M. D. Anderson Cancer Center; Adjunct Assistant Professor of Integrative Biology and Pharmacology, University of Texas Health Science Center, Houston, Texas*

Douglas C. Shook, MD *Instructor, Department of Anesthesia, Harvard Medical School; Program Director, Cardiothoracic Anesthesia Fellowship, Department of Anesthesiology, Perioperative and Pain Medicine, Brigham and Women's Hospital, Boston, Massachusetts*

George Shorten, MD, PhD, FRCA, FCA(RCSI) *Professor, Department of Anesthesia and Intensive Care Medicine, University College Cork; Consultant Anesthetist, Department of Anesthesia and Intensive Care Medicine, Cork University Hospital, Wilton, Cork, Ireland*

Stephen D. Small, MD *Assistant Professor, Director, Center for Simulation and Safety in Healthcare, Department of Anesthesia and Critical Care, University of Chicago, Chicago, Illinois*

Juraj Sprung, MD, PhD *Professor, Department of Anesthesiology, Mayo Clinic College of Medicine; Consultant, Department of Anesthesiology, Mayo Clinic College of Medicine, Rochester, Minnesota*

BobbieJean Sweitzer, MD *Associate Professor, Department of Anesthesia and Critical Care, University of Chicago; Director, Anesthesia Perioperative Medicine Clinic, University of Chicago Medical Center, Chicago, Illinois*

Ann T. Tong, MD *Director, Echocardiography Laboratory, Department of Cardiology, Southwest Medical Associates, Los Vegas, Nevada*

Avery Tung, MD *Associate Professor, Department of Anesthesia and Critical Care, University of Chicago; Director, Quality Assurance for Anesthesia, Department of Anesthesia and Critical Care, University of Chicago Medical Center, Chicago, Illinois*

William J. Vernick, MD *Assistant Professor, Department of Anesthesia and Critical Care, Hospital of the University of Pennsylvania; Director of Cardiac Anesthesia, Penn-Presbyterian Medical Center, Philadelphia, Pennsylvania*

David O. Warner, MD *Professor, Department of Anesthesiology, Mayo Clinic College of Medicine; Consultant in Anesthesiology, Mayo Clinic Rochester, Rochester, Minnesota*

Preface

As increasing numbers of patients with complex, advanced conditions undergo surgery and anesthesia, providers of preoperative evaluation must be familiar with a number of comorbidities such as those presented in this book. Virtually all diseases have a direct impact on patients and their care perioperatively. The second edition of *Preoperative Assessment and Management* builds on the first edition (*Handbook of Preoperative Assessment and Management*). Material on the cardiac evaluation of patients for noncardiac surgery has been updated; risk assessment has been expanded with an exploration of the psychology behind clinicians' decision-making; and new or revised case studies are intended to foster discussion for a greater understanding of the challenges faced by the caregivers who evaluate patients for anesthesia and surgery. There are new chapters on the assessment of pregnant patients and the evaluation and selection of patients for procedures outside of conventional hospital-based sites; for ambulatory surgery; and for procedures that require special perioperative treatment.

Some of the presented topics may challenge the typical practitioner. People living longer with advanced diseases (e.g., renal, heart, pulmonary failure) may require surgery for incidental conditions (e.g., cholelithiasis, fractures). As we advance technologies (e.g., minimally invasive or robotic procedures), surgical risk should be reduced to levels acceptable for even frail, elderly, or very ill individuals in advanced stages of disease who need transplants, cancer surgeries, or joint replacements. Ambulatory procedures, including those in offices or gastroenterology and radiology suites, continue to outpace inpatient procedures. All care has become fragmented and superspecialized, and issues of communication and information technology continue to defy easy fixes.

How do caregivers provide efficient, economically feasible, and comprehensive preoperative care? I believe such care begins with attempts to define problems, develop knowledge, gain expertise, formulate guidelines, and distribute this information in easy-to-access ways, such as this text attempts to do. Mechanisms to foster collaboration and sharing of best practices are essential. To this end, the newly formed Society for Perioperative Assessment and Quality Improvement (SPAQI), a nonprofit, international organization, aims to bring together a variety of healthcare professionals of various disciplines to collaborate and share expertise and resources to advance perioperative medicine. Their mission is "to provide evidence of best practice and help both community and academic institutions share findings and benchmarks; to provide international, multidisciplinary professionals with networking opportunities and shared learning; to communicate national and international practice by publishing work, research, proposed algorithms, and guidelines in the format of newsletters and conferences." More information can be found at *www.SPAQI.org*.

The writers of this text hope it has given its readers a foundation to develop and implement comprehensive and excellent preoperative care.

Acknowledgments

I am indebted to the contributors who gave their time and expertise to this project. Their knowledge and efforts are the foundation for this compilation of preoperative medical information and practice guidelines. I am grateful to my patients who have allowed me to "practice" medicine on and with them. They have motivated me to try to improve perioperative care. My students and colleagues throughout my medical career, but especially at Massachusetts General Hospital and now at the University of Chicago, have challenged and stimulated me with their questions and discussions. Much of this book was developed from those interactions.

Without Craig Percy, formerly of Lippincott Williams & Wilkins, the first edition of this book would not have happened. Brian Brown, senior acquisitions editor, and the wonderful Nicole Dernoski, managing editor, and Rosanne Hallowell, production editor at Lippincott Williams & Wilkins; and Stephanie Lentz and Renee Redding, project managers at Aptara, contributed to this second edition.

My secretary, Katherine Chapton, and Sally Kozlik, editor in the department of Anesthesia and Critical Care at the University of Chicago, spent countless hours assisting me and persisted, even when I was most demanding. Lastly, my department chairman, Jeffrey Apfelbaum, MD, has provided me the opportunity to practice preoperative medicine in a setting that fosters scholarship and creativity and has supported and encouraged my career.

BobbiJean Sweitzer, MD

Acknowledgments

Risk Reduction and Risk Assessment

Avery Tung

"It is a fact that to anesthetize a human being, to deprive him of consciousness outright, is to take a considerable step along the road to killing him."
—*W.G. Hawkins, 1957*

DEFINITION

The word *risk* can be a noun or verb (1). As a noun, *risk* is a "hazard, danger, or exposure to peril"; as a verb, *to risk* incorporates an element of uncertainty: "to expose to the chance of injury or loss." In a medical context, both hazard and uncertainty are relevant. Medical care has always involved both the real potential for an undesired outcome and an irreducible uncertainty in assessing that potential. Among medical specialties, however, anesthesiology is unique in its relationship to risk. Unlike most other physicians, anesthesiologists routinely and intentionally expose the patient to risk for no direct gain to facilitate a desired surgical outcome. Anesthesia is only rarely an end in itself. Taken together, these factors increase the importance of accurate risk assessment in anesthetic practice.

Four broad sources of risk can be defined in the perioperative period. The first involves technical, systems-related aspects of health care delivery. Examples of such issues include specialization of nurses and/or equipment, quality of information systems, appropriateness of postoperative monitoring, staffing patterns, and environment such as specialty versus general hospital or inpatient versus outpatient setting. These factors can, and do, determine the likelihood of adverse health care outcomes. Data to reliably assess their impact on outcomes, however, are generally lacking. Publication bias tends to report the successes of streamlined care systems over elaborate ones, thus prioritizing more specialized, outpatient environments over costly inpatient surgery. Data relating specific organizational practices to perioperative risk may not be generalizable from one location to another. Anesthesiologists may be less able to assess organizational factors such as the specifics of floor care and/or intensive care unit (ICU) triage. Finally, models for efficient and safe delivery of health care continuously evolve, making observations obsolete after just a few years. Although some systems issues (sterile barriers and handwashing for line placement) have clearly and consistently improved outcomes when studied (2), others (production pressure, staffing ratios, routine ICU admission for suspected sleep apnea) have not shown such clear benefit (3). Assessment of risk in this domain must therefore be individualized from one hospital environment to another.

The second source of risk is anesthetic management. Factors in this category include technical difficulties with airway management, risks with specific positions, choice of anesthetic (regional, general anesthesia, or sedation), choice of monitoring, use of adjuvant drugs (narcotics or muscle relaxants), postoperative extubation, and pain management. This category incorporates elements of systems-based practice typical of the first category, but also anesthesia-specific issues that modify perioperative risk. Accurately assessing this type of risk, however, is extremely difficult. Variability in individual practice patterns, difficulties in quantitating the relationship between man and machine, and the low baseline rate of adverse anesthesia-related events combine to increase the difficulty in relating outcome benefits from specific anesthetic strategies. Although extensive clinical experience and pathophysiology provide subjective support for many anesthetic strategies, few outcome effects have clearly demonstrated the superiority of one technique or strategy over another. The use of specific monitors, anesthetics, or adjuvant regional anesthesia, for example, has only rarely been shown to impact outcomes. Nevertheless, a large clinical experience indicating that such decisions impact patient outcomes keeps these anesthesia-specific factors relevant to perioperative risk.

The third category of risk lies in the medical factors that make an adverse perioperative event likely. These factors do not depend on practice location or on anesthetic technique, but rather are found in the patient and the procedure. For many preoperative medical conditions, a robust literature exists to define the effect of a particular procedure or risk profile on outcome. The means for evaluating the effect of coronary artery disease on perioperative risk, for example, are based firmly on data from large-scale clinical trials, with only a small contribution from clinical experience (4). In contrast, for preoperative medical conditions such as obstructive lung disease, risk assessment is much less precise (5). For many of the risk decisions in this category, extensive tools have been developed to assist clinicians to apply the results of medical research to decisions involving perioperative risk.

Finally, risk depends on the severity of the surgical procedure. Extremely complex procedures or those affecting vital structures are more risky than those on peripheral areas. As with patient comorbidities, this category of risk is well described, and decisions in this domain can usually be firmly data based.

This chapter reviews the goals and history of anesthesia risk assessment, defines the two most commonly used classifications for perioperative risk, identifies applications of risk assessment to perioperative care, and considers the challenges in risk assessment when insufficient data require subjective assessments.

GOALS OF RISK ASSESSMENT

Accurately assessing perioperative risk has two goals. The first is to assess the potential risk in performing the desired procedure on a specific patient. Because most surgery is nonemergent, the decision to shoulder the increased risk of anesthesia and surgery is not automatic. The risk can be deferred, avoided altogether if it is severe, or effectively reduced with intervention. Thus, accurate risk assessment is meaningful because it leads to a decision to proceed, postpone, or cancel surgery. Emergent or life-saving procedures must be performed, regardless of the degree of perioperative risk, and some purely cosmetic surgeries may be postponed indefinitely. But surgical procedures such as prostatectomy, cholecystectomy, and joint replacement lie in a gray zone because postponement carries real long-term risk. Accurate preoperative assessment of perioperative risk facilitates a decision about procedures in the gray zone.

The second goal is to identify modifiable risk factors. Although many factors that increase the risk of surgery and anesthesia are static, the impact of others can be lessened, eliminated, or adjusted. Treatment of ongoing pneumonia, coronary revascularization, and control of essential hypertension are examples of types of modifiable risk. It is in this realm that the anesthesiologist may make the largest impact with accurate preoperative risk assessment. By not only assessing risk but also identifying risk factors most amenable to treatment and recommending appropriate modification of those risk factors, the balance of risk and reward may be changed considerably.

Our knowledge of the factors that constitute modifiable or fixed risk is not homogenous across all types of risk. The calculation of risk and reward for cardiac revascularization before noncardiac surgery, for example, is more completely understood than that for preoperative treatment of obstructive sleep apnea. Nevertheless, knowledge of what risk factors are modifiable and the degree to which they can be modified can dramatically influence the decision to undergo a surgical procedure.

HISTORICAL BACKGROUND

Identifying the factors that alter perioperative risk and understanding the factors that may be modified to reduce the risk of surgery have long been part of the medical specialty of anesthesiology. Attempts to evaluate perioperative risk began with an effort by the American Society of Anesthesiologists (ASA) in 1941 to organize and analyze statistical data relating to anesthesia outcomes. The committee formed at that time concluded that calculation of overall operative risk would be "useless from several standpoints: the excessive number of variables to be considered, the tremendous degree of variation in different clinics and different physicians and the complete lack of agreement as to definition of terms" (6). It was immediately clear at that time that perioperative risk assessment required not only an assessment of patient health, but also, at a minimum, a measure of the severity of the planned surgery and of the hospital's familiarity with the demands of perioperative care. The ASA developed a scale for the patient's physical state, a process that eventually led to the ASA physical status classification used today (7). Well known to almost all practicing anesthesiologists, the ASA physical status score classifies patients on the basis of existing disease only, defining a spectrum where class I represents a patient with no systemic disease and class V represents a moribund patient not expected to survive without the operation (Table 1.1).

Subsequent observations have supported the ASA concept that an overall assessment of perioperative risk is a multifactorial process only partly dependent on anesthesia. In 1954, Beecher and

Table 1.1. American Society of Anesthesiologists physical status classification

1	Healthy patient without medical problems
2	Mild, well-controlled systemic disease
3	Severe systemic disease (not incapacitating)
4	Severe systemic disease (constant threat to life)
5	Moribund (not expected to live 24 hours regardless of operation)
6	Organ donor

From ASA physical status classification system. Available at: http://www.asahq.org/clinical/physicalstatus.htm. Accessed April 12, 2007.

Todd reviewed 599,548 anesthetics administered over 4 years at ten institutions (8). When the cause of perioperative death was assessed by both a surgeon and an anesthesiologist, the responsibility for mortality was distributed among anesthesiologist (1 in 2,680 cases), surgeon (1 in 420 cases), and patient comorbidity (1 in 95 cases). The primary finding in this study, that patient comorbidity was the most common contributor to perioperative mortality, has since been replicated by a 1987 study, which found that patient disease was a major contributor to 30-day mortality in up to 67% of 485,850 operations analyzed (9). Taken together, these two studies confirm that perioperative risk is multifactorial, that anesthesia management affects outcome, but that patient comorbidity appears to be the most important factor in assessing the likelihood of an adverse outcome.

The ASA physical status score differs in two important ways from an overall perioperative risk index. A comprehensive perioperative risk index assigns less risk to a cataract replacement than a total gastrectomy. The ASA physical status score is independent of the operation and would be the same for both procedures in two patients of similar health. A comprehensive risk index should be based on real associations elucidated from prospective data. The ASA physical status, however, was not derived from systematic data analysis, but from subjective physician assessments of comorbid medical conditions in patients considered relevant to preoperative outcome. It is easy to see, for example, how a more experienced anesthesiologist might assign an ASA class different from that assigned by a less experienced anesthesiologist. It is also easy to see how anesthesiologists accustomed to caring for patients with a high degree of baseline comorbidity might assign an ASA class different from that assigned by anesthesiologists caring for healthy patients. An ASA class is a "potential" and subjective approach to risk assessment.

The authors of the ASA physical status classification realized that even though it was not intended to be an overall risk index for surgical intervention, it would be treated as such. In fact, the authors observed that the anesthesiologist is subconsciously likely "to allow his knowledge of the contemplated surgical procedure to influence him in his grading of patients" (6). Evidence that different physicians assign different ASA scores to the same patient

Table 1.2.   Johns Hopkins risk classification system

Category 1	Minimally invasive procedure; little or no blood loss. Often done in an office setting. Minimal risk to patient independent of anesthesia
Category 2	Minimal to moderately invasive procedure. Blood loss <500 mL. Mild risk to patient independent of anesthesia
Category 3	Moderately to significantly invasive procedure. Blood loss potential 500–1,500 mL. Moderate risk to patient independent of anesthesia
Category 4	Highly invasive procedure. Blood loss >1,500 mL. Major risk to patient independent of anesthesia
Category 5	Highly invasive procedure. Blood loss >1,500 mL. Critical risk to patient independent of anesthesia. Usual postoperative intensive care unit stay with invasive monitoring

From Pasternak LR. Risk assessment in ambulatory surgery: challenges and new trends. *Can J Anaesth.* 2004;51:R4.

underscores this possibility (10–12). Nevertheless, the ASA classification has performed surprisingly well as an overall risk assessment tool when mortality is the undesired outcome. Several large-scale studies have documented death rates for ASA class 4 patients up to 100 times greater than those for ASA class 1 (13). When outcomes other than death are considered, however, the ASA class is a less good predictor. The ASA class correlates well with perioperative complications such as hypotension and aspiration; it is less good at predicting cancellations or unplanned admissions after outpatient surgery (14).

Other risk indexes consider different aspects of the perioperative period. The Johns Hopkins risk classification system (15), for example, focuses primarily on the severity of the surgery and degree of blood loss (Table 1.2). Under this classification, risk is categorized on the basis of severity of planned surgery, degree of invasiveness, and amount of anticipated blood loss.

The Johns Hopkins system suffers from many of the same limitations as the ASA physical status score. Limited to the severity of the proposed surgery, this tool fails to consider either patient comorbidity or anesthetic difficulty. Moreover, like the ASA physical status score, the Johns Hopkins system was not developed prospectively but on theoretical models of factors that affect the degree of surgical risk. The actual degree of surgical severity and amount of blood loss can only be estimated beforehand and may differ dramatically from the estimates. Nevertheless, an assessment of surgical severity is integral to any measure of perioperative risk.

Although no comprehensive algorithmic risk scale yet exists that integrates patient physical status and surgical severity, risk assessment scales that first assess patient comorbidity and then evaluate specific procedural risks have been proposed (Fig. 1.1).

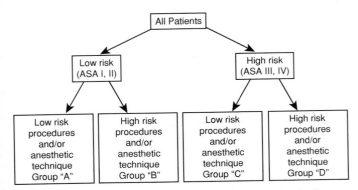

Figure 1.1. Example of a risk classification incorporating both patient comorbidity and surgical severity. ASA, American Society of Anesthesiologists. (From Pasternak LR. Risk assessment in ambulatory surgery: challenges and new trends. *Can J Anaesth.* **2004;51:R4.)**

The American College of Cardiology/American Heart Association (ACC/AHA) guideline for preoperative cardiac evaluation of patients undergoing noncardiac surgery is one example of a scale integrating both patient and surgical factors (16) (Fig. 1.2). This algorithm was initially developed to assess the risk of an adverse perioperative cardiac event, and to identify patients for whom further evaluation of cardiac disease and risk modification would be beneficial. Although elements of the guideline are likely to undergo revision as testing and revascularization strategies evolve, the basic model of a risk stratification risk modification algorithm derived from clinical trials and including both patient and surgical factors is likely to remain constant.

The first part of the ACC/AHA algorithm assesses the likelihood of coronary artery disease. The second part assesses risk from the surgical procedure. This risk was defined as the propensity for the surgery and its aftermath to induce prolonged, high-stress recovery and large fluid shifts. By integrating both surgical and patient-related risk factors, these guidelines sought to identify patients most likely to require preoperative cardiac evaluation. A recent update makes recommendations for perioperative beta blockers (17).

As one of the only preoperative risk assessment tools incorporating both patient and surgical factors, the ACC/AHA guidelines provide a model for algorithm-based, data-driven risk evaluation. Unfortunately, the need to include patient- and surgery-specific indicators, as well as a stepped approach to testing, makes the guidelines sufficiently complex (as can be seen in the figure) that applying them can be problematic. In one study of 138 patients (18), researchers found disagreement between the guidelines of the American College of Physicians and those of the ACC/AHA with respect to noninvasive stress testing, "extreme" differences in final recommendations in 7% of actual cases, and more frequent

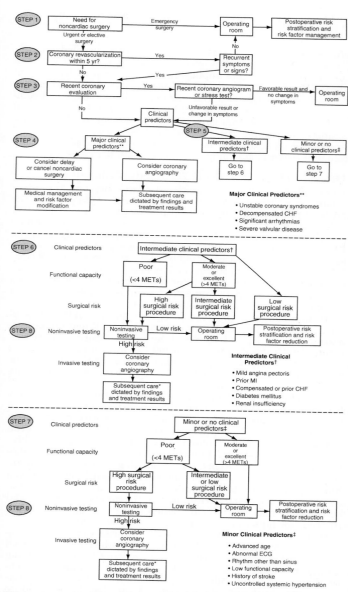

Figure 1.2. 2001 American College of Cardiology/American Heart Association guideline for perioperative cardiovascular evaluation for noncardiac surgery. CHF, congestive heart failure; ECG, electrocardiogram; METs, metabolic equivalents; MI, myocardial infarction. (From Eagle KA, Berger PB, Calkins H, et al. American College of Cardiology/American Heart Association Task Force on Practice Guidelines. ACC/AHA guideline update for perioperative cardiovascular evaluation for noncardiac surgery. *Circulation.* 2002;105:1257–1267.)

orders for noninvasive stress testing than were specified in either guideline. Such "guideline chaos" identifies a conflict between comprehensiveness and applicability well known to decision analysts (19). Because decisions are often complex, algorithms addressing all possible situations are unavoidably large and computationally intense. Under conditions in which time, risk, and uncertainty are relevant variables, the time required to compute complex algorithmic solutions may not be available. The inability to use such algorithms in practice is one reason that physician compliance with externally promulgated guidelines is poor.

TRANSLATING RESEARCH TO CLINICAL MEDICINE

The conflict between computational complexity and the applicability of a risk assessment algorithm represents perhaps the greatest difficulty in applying clinical research to perioperative risk assessment. The ACC/AHA guidelines, which consider only preoperative cardiac evaluation, are already relatively complex. Factoring in risk elements from pulmonary, renal, endocrine, and hematologic diseases would be likely to increase complexity. When trial results are superseded by new studies or when unanticipated events materialize after research-based care strategies are implemented widely, human judgment is frequently required to supplement existing risk assessment tools.

So how should physicians integrate human judgment and research-based algorithms for assessing risk? When human assessment of perioperative risk differs from algorithmic assessments, which should prevail? In light of known inconsistencies in subjective human judgment, should all subjectivity be eliminated from perioperative risk assessment to be replaced by strict adherence to guidelines?

Few data exist to answer these three questions. Comparisons between research-driven algorithms and human judgment are lacking in the medical literature. In social science domains, however, retrospectively applied algorithms have frequently been compared to prospective human judgment in tasks such as forecasting suicide risk in depressed individuals, assessing the likelihood of parole violations, and predicting success in graduate school. In all cases, algorithmic models consistently outperformed human judgment (20). But these studies do not account for the continuously changing environment or the complexity of tests and outcomes in modern medicine. When these variables are added, the need for human judgment may become more apparent.

There are strengths and weaknesses in the two methods of assessing perioperative risk. The strengths of objective, data-based approaches are clear. Objective data are generated by sampling a large number of subjects under controlled circumstances, observing results, and calculating probabilities of measured outcomes. Standardizing all nonmeasured variables helps to reduce the likelihood of a previously unconsidered factor that can skew outcomes. Finally, the results are usually unambiguous and reported using standard formats (21).

The weaknesses of data-based strategies are slightly less clear. Because data are collected in controlled environments, results may not be the same under different conditions. Widespread Canadian implementation of spironolactone therapy for congestive heart failure, for example, led to a sixfold rise in the need for hospitalization from dangerous hyperkalemia (22). Even the results of highly cited trials may not be replicated in subsequent trials, casting doubt on their veracity. In one review, fully 30% of "highly cited" clinical trials either demonstrated overly large treatment effects or were refuted by subsequent trials (23). Recent information regarding the duration of antiplatelet therapy for drug-eluting coronary stents (24) and the use of aprotinin for cardiac surgery (25) are examples of initially validated therapies subsequently found on large-scale use to have previously unrecognized side effects. Because large-scale trials are expensive, bias driven by the funding source is difficult to avoid (26). Finally, the time lag between data collection and publication can accelerate the clinical obsolescence of research results.

Other weaknesses of risk assessment tools based solely on research findings are slightly more subtle. Because medical practice is fluid, findings true at one point in time may not be true subsequently. When change is pronounced, research findings are devalued and the potential for cognitive mishaps increases. Examples of changes in pretest probability that may alter risk assessment include the dramatically rising rate of both peanut (27) and heparin (28) allergy and the falling incidence of death from acute respiratory distress syndrome. By uniformly applying rules derived from clinical trials, physicians may be deterred from developing new, potentially valuable strategies.

Human judgment also has strengths and weaknesses well documented by economists and psychologists. Such research, for example, documents that human decision making about irreducible risk and uncertainty frequently produces cognitive behavior that deviates from rationality. Several of the cognitive behaviors are relevant to perioperative risk assessment. Humans process information both consciously using well-described analytical processes and unconsciously using a parallel, "intuitive" approach (29), which processes complex, poorly quantitatable information rapidly and is an indispensable factor in expert behavior. Intuitive processing, however, is frequently susceptible to cognitive illusions that distort accurate decision making. One example of this type of illusion is a tendency to consider events likely if they are memorable or plausible more than whether they happen frequently (30). Consider the following simple example:

Which of the following is a more likely statement?

1. *Mr. F has had one or more heart attacks.*
2. *Mr. F is over 55 years old and has had one or more heart attacks.*

Item 2 is a subset of item 1 and thus must be less likely; yet item 2 sounds more plausible (particularly to physicians) and at least initially is often chosen as the more likely event.

Judging the frequency of events based on their resonance in memory is a generally successful approach to risk assessment. When highly memorable events are vanishingly rare, however, the human tendency to overweight their likelihood can lead to misassessment of risk.

Another characteristic of intuitive processing is a strong aversion to ambiguity or uncertainty. Humans prefer certainty, to such a degree that they make inferior choices to avoid uncertainty.

Consider the following example, first proposed by the mathematician Maurice Allais in 1952 (31):

Which gamble would you choose?

a. *Receiving $1 million in cash*
b. *A 10% chance of $5 million, 89% chance of $1 million, and 1% chance of nothing*

When given the above choice, most would choose a. But now consider the following choices:

c. *An 11% chance of winning $1 million and 89% chance of winning nothing*
d. *A 10% chance of winning $5 million and 90% chance of winning nothing*

In this case, most would choose d. Upon closer inspection, however, the two pairs are equal except for the degree of certainty. This can be seen if a case is recast as an 11% chance of winning $1 million and an 89% chance of winning $1 million. Then, by switching an 89% chance of winning $1 million to an 89% chance of winning nothing (in both cases), choices a and b can be converted to c and d, respectively.

The aversion to ambiguity has several important consequences for risk assessment. First, most risk assessment protocols based on findings in the medical literature explicitly acknowledge the possibility of individual failure and are designed to maximize the overall group outcome. Physicians, however, generally approach every patient with the goal of success. As a result, when protocol failures result, the cognitive dissonance is not only memorable (which diminishes the perceived utility of the protocol), but also frustrating. Cognitive studies demonstrate that when given a choice between a protocol with a finite, nonzero failure rate and making individual subjective judgments, both motivation and training correlate with the desire to avoid preset protocols (32).

Secondly, a desire for certainty can lead to more testing than is appropriate or cost effective. In addition to the cost of increased testing, performing a test when not supported by pretest probability or predictive value may result in false-positive results that trigger even more testing and diagnosis.

Finally, humans consistently overassess their own abilities when compared to those of others and incorporate imagined regret from potential adverse outcomes into future decisions (33). Thus, using a monitor specifically to avoid decision regret may distort objective calculation. Data suggesting that a particular strategy does not benefit other practitioners may be discounted on the basis that inferior operator skill caused the lack of benefit.

It is easy to see how these cognitive effects can alter risk assessment. Making decisions with an eye toward regret if outcomes are undesired may lead to overly cautious, conservative choices. A sense that one's own abilities surpass those of one's peers may also reduce compliance with existing guidelines and lead to decisions that fail to adequately account for difficulties in patient management.

Benefits of intuitive, subjective human judgment are less well appreciated but critical to expert medical practice. Human intuitive processing is much more rapid than analytical methods and plays a critical role when time is an important factor. Humans can also process visual and audio information not well quantified by research methods. The human ability to pattern-match allows ready diagnosis of extremely complex event sequences, and equally as important, allows the expert to identify factors that "do not fit," thus potentially signifying an incorrect diagnosis or treatment (34). Humans are extremely sensitive to the frequency of observed events, so much so that the correlations between human and actual measurements of word frequency in English are extremely close (35).

SUMMARY

Accurately assessing perioperative risk is a critical tool in the anesthesiologist's repository. Although the list of adverse or undesired perioperative outcomes is immense, four broad categories of risk factors can be identified: Practice environment, anesthesia-related factors, patient-related factors, and surgery-related factors. Of these, the most difficult to quantify accurately is the impact of the practice environment, and the category most thoroughly studied (and the one found to have the greatest impact on perioperative outcomes) is that of patient comorbidities.

No comprehensive risk scale is in wide use today. The ASA physical status class, frequently used as a proxy for perioperative risk, lacks prospective validation, fails to account for surgical complexity or environmental factors, and is subjective. The Johns Hopkins risk classification system, which focuses on surgical risk factors, also lacks prospective validation. The ACC/AHA guidelines for preoperative evaluation for noncardiac surgery effectively integrate both patient and surgical factors, but their complexity make them difficult to use, and their application is to cardiac risk only.

The tradeoff in the development of better risk assessment tools is between usability and complexity. Because of complexity and ongoing change in the clinical environment, it is unlikely that readily usable, comprehensive perioperative risk algorithms will be developed in the near future.

In the meantime, physicians must integrate clinical experience-based intuition and research data to make the best possible risk assessments. Positives and negatives of data-derived algorithms are relatively clear; good and bad attributes of intuition-based decision making are less so. Several pitfalls that require constant attention include representativeness, regret, preferences for certainty, and ego. Conversely, when applied properly, human intuition, which is tremendously powerful, fast, and superior to analytical techniques, is at the root of all expert performance.

Situations in which intuition and literature findings perform best should be recognized. When time is short, data are perceptually based, human preferences must be considered, and complexity is high, intuitive decision processes should be emphasized. When time is ample, data are numerical, and decisions and the environment are relatively simple, literature findings may be emphasized. Further research is required to learn the best methods to integrate experience and evidence for assessment of perioperative risk.

REFERENCES

1. *Compact Oxford English Dictionary of Current English*. 3rd ed. Oxford: Oxford University Press; 2005.
2. Pronovost P, Needham D, Berenholtz S, et al. An intervention to decrease catheter-related bloodstream infections in the ICU. *N Engl J Med*. 2006;355:2725–2732.
3. Terris DJ, Fincher EF, Hanasono MM, et al. Conservation of resources: indications for intensive care monitoring after upper airway surgery on patients with obstructive sleep apnea. *Laryngoscope*. 1998;108:784–788.
4. Barak M, Ben-Abraham R, Katz Y. ACC/AHA guidelines for preoperative cardiovascular evaluation for noncardiac surgery: a critical point of view. *Clin Cardiol*. 2006;29:195–198.
5. Smetana GW, Lawrence VA, Cornell JE; American College of Physicians. Preoperative pulmonary risk stratification for noncardiothoracic surgery: systematic review for the American College of Physicians. *Ann Intern Med*. 2006;144:581–595.
6. Saklad M. Grading of patients for surgical procedures. *Anesthesiology*. 1941;2:281–284.
7. ASA physical status classification system. Available at: http://www.asahq.org/clinical/physicalstatus.htm. Accessed April 12, 2007.
8. Beecher HK, Todd DP. A study of the deaths associated with anesthesia and surgery: based on a study of 599,548 anesthesias in ten institutions 1948–1952, inclusive. *Ann Surg*. 1954;140: 2–35.
9. Lunn JN, Devlin HB. Lessons from the confidential enquiry into perioperative deaths in three NHS regions. *Lancet*. 1987;2:1384–1386.
10. Owens WD, Felts JA, Spitznagel EL Jr. ASA physical status classifications: a study of consistency of ratings. *Anesthesiology*. 1978;49:239–243.
11. Mak PH, Campbell RC, Irwin MG. The ASA physical status classification: inter-observer consistency. *Anaesth Intensive Care*. 2002;30:633–640.
12. Jacqueline R, Malviya S, Burke C, et al. An assessment of interrater reliability of the ASA physical status classification in pediatric surgical patients. *Paediatr Anaesth*. 2006;16: 928–931.
13. Vacanti CJ, VanHouten RJ, Hill RC. A statistical analysis of the relationship of physical status to postoperative mortality in 68,388 cases. *Anesth Analg*. 1970;49:564–566.
14. Meridy HW. Criteria for selection of ambulatory surgical patients and guidelines for anesthetic management: a retrospective study of 1553 cases. *Anesth Analg*. 1982;61:921–926.
15. Pasternak LR. Risk assessment in ambulatory surgery: challenges and new trends. *Can J Anaesth*. 2004;51:R4.
16. Fleisher LA, Beckman JA, Brown KA, et al. ACC/AHA guidelines on perioperative cardiovascular evaluation and care for noncardiac surgery. *J AM Coll Cardiol*. 2007;50:e159–241. www.acc.org.
17. Fleisher LA, Beckman JA, Brown KA, et al. ACC/AHA committee to update the 2002 Guidelines on Perioperative Cardiovascular Evaluation for Noncardiac Surgery. *Circulation*. 2006;113:2662–2674.

18. Gordon AJ, Macpherson DS. Guideline chaos: conflicting recommendations for preoperative cardiac assessment. *Am J Cardiol*. 2003;91:1299–1303.
19. Simon HA. A behavioral model of rational choice. *Quart J Econ*. 1955;69:99–118.
20. Dawes RM, Faust D, Meehl PE. Clinical vs actuarial judgment. *Science*. 1989;243:1668–1674.
21. Sackett DL, Straus SE, Richardson WS, et al., eds. *Evidence-Based Medicine: How to Practice and Teach EBM*. 2nd ed. Edinburgh: Churchill Livingstone; 2000.
22. Juurlink DN, Mamdani MM, Lee DS, et al. Rates of hyperkalemia after publication of the Randomized Aldactone Evaluation Study. *N Engl J Med*. 2004;351:543–551.
23. Ioannidis JP. Contradicted and initially stronger effects in highly cited clinical research. *JAMA*. 2005;294:218–228.
24. Shuchman M. Trading restenosis for thrombosis? New questions about drug-eluting stents. *N Engl J Med*. 2006;355:1949–1952.
25. Mangano DT, Tudor IC, Dietzel C. The Multicenter Study of Perioperative Ischemia Research Group and the Ischemia Research and Education Foundation. The risk associated with aprotinin in cardiac surgery. *N Engl J Med*. 2006;354:353–365.
26. Patsopoulos NA, Ioannidis JP, Analatos AA. Origin and funding of the most frequently cited papers in medicine: database analysis. *BMJ*. 2006;332:1061–1064.
27. Sicherer SH, Munoz-Furlong A, Sampson HA. Prevalence of peanut and tree nut allergy in the United States determined by means of a random digit dial telephone survey: a 5-year follow-up study. *J Allergy Clin Immunol*. 2003;112:1203–1207.
28. Warkentin TE. Heparin-induced thrombocytopenia: a ten-year retrospective. *Ann Rev Med*. 1999;50:129–147.
29. Kahneman D. A perspective on judgment and choice: mapping bounded rationality. *Am Psychol*. 2003;58:697–720.
30. Tversky A, Kahneman D. Extensional versus intuitive reasoning: the conjunction fallacy in probability judgment. *Psychol Rev*. 1983;90:293–315.
31. Allais M. Le comportement de l'homme rationnel devant le risque: critique le Postulats et Axiomes de L'École Américaine. *Econometrica*. 1953;21:503–546.
32. Arkes HR, Dawes RM, Christensen C. Factors influencing the use of a decision rule in a probabilistic task. *Org Behav Hum Dec Proc*. 1986;37:93–110.
33. Dunning D, Heath C, Suls JM. Flawed self-assessment: implications for health, education, and the workplace. *Psychol Sci Public Interest*. 2004;5:69–106.
34. Klein G. *Sources of Power: How People Make Decisions*. Cambridge: MIT Press; 1998.
35. Hasher L, Zacks RT. Automatic processing of fundamental information. *Am Psychol*. 1984;39:1372–1388.

Overview of Preoperative Evaluation and Testing

BobbieJean Sweitzer

OVERVIEW

As the scope of surgery and anesthesia has moved into the outpatient arena with the majority of patients coming to the hospital shortly before undergoing a procedure, anesthesiologists have struggled with how best to accomplish their preoperative evaluation. Preoperative assessment and management continue to change as more procedures are performed in settings outside traditional hospital-based operating rooms. With technologic improvements, minimally invasive and less risky surgical procedures can be performed on patients with advanced comorbidities or on elderly, frail individuals. Likewise, nonsurgical specialists such as gastroenterologists, radiologists, and cardiologists are performing interventions that require anesthesia services. Clinicians are called upon to develop innovative methods to care for patients as the practice of medicine evolves.

Traditionally surgical risk has been considered more important than anesthetic risk. Now a general anesthetic requiring instrumentation of the airway with associated significant physiologic perturbations may pose a significant and greater risk than surgery itself to some extremely fragile individuals. Often patients have multiple, complex problems that require advanced and diverse skills of their caregivers. The sub–subspecialization of medicine results in fragmentation of care and silos of interventions, information, and skill sets. The task of gathering the necessary information and sharing that information among the various providers can be challenging. All this comes as medicine strives to become more outcome driven and cost conscious.

Evidence suggests that the perioperative period (choices of drugs, depth of anesthesia, adverse events) may have long-term health consequences. The preoperative evaluation may be a "window of opportunity" for preventive care and improvement in chronic therapies as well as a motivating, life-altering period for patients, so physicians and perioperative caregivers must expand and develop processes with this in mind (1,2). Health care providers evaluating and preparing patients who will undergo anesthesia, surgery, and increasingly varied interventions face a challenge as new methods are created and implemented. As longevity increases, patients with complex chronic multiple diseases come to us for care.

The goals of preoperative assessment include the following:

1. To assess medical conditions that may impact perioperative care

2. To manage and improve comorbidities that may impact perioperative care
3. To assess the risk of anesthesia and surgery and lower the risk by altering planned procedures or by improving patients' condition(s)
4. To identify patients who may require special anesthetic techniques or postoperative care
5. To establish baseline results to aid perioperative decisions
6. To educate patients and families about anesthesia and postoperative events
7. To obtain informed consent
8. To facilitate timely care and avoid cancellations on the day of surgery
9. To motivate patients to commit to preventive care (e.g., stop smoking, lose weight, or adhere to care plans)
10. To investigate, develop, and disseminate evidence-based practices
11. To train personnel in the art and science of preoperative assessment and to optimize patient conditions that may impact the procedure

The Australian Incident Monitoring Study (AIMS) database found that 11% of reports identified inadequate or incorrect preoperative *assessment* (478 of 6,271) or preoperative *preparation* (248 of 6,271) (3). Of adverse events 3.1% (197) were indisputably related to inadequate or incorrect preoperative assessment or preparation. In these 197 patients morbidity was major in 23 and 7 patients died. The investigators concluded that patient factors contributed only 1% of the time. More than half of incidents were preventable; an additional 21% were possibly preventable. Unpreventable events made up only 5% of cases. Almost one quarter of the time, communication failures were cited as the most significant factor. An analysis of the first 2,000 reports to AIMS found a sixfold increase in mortality in patients who were inadequately assessed preoperatively (4).

In a different study of anesthetic-related perioperative deaths, 53 of 135 deaths involved inadequate preoperative assessment and management (5). Delays, complications, and unanticipated postoperative admissions can be significantly reduced by preoperative screening and patient contact (6). Preoperative health status predicts operative clinical outcomes and resource utilization. Preoperative preparation and education can facilitate recovery and reduce postoperative morbidity. Anxiety, postoperative pain, and length of stay are positively affected by comprehensive preoperative care. In a study conducted in Canada and Scotland, patients rated meeting the anesthesiologist as the highest priority, above that of information on pain relief, alternative methods of anesthesia, and complications (7).

Many anesthesiologists perform preoperative evaluations, review diagnostic studies (chosen and ordered by someone else), discuss anesthetic risks, and obtain informed consent moments before patients undergo major, potentially life-threatening or disfiguring procedures. This choice offers little opportunity to optimize comorbid conditions or alter risk. Legally, morally, and psychologically, anesthesiologists and patients are in awkward and often unpleasant situations. The effects of extensive disclosure are stressful for patients and families at a time when they may be ill prepared to consider the implications rationally. An increase in preoperative anxiety likely affects postoperative outcomes because increased anxiety correlates with increased postoperative analgesic requirements and prolonged recovery and hospital stay. Anxiety impairs retention of information, with attendant medicolegal implications because of inadequate communication or discussion of the risks of anesthesia.

Preoperative evaluation must be convenient and efficient for both patients and medical personnel. It can be cost effective and reduce turnover times, cancellations, length of hospital stays, and postoperative complications (6). Preoperative visits should be comprehensive and include plans for postdischarge care. Anesthesiologists must adapt practices to provide patients with the best preoperative services.

At a minimum, the guidelines of the American Society of Anesthesiologists (ASA) indicate that a preanesthesia visit should include the following (8):

- An interview with the patient or guardian to review medical, anesthesia, and medication history
- An appropriate physical examination
- Review of diagnostic data (laboratory, electrocardiogram, radiographs, consultations)
- Assignment of ASA physical status score (ASA-PS) (Table 2.1)

Table 2.1.   American Society of Anesthesiologists (ASA) physical status classification[a]

ASA 1	Healthy patient without organic, biochemical, or psychiatric disease
ASA 2	A patient with mild systemic disease (e.g., mild asthma or well-controlled hypertension). No significant impact on daily activity. Unlikely impact on anesthesia and surgery
ASA 3	Significant or severe systemic disease that limits normal activity (e.g., renal failure on dialysis or class 2 congestive heart failure). Significant impact on daily activity. Likely impact on anesthesia and surgery
ASA 4	Severe disease that is a constant threat to life or requires intensive therapy (e.g., acute myocardial infarction, respiratory failure requiring mechanical ventilation). Serious limitation of daily activity. Major impact on anesthesia and surgery
ASA 5	Moribund patient who is equally likely to die in the next 24 hours with or without surgery
ASA 6	Brain-dead organ donor

[a]"E" added to the classifications indicates emergency surgery.
From http://www.asahq.org/clinical/physicalstatus.htm. Accessed April 13, 2007.

- A formulation and discussion of anesthesia plans with the patient or a responsible adult

As early as 1949 the concept of an anesthesia-based outpatient clinic was proposed. Some clinics do no more than gather information provided by the patient, the medical record, or others who have seen the patient. Some anesthesiologists rely on other physicians to prepare patients for surgery, either based on anesthesia-derived guidelines or not. These practitioners may have no expertise in preoperative assessment and little understanding of the proposed surgery and anesthesia. The use of primary care physicians, internists, or specialists to "clear" patients or manage comorbid conditions is common. This reliance may be appropriate for a few, very select diseases and patients, or for the management of conditions of everyday life. To reduce long-term complications from the stresses of a surgical procedure and anesthesia is very different. Many anesthesia practices simply review information that is provided to them but have little direct oversight of the process. At a minimum, anesthesiologists must develop guidelines to direct testing, determine evaluation processes, and establish preoperative medication and fasting instructions. Examples of guidelines are shown in Tables 2.2 and 2.3 and Figure 2.1.

Table 2.2. Preoperative testing guidelines for healthy patients (American Society of Anesthesiologists physical status 1)

Procedure Type	Invasive Status	Tests[a−c]
Low risk (i.e., breast biopsy, knee arthroscopy, cataracts)	Minimal	Baseline creatinine if procedure involves injection of contrast dye
Intermediate risk (i.e., inguinal hernia or lumbar laminectomy)	Moderate	Baseline creatinine if procedure involves injection of contrast dye or patient >55 yr of age
High risk (i.e., procedures with significant blood loss)	High	CBC; baseline creatinine if procedure involves injection of contrast dye or patient >55 yr of age

CBC, complete blood count.

[a] Results from laboratory tests within 6 months of surgery are acceptable unless major abnormalities are present or a patient's condition has changed.

[b] A routine pregnancy test before surgery is not recommended before the day of surgery. A careful history and local practice determine whether a pregnancy test is indicated.

[c] Age alone is not an indication for an electrocardiogram (ECG). Reimbursement for an ECG depends on indication (pallor, dizziness, hypertension) or a diagnosis documented by history or physical examination. No new ECG is needed if results from an ECG within 6 months of surgery are normal and the patient's condition has not changed.

Table 2.3. Preoperative testing guidelines based on comorbid conditions

Disease-based indications

Alcohol abuse	CBC; ECG; electrolytes; LFTs; platelet count; PT
Anemia	CBC
Bleeding disorder (personal or family)	CBC; LFTs; platelet count; PT; PTT
Cardiovascular disease	CBC; creatinine; chest radiograph[a]; ECG; electrolytes
Cerebrovascular disease	Creatinine; glucose; ECG
Diabetes	Creatinine; electrolytes; glucose; ECG
Hepatic disease	CBC; creatinine; electrolytes; LFTs; platelet count; PT
Hepatitis exposure (recent)	LFTs
Hypercoagulable condition	PTT
Intracranial disease	Electrolytes; glucose; ECG
Malignancy	CBC; platelet count; chest radiograph[a,b]
Malnutrition; Malabsorption	Albumin; CBC; ECG; electrolytes; PT
Morbid obesity	Glucose; ECG
Peripheral vascular disease	Creatinine; ECG
Poor exercise tolerance	CBC; ECG
Possible pregnancy	β-hCG
Pulmonary disease	CBC; ECG; chest radiograph[a]
Renal disease	CBC; creatinine; electrolytes; ECG
Rheumatoid arthritis	CBC; ECG; chest radiograph[a]
Sleep apnea	CBC; ECG
Smoking >40 pack-years	CBC; ECG; chest radiograph[a]
Systemic lupus erythematosus	Creatinine; ECG; chest radiograph[a]
Thyroid disease	TFTs
UTI (or suspected)	U/A

Therapy-based indications

Radiation therapy	CBC; ECG[b]; chest radiograph[b]
Use of warfarin	PT
Use of digoxin	Electrolytes; ECG
Use of diuretics	Creatinine; electrolytes; ECG
Use of steroids	Glucose; ECG

Procedure-based indications

Procedure with significant blood loss	CBC; T&S
Radiographic dye injection	Creatinine

CBC, complete blood count; ECG, electrocardiogram; β-hCG, pregnancy test; LFTs, liver function tests (alkaline phosphatase, alanine aminotransferase [AST], aspartate aminotransferase [AST], albumin, bilirubin); PT, prothrombin time; PTT, partial thromboplastin time; T&S, type and screen; TFTs, thyroid function tests (thyroid stimulating hormone [TSH], T3, T4); U/A, urinalysis.

All tests are valid for 6 months before surgery unless abnormal or patient's condition has changed, with the exception of β-hCG for pregnancy. Guidelines may not apply for low-risk procedures where testing is only indicated if the medical condition is newly diagnosed or unstable.

[a] For active, acute process or significant dyspnea with chronic process.

[b] Only if radiation to breasts, chest, lungs, or thorax.

Simplified Cardiac Evaluation for Noncardiac Surgery

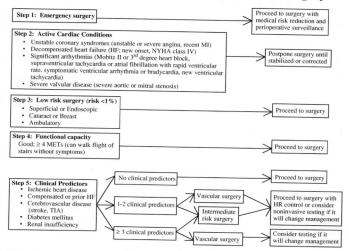

Figure 2.1.   **Based on Fleisher LA, Beckman JA, Brown KA, et al. ACC/AHA 2007 guidelines on perioperative cardiovascular evaluation and care for noncardiac surgery.** *J Am Coll Cardiol.* **2007;50:e159–241. http://www.acc.org/quality and science/clinical/guidelines/Periop_Fulltext_2007.pdf. Accessed September 28, 2007.**

PREOPERATIVE EVALUATION

Many surgeons and anesthesiologists rely on routine or screening batteries of tests when preparing patients for surgery. This practice may be based on institutional policies or on the mistaken belief that screening batteries of tests can substitute for taking a history or performing a comprehensive physical examination. Preoperative tests without specific indications lack clinical utility and may actually lead to patient injury because they prompt further testing to evaluate abnormal results, unnecessary interventions, delay of surgery, anxiety, and perhaps even inappropriate therapies. The history is responsible for diagnoses 75% of the time and is more important than the physical examination and laboratory investigations combined. In addition, the evaluation of abnormal test results is costly.

Many studies have evaluated the benefits of procedure- or disease-indicated testing versus screening batteries of tests. Few abnormalities detected by nonspecific testing resulted in changes in management and rarely have such changes had a beneficial patient effect (9). At most 1 in 1,000 patients has benefited from findings derived from unindicated testing (10). Of tests without specific indications, only 0.4% provided useful clinical information (9). However, 1 in 2,000 preoperative tests resulted in patient harm from pursuit of abnormalities detected by those tests; only 1 in 10,000 was of benefit to the patient (11).

Preoperative diagnostic tests ordered because of a condition suspected from a finding on the history or physical examination are much more likely to be abnormal (12). Equally important is the finding that a previously abnormal result is associated with new or persistent abnormalities (13).

Preoperative evaluation is an ideal opportunity to evaluate patients not simply for the pending procedure, but from a broader perspective. Primary care providers evaluating patients preoperatively may find this period an opportune time to provide other care.

Very few diagnostic tests not based on complaints or physical findings have utility to screen for disease (14). The ideal screening test must be highly specific (to avoid false-positive results) and sensitive (to avoid false-negative results), pose little risk to the patient, and be inexpensive. The condition being screened for must be common in the examined population, and there must be effective interventions or benefits from establishing a diagnosis. Processes should be in place for follow-up of test results. Some examples of beneficial screening tests include lipid profiles, the test for prostate-specific antigen (PSA), mammography, and colonoscopy. It is unlikely that anesthesiologist-directed clinics are a good place to offer this type of service. Before any further discussion of diagnostic testing, we must consider the clinical encounter to identify morbidities based on the history and physical examination and the planned procedure.

DETECTING DISEASE

Repeatedly it has been shown that the history and physical examination (H&P), commonly referred to as the *clinical examination*, often is all that is required for a diagnosis or elimination of alternative hypotheses.

A study of patients in a general medical clinic found that 56% of correct diagnoses were made with the history alone; the percentage increased to 73% with the physical examination. In patients with cardiovascular disease, the history establishes the diagnosis two thirds of the time, and the physical examination contributes to one quarter of diagnoses (15). Diagnostic tests, such as chest radiographs and electrocardiograms (ECGs), helped with only 3% of diagnoses, and special tests (e.g., exercise ECGs) assisted with 6%. In respiratory, urinary, and neurologic conditions, history has also been shown to be the most important diagnostic method. The skill of performing a clinical examination derives from pattern recognition learned by listening to and seeing patients and assimilating the stories and outcomes of their illnesses. The diagnostic acumen of the physician is a result of the ability to integrate and develop an overall impression rather than to just review a compilation of facts.

Importance of the Medical History

The variability of the medical history and the different words that patients and physicians use to describe symptoms are a common problem. Using lay language and recording symptoms in ordinary words leads to greater interobserver agreement between practitioners and can lessen communication errors, which are common obstacles in medical care. Common errors occur when diagnostic labels such as "angina" are written in the record when the patient actually complained of "chest pain." Conversely, true angina or cardiac ischemia/infarction is rarely described by a patient as "chest pain." More likely the patient will complain of tightness or squeezing, often in the upper abdomen, shoulder, or neck. Therefore, medical interviewers should not be surprised that patients may deny ever having chest pain when these are the only words used to inquire about symptoms of angina. Obtaining a history is not simply asking questions, but asking the right questions, often in a variety of ways, and interpreting and carefully recording the answers. Complete and thorough histories, which assist in planning appropriate and safe anesthesia care, are more accurate and cost effective in establishing diagnoses than screening laboratory tests.

Components of the Medical History

The important components of the anesthesia history are shown in Figure 2.2. The form can be completed by the patient in person, on paper or via an electronic version, Web-based programs, or a telephone interview, or by anesthesia staff.

The classic "history of present illness" (HPI) as it relates to the anesthesia H&P starts with the reason the patient is having the planned procedure. How the surgical condition developed and any prior therapies related to this problem are noted. Current and past medical problems, previous surgeries and types of anesthesia, and any anesthesia-related complications also are noted. Rarely is simply a notation of diseases or symptoms such as hypertension (HTN), diabetes mellitus (DM), coronary artery disease (CAD), shortness of breath (SOB), or chest pain (CP) sufficient. The presence of a disease and its severity are established, as are current or recent exacerbations, the stability and prior treatment of the condition, or planned interventions. The extent, degree of control, and activity-limiting nature of the problems are determined. The patient's medical problems, previous surgeries, and responses to questions set the framework for further inquiry to establish a complete history.

Prescription and over-the-counter medications, including supplements and herbals, along with dosages and schedules are carefully recorded, as are any recent but currently interrupted medications, often a clue to recent disease fluctuations. It is necessary to inquire about allergies to medicines and substances such as latex or radiographic dye with special emphasis on the specifics of the patient's response to the exposure. Often patients claim an allergy to a substance when in reality the reaction(s) is a common, expected side effect. Use of tobacco, alcohol, or illicit drugs is documented.

A history of malignant hyperthermia (MH) or a suggestion of it (hyperthermia or rigidity during anesthesia) either in a patient or family member is documented so that appropriate arrangements can be made before the day of surgery. A personal or family history of pseudocholinesterase deficiency should be identified preoperatively. Records from previous anesthetics may clarify an uncertain history.

Patient's Name _____ Age____ Sex _____ Date of Surgery_____

Planned Operation_____ Surgeon_____

Primary care doctor/phone #_____ Other physicians/phone #s_____

1. Please list **all operations** (and approximate dates)

a.	d.
b.	e.
c.	f.

2. Please list any **allergies** to medicines, latex or other (and your reactions to them)

a.	c.
b.	d.

3. Please list **all medications** you have taken in the last month (include over-the-counter drugs, inhalers, herbals, dietary supplements and aspirin)

Name of Drug	Dose and how often	Name of Drug	Dose and how often
a.		f.	
b.		g.	
c.		h.	
d.		i.	
e.		j.	

(Please check YES or NO and circle specific problems)   YES   NO

4. Have you taken steroids (prednisone or cortisone) in the last year?   ☐ ☐
5. Have you *ever* smoked? (Quantify in ___ packs/day for ___ years)   ☐ ☐
   Do you still smoke?   ☐ ☐
   Do you drink alcohol? (If so, how much?) _____   ☐ ☐
   Do you use or have you ever used any illegal drugs? (we need to know for your safety)   ☐ ☐
6. Can you walk up one flight of stairs without stopping?   ☐ ☐
7. Have you had any problems with your heart? **(circle)** (chest pain or pressure, heart attack, abnormal ECG, skipped beats, heart murmur, palpitation, heart failure [fluid in the lungs], require antibiotics before routine dental care)
8. Do you have high blood pressure?   ☐ ☐
9. Have you had any problems with your lungs or your chest? **(circle)** (shortness of breath, emphysema, bronchitis, asthma, TB, abnormal chest x-ray)   ☐ ☐
10. Are you ill now or were you recently ill with a cold, fever, chills, flu or productive cough?   ☐ ☐
    Describe recent changes
11. Have you or anyone in your family had serious bleeding problems? **(circle)** (prolonged bleeding from nosebleed, gums, tooth extractions, or surgery)   ☐ ☐
12. Have you had any problems with your blood (anemia, leukemia, sickle cell disease, blood clots, transfusions)?   ☐ ☐
13. Have you ever had problems with your: **(circle)**
    Liver (cirrhosis, hepatitis, jaundice)?   ☐ ☐
    Kidney (stones, failure, dialysis)?   ☐ ☐
    Digestive system (frequent heartburn, hiatus hernia, stomach ulcer)?   ☐ ☐
    Back, neck or jaws (TMJ, rheumatoid arthritis)?   ☐ ☐
    Thyroid gland (underactive or overactive)?   ☐ ☐
14. Have you ever had: **(circle)**
    Seizures, epilepsy, or fits?   ☐ ☐
    Stroke, facial, leg or arm weakness, difficulty speaking?   ☐ ☐
    Cramping pain in your legs with walking?   ☐ ☐
    Problems with hearing, vision or memory?   ☐ ☐
15. Have you ever been treated for cancer with chemotherapy or radiation therapy? **(circle)**
16. Women: Could you be pregnant?   ☐ ☐
    Last menstrual period began: _____
17. Have you ever had problems with anesthesia or surgery? **(circle)** (severe nausea or vomiting, malignant hyperthermia (in blood relatives or self), prolonged drowsiness, anxiety, breathing difficulties, or problems during placement of a breathing tube)   ☐ ☐
18. Do you have any chipped or loose teeth, dentures, caps, bridgework, braces, problems opening your mouth, swallowing or choking? **(circle)**   ☐ ☐
19. Do your physical abilities limit your daily activities?   ☐ ☐
20. Do you snore?   ☐ ☐
21. Please list any medical illnesses not noted above: _____
_____
_____

22. Additional comments or questions for nurse or anesthesiologist?
_____
_____

Figure 2.2.   Sample patient preoperative history.

A screening review of systems (ROS) is especially useful to uncover symptoms that may suggest previously undiagnosed conditions. An ROS for anesthesia purposes checks for airway abnormalities; personal or family history of adverse events related to anesthesia; and cardiovascular, pulmonary, hepatic, renal, endocrine, or neurologic symptoms (Fig. 2.2). Responses to questions about snoring and daytime somnolence may suggest undiagnosed sleep apnea, which has implications for anesthesia management. The Berlin Questionnaire is useful to identify patients with undiagnosed sleep apnea (16). The presence of any two of the following is considered a high risk for sleep apnea: snoring, daytime sleepiness, hypertension, or obesity.

A significant history of heartburn, especially with associated reflux or after a period of fasting comparable to that expected preoperatively, is noted. Women of childbearing age are prompted to recall their last normal menstrual period and the likelihood of being pregnant. The response is more reliable if the female, especially if a minor child, is questioned in privacy.

A determination of the patient's cardiorespiratory fitness or functional capacity is useful in guiding additional preanesthetic evaluation and predicting outcome and perioperative complications (17,18). Exercise or work activity can be quantified in metabolic equivalents (METs), a measure of the volume of oxygen consumed during an activity (Table 2.4). Better fitness decreases mortality through improved lipid and glucose profiles and reduction in blood pressure (BP) and obesity. Lack of exercise increases the risk of developing cardiac disease. Conversely, an inability to exercise may be a *result* of cardiopulmonary disease. Patients with peripheral vascular disease (PVD) are limited by claudication and those with ischemic heart disease may complain of shortness of breath or chest discomfort with exertion. Patients

Table 2.4.   Metabolic equivalents (METs) of functional capacity

MET	Functional Levels of Exercise
1	Eating, working at computer, dressing
2	Walking down stairs or in your house, cooking
3	Walking one to two blocks
4	Raking leaves, gardening
5	Climbing one flight of stairs, dancing, bicycling
6	Playing golf, carrying clubs
7	Playing singles tennis
8	Rapidly climbing stairs, jogging slowly
9	Jumping rope slowly, moderate cycling
10	Swimming quickly, running or jogging briskly
11	Skiing cross country, playing full-court basketball
12	Running rapidly for moderate to long distances

1 MET = consumption of 3.5 mL O_2/min/kg of body weight.
Adapted from Jette M, Sidney K, Blumchen G. Metabolic equivalents (METs) in exercise testing, exercise prescription, and evaluation of functional capacity. *Clin Cardiol.* 1990;13:555–565.

may not volunteer this information unless asked if they can walk more than a certain distance or climb stairs. Several studies have shown that inability to perform average levels of exercise (4 to 5 METs) identifies patients at risk of perioperative complications (17) (Fig. 2.1).

Medical History of Specific Conditions

The following is an overview of the basic points for most preoperative patient assessments. Detailed discussions for evaluation of specific diseases are found in the chapters of this text.

Cardiovascular

Cardiovascular complications are the most common cause of significant adverse events in the perioperative period. It is estimated that 1% to 5% of unselected noncardiac surgical patients will suffer a cardiac morbidity. Perioperative interventions have been shown to modify cardiovascular morbidity and mortality (17). Therefore, a very careful cardiovascular history of the patient and the family is of utmost importance. The evaluator inquires about chest discomfort (pain, pressure, tightness), duration of discomfort, precipitating factors, associated symptoms, or methodologies of relief. Diagnoses, diagnostic tests, therapies, and names of treating physicians are noted, as is shortness of breath with exertion or when lying flat (orthopnea) or peripheral edema.

A history of heart murmurs and whether patients with murmurs have been evaluated or given prophylaxis for subacute bacterial endocarditis (SBE) are elicited. The cardinal symptoms of severe aortic stenosis are angina, heart failure, and syncope, although patients are much more likely to complain of a decrease in exercise tolerance and exertional dyspnea.

Pulmonary

A history of asthma, chronic obstructive pulmonary disease (COPD), or other respiratory disease prompts further questioning about shortness of breath, recent exacerbations, therapy, the use of steroids (especially within the previous year) or oxygen, hospitalizations, and intubations. The patient's best exercise level is important information for risk assessment.

Hematologic

The goal in the preoperative clinic is to determine the etiology, duration, and stability of anemia, related symptoms, and therapy (especially transfusions). The extent and type of surgery are considered as well as the anticipated blood loss and the patient's comorbid conditions that may impact oxygenation, such as pulmonary, cerebrovascular, or cardiovascular disease. Inquiries are made about a personal or family history of bleeding or hypercoagulable disorders.

Neurologic

For a patient with neurologic disease (e.g., stroke, seizure disorder, multiple sclerosis), a detailed history focuses on recent events, exacerbations, deficits, or evidence of poor control of the medical condition. Information about previous investigations or therapy is recorded. The type of seizure (e.g., grand mal or petit mal) and symptoms such as staring or focal findings alert care-givers to the manifestations of the seizure.

Hepatic

Issues to explore include the cause and degree of hepatic dysfunction. Patients with severe liver disease have increased perioperative morbidity and mortality. The presence of encephalopathy, coagulopathy, ascites, volume overload, and infectivity are determined preoperatively. Any previous test results can be useful.

Renal

The type and degree of impairment are noted. Patients with renal dysfunction have many associated comorbidities, generally related to the accompanying vasculopathy. Hypertension, cardiovascular disease, and electrolyte disturbances are most common. Renal insufficiency (creatinine >2.0 mg/dL) or failure is a significant risk factor for ischemic heart disease. Such patients are at risk equal to that of a patient with angina or myocardial infarction (MI) (17) (Fig. 2.1). Renal replacement therapy (dialysis) schedules need to be determined. Ideal timing of surgery is within 24 hours after dialysis.

Musculoskeletal

Deformities and chronic inflammation are key components of many musculoskeletal disorders. The deformities may present potential challenges in airway and regional anesthesia management. Chronic inflammation and associated vasculopathy of diseases such as rheumatoid arthritis, systemic lupus erythematosus (SLE), and scleroderma often result in multiorgan dysfunction. The cardiovascular, pulmonary, renal, hematologic, integumentary, gastrointestinal, central, and peripheral nervous systems can be involved.

Endocrine

Diabetes and thyroid disease are among the most commonly encountered endocrinopathies in the perioperative period. Diabetics are at risk for multiorgan dysfunction, with renal insufficiency, strokes, peripheral neuropathies, and cardiovascular disease most prevalent. Diabetes is a significant risk factor for ischemic heart disease, so these patients are evaluated just as a patient with angina or MI would be (17) (Fig. 2.1).

Cancer

Patients with a history of cancer may have conditions related to the disease or the treatment. Preoperative evaluation focuses on evaluation of the heart, lungs, and neurologic and hematologic systems. Previous head and neck irradiation may cause carotid artery disease, hypothyroidism, or difficulty with airway management (19). Mediastinal, chest wall, or left breast irradiation can cause conduction abnormalities, cardiomyopathy, valvular abnormalities, and premature CAD even without traditional risk factors (20).

The Elderly

Chronologic age is a less important determinant of operative outcome than are comorbid conditions and physiologic age. Age older than 70 years is an independent predictor of postoperative mortality, cognitive dysfunction, major perioperative complications, and longer hospital stays (21). Organ function declines in the elderly, who respond differently to medications and have a greater number of comorbid conditions than their younger counterparts. One study found coexisting disease in 95% of geriatric patients scheduled for surgery. Postoperatively 35% of patients had cardiac or pulmonary complications that were associated with comorbid conditions, and many conditions could have been predicted preoperatively (22). Other studies have found that the rate of perioperative complications among the very elderly (>85 years) does not prohibit surgery (21).

Substance Abuse

Patients who use alcohol to excess or illicit drugs may not give a reliable history. Addicts may be at risk for myriad perioperative complications including withdrawal, acute intoxication, an altered tolerance to anesthetic and opioid medications, infections, or end-organ damage. Intravenous drug use should prompt an evaluation for cardiovascular, pulmonary, neurologic, and infectious complications. Alcoholics need assessment of cardiovascular, hepatic, and neurologic alterations. If and for how long patients can stop consuming alcohol or addictive drugs are determined. When they do stop, do they develop delirium tremens or have seizures or other signs of withdrawal? Preanesthesia clinic staff should be prepared to refer patients to addiction specialists or programs or prescribe medications to prevent withdrawal in the preoperative period if patients agree to abstinence.

Physical Examination

At a minimum, the preanesthetic examination should include vital signs (e.g., BP, heart rate [HR], respiratory rate [RR], oxygen saturation), height, and weight. Body mass index (BMI) is one of many factors associated with development of chronic diseases such as heart disease, cancer, or diabetes, and can be calculated from the height and weight (23). The formulas for calculating the BMI are as follows:

English formula:

$$BMI = \left(\frac{\text{Weight in pounds}}{(\text{Height in inches}) \times (\text{Height in inches})} \right) \times 703$$

Metric formula:

$$BMI = \frac{\text{Weight in kilograms}}{(\text{Height in meters}) \times (\text{Height in meters})}$$

or

$$BMI = \left(\frac{\text{Weight in kilograms}}{(\text{Height in centimeters}) \times (\text{Height in centimeters})} \right) \times 10,000$$

A BMI ≥40 defines extreme obesity; obesity is defined as a BMI of 30 to 39.9. An overweight person has a BMI of 25 to 29.9. Table 2.5 gives the BMI categories for children and adults.

Table 2.5. Body Mass Index (BMI)

For adults over 20 years old	
BMI	**Weight status**
Below 18.5	Underweight
18.5–24.9	Normal
25.0–29.9	Overweight
30.0 and above	Obese
For children and teens	
Underweight	BMI-for-age <5th percentile
Normal	BMI-for-age 5th percentile to <85th percentile
At risk of overweight	BMI-for-age 85th percentile to <95th percentile
Overweight	BMI-for-age ≥95th percentile

From www.cdc.gov

Not infrequently patients will have elevated BP during the preoperative visit, even without a history of hypertension. Elevated BP may be caused by anxiety or missing doses of drugs as often patients do not take their medications before an appointment or procedure. A BP reading in this setting likely does not reflect their usual control. The BP measurement should be repeated, especially after administration of anxiolytics if this is planned, or previous readings are obtained either from medical records or by asking the patient.

Inspection of the airway may be the single most important component of the physical examination from an anesthesiologist's perspective. Without specialized training in airway evaluation and management, including advanced techniques such as fiberoptic intubation (FOI), it is unlikely that nonanesthesiologists are capable of performing an adequate assessment. See Table 2.6 for components of the airway examination.

The documentation of an airway examination includes the Mallampati score, status of teeth, range of motion of the neck,

Table 2.6. Components of the airway examination

Length of upper incisors
Condition of the teeth
Relationship of upper (maxillary) incisors to lower (mandibular) incisors
Ability to protrude or advance lower (mandibular) incisors in front of upper (maxillary) incisors
Interincisor or intergum (if edentulous) distance
Visibility of the uvula
Presence of heavy facial hair
Compliance of the mandibular space
Thyromental distance
Length of the neck
Thickness or circumference of the neck
Range of motion of the head and neck

neck circumference (increasing size predicts difficulty with laryn-goscopy), thyromental distance, body habitus, and pertinent de-formities (24,25). Because of the relatively frequent incidence of dental injuries during anesthesia, a thorough documentation of pre-existing tooth abnormalities is useful. Either a tooth chart (Table 2.7) or standard nomenclature (Fig. 2.3) can be helpful. After the examination is a good time to discuss with patients the options of airway management or techniques other than general anesthesia. If awake FOI is anticipated, patients are prepared for the possibility. When challenging airways are identified, advance planning ensures that necessary equipment and skilled person-nel are available.

An evaluation of the heart, lungs, skin, and organ systems involved with disease reported by the patient is necessary.

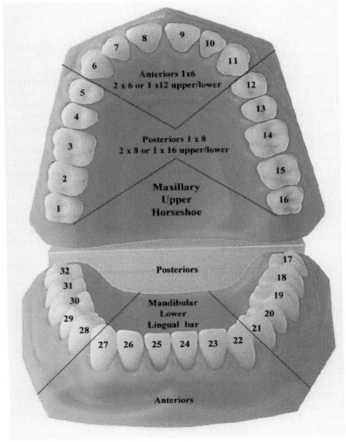

Figure 2.3. Standard dental nomenclature.

Table 2.7. Tooth classification (examples)

Top, left central incisor	Tooth #9
Top, right central incisor	Tooth #8
Bottom, left central incisor	Tooth #24
Bottom, right central incisor	Tooth #25
Top, left lateral incisor	Tooth #10
Top, left bicuspid	Tooth #11
Top, left first molar	Tooth #12
Top, left second molar	Tooth #13
Top, left third through fifth molars	Teeth #14 through 16

Auscultation of the heart for murmurs, rhythm disturbances, and signs of volume overload; inspection of the pulses and peripheral and central veins; and the presence of edema in the extremities are important diagnostically and for risk assessment. The patient is examined for third (S_3) or fourth (S_4) heart sounds, rales, jugular venous distention (JVD), ascites, hepatomegaly, and edema.

The quandary in the preoperative clinic is to determine the etiology of cardiac murmurs and to distinguish between significant murmurs and clinically unimportant ones. Diastolic murmurs are always pathologic and require further evaluation. Aortic stenosis (AS) causes a systolic ejection murmur, best heard in the right upper sternal border and often radiating to the neck. Aortic stenosis is the most common valvular lesion in the United States, affecting 2% to 4% of adults older than 65 years of age; severe stenosis is associated with a high risk of perioperative complications (17).

Observing whether the patient can walk up one to two flights of stairs can predict a variety of postoperative complications including pulmonary and cardiac events and mortality and aid in decisions regarding the need for further specialized testing such as pulmonary function tests (PFTs) or noninvasive cardiac stress testing (26) (Fig. 2.1).

The pulmonary examination includes auscultation for wheezing and decreased or abnormal breath sounds. Cyanosis or clubbing, the use of accessory muscles, and the effort of breathing are noted.

A basic neurologic examination documents deficits in mental status, speech, cranial nerves, gait, and motor and sensory function. For patients with deficits or disease or those undergoing neurologic surgery, a more extensive neurologic examination searches for specific pre-existing abnormalities that may aid in diagnosis, interfere with positioning, serve as a basis for postoperative evaluation of new deficits, and establish a baseline to defend against potential malpractice claims.

Obesity, HTN, and large neck circumference predict a greater chance of obstructive sleep apnea (OSA) (27). Intravenous access sites are noted. If sites are limited, possible central line placement is discussed with the patient or arrangements are made for assistance from interventional radiology. Auscultation for bruits is performed in patients with a history of head and neck irradiation, strokes, or transient ischemic attacks (TIAs).

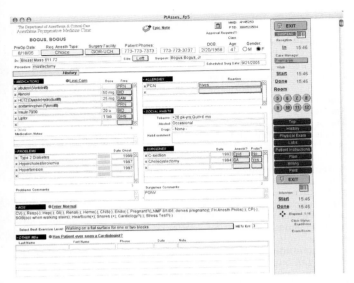

Figure 2.4. Computerized patient history.

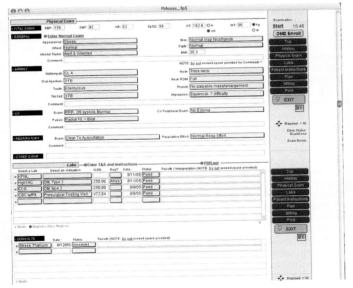

Figure 2.5. Computerized patient physical examination.

DOCUMENTATION

Frequently, preoperative evaluations are performed at locations and times remote from the delivery of anesthesia by a provider who will not preside over the anesthetic. Therefore, good methods of communication are needed. Communication issues are common problems in the perioperative period. Modern, up-to-date information systems streamline acquisition, storage, and transfer of patient data among primary care providers, the laboratory, consultants, surgeons, and operating room (OR) and clinic personnel. Many institutions have developed their own computer-based programs (Figs. 2.4 and 2.5) and a variety of commercial products are available. These products can be as simple as a questionnaire or as advanced as complex systems with decision support tools for diagnostic testing or consultations, physician computer order entry, direct links to laboratory databases, and the capability of printing patient instructions (Fig. 2.6) and a summary of the evaluation.

PREOPERATIVE TESTING

Diagnostic tests can aid in the assessment of the risk of anesthesia and surgery, guide medical intervention to lower risk, and provide baseline results to direct intra- and postoperative decisions. The choice of laboratory tests depends on the probable impact of the test results on the differential diagnosis and on patient management. Preoperative testing may be necessary to establish baseline values (but have limited usefulness for this purpose), evaluate existing medical conditions, and establish diagnoses in asymptomatic individuals with known risk factors for a disease. A test should be ordered only if the results will inform the decision to proceed with the planned procedure or alter the care plans. The results of the history and physical examination direct test ordering. Table 2.2 contains recommendations for testing based on specific medical conditions and procedures.

Healthy patients, regardless of age, who will undergo low- or intermediate-risk procedures without expected significant blood loss are unlikely to benefit from any tests. Exceptions are a procedure with the injection of contrast dye or a patient >55 years, in whom a screening creatinine level is indicated. When there is a possibility of pregnancy, a pregnancy test should be ordered. Table 2.3 lists recommendations for tests for healthy patients. In general, tests are recommended only under the following conditions, when results:

- Confirm an abnormality suspected from the history or physical examination
- Change, cancel, or postpone the surgical procedure
- Change anesthesia and medical management
- Change monitoring or intra- or postoperative care

The ASA task force found that test results are valid for up to 6 months before surgery if the medical history has not substantially changed (8).

Electrocardiograms

ECGs are one of the most frequently ordered preoperative tests. Some ECGs are ordered without a clear understanding of their

Patient Instructions For: **Bogus Patient 5/13/2003**   MHID#: 9999999

The day before your surgery you should take your regular medications, unless instructed otherwise. On the morning of surgery, please take only the requested medications as shown below, with water.

MEDICATIONS	
Medication	**Instruction**
Labetalol	Take morning of surgery
Minoxidil	Take morning of surgery
Procardia	Take morning of surgery
Vasotec	Take morning of surgery
Calcium	DO NOT take the morning of surgery
Renegel	DO NOT take the morning of surgery

OTHER SPECIAL INSTRUCTIONS:

NOTHING to eat or drink after MIDNIGHT the night before your surgery, except TAKE MEDICATIONS AS DIRECTED with a small amount of water.

Today, the anesthesiologist or the physician's assistant talked to you about different kinds of anesthesia that are <u>possible</u> **options for you. However, the choice of anesthesia is not made until the day of your procedure with the anesthesiologist who will be taking care of you. You will have an opportunity to meet your anesthesiologist on the day of your procedure to ask questions and make a final decision.**

Please come to the surgical waiting area at least one hour before the start of your scheduled surgery time unless you are informed to do otherwise.

You must have an escort home that is here with you or readily available if you are receiving anesthesia the day of your surgery. A taxi driver is not an escort. You will not be able to drive youself home, walk home, or take a bus after receiving anesthesia.

If you have a child who is having surgery, please do not leave the building! Your child will need you when he/she wakes up from surgery.

Please leave all jewelry, cash and other valuables at home. <u>Note</u>: this includes rings in your belly button, ears, nose, tongue, and/or face. Please do not wear make-up to the hospital.

After the nurse has completed your assessment and your intravenous line has been placed you will be allowed to have one visitor in the pre-op area.

No food or drinks are allowed in the pre-op area.

Today you met with Dr. Anesthesia to discuss plans for anesthesia. You will be contacted if any follow-up work needs to be done. We have the following telephone number(s) to contact you: 666–666–6666

If you have questions regarding anesthesia or your medications call your Anesthesia Manager, Nurse RN at the Anesthesia Perioperative Clinic (773) 834-7255.

If you have questions about surgery (time, place, type of surgery) call your surgeon:

Surgeon, Doctor

The University of Chicago • Department of Anesthesia & Critical Care
5841 S. Maryland Avenue, MC 4028, Chicago, Ilinois 60637   **Tel: (773) 834-7255**
                                                  Fax: (773) 834-7137

Figure 2.6. Sample of patient instructions.

usefulness. A normal ECG adds little to preoperative evaluation, and abnormal tracings are quite common. Few abnormalities on a preoperative resting ECG are likely to change management. Preoperative ECGs may establish a baseline for comparison postoperatively. This is likely the most important reason to order a preoperative ECG, but this has never been studied. Cardiovascular complications are among the most common serious adverse events intra- and postoperatively and an ECG is necessary in evaluating patients suspected of such events. Because patients at risk for cardiovascular complications are less likely to have a normal tracing preoperatively, having a comparison ECG may be useful. A preoperative ECG is needed on patients who are likely to have an abnormal ECG *and* who have risk factors for perioperative cardiac complications. Conditions for which an ECG needs to be ordered are listed in Table 2.3.

Another reason to obtain a preoperative ECG is to detect occult heart disease. Heart disease is common in a middle-aged population and increases with age. Pre-existing heart disease increases perioperative risk. A resting ECG is not a reliable screen for CAD and is a poor predictor of heart disease without a supporting history in nonsurgical patients. Symptoms and risk factors are much better predictors of heart disease.

Many abnormalities may have implications for anesthesia care beyond the detection of CAD. Arrhythmias such as atrial fibrillation, which should be detected on physical examination and confirmed by ECG; conduction abnormalities; or left ventricular hypertrophy (LVH) may alter anesthesia plans.

Some ECG abnormalities, such as new Q waves and arrhythmias, are important in the perioperative period. One study found that only 2% of patients had one or both of these abnormalities (28). It has been estimated that the frequency of silent Q-wave infarctions found only by ECG in men 75 years or older (the highest-risk group) is 0.5%. In ambulatory surgical patients, the incidence of abnormal ECGs was 43% in a population in which only 1.6% of patients had an adverse perioperative cardiac event. The preoperative ECG was of potential value in only half (6 of 751) of those suffering a morbid event (29).

Unfortunately, the specificity of an ECG abnormality for predicting postoperative cardiac complications is only 26%; therefore, a normal ECG does not exclude cardiac disease (30). According to American College of Cardiology/American Heart Association (ACC/AHA) guidelines, ECG abnormalities other than Q waves are a minor predictor of complications (17). History is a far better predictor. An abnormal ECG will be found in 62% of patients, in 44% of patients with strong risk factors for ischemic heart disease and in 7% of patients >50 years with no risk factors. Results are abnormal in only 3% of patients between 50 and 70 years of age without risk factors for heart disease (31). Routine preoperative ECG testing is not indicated in patients without a history of cardiovascular disease or significant risk factors (32). In summary, the prevalence of abnormalities on ECG may incur costly evaluation (the yield of which is quite low) and delay necessary surgery. Another option is to obtain a 12-lead ECG for baseline comparison only for patients with abnormalities on tracings when monitors are placed in the preoperative area or the OR on the day of surgery. This method limits the expense of unnecessary 12-lead ECGs in patients with normal tracings.

The Center for Medicare and Medicaid Services (CMS) does not reimburse for "routine" or "preoperative" ECGs without an appropriate International Classification of Diseases (ICD-9) code (33).

Hematology

Hemoglobin (Hgb) and hematocrit (Hct) levels are frequently borderline abnormal in otherwise healthy patients of any age but rarely impact anesthetic care or management unless the planned procedure involves the potential for significant bleeding. Preoperative Hct, surgical procedure, and surgeon can predict the need for perioperative transfusion and can guide type and screen (T&S) or crossmatch (T&CM) ordering or blood conservation strategies (34). The incidence of abnormalities in Hgb or Hct ranges from 0.3% to 10.5% in published studies, with elderly patients accounting for most abnormal values (35,36). Low Hgb can be predicted from the likelihood of anemia in underlying disease (e.g., 75% of patients with Duke's stage D colon cancer) (37). Consequences from moderate levels of anemia and Hgb levels ≥ 6.0 g/dL in patients without CAD are minimal. According to the ASA guidelines for perioperative blood transfusion, transfusion is rarely required for patients with Hgb >10 g/dL (38). In nonoperative settings in populations with critical illness or chronic disease states associated with known CAD or risk factors for CAD, Hct levels $>33\%$ are associated with adverse outcomes (39,40). Patients with OSA, significant pulmonary disease, smoking history, or congenital heart disease are at risk for polycythemia.

Preoperative Hgb should be obtained based on the likelihood of abnormalities of anemia or polycythemia and the likelihood of significant intraoperative blood loss.

White Blood Cell Count

Abnormal white blood cell (WBC) counts have a very low yield in preoperative screening with a prevalence of $<1\%$ (41). WBC determination is indicated if one suspects an infection, a myelodysplastic syndrome, leukocytosis, or leucopenia. Many institutions include a WBC count with a complete blood count (CBC), so an abnormal test result may need further evaluation. As with most unexpected abnormalities, the test needs to be repeated. If results are still abnormal, drugs (corticosteroids are a common cause of an elevated WBC count) or diseases found by history and physical examination should be considered.

Platelet Count

The reported incidence of abnormal platelet counts is 0.0% to 2.0% (36,42). In one study, 8% of tests were abnormal, and all the patients had slight thrombocytosis (43). No study in the literature has used a platelet count of $<100,000$ (the level that increases risk of bleeding with centroneuraxial anesthesia) or of $<50,000$ (the level that increases surgical bleeding) to determine the prevalence of abnormal platelet counts. The likelihood of finding a value this low without a history of significant bruising or bleeding, a myelodysplastic disorder, or exposure to drugs or chemotherapeutic agents known to cause thrombocytopenia is rare. Spurious thrombocytopenia from platelet clumping caused by ethylene-diaminetetraacetic acid (EDTA, a chelating agent used in test tubes for CBC determinations) is a possibility, so in addition to repeating the test, examination of the peripheral blood smear is warranted. Platelets are "acute phase reactants" and levels transiently rise with various stressors.

Coagulation Studies

Coagulation studies (prothrombin, activated partial thrombo-plastin time, bleeding time) are not recommended unless the patient history suggests a coagulation disorder or the patient is taking anticoagulants. If the history is negative for a bleeding disorder, the cost of screening coagulation tests before minor surgery outweighs the benefit. Many practitioners mistakenly believe that a *screening* prothrombin time (PT) is more likely to be abnormal because of the numbers of patients with liver disease, malnutrition, or warfarin use, conditions that should be readily identified by the history. If *screening* tests (not based on history) are ordered, a platelet count and activated partial thromboplastin time (aPTT) are most beneficial to detect the uncommon patient with thrombocytopenia, an acquired anticoagulant (e.g., lupus anticoagulant), or a reduced level of a contact activation factor (e.g., von Willebrand disease or deficiencies in factors VIII, IX, XI, or XII) (43,44). The most common congenital coagulopathy is von Willebrand disease, estimated to be present in 1% of the population.

Acquired anticoagulants (e.g., lupus anticoagulant, anticardi-olipin antibody) cause a prolonged aPTT but actually increase the risk of deep venous thrombosis (DVT) and pulmonary emboli (PE), not bleeding. Therefore, both *hypo*coagulable and *hyper*coagulable states can result in a prolonged aPTT, making accurate preoperative diagnosis necessary because the treatment for each condition is different. Just as with a prolonged aPTT, a *short* aPTT may increase the risk of thromboembolism.

The CMS does not reimburse for "routine" or "preoperative" PT/aPTT without an appropriate ICD-9 code (33).

Bleeding times are poor predictors of perioperative bleeding (46,47). They are extremely operator dependent and have poor reproducibility. Many institutions no longer even offer this test.

Blood Typing

Type and screen (T&S) testing before the day of surgery and planning for the availability of blood avoid delay of the procedure (48). A "type" is done for the ABO group and Rh type and the "screen" is for significant red blood cell (RBC) antibodies. If the antibody screen is positive, the target antigen must be determined. Approximately 2% to 3% of patients will have unusual antibodies detected by the T&S, which makes finding matching blood difficult. Hours or weeks may be needed depending on the rarity of the antigen and the inventory of available blood products.

Traditionally blood for the T&S was collected on patient admission to the hospital. Now same-day admission for surgery means that blood banks have little time to test and obtain blood. A T&S ahead of time can ease the burden on the blood bank personnel for same-day admission or outpatient surgery and potentially decrease errors. Minimizing time constraints may prevent the clerical mistakes that are the most common cause of transfusion reactions. One fourth of the time a T&S collected on the day of surgery is not complete until after the start of the procedure (49). A common misconception is that O-negative blood is a "universal donor," but it is not appropriate for the subset of patients with alloantibodies against non-ABO antigens.

A T&S may be all that is needed if the probability of a transfusion is low. A T&S is the first step when the need for blood products and a type and crossmatch (T&CM) is anticipated. Crossmatching blood that is not transfused is costly (personnel, inventory) and increases waste (blood reserved that then becomes outdated). The Federal Drug Administration (www.fda.gov) regulates how far in advance T&S and T&CM can be obtained, and factors such as previous transfusions and pregnancy (within 3 months) further limit this time. A protocol can be instituted with the departments of surgery and anesthesia and the blood bank based on the likelihood of requiring blood replacement depending on the type of surgery (i.e., maximum surgical blood ordering schedule [MSBOS]) (34,50). Institutions with specific protocols to collect T&S samples before hospital admission are successful in doing so 75% of the time (48).

A T&S should be obtained (within the expiration timeframe) when there is a reasonable likelihood the patient will require a transfusion.

Chemistries

Creatinine

Preoperative renal insufficiency increases the risk of perioperative cardiac complications (an intermediate risk factor on par with known CAD), worsening renal function and mortality (17). Mild to moderate renal insufficiency is unlikely to be associated with symptoms or physical findings to suggest this diagnosis. A screening study targeting people with diabetes, hypertension, or age >55 years found one case of renal insufficiency (defined as a glomerular filtration rate [GFR] <60 mL/min/1.73 m^2) for each 8.7 persons screened (51). A creatinine should be obtained for patients with known kidney disease or with risk factors for renal dysfunction (age >55 years, diabetes, vascular disease, lupus) use of diuretics, or planned use of radiographic dye.

Electrolytes

Not unexpectedly, the incidence of electrolyte abnormalities in preoperative screening studies is 0.2% to 81.2%, depending on the criteria for abnormal values and the screened population, which has fueled the advocacy for performing these tests (12,52). Preoperative hypokalemia (arguably the most important electrolyte perioperatively) was not associated with arrhythmias, and most abnormalities could have been predicted by the patient history (35,53,54). Preoperative electrolytes should be obtained for patients with a history of renal disease, malnutrition, gastric bypass procedures, or use of digoxin or diuretics.

Glucose

There are approximately 20 million persons in the United States with diabetes and 1 million new cases are diagnosed each year.

Many patients have undiagnosed disease, newly discovered in one third after diabetes-related complications. Diabetes markedly increases the risk of vascular (cerebral, renal, coronary, and peripheral) disease and perioperative complications (17,55). Symptoms of diabetes are nonspecific, making history (other than family history of the disease) less reliable in screening at-risk patients. Tight perioperative management of glucose in stroke, coronary bypass surgery, or critically ill individuals improves outcomes (55). If future studies extend this finding to a broader surgical population or to those with a high rate of diabetes-related complications (e.g., infections in joint replacement surgeries in obese individuals), then future diabetes *screening* may be warranted. Glucose should be measured in patients with diabetes, obesity, a family history of diabetes, cerebrovascular or intracranial disease, or poor exercise tolerance (which may be associated with coronary disease and inability to monitor symptoms) or in those taking steroids.

HbA1c

Glycosylated hemoglobin (HbA1c) is a measure of long-term (3 months) glucose control and is a much better assessment of adequacy of therapy than a fasting or random blood glucose measurement. Currently, the American Diabetes Association recommends a target of <7% for patients with type 2 diabetes. Lower levels of HbA1c are associated with reduced microvascular and neuropathic complications. An elevated HbA1c is associated with an increased risk for cardiovascular events, postoperative infections, and fasting gastric fluid volumes (56,57,58). Obtaining an HbA1c level preoperatively can guide glucose management to intensify therapy before a procedure (59). An argument can be made for obtaining an HbA1c for all diabetics before surgery.

Liver Tests

Patients with acute hepatitis, significant liver dysfunction, or cirrhosis are at increased risk for perioperative complications and death. No data, however, suggest that patients with asymptomatic elevations of transaminases, bilirubin, or PT have adverse perioperative events. One study in veterans who had major noncardiac surgery, a serum albumin <2.1 mg/dL was a strong predictor of mortality (60). An albumin level should be measured preoperatively in patients with malnutrition or malabsorption or at risk for such conditions (e.g., gastric bypass patients).

Thyroid Function Tests

There is no evidence that patients with mild or moderate thyroid disease have a greater risk of major perioperative complications. Surgery, stress, or illness can precipitate myxedema or thyroid storm in patients with untreated or severe thyroid dysfunction (61). It is reasonable to order thyroid stimulating hormone (TSH), T4, and T3 tests if patients have a history of hyper- or hypothyroidism, whether treated or not, if such tests were not obtained within the last 6 to 12 months before surgery.

Pregnancy Testing

There is much controversy and no consensus for routine pregnancy testing. Surveys have shown that 30% to 50% of practitioners mandate testing in females of childbearing age, primarily because of the unreliability of the history, especially from minors, and the concern over the potential harm to the pregnancy or fetus from anesthesia and surgery, with the attendant medicolegal implications (62). Opponents of mandatory testing cite the false-positive rate, the cost, the belief that history is reliable if taken in privacy, and the paucity of data establishing risks of anesthesia in early pregnancy. When minors are pregnant, their privacy is governed by state laws. One must be familiar with local statutes and how unexpected positive pregnancy results will be handled.

Some practices and facilities provide patients with information about the potential risks of anesthesia and surgery on pregnancy but allow them to decline testing. If medicolegal concerns are paramount, a signed waiver of the right to sue over a denied and undetected pregnancy can be obtained (63). Other practices mandate that all females of childbearing age undergo a urine pregnancy test on the day of surgery. It has been suggested that if a mandatory testing policy is utilized that patients be informed that consent to surgery or anesthesia includes consent for pregnancy testing. This policy may prevent conflicts in which patients or legal guardians refuse to pay charges or even threaten lawsuits over undesired testing (63).

With the high reliability of urine testing for pregnancy, it is best to delay testing until the day of surgery, unless the patient herself suspects pregnancy or the menstrual period is delayed. Negative test results days before surgery may be positive on the day of surgery. In its Preoperative Evaluation Practice Advisory, the ASA recognized that the literature "is insufficient to inform patients or physicians whether anesthesia causes harmful effects on early pregnancy." The advisory suggests that pregnancy testing be offered to women if the test result would alter patient management (8).

Therapeutic Drug Levels

Routinely ordering tests for serum levels of certain drugs (e.g., seizure medications, digoxin, theophylline) is not indicated unless toxicity is a concern or one suspects that the patient is not compliant or not optimally treated. Many conditions are adequately treated even with subtherapeutic levels of medications. For most drugs the effective target is based on the trough level. Therefore, if blood levels are drawn, when the patient ingested the drug, any missed doses within the previous days, and the exact time the blood sample was obtained are documented.

Arterial Blood Gases

Arterial blood gas (ABG) measurement is useful in hypoxic patients (oxygen saturation by pulse oximetry ≤90% to 91%) and patients with severe lung disease, decompensated congestive heart failure (CHF), or musculoskeletal disorders that impact ventilation. ABGs are not useful in predicting pulmonary complications in patients undergoing non–lung resection surgeries (64). ABGs are useful in predicting pulmonary function after lung resection surgery but not risk for complications.

Chest Radiographs

Abnormal results on preoperative chest radiographs range from 7% to 60%, with higher rates in elderly populations (65,66). In one meta-analysis of the value of preoperative chest radiographs, 10% were abnormal, 1.3% showed new unanticipated problems, and only 0.1% changed perioperative care (67). Chest radiographs have not been shown to predict postoperative pulmonary complications (64). Chest radiographs are indicated only in patients with cardiovascular or pulmonary signs or symptoms of undetermined cause or severity.

Pulmonary Function Tests

Pulmonary function tests (PFTs) may be indicated to diagnose disease (*is dyspnea caused by lung disease or CHF?*) or assess management (*can dyspnea or wheezing be improved further?*) but *not* as a risk assessment tool or to deny a beneficial procedure (68). The degree of airway obstruction, measured by the forced expiratory volume in 1 second (FEV_1), does not predict pulmonary complications (64,69).

Traditionally PFTs have been obtained for patients before lung resection. A preoperative FEV_1 <2 L or 50% of predicted, a maximal voluntary ventilation <50% predicted, or diffusing capacity for carbon monoxide (DL_{CO}) <60% of predicted increases the risk of postoperative respiratory insufficiency or death in patients undergoing pneumonectomy (70). PFTs are also used to estimate postresection pulmonary reserve in patients scheduled for lung resection. Spirometry with determination of FEV_1 is the first step. If there is a significant reduction in FEV_1, a radionuclide quantitative lung scan (V/Q) can evaluate functional capacity of the proposed residual lung (71). A calculated predicted postoperative FEV_1 ≥0.8 L or ≥40% of normal suggests that the patient will tolerate the procedure with acceptable risks (72). See Chapter 5 for a more detailed discussion of this topic.

Urinalysis

The reported incidence of abnormal urinalysis in the literature ranges from 0.8% to 39%. The number of abnormalities that influenced management, were not predicted by history, or were not caused by contamination averages <2%. Urinalysis is needed preoperatively only if a urinary tract infection (UTI) is suspected.

Age-based Testing

Testing should be determined from disease and procedure indications, not age alone. No correlation has been established independent of coexisting disease, a positive history, or findings on physical examination between age and abnormalities in Hgb, electrolytes, radiographs, or PFTs (10,12,73). In a screening of the general population for renal insufficiency (defined as a GFR <60 mL/min/1.73 m^2), age >55 years was highly predictive (51). Because renal insufficiency, until very advanced, produces few symptoms or physical signs and yet is strongly associated with perioperative adverse events (progression of renal dysfunction, cardiovascular complications, and mortality), there is an argument for obtaining a preoperative creatinine based on age (17).

Even though ECG abnormalities are more common with advanced age, abnormalities alone do not predict postoperative cardiac complications in the elderly (29,30). Significant abnormalities that impact care are rare in the absence of a history or symptoms of cardiac disease (29). The ASA Practice Advisory for Preanesthesia Evaluation recognizes "that age alone may not be an indication for an electrocardiogram" (8). CMS will not pay for age-based ECGs or those ordered as a preoperative test; a supporting diagnosis with an acceptable ICD-9 code is required (45).

Cataract Surgery

In a study of more than 18,000 patients randomly allocated to no *routine* testing before cataract surgery or a battery of tests including ECG, CBC, electrolytes, blood urea nitrogen (BUN), creatinine, and glucose levels, no differences in postoperative adverse events were found between the two groups (74). However, the results of this study do not suggest that patients undergoing cataract surgery require no laboratory testing (74). This study of patients having the most minimal of surgeries showed that it was safe to eliminate *routine* tests, not tests indicated for a new or worsening medical problem. *All* patients underwent a *preoperative medical assessment*. The group that crossed over from no testing to some testing had significantly more coexisting illness and poor self-reported health status. More than 85% of enrollees reported good to excellent health status; almost 25% reported no coexisting illnesses such as hypertension, anemia, diabetes, or heart or lung disease; almost 30% were <70 years old; and 65% had an ASA-PS 1 or 2 score, suggesting a fairly healthy group. Exclusion criteria for the study were general anesthesia or a MI within 3 months (74).

If patients are comparable to those in the study, are routinely evaluated by primary care physicians, have stable mild disease, and will undergo cataract surgery under topical or bulbar block, then no special testing is required because of cataract surgery. The study by Schein et al. (74) suggests that a preoperative care provider needs to evaluate patients before surgery. Poorly controlled, serious conditions must be normalized, and selective testing suggested by history and physical examination may be necessary. Rarely is testing necessary *because* of cataract surgery, but patients with limited access to health care services may benefit from medical evaluation.

THE ECONOMICS OF TESTING

Diagnostic testing is expensive. The cost of routine medical testing before cataract surgery alone is estimated at $150 million annually. Routine urinalyses before knee surgery in the United States cost $1.5 million in 1989 to prevent one wound infection (75). One study found that 50% more routine ECGs and 40% more chest radiographs were ordered in a fee-for-service versus a prepaid practice (76).

Many facilities have developed diagnostic testing guidelines to improve patient care, standardize clinical practice, improve efficiency, and reduce costs. With implementation of guidelines, one facility reduced tests ordered by 60%, improved testing by 81%, and saved almost $80,000 per year (77). The Mayo Clinic reduced preoperative testing and associated costs without a change in outcomes (52). A computerized preanesthetic evaluation system can increase hospital (not just preoperative clinic) reimbursement by improved documentation of diagnosis-related group (DRG) codes when ICD-9 codes are changed (78).

Physicians working in or administering preanesthetic clinics in the United States must familiarize themselves with the CMS Advance Beneficiary Notice (ABN) billing rules (33). These rules govern whether physicians and other part B providers can bill beneficiaries directly if Medicare will not pay for services for lack of medical necessity. In the past, under Medicare, liability for uncovered services was the responsibility of the beneficiary. Changes to the rules relieve beneficiaries from financial liability if the provider failed to disclose that the service was not reimbursed by CMS. Unless the physician or facility has followed the ABN rules, payment may not be sought from the patient. ABN rules apply only to outpatient services. Additional information can be obtained from http://www.cms.hhs.gov.

TIMING OF ASSESSMENT

The Practice Advisory for Preanesthesia Evaluation commissioned by the ASA determined that the timing of the preanesthesia assessment depends on the patient's condition, the type of procedure, the health care system, and the patient's access to care providers (8). The recommendations, the opinions of experts and randomly selected ASA members, favored assessments on the day of surgery or before for low to medium invasive procedures. Assessments were recommended before the day of surgery for highly invasive procedures or for patients with severe disease. For selected patients, evaluations on the day of surgery can be safe and effective.

It has been suggested that the importance of a visit to the preoperative clinic before a surgical procedure cannot be overestimated (79). A Canadian survey found that more than 60% of patients thought it important to see an anesthesiologist preoperatively; more than 30% thought it was extremely important; and more than half indicated the visit should be before the day of surgery (80). Anesthesiologists at Massachusetts General Hospital showed that a preoperative visit before the day of surgery was as good as or better than medication in reducing preoperative anxiety and postoperative pain (81).

Table 2.8 outlines the criteria and medical conditions of patients likely to benefit from evaluation in a preanesthesia clinic before the day of surgery.

PATIENT MANAGEMENT

Management of comorbid conditions and interventions to reduce risk are as important as identification and diagnosis of medical disease. If anesthesiologists do not intervene to improve new or chronic disease states, then close collaboration with primary care physicians, specialists, and surgeons is essential. Far too many anesthesia practices collect information without processes in place for follow through to manage risk, optimize outcomes, and reduce adverse events.

Table 2.8. Situations for which preoperative evaluation before the day of surgery is recommended

Airway
Previous airway surgery
Unusual airway anatomy
Airway tumor or obstruction

Anesthesia-related
Patient has had previous difficult intubation or paralysis or nerve damage during surgery
Patient or family has had elevated temperature during anesthesia, malignant hyperthermia, allergy to succinylcholine, or pseudocholinesterase deficiency

Cardiovascular
Angina
Coronary artery disease
History of myocardial infarction
Symptomatic arrhythmias
Congestive heart failure
Pacemaker
Implantable cardioverter defibrillator (ICD)
Poorly controlled hypertension SBP >180 mm Hg or DBP >110 mm Hg

Endocrine/metabolic
Diabetes
Adrenal disorders
Active thyroid disease
Obesity >140% ideal body weight

General
Normal activity severely inhibited
Monitoring or medical assistance at home within 6 mo
Hospital admission within 2 mo

Language
Patient or parent/guardian cannot hear, speak, or understand English

Neuromuscular
Seizure disorder
CNS disease (i.e., multiple sclerosis, CVA)
Myopathy, myasthenia gravis, or other muscle disorders

Oncology
Chemotherapy (within 6 mo)
Radiation (within 6 mo)
Significant physiologic compromise

Pregnancy
Patient is pregnant (unless the procedure is termination of pregnancy)

Procedure-Related
Intraoperative blood transfusion likely
ICU admission likely
High-risk surgery

Renal
Renal insufficiency or failure

CNS, central nervous system; CVA, cerebrovascular accident; DBP, diastolic blood pressure; ICU, intensive care unit; SBP, systolic blood pressure.
The medical condition portion of this table has been adapted with permission from Pasternak LR. Preoperative evaluation of the ambulatory surgery patient. Ambulatory surgery. *Anesthesiol Rep.* 1990;3(1):8.

Dear Colleague:

_____ **is scheduled for** __(type of surgery)__ . **Please evaluate for the following:**

( ) Coronary artery disease

( ) Review of previous stress test, echo or catheterization

( ) Prophylactic preoperative beta blocker therapy

( ) Poorly controlled CHF

( ) Murmur requiring identification &/or recommendations for management

( ) Poorly controlled hypertension

( ) Poorly controlled asthma, COPD or other pulmonary condition

( ) Carotid bruit

( ) Poorly controlled diabetes

( ) Abnormal liver function

( ) Blood dyscrasia

( ) Other _____

Pertinent Information: _____
_____
_____
_____

_____,M.D. Pager #_____

Please fax your notes *and* **all test results to** _____ **or call** _____ **with questions.** *This is not a request from the surgeon's office.* **Please do NOT send us a** *"clearance letter"* **without supporting documentation or a summary of the patient's condition**

Figure 2.7. Consultation request sample.

Consultations

Collaborative care of patients is often necessary and beneficial. Consultation initiated by the preoperative physician seeks specific advice regarding diagnosis and status of the patient's condition(s) (Fig. 2.7). Asking specific questions such as "Does this patient have CAD?" or "Is this patient in the best medical condition for planned thoracotomy with lung resection under general anesthesia?" is the first step. Letters or notes stating "cleared for surgery" are rarely sufficient to design a safe anesthetic. A letter summarizing the patient's medical problems and condition, along with the results of diagnostic tests, is necessary.

Close coordination and good communication among the preoperative anesthesiologist, surgeon, primary care physician, and consultant are vital. Miscommunication among care providers was central to most reported incidents in the AIMS whenever preoperative assessment was implicated (3).

In many practices, the cardiology service is most frequently consulted perioperatively. In one survey, however, the utility of such consultations was questioned by anesthesiologists. Only

17% of anesthesiologists felt obligated to follow the consulting cardiologist's recommendations. Forty percent of the consultations contained only the recommendation to "proceed with the case," "cleared for surgery," or "continue with current medications." Recommendations regarding intraoperative monitoring or cardiac medications were largely ignored (82). Part of this responsibility lies with the consulting physicians (whether surgeons or anesthesiologists) and the longstanding practice of asking for or receiving cardiac "clearance." This request is vague and a response (often scribbled on a prescription pad) simply stating "low risk" or "cleared for surgery" is meaningless and unhelpful. In general, preoperative consultations should be sought for the following:

- Diagnosis, evaluation, and improvement of a new or poorly controlled condition
- Creation of a clinical risk profile that the patient, anesthesiologist, and surgeon use to make management decisions

Detailed discussions and communication, preferably oral, are essential for the best management of complicated patients. Copies of diagnostic studies that accompany the consultation letter help the anesthesiologist to make an independent decision about patient risk and to plan anesthetic care.

Medicolegal Culpability

As anesthesiologists broaden their scope of practice and responsibilities, concerns over medical liability arise. Professional negligence or malpractice is generally characterized as a failure on the part of the physician to possess or exercise reasonable skill or diligence in the diagnosis or treatment of a patient. The essential elements of a medical malpractice claim include a duty toward the patient, a breach of that duty, and an injury because of a breach of duty. A physician's responsibility is to act in accordance with *national* standards of care established by the profession, which are defined in terms of care delivered by an average practitioner, not the *best* practitioner.

Duties of the preoperative physician include examination of the patient and referral to a specialist if necessary. Part of the examination requires the use of diagnostic tests or techniques that an average, reasonable practitioner would use in similar circumstances.

Often physicians are concerned about failure to diagnose a condition by failing to order a diagnostic screening test. The traditional system of ordering preoperative tests routinely evolved from the mistaken belief that more information, no matter how irrelevant or expensive, will improve care, enhance safety, and decrease liability. In reality, nonselective screening may increase legal culpability. Unanticipated abnormalities on laboratory test results are uncommon. The relationship between these abnormalities and surgical and anesthetic morbidity is weak at best. More than half of all abnormal test results obtained in routine preoperative screening are ignored or not noted in the medical record, which is the document of interest to the courts. It has been suggested that not following up on an abnormal result is a greater medicolegal risk than failure to order the test in the first place or not identifying the abnormality to begin with.

Practice Guidelines

An important element for a successful preoperative evaluation system is a uniform, consistent method for assessment and management. Even though individual judgment is necessary, guidelines and policies for the group should be developed. Cancellations, delays, or demands for additional diagnostic testing on the day of surgery after a patient has been evaluated and deemed acceptable for anesthesia by the preoperative clinic is detrimental to the success of a preoperative assessment program.

Practice guidelines to improve the process of preoperative evaluation and management can affect surgical outcomes. Guidelines minimize variation in clinical practice and make good use of resources. They may help to avoid cancellations or delays on the day of surgery when the anesthesiologist in the preanesthetic clinic and the one performing the anesthetic have differences of opinion about the patient's fitness for surgery. This will prevent patient inconvenience and disappointment and surgeon dissatisfaction. Guidelines synthesized from the best, most current sources help practitioners stay up to date with recommendations in the literature. Guidelines can be as simple as an organization of the type and timing of care delivered to typical, uncomplicated patients or as complex as instructions for dealing with a specific issue expressed by decision trees in branching logic format (83). When disease-specific algorithms are developed and agreed upon by all stakeholders, acceptance is more likely. The intent is not to design inflexible standards but to provide a consistent, straightforward method to evaluate a particular disease, such as hypertension or CAD (Fig. 2.1); a finding such as a murmur; or a symptom such as chest pain. Practice guidelines recommend care based on scientific evidence and broad consensus but leave room for justifiable variations in practice.

Practice guidelines typically rely on evidence-based medicine that examines the data from clinical research. Intuition, personal clinical experience, and pathophysiologic rationale are less important. The practice and teaching of evidence-based medicine requires skills that are not part of traditional medical training. Precisely defining a problem and the information required to resolve it are the first steps. The pertinent studies from a well-conducted literature search are selected and applied to the treatment of medical conditions found in patients.

THE FUTURE

Preoperative assessments in the future may involve taking a blood sample to identify a patient with genetic polymorphisms linked to perioperative adverse outcomes. Theoretically, this information would allow caregivers to design pharmacologic interventions and management to directly alter morbidity and mortality (84). Molecular biology, which is rapidly increasing our ability to identify genetic variability and its effects on diseases and responses to therapies, could dramatically alter risk assessment and management plans. Reliance on population studies may be supplanted by treatments based on individual patient characteristics. Pharmacogenetics may eventually lead to genetic screening tests to identify patients at risk for adverse perioperative outcomes. These include the classic examples of pseudocholinesterase deficiency, halothane hepatitis, susceptibility to malignant hyperthermia, and pain tolerance, and the less familiar traits associated with the duration and response to benzodiazepines, opioids, anesthetics, and nonsteroidal anti-inflammatory drugs (85).

CONCLUSION

In the AIMS study perioperative morbidity and mortality were attributed to poor assessment and management of patients in the preoperative period (3). One of the deficiencies noted was that the anesthesiologist delivering the anesthetic did the preoperative evaluation in only 77% of the cases. The authors concluded that this had a potentially negative effect. However, another view would hold that if preoperative assessment and management require expert knowledge and skills that the average care provider without advanced training in the field possesses, then harm may be a result of a failure to appreciate opportunities for interventions to lower risk.

REFERENCES

1. Maze M, Todd MM. Special issue on postoperative cognitive dysfunction. Selected reports from the journal-sponsored symposium. (editorial) *Anesthesiology.* 2007;106:418–420.
2. Mangano DT. Assessment of the patient with cardiac disease: an anesthesiologist's paradigm. *Anesthesiology.* 1999;91:1521–1530.
3. Kluger MT, Tham EJ, Coleman NA, et al. Inadequate preoperative evaluation and preparation: a review of 197 reports from the Australian incident monitoring study. *Anaesthesia.* 2000;55:1173–1178.
4. Runciman WB, Webb RK. *Austr Soc Anaesth Newsl.* 1994; 94:15–17.
5. Davis NJ, ed. *Anaesthesia-Related Mortality in Australia 1994–1996.* Melbourne: Capital Press; 1999.
6. Ferschl MB, Tung A, Sweitzer BJ, et al. Economic impact of a preoperative clinic on operating room efficiency. *Anesthesiology.* 2005;103:855–859.
7. Lonsdale M, Hutchison GL. Patients' desire for information about anaesthesia; Scottish and Canadian attitudes. *Anaesthesia.* 1991;46:410–412.
8. American Society of Anesthesiologists Task Force on Preanesthesia Evaluation. Practice advisory for preanesthesia evaluation: a report by the American Society of Anesthesiologists Task Force on Preanesthesia Evaluation. *Anesthesiology.* 2002;96:485–496. Available at: http://www.asahq.org. Accessed March 11, 2007.
9. Blery C, Szatan M, Fourgeaux B, et al. Evaluation of a protocol for selective ordering of preoperative tests. *Lancet.* 1986;18:139–141.
10. O'Connor ME, Drasner K. Preoperative laboratory testing of children undergoing elective surgery. *Anesth Analg.* 1990;70:176–180.
11. Apfelbaum JL. Preoperative evaluation, laboratory screening, and selection of adult surgical outpatients in the 1990s. *Anesth Rev.* 1990;17(Suppl 2):4–12.
12. Charpak Y, Blery C, Chastang C, et al. Usefulness of selectively ordered preoperative tests. *Med Care.* 1988;36:95–104.

13. Macpherson DS, Snow R, Lofgren RP. Preoperative screening: value of previous tests. *Ann Intern Med*. 1990;113:969–973.
14. Fletcher RH, Fletcher SW, Wagner EH. *Clinical Epidemiology. The Essentials*. 3rd ed. Baltimore: Williams & Wilkins; 1996.
15. Sandler G. The importance of the history in the medical clinic and the cost of unnecessary tests. *Am Heart J*. 1980;100:928–931.
16. Netzer NC, Stoohs RA, Netzer CM, et al. Using the Berlin Questionnaire to identify patients at risk for the sleep apnea syndrome. *Ann Intern Med*. 1999;3:485–491.
17. Fleisher LA, Beckman JA, Brown KA, et al. ACC/AHA guidelines for perioperative cardiovascular evaluation and care for noncardiac surgery. *J Am Coll Cardiol*. 2007;50:e159–241. Available at: http://www.acc.org. Accessed September 28, 2007.
18. Hlatky MA, Boineau RE, Higginbotham MB, et al. A brief self-administered questionnaire to determine functional capacity (the Duke Activity Status Index). *Am J Cardiol*. 1989;64:651–654.
19. Cameron EH, Lipshultz SE, Tarbell NJ, et al. Cardiovascular disease in long-term survivors of pediatric Hodgkin's disease. *Circulation*. 1998;8:139–144.
20. Adams MJ, Hardenbergh PH, Constine LS, et al. Radiation-associated cardiovascular disease. *Crit Rev Oncol Hematol*. 2003; 45:55–75.
21. Polanczyk CA, Marcantonio E, Goldman L, et al. Impact of age on perioperative complications and length of stay in patients undergoing noncardiac surgery. *Ann Intern Med*. 2001;134:637–643.
22. National Confidential Enquiry into Patient Outcome and Death. Extremes of Age. Available at: http://www.ncepod.org.uk. Accessed March 11, 2007.
23. Calle EE, Rodriquez C, Walker-Thurmond K, et al. Overweight, obesity, and mortality from cancer in a prospectively studied cohort of U.S. adults. *N Engl J Med*. 2003;348:1625–1638.
24. Brodsky JB, Lemmens HJ, Brock-Utne JG, et al. Morbid obesity and tracheal intubation. *Anesth Analg*. 2002;94:732–736.
25. Mallampati SR, Gatt SP, Gugino LD, et al. A clinical sign to predict difficult tracheal intubation: a prospective study. *Can Anaesth Soc J*. 1985;32:429–434.
26. Girish M, Trayner E, Dammann O, et al. Symptom-limited stair climbing as a predictor of postoperative complications after high-risk surgery. *Chest*. 2001;120:1147–1151.
27. Katz I, Stradling J, Slutsjy AS, et al. Do patients with obstructive sleep apnea have thick necks? *Am Rev Respir Dis*. 1990;141: 1228–1231.
28. Rabkin SW, Horne JM. Preoperative electrocardiography: its cost-effectiveness in detecting abnormalities when a previous tracing exist. *Can Med Assoc J*. 1979;121:301–306.
29. Gold BS, Young ML, Kinman JL, et al. The utility of preoperative electrocardiograms in the ambulatory surgical patient. *Arch Intern Med*. 1992;152:301–305.
30. Liu LL, Dzankic S, Leung JM. Preoperative electrocardiogram abnormalities do not predict postoperative cardiac complications in geriatric surgical patients. *J Am Geriatr Soc*. 2002;50:1186–1191.
31. Callaghan LC, Edwards ND, Reilly CS. Utilization of the preoperative ECG. *Anaesthesia*. 1995;50:488–490.

32. Tait AR, Parr HG, Tremper KK. Evaluation of the efficacy of routine preoperative electrocardiograms. *J Cardiothorac Vasc Anesth*. 1997;11:752–755.

33. Centers for Medicare and Medicaid Services. Available at: http://www.cms.hhs.org. Accessed March 11, 2007.

34. Palmer T, Wahr JA, O'Reilly M, et al. Reducing unnecessary cross-matching: a patient-specific blood ordering system is more accurate in predicting who will receive a blood transfusion than the maximum blood ordering system *Anesth Analg*. 2003;96:369–375.

35. Kaplan EB, Sheiner LB, Boeckmann AJ, et al. The usefulness of preoperative laboratory screening. *JAMA*. 1985;253:3576–3581.

36. Dzankic S, Pastor D, Gonzalez C, et al. The prevalence and predictive value of abnormal preoperative laboratory tests in elderly surgical patients. *Anesth Analg*. 2001;93:301–308.

37. Shander A, Knight K, Thurer R, et al. Prevalence and outcomes of anemia in surgery: a systematic review of the literature. *Am J Med*. 2004;116(Suppl 7A):58S–69S.

38. Practice guidelines for perioperative blood transfusion and adjuvant therapies. An updated report by the American Society of Anesthesiologists task force on perioperative blood transfusion and adjuvant therapies. *Anesthesiology*. 2006;105:198–208. Available at: http://www.asahq.org. Accessed March 11, 2007.

39. Hebert PC, Wells G, Blajchman MA, et al. A multicenter randomized controlled clinical trial of transfusion requirements in critical care. *N Engl J Med*. 1999;340:409–417.

40. Singh AK, Szczech L, Tang KL, et al. Correction of anemia with epoetin alfa in chronic kidney disease. *N Engl J Med*. 2006;355:2085–2098.

41. Perez A, Planell J, Bacardaz C, et al. Value of routine preoperative tests: a multicentre study in four general hospitals. *Br J Anaesth*. 1995;74:250–256.

42. Turnbull JM, Buck C. The value of preoperative screening investigation in otherwise healthy individuals. *Arch Intern Med*. 1987;147:1101–1105.

43. Rohrer M, Mechelotti M, Nahrwold D. A prospective evaluation of the efficacy of preoperative coagulation testing. *Ann Surg*. 1988;208:554–557.

44. Eckman MH, Erban JK, Singh SK, et al. Screening for the risk for bleeding or thrombosis. *Ann Intern Med*. 2003;138:15–24.

45. Michiels JJ, Gadisseur A, Budde U, et al. Characterization, classification, and treatment of von Willebrand diseases: a critical appraisal of the literature and personal experiences. *Semin Thromb Hemost*. 2005;31:577–601.

46. Peterson P, Hayes TE, Arkin CF, et al. The preoperative bleeding time test lacks clinical benefit. College of American Pathologists' and American Society of Clinical Pathologists' position article. *Arch Surg*. 1998;133:134–139.

47. Rodgers R, Levin J. A critical appraisal of the bleeding time. *Sem Thromb Hemost*. 1990;16:1–20.

48. Friedberg RC, Jones BA, Walsh MK. Type and screen completion for scheduled surgical procedures. *Arch Pathol Lab Med*. 2003;127:533–540.

49. Dzik WH, Corwin H, Goodnough LT, et al. Patient safety and blood transfusion: new solutions. *Transfus Med Rev*. 2003;17: 169–180.
50. Foley CL, Mould T, Kennedy JE, et al. A study of blood cross-matching requirements for surgery in gynecological oncology: improved efficiency and cost saving. *Int J Gynecol Cancer*. 2003; 13:889–893.
51. Hallan SI, Dahl K, Oien CM, et al. Screening strategies for chronic renal disease in the general population: follow-up of cross sectional health survey. *BMJ*. 2006;333:1047–1050.
52. Narr BJ, Hansen TR, Warner MA. Preoperative laboratory screening in healthy Mayo patients: cost-effective elimination of tests and unchanged outcomes. *Mayo Clin Proc*. 1991;66:155–159.
53. Hirsch IA, Tomlinson DL, Slogoff S, et al. The overstated risk of preoperative hypokalemia *Anesth Analg*. 1988;67:131–136.
54. Nally BR, Dunbar SB, Zellinger M, et al. Supraventricular tachycardia after coronary artery bypass grafting surgery and fluid and electrolyte variable. *Heart Lung*. 1996;25:31–36.
55. Moitra VK, Meiler SE. The diabetic surgical patient. *Curr Opin Anaesthesiol*. 2006;19:339–345.
56. Selvin E, Marinopoulos S, Berkenblit G, et al. Meta-analysis: glycosylated hemoglobin and cardiovascular disease in diabetes mellitus. *Ann Intern Med*. 2004;141:421–431.
57. Dronge AS, Perkal MF, Kancir S, et al. Long-term glycemic control and postoperative infectious complications. *Arch Surg*. 2006;141:375–380.
58. Jellish WS, Kartha V, Fluder E, et al. Effect of metoclopramide on gastric fluid volumes in diabetic patients who have fasted before elective surgery. *Anesthesiology*. 2005;102:904–909.
59. Moitra V, Greenberg J, Sweitzer BJ. The sweet truth of diabetics scheduled for surgery. *Anesthesiology*. 2005;103:A654.
60. Gibbs J, Cull W, Henderson W, et al. Preoperative serum albumin level as a predictor of operative mortality and morbidity. *Arch Surg*. 1999;134:36–42.
61. Weinberg AD, Brennan MD, Gorman CA, et al. Outcome of anesthesia and surgery in hypothyroid patients. *Arch Intern Med*. 1983;143:893–897.
62. Hennrickus WL, Shaw BA, Gerardi JA. Prevalence of positive preoperative pregnancy testing in teenagers scheduled for orthopedic surgery. *J Pediatr Orthop*. 2001;21:677–679.
63. Bierstein K. Preoperative pregnancy testing: mandatory or elective? *Am Soc Anesthesiol Newsl*. 2006;70:37.
64. Qaseem A, Snow V, Fitterman N, et al. Risk assessment for and strategies to reduce perioperative pulmonary complications for patients undergoing noncardiothoracic surgery: a guideline from the American College of Physicians. *Ann Intern Med*. 2006;144:575–580.
65. Gagner M, Chiassdon A. Preoperative chest x-ray films in elective surgery: a valid screening tool. *Can J Surg*. 1990;33:271–274.
66. Seymour DG, Pringle R, Shaw JW. The role of the routine preoperative chest x-ray in the elderly general surgical patient. *Postgrad Med J*. 1982;58:741–745.
67. Archer C, Levy AR, McGregor M. Value of routine preoperative chest x-rays: a meta-analysis. *Can J Anaesth*. 1993;40:1022–1027.

68. De Nino LA, Lawrence VA, Averyt EC, et al. Preoperative spirometry and laparotomy: blowing away dollars. *Chest*. 1997;111: 1536–1541.

69. Warner DO, Warner MA, Offord KP, et al. Airway obstruction and perioperative complications in smokers undergoing abdominal surgery. *Anesthesiology*. 1999;90:372–379.

70. Celli BR, MacNee W. Standards for the diagnosis and treatment of patients with COPD: a summary of the ATS/ERS position paper. *Eur Respir J*. 2004;23:932–946.

71. Wyser C, Stulz P, Soler M, et al. Prospective evaluation of an algorithm for the functional assessment of lung resection candidates. *Am J Respir Crit Care Med*. 1999;159:1450–1456.

72. Schuurmans MM, Diacon AH, Bolliger CT. Functional evaluation before lung resection. *Clin Chest Med*. 2002;23:159–172.

73. Zibrak JD, O'Donnell CR, Marton K. Indications for pulmonary function testing. *Ann Intern Med*. 1990;112:763–771.

74. Schein OD, Katz J, Bass EB, et al. The value of routine preoperative medical testing before cataract surgery. *N Engl J Med*. 2000;342:168–175.

75. Lawrence VA, Gafni A, Gross M. The unproven utility of the preoperative urinalysis: economic evaluation. *J Clin Epidemiol*. 1989;42:1185–1192.

76. Epstein AM, Begg CB, McNeil BJ. The use of ambulatory testing in prepaid and fee-for service group practices. *N Engl J Med*. 1986;314:1089–1094.

77. Nardella A, Pechet L, Snyder LM. Continuous improvement, quality control, and cost containment in clinical laboratory testing. *Arch Pathol Lab Med*. 1995;119:518–522.

78. Gibby GL, Paulus DA, Sirota DJ. Computerized pre-anesthetic evaluation results in additional abstracted comorbidity diagnoses. *J Clin Monit*. 1997;13:35–41.

79. Roizen MF, Klock PA, Klafta J. How much do they really want to know? Preoperative patient interviews and the anesthesiologist. *Anesth Analg*. 1996;82:443–444.

80. Matthey P, Finucane BT, Finegan BA. The attitude of the general public towards preoperative assessment and risks associated with general anesthesia. *Can J Anaesth*. 2001;48:333–339.

81. Egbert LD, Battit GE, Turndorf H, et al. The value of the preoperative visit by an anesthetist. A study of doctor-patient rapport. *JAMA*. 1963;185:553–555.

82. Katz RI, Barnhart JM, Ho G, et al. A survey on the intended purposes and perceived utility of preoperative cardiology consultations. *Anesth Analg*. 1998;87:830–836.

83. Maurer WG, Borkowski RG, Parker BM. Quality and resource utilization in managing preoperative evaluation. *Anesthesiol Clin North Am*. 2004;22:155–175.

84. Ziegeler S, Tsusaki BE, Collard CD. Influence of genotype on perioperative risk and outcome. *Anesthesiology*. 2003;99:212–219.

85. Palmer SN, Giesecke NM, Body SC, et al. Pharmacogenetics of anesthetic and analgesic agents. *Anesthesiology*. 2005;102:663–671.

Ischemic Heart Disease

William Vernick and Lee A. Fleisher

The high-risk patient who needs noncardiac surgery continues to represent a dilemma with respect to the appropriate degree of preoperative diagnostic testing. In patients with known cardiovascular disease (CVD), information on its extent and stability and on ventricular function may be beneficial in directing perioperative management. Many patients, particularly those who will undergo major vascular surgery, may be asymptomatic, and no prior or recent evaluations may have been performed; however, the probability of extensive coronary artery disease (CAD) may be high.

Numerous investigators have advocated the use of preoperative evaluation and perioperative interventions to reduce complications for high-risk patients undergoing major surgical procedures. The underlying premise is that identifying patients with significant CAD and areas at risk for myocardial ischemia leads to interventions that reduce perioperative risk. Despite this belief, multiple studies have been unable to demonstrate a benefit to testing and coronary revascularization through surgery or percutaneous coronary interventions (PCIs). A good preoperative database will help dictate management, but further invasive diagnostic testing should only be performed if it impacts care. The approach we advocate balances the value of preoperative testing that prompts perioperative and long-term interventions to improve a patient's health with economic concerns. It focuses on guidelines from the American College of Cardiology/American Heart Association (ACC/AHA) for risk stratification and appropriate use of diagnostic testing (1). Both a short-term (perioperative) and long-term perspective are taken.

PATHOPHYSIOLOGY OF PERIOPERATIVE CARDIAC MORBIDITY

The etiology of perioperative myocardial infarction (PMI) is complex. Infarction typically occurs within the first 24 to 48 hours after surgery and is often preceded by prolonged periods of ST-segment depression indicative of ischemia (2,3). In the majority of cases a non–Q-wave MI with complete resolution of ischemic electrocardiographic (ECG) changes after the initial event results in a mortality of 10% to 15% (4). In most, the infarction is silent. Patients who suffer a PMI are likely to be older with more extensive pre-existing CAD. In a study of patients who needed major vascular surgery, troponin levels rose during or shortly after periods of postoperative ischemia >100 minutes long and peak troponin level was associated with the length of ischemia (3). Ischemia was related to postoperative tachycardia. The pattern of troponin release is typically as follows: A low-level release during the first 8 to 24 hours postoperatively before peak levels over the next 12 to 48 hours. In two separate small pathologic studies, plaque rupture was found in 7% of patients in one study and in 46% in the other; intracoronary thrombus was found in only 28% and 27%, respectively (5,6). These findings have led many to believe that PMI is solely the result of stress-induced ischemia from supply:demand mismatch, most frequently from postoperative tachycardia, anemia, hypothermia, hypotension, or stress-induced hypertension.

These same perioperative sympathetic surges also increase shear forces on coronary plaque. Endothelial and systemic inflammation in combination with increased shear forces can promote plaque destabilization, leading to either rupture or fissuring (7). The formation of intracoronary thrombosis on such plaque lesions is further promoted by the hypercoagulable state induced by surgery.

Given the complexity of PMI, preoperative evaluation may be limited for predicting perioperative cardiac events. Stress testing can identify the presence as well as the severity of CAD but not which plaques are vulnerable, the impact of perioperative inflammation and hypercoagulability, or the effect of perioperative medical interventions. The same limitations also apply to cardiac catheterization. These issues are critical in defining the extent of diagnostic testing of the patient.

The evaluation of the patient with known CVD or risk factors for CVD requires an understanding of the extent and stability of the disease and ventricular function. If the anesthesiologist has sufficient information regarding these factors, then no further consultation is required. Frequently, a simple phone call to the primary physician or the patient's cardiologist suffices. If the information is not easily obtainable from the patient or the medical record, then a formal consultation may be required. The focus of the consultation should be to ask *specific* questions regarding the cardiovascular status that are important to perioperative management. Such an approach is advocated in the ACC/AHA guidelines.

RISK STRATIFICATION SYSTEMS

The original stratification system for perioperative risk assessment, the Dripps Index of the American Society of Anesthesiology (ASA), published in 1961, remains in clinical use today (8). A patient's physical status (PS) is ranked from 1 to 5, with class 1 being a completely healthy patient and class 5 being a patient considered moribund with surgery as a last resort. The ASA-PS score is a subjective index that has not been found to be predictive of cardiac complications. In 1977 Goldman et al. published a landmark article after studying 1,001 patients who had noncardiac surgery, excluding transurethral resection of the prostate (9). Goldman's Cardiac Risk Index (CRI) was the first validated multivariate model used in noncardiac surgery to predict cardiac morbidity and mortality. Nine risk factors were identified and weighted based on their ability to predict postoperative cardiac death, MI, congestive heart failure (CHF), or ventricular tachycardia (VT). A previous MI or the presence of an S_3 gallop was the most predictive for an adverse event. A patient's CRI score was calculated from the number and corresponding weight of risk factors, and scores ranged from 1 to 4, with a score of 4 representing

Table 3.1. Revised cardiac risk index

- High-risk surgery: Intraperitoneal, intrathoracic, or suprainguinal vascular procedures
- Ischemic heart disease
- Congestive heart failure
- Cerebrovascular disease
- Insulin therapy for diabetes
- Creatinine >2.0 mg/dL

From Lee TH, Marcantonio ER, Mangione CM, et al. Derivation and prospective validation of a simple index for prediction of cardiac risk of major noncardiac surgery. *Circulation.* 1999;100:1043–1049.

the highest risk. A major limitation of the CRI was that it did not take into account the type of surgery. To improve the predictive accuracy for patients undergoing major vascular surgery, Detsky et al. modified the CRI in 1986 (10). Significant angina was added as a new variable and an old MI was differentiated from a recent MI. Scoring was simplified by decreasing the number of risk classes from four to three. The CRI and modified CRI have been validated for predicting cardiac complications in patients with high scores; however, after both vascular and nonvascular surgery, a significant number of patients identified at low risk sustained cardiac events. The applicability of these indices today may be questioned, given the advances in medical therapy for cardiac disease as well as improvements in anesthetic and surgical techniques.

More recent risk-scoring systems have been developed by Eagle et al. (11) and Lee et al. (12). Both systems use multivariate analysis to identify preoperative clinical factors predictive of perioperative cardiac events and consist of six similar risk factors. The Revised Cardiac Risk Index (RCRI) published in 1999 by Lee et al. is the most widely used scoring system today (Table 3.1). It assigns one point each for the presence of six independent risk factors for major cardiac complications in patients having nonemergency surgery. The incidence of major cardiac events in patients with zero, one, two, or three risk factors was 0.4%, 0.9%, 7%, and 11%, respectively, in the validation cohort. This risk stratification system predicts outcome, but also identifies patients who need additional testing or medical interventions.

CLINICAL EVALUATION FOR CORONARY ARTERY DISEASE

Frequently, the preoperative evaluation represents an opportunity to evaluate patients who rarely access the health care system otherwise and are not currently being treated for CVD. In evaluating the patient, the first step is to identify the presence of unstable symptoms. Many patients scheduled for vascular surgical procedures may have coexisting diabetes mellitus or a limitation of activity that masks cardiac symptoms. In patients with symptomatic CAD, the preoperative evaluation may lead to the recognition of a change in the frequency or pattern of anginal symptoms. The presence of unstable angina has been associated with a high risk of PMI. The perioperative period is associated with a hypercoagulable state and surges in levels of endogenous catecholamines, both of which may exacerbate unstable angina, increasing the risk of PMI. The anesthesiologist can influence a patient's short- and long-term health by referring patients with unstable angina for further medical or coronary interventions.

Stable angina represents a continuum from mild angina with extreme exertion to dyspnea or angina after climbing a few stairs. The patient with angina only after strenuous exercise and no signs of left ventricular (LV) dysfunction is low risk. In contrast, a patient with dyspnea on minimal exertion is at high risk for developing perioperative LV dysfunction, myocardial ischemia, and possible MI. Extensive CAD is highly probable in these patients who may need additional monitoring or cardiovascular testing, depending on the surgical procedure and institutional factors.

In virtually all studies, the presence of active CHF preoperatively has been associated with an increased incidence of perioperative cardiac morbidity. LV function should be stabilized and pulmonary congestion is treated before elective surgery (see Chapter 4). The cause of the CHF should be determined. Congestive symptoms may be caused by nonischemic cardiomyopathy, mitral or aortic insufficiency, or stenosis. The type of perioperative monitoring and treatments depends on clarifying the cause of cardiac congestion.

Most patients with a prior MI have CAD, although a small group of them may sustain an MI from a nonatherosclerotic mechanism. Traditionally, risk assessment for noncardiac surgery was based on the time interval between the MI and surgery. Multiple studies have demonstrated an increased incidence of reinfarction if the MI was within 6 months of surgery (13,14).

With improvements in perioperative care such as thrombolytics, percutaneous transluminal coronary angioplasty (PTCA), and risk stratification after an acute MI, the intervening time interval may no longer be important. Although many patients with an MI may continue to be at risk for subsequent ischemia and infarction, other patients may have either totally occluded or widely patent coronary stenoses. For example, the use of PTCA is associated with a lower incidence of death or reinfarction within 6 months than is traditional medical therapy or the use of thrombolytics. Therefore, patients should be evaluated from the perspective of their risk for ongoing ischemia. The ACC/AHA has advocated (without objective evidence) that patients who have had an acute MI (MI within 7 days) or a recent MI (within 8 to 30 days) with ischemic risk by history or noninvasive testing be considered high risk. An MI that occurred longer ago than 30 days is considered an intermediate-risk predictor.

PATIENTS AT RISK FOR CORONARY ARTERY DISEASE

For those patients without overt symptoms or history, the probability of CAD varies with the type and number of atherosclerotic risk factors. Peripheral vascular disease (PVD) has been associated with CAD in multiple studies. Among 1,000 consecutive patients scheduled for major vascular surgery, approximately 60% had at least one coronary artery with a critical stenosis (15). Therefore, the patient with PVD should be evaluated further for evidence of CAD.

Patients with diabetes mellitus have a higher probability of CAD than do nondiabetic patients. Diabetes mellitus is an independent risk factor for perioperative cardiac morbidity (12). Time since diagnosis and other associated end-organ dysfunction are considered to determine degree of probability. Autonomic neuropathy is the best predictor of silent CAD. Because diabetic patients are at high risk for a silent MI, an electrocardiogram (ECG) should be evaluated for the presence of Q waves.

Renal insufficiency is associated with cardiac disease and CVD events. Patients with both diabetes and renal impairment have particularly elevated risk. Creatinine levels >2.0 mg/dL are a significant independent risk factor for perioperative cardiac complications.

Hypertension has been associated with an increased incidence of myocardial ischemia and infarction. Those hypertensive patients with left ventricular hypertrophy (LVH) who need noncardiac surgery are at a higher perioperative risk than nonhypertensive patients. The presence of a strain pattern on ECG (LVH with ST-T–wave changes) suggests a chronic ischemic state. Therefore, the probability of CAD and cardiovascular morbidity is increased, and further evaluation is warranted if the pattern is a new finding.

Atherosclerotic processes associated with tobacco use and hypercholesterolemia increase the probability of CAD, but not perioperative cardiac risk. To determine the overall probability of disease, the number and severity of the risk factors are considered.

PHYSICAL EXAMINATION OF THE PATIENT WITH CARDIOVASCULAR DISEASE

During the complete physical examination, auscultation of the heart can reveal a previously undiagnosed murmur or additional heart sounds. An S_3 gallop is associated with CHF. Frequently, a murmur is detected on the day of surgery, and the value of further testing must be balanced against the disadvantages of delaying the procedure. The nature of the murmur and concomitant symptoms can provide important information regarding the underlying pathophysiology. Auscultation of the lungs should include evaluation for findings of CHF and pulmonary disease. Wheezing, which may reflect bronchospastic disease, may also signify CHF as do crackles or rales. In addition to signs of left heart failure, patients at risk for CVD should be evaluated for hepatomegaly, lower extremity edema, and jugular venous distension (JVD), which are signs of right heart failure.

Blood pressure (BP) and heart rate (HR) are determined in supine and standing positions to assess intravascular volume or autonomic dysfunction. Patients with PVD need BP measured in both arms because significant differences may exist. Peripheral arterial pulses may suggest valvular disease or the presence of atherosclerotic disease.

Risk factors may also aid in the interpretation of noninvasive tests. Eagle et al. evaluated the implications of the prior probability of disease based on clinical criteria in determining the value of preoperative testing. Patients without clinical risk factors (angina, Q waves, ventricular ectopic activity requiring treatment, diabetes mellitus, age >70 years) had only a 3% incidence of perioperative morbidity, and noninvasive testing could not further stratify risk. Similarly, patients with three or more risk factors had a 50% morbidity, and noninvasive testing did not further discriminate risk. Preoperative dipyridamole-thallium imaging (DTI), however, was useful in the group at moderate risk (one to two risk factors) (11).

Paul et al. (16) evaluated the ability of clinical risk factors to predict the angiographic severity of CAD in patients who needed vascular surgery. Using a cohort of patients at the Cleveland Clinic who underwent angiography, they demonstrated that critical three-vessel or left main disease was present in 5% of low-risk patients (zero risk factors) but was found in 43% of high-risk patients (more than two risk factors). The absence of angina, prior MI, or history of CHF seemed to predict with 94% accuracy freedom from critical CAD.

Two studies illustrate the reduced value of noninvasive testing. When 60 consecutively treated patients undergoing vascular surgery were studied, DTI had a positive predictive value of 27% for adverse cardiac events, a negative predictive value of 82%, and no net discriminative ability (17). In 457 consecutive patients who had abdominal aortic surgery, an association was found between thallium redistribution and perioperative cardiac morbidity (18). Both studies illustrate the low positive predictive value of testing and significant incidence of morbidity in patients with negative test results when consecutively treated patients are studied.

L'Italien et al. (19) incorporated clinical risk factors and the results of DTI. The pretest (baseline) probability of an event was calculated similarly to Goldman's CRI, whereby risk factors are weighted to determine overall risk. The results of DTI can then be used to modify the risk and determine the posttest probability of an event. Poldermans et al. also demonstrated that risk factors could determine the value of preoperative testing in patients undergoing dobutamine stress echocardiography (DSE) (20).

The additive value of diagnostic testing was best illustrated by Vanzetto et al., who followed a cohort of consecutively treated patients who had abdominal aortic surgery. DTI was performed in patients with two or more clinical or ECG risk factors. Among patients with reversible defects, 23% had major cardiac events; only 1% of patients without reversible defects had cardiac events. Thallium single photon emission computed tomography for high-risk patients had significantly greater prognostic value for cardiac events than that provided by clinical variables alone.

GUIDELINES FOR PREOPERATIVE TESTING FOR CORONARY ARTERY DISEASE

Table 3.2 lists the indications for obtaining a preoperative rest electrocardiogram. In 1996 the ACC and AHA published a consensus statement on the preoperative cardiac evaluation of patients who needed noncardiac surgery. The consensus statement included an algorithm for identifying patients for cardiac testing before surgery (Fig. 3.1). The consensus statement was later updated in 2002 (1) and revised in 2007 (1A). The algorithm, based on expert opinion given the limited number of randomized studies in the operative setting, not only incorporates the

Table 3.2.   Recommendations for preoperative resting 12-lead ECG

Class I
1. Preoperative resting 12-lead ECG is recommended for patients with at least 1 clinical risk factor* who are undergoing vascular surgical procedures. *(Level of Evidence: B)*
2. Preoperative resting 12-lead ECG is recommended for patients with known CHD, peripheral arterial disease, or cerebrovascular disease who are undergoing intermediate-risk surgical procedures. *(Level of Evidence: C)*

Class IIa
1. Preoperative resting 12-lead ECG is reasonable in persons with no clinical risk factors who are undergoing vascular surgical procedures. *(Level of Evidence: B)*

Class IIb
1. Preoperative resting 12-lead ECG may be reasonable in patients with at least 1 clinical risk factor who are undergoing intermediate-risk operative procedures. *(Level of Evidence: B)*

Class III
1. Preoperative and postoperative resting 12-lead ECGs are not indicated in asymptomatic persons undergoing low-risk surgical procedures. *(Level of Evidence: B)*

From Lee TH, Marcantonio ER, Mangione CM, et al. Derivation and prospective validation of a simple index for prediction of cardiac risk of major noncardiac surgery. *Circulation.* 1999;100:1043–1049.

patient's medical history and the risks associated with the planned surgery, but also considers previous cardiac evaluations and interventions. In one small study, use of the algorithm reduced unnecessary cardiac stress testing without increasing cardiac complications (21).

The first step in the algorithm is to define patient-specific risk based on medical history. Patients are divided into high, intermediate, and low risk of PMI, CHF, or death based on the presence of active cardiac condition and clinical risk factors. The clinical risk factors were drawn from the revised cardiac risk index (Table 3.1). Active cardiac conditions justify cancellation or delay and mandate intensive medical management. Based on consensus of the ACC/AHA committee, an acute (within 7 days) or recent (8 to 30 days) MI with evidence of ischemic risk by clinical symptoms or noninvasive studies is a major clinical predictor. The ACC/AHA committee still recommends waiting 4 to 6 weeks before surgery if possible, as a precaution.

The decision to perform additional cardiac testing in patients with clinical risk factors requires an assessment of the patient's functional status, the risk of the planned surgery, and previous cardiac evaluations and interventions (Tables 3.4 and 3.5). A thorough search for signs of ischemia must be made to identify active cardiac conditions because many patients may have a low activity level that rarely provokes ischemia. Atypical signs of

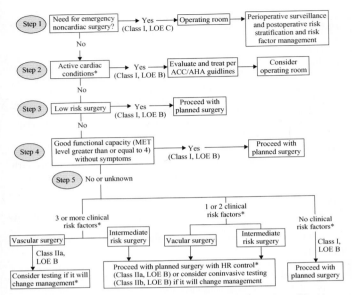

Figure 3.1. The American College of Cardiology/American Heart Association 2007 guidelines on perioperative cardiovascular evaluation and care for noncardiac surgery proposed an algorithm for decisions regarding the need for further evaluation. *Active cardiac conditions (Table 3.3), Exercise tolerance (Table 3.4), Clinical risk factors (Table 3.1 excluding surgical procedure as a risk factor), and Surgical risk (Table 3.5). Reproduced with permission from reference 1A.

ischemia include shortness of breath or dyspnea on exertion, and jaw pain. Silent ischemia is particularly common in diabetics, with diabetic neuropathy the best predictor. Some patients may never have had symptoms of ischemia if their CAD was diagnosed with noninvasive testing done routinely or for previous surgery. If patients have never had symptoms, recurrence cannot be relied upon as a valid marker of ischemia.

It may be prudent to be suspicious of older favorable coronary test results in patients with a low functional status. A decreased functional capacity, defined as the inability to walk four blocks or climb two flights of stairs, has been shown to be an independent predictor of perioperative cardiac events (22). Functional capacity is typically expressed in metabolic equivalents (METs) with 1 MET equivalent to oxygen consumption when a 70-kg, 40-year-old male is resting, and 10 METs equivalent to strenuous sports like swimming or basketball. A low capacity is typically defined as 4 METs of activity or less. Examples of activities >4 METs include running a short distance or walking on level ground at 4 mph; light work around the house or walking at 2 to 3 mph are considered <4 METs.

Clinical risk factors were derived from the RCRI risk factors: Stable, mild angina; MI (by history or Q wave) >30 days ago;

Table 3.3. Active cardiac conditions for which the patient should undergo evaluation and treatment before noncardiac surgery (Class I, level of evidence: B)

Condition	Examples
Unstable coronary syndromes	Unstable or severe angina[a] (CCS class III or IV)[b] Recent MI[c]
Decompensated HF (NYHA functional class IV; worsening or new-onset HF)	
Significant arrhythmias	High-grade atrioventricular block Mobitz II atrioventricular block Third-degree atrioventricular heart block Symptomatic ventricular arrhythmias Supraventricular arrhythmias (including atrial fibrillation) with uncontrolled ventricular rate (HR greater than 100 bpm at rest) Symptomatic bradycardia Newly recognized ventricular tachycardia
Severe valvular disease	Severe aortic stenosis (mean pressure gradient greater than 40 mm Hg, aortic valve area less than 1.0 cm^2, or symptomatic) Symptomatic mitral stenosis (progressive dyspnea on exertion, exertional presyncope, or HF)

CCS indicates Canadian Cardiovascular Society; HF, heart failure; HR, heart rate; MI, myocardial infarction; NYHA, New York Heart Association.
[a]According to Campeau (10).
[b]May include "stable" angina in patients who are unusually sedentary.
[c]The American College of Cardiology National Database Library defines recent MI as more than 7 days but less than or equal to 1 month (within 30 days). Reproduced with permission from Fleisher LA, Beckman JA, Brown KA, et al. ACC/AHA 2007 guidelines on perioperative cardiovascular evaluation and care for noncardiac surgery: A report of the American College of Cardiology/American Heart Association Task Force on Practice Guidelines (Writing Committee to Revise the 2002 Guidelines on Perioperative Cardiovascular Evaluation for Noncardiac Surgery). *J AM Coll Cardiol* 2007;50:e159–241.

a history or presence of compensated CHF; diabetes mellitus; and chronic renal insufficiency (CRI) defined by a serum creatinine >2.0 mg/dL. According to the ACC/AHA guidelines, no further cardiac testing is needed for patients with clinical risk factors who can achieve >4 METs without symptoms. Patients with three or more clinical risk factors undergoing vascular surgery, noninvasive testing should be considered if it will change management. In patients with one or two clinical risk factors undergoing

Table 3.4. Estimated energy requirement for various activities[a]

1 MET	Can you take care of yourself?	4 METs	Climb a flight of stairs or walk up a hill?
	Eat, dress, or use the toilet?		Walk on level ground at 4 mph or 6.4 km/h?
	Walk indoors around the house?		Run a short distance?
	Walk a block or two on level ground at 2–3 mph or 3.2–4.8 km/h?		Do heavy work around the house like scrubbing floors or lifting or moving heavy furniture?
	Do light work around the house like dusting or washing dishes?		Participate in moderate recreational activities like golf, bowling, dancing, doubles tennis, or throwing a baseball or football?
4 METs		>10 METs	Participate in strenuous sports like swimming, singles tennis, football, basketball, or skiing?

MET, metabolic equivalent.
[a] Adapted from the Duke Activity Status Index and American Heart Association Exercise Standards.
Reproduced with permission from Eagle KA, Berger PB, Calkins H, et al. ACC/AHA guideline update for perioperative cardiovascular evaluation for noncardiac surgery-executive summary: a report of the American College of Cardiology/American Heart Association Task Force on Practice Guidelines (committee to update the 1996 Guidelines on Perioperative Cardiovascular Evaluation for Noncardiac Surgery). *J Am Coll Cardiol.* 2002;39:542–553.

intermediate risk as vascular surgery or three or more clinical risk factors undergoing intermediate risk surgery, either proceeding with the planned surgery with heart rate control or performing noninvasive testing if it will change management are appropriate approaches. Coronary revascularization may not benefit this group, and therefore the value of testing may be very limited (23). High-risk surgery are procedures associated with a >5% incidence of cardiac complications. Prolonged major vascular, abdominal, or thoracic surgeries associated with large fluid shifts or blood loss are considered high risk. The high incidence of complications is caused not only by the hemodynamic stress associated with the surgery, but also by underlying CAD in

Table 3.5. Cardiac risk[a] stratification for noncardiac surgical procedures

Risk Stratification	Procedure Examples
Vascular (reported cardiac risk often more than 5%)	Aortic and other major vascular surgery
	Peripheral vascular surgery
Intermediate (reported cardiac risk generally 1% to 5%)	Intraperitoneal and intrathoracic surgery
	Carotid endarterectomy
	Head and neck surgery
	Orthopedic surgery
	Prostate surgery
Low[b] (reported cardiac risk generally less than 1%)	Endoscopic procedures
	Superficial procedure
	Cataract surgery
	Breast surgery
	Ambulatory surgery

[a]Combined incidence of cardiac death and nonfatal myocardial infarction.
[b]These procedures do not generally require further preoperative cardiac testing.

patients. For example, Hertzer et al. found a 60% incidence of critical stenosis in at least one coronary artery in patients who had major vascular surgery (15). Patients without active cardiac conditions undergoing low-risk surgery should proceed without further cardiac testing, regardless of their functional capacity. Low-risk procedures carry a risk of serious cardiac complications of <1%. Examples include cataract surgery, endoscopic procedures, or superficial procedures.

TESTS TO CONFIRM THE DIAGNOSIS AND DETERMINE THE EXTENT OF CORONARY ARTERY DISEASE

Noninvasive diagnostic tests have been proposed to evaluate the extent of CAD before noncardiac surgery (Table 3.6). Exercise ECG has been the traditional method of evaluating individuals

Table 3.6. Sensitivity and specificity of various diagnostic tests for detecting coronary artery disease

Test	Sensitivity (%)	Specificity (%)
Exercise electrocardiography	81	66
Exercise thallium imaging		
Qualitative planar	84	87
Quantitative planar	89	89
Single photon emission computed tomography	94	82
Dipyridamole-thallium imaging (DTI)	85	90
Stress echocardiography	80–90	80–90
Stress radionuclide angiography	70–80	70–80

for the presence of CAD. It represents the least invasive and most cost-effective method of detecting ischemia, with a reasonable sensitivity (68% to 81%) and specificity (66% to 77%) for identifying CAD. The goal of the test is to provoke ischemia through exercise by increasing myocardial oxygen demand relative to myocardial oxygen supply. ECG signs of myocardial ischemia and clinical signs of LV dysfunction are considered positive. Patients with a good exercise tolerance rarely benefit from further testing. Therefore, information regarding maximal HR (i.e., an adequate test is 85% of predicted maximum HR, which is defined as 220 − age) exercise level, and BP during the test must be provided.

Many high-risk patients are unable to exercise. In vascular surgical patients, this contraindication is most evident in patients with claudication or PVD who have a high rate of perioperative cardiac morbidity. Therefore, pharmacologic stress testing has become popular as a preoperative test for vascular surgery patients.

Pharmacologic stress tests for the detection of CAD dilate coronary arteries or increase myocardial oxygen demand. Examples of coronary vasodilators are dipyridamole and adenosine. Dipyridamole blocks adenosine reuptake and increases adenosine concentration in the coronary vessels. Adenosine is a direct coronary vasodilator. After infusion of the vasodilator, flow is preferentially distributed to areas distal to normal coronary arteries and minimized to areas distal to a coronary stenosis. A radioisotope such as thallium chloride Tl 201 or technetium Tc 99m sestamibi is then injected. Normal myocardium shows up on initial imaging; myocardial necrosis or areas distal to a significant coronary stenosis demonstrate a defect. After a delay of several hours, or after infusion of a second dose of technetium Tc 99m sestamibi, the myocardium is again imaged. Initial defects that remain defects are consistent with old scar. Defects that demonstrate normal activity on subsequent imaging are at risk for myocardial ischemia. A redistribution defect on DTI or technetium imaging in patients who will undergo peripheral vascular surgery predicts postoperative cardiac events (Fig. 3.2).

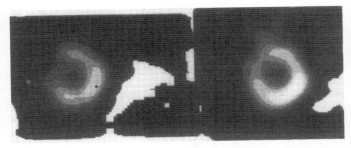

Figure 3.2. Example of dipyridamole-thallium imaging showing both a stress image (*left*) and a rest image (*right*.) A defect is seen on the initial stress image that fills in on the subsequent rest imaging. The presence of a reversible defect has been associated with an increased incidence of perioperative cardiac morbidity.

To increase the predictive value of the test, several strategies have been suggested. The redistribution defect can be quantified, with larger areas of defect associated with increased risk. Both increased uptake in the lungs and dilation of the LV cavity are markers of LV dysfunction with ischemia. Fleisher et al. demonstrated that the delineation of low and high risk via DTI (the latter showing a larger area of defect, increased uptake in the lungs, and dilation of the LV cavity) markedly improved the test's predictive value (26). Only patients with high-risk DTI were at increased risk for perioperative morbidity and long-term mortality.

During dobutamine stress echocardiography (DSE) patients are given an infusion of dobutamine to increase both HR and inotropy. If HR cannot be raised to >85% of the age-predicted maximum, atropine is given. The ECG is monitored continuously for ST-segment changes. The echocardiogram is also monitored at discrete time points for the appearance of new or worsened regional wall-motion abnormalities (WMAs), which indicates a positive test and areas at risk for myocardial ischemia. The advantage of DSE is that it is a dynamic assessment of the ability to provoke myocardial ischemia in response to increased HR, similar to that which might be expected during the perioperative period. As with DTI, DSE can be further quantified with WMAs in >4 of 16 segments denoting increased perioperative risk. The presence of WMAs at low HR is also a strong predictor of increased perioperative risk.

The question remains regarding the choice of diagnostic tests for a given patient. Beattie et al. performed a meta-analysis of 68 studies and 10,278 patients who had noncardiac surgery from 1985 to 2003 (Table 3.6) (27). The likelihood ratio of a positive DSE in predicting a cardiac complication was twice that of DTI, 4.09 (95% confidence interval [CI], 3.21 to 6.56) versus 1.83 (95% CI, 1.59 to 2.10). There was no difference in the ability of either test to predict complications in patients with moderate to large perfusion defects or regions of WMAs. The likelihood of false negatives was also higher for DTI than for DSE, with a likelihood ratio of 0.44 (95% CI, 0.36 to 0.54) versus 0.23 (95% CI, 0.17 to 0.32). In the seven studies directly comparing these two tests, no statistically significant difference in likelihood ratios could be found for either positive or negative tests. Over a third of the complications that were found in their meta-analysis occurred in patients with a negative stress test. In summary, given the large overlap in predictive value between the tests, the best choice of test is left to the individual center.

PERIOPERATIVE INTERVENTIONS TO REDUCE RISK

Modification of perioperative care based on the preoperative evaluation can take the form of medical and coronary interventions performed preoperatively, changes in anesthetic technique, aggressive treatment of hemodynamic perturbations, and utilization of expensive resources such as treatment in the intensive care unit (ICU), ST-segment telemetry, or invasive monitoring. Based on the accumulated data, no one anesthetic technique appears to be best; however, information from the preoperative evaluation is taken into account in designing an anesthetic plan.

Although insufficient evidence exists to determine the value of postoperative ICU care or invasive monitoring for the patient with active CVD, both are routinely used for high-risk patients who have extensive surgery. The evidence, however, suggests that more intensive monitoring is not needed *in the absence* of active CVD (i.e., negative history or negative results on a noninvasive test). Therefore, screening can be used to define the population of patients who would not benefit from intensive monitoring. In an era of rationing of expensive medical resources, the costs of screening may be easily offset by the savings from lower utilization of postoperative resources, such as not placing the patient in the ICU. Identification of high-risk patients (e.g., those with extensive CAD or LV dysfunction) would allow for rational utilization of these intensive resources for extended periods. Table 3.7 lists some perioperative interventions to reduce risk.

CORONARY REVASCULARIZATION

The Coronary Artery Revascularization Prophylaxis (CARP) study was the first randomized trial to explore the usefulness of revascularization before noncardiac surgery (25). The patients needed repair of abdominal aortic aneurysm (AAA) or lower extremity revascularization and were evaluated for high risk for postoperative cardiac complications by a cardiologist based on medical history. For those considered at high risk, a screening angiogram was performed. Patients were eligible for the study if coronary stenosis was $\geq$70% in at least one major coronary vessel suitable for revascularization. Exclusion criteria included the presence of severe coexisting illness or the finding of a >50% stenosis of the left main coronary artery, severe aortic stenosis, or an LV ejection fraction <20%. A total of 510 patients were randomized to either revascularization or intensive medical therapy perioperatively. The incidence of death or MI within 30 days of the vascular procedure was high but similar: 14.7% versus 17.7% for revascularization and medical therapy, respectively. Perioperative medical therapy was similar in both groups and included beta blockers (85%), aspirin (72%), statins (53%), intravenous nitroglycerin (33%), and heparin (93%). At a median follow-up of 2.7 years long-term mortality was high but similar between the groups, averaging 22.5%.

Shortly after the publication of the CARP trial, further evidence supporting a more conservative treatment strategy for patients at risk for cardiac complications after noncardiac surgery was presented by Poldermans et al. (23). In this study, 770 patients needed major vascular surgery and had intermediate cardiac risk, defined as the presence of one or two cardiac risk factors (age >70 years, angina, history of MI, a history of or compensated CHF, diabetes, creatinine >2.0 mg/dL, or previous transient ischemic attack or cerebrovascular accident) were randomized to either undergo further risk stratification with DSE or proceed to surgery. Patients with three or more risk factors were excluded from the study and considered for further risk stratification. All patients received preoperative bisoprolol initiated before and continued after surgery with a targeted HR of 60 to 65 bpm. In the tested group, 74% had no ischemia, 17% had limited ischemia, and 8.8% had extensive ischemia. Physicians were not blinded to

Table 3.7. Strategies to reduce cardiac risk of noncardiac surgery

	Recommendations
Coronary revascularization	• Prophylactic revascularization in asymptomatic patients without extensive ischemia on testing or positive stress tests with Revised Cardiac Risk Index scores <3 has not been shown to have a benefit over intensive medical therapy. • In patients who undergo revascularization, the completeness of vascularization in CABG appears to provide a protective advantage over stenting.
Stents	• Elective surgery should be delayed for 1 year if possible in patients with drug-eluting stents, and dual antiplatelet therapy should be continued. • In patients with bare-metal stents, elective surgery should be delayed at least 4 weeks to allow for dual antiplatelet therapy. • In patients with a drug-eluting or bare-metal stent, for whom clopidogrel was prematurely discontinued before surgery it should be restarted as soon as possible. • Strong consideration should be given to continuation of aspirin perioperatively. • Strong consideration should be given to placing a bare-metal stent in patients expected to need surgery within 1 year of placement.
Beta blockers	• Patients with ischemia on stress testing or with class I indications for chronic beta blocker therapy should receive beta blockers perioperatively. • Beta blockers should be started as soon as possible and titrated to heart rate with a goal of 70 bpm. • Long-acting agents are preferable. • Chronic therapy should not be discontinued perioperatively.
Statins	• The perioperative discontinuation of statins may be harmful. • In patients with known CAD or multiple risk factors for CAD, the use of statins is part of optimal perioperative medical therapy
Antiplatelet agents	• Patients taking aspirin for primary or secondary protection should continue to take aspirin perioperatively, as the risk of bleeding in most surgeries is outweighed by an increased risk of cardiovascular thrombosis.

CABG, coronary artery bypass surgery; CAD, coronary artery disease.

the results of DSE, and HR was kept below the ischemic threshold with tight perioperative beta blocker control. Of the 34 patients who were considered for revascularization because of extensive ischemia on DSE, 12 underwent revascularization (10 PCI and two had coronary artery bypass grafting [CABG]) with complete revascularization in only six. The 30-day incidence of cardiac death and nonfatal MI was similar in both groups (1.8% in the no-testing group vs. 2.3% in the tested group). Those in the no-test group had surgery almost 3 weeks sooner than those who were tested. The conclusion of the authors was that further risk stratification in this group of patients considered at intermediate risk based on clinical history alone was unnecessary as long as perioperative beta blockers were used. Testing only delayed necessary vascular surgery.

The results of the CARP trial and the study by Poldermans et al. suggest no benefit to revascularization, yet several study limitations with the CARP trial must be considered. It was unclear what percent of patients received a bare-metal stent (BMS) or PCI without stent. The effect of inadequate antiplatelet therapy was unclear as was the impact of a vascular surgery without the recommended delay of 6 weeks after BMS placement. The authors stated that the "majority" of patients remained on antiplatelet therapy throughout the perioperative period, but the type of therapy or its duration was not given.

CABG for triple vessel disease may be beneficial. When Ward et al. reanalyzed the CARP data, they reported fewer PMIs after the vascular operation in CABG patients (6.6%) than in PCI patients (16.8%), despite more diseased vessels in the CABG group (28). Landesberg et al. reported improved long-term survival in patients with intermediate clinical risk factors who had stress testing and coronary revascularization (29). Therefore, revascularization by CABG for selected patients with extensive disease may show benefit.

Coronary Stents

Reports of stent thrombosis during the perioperative period have been published, although the actual number of patients described remains low. Kaluza et al. found a 17.5% incidence of presumed stent thrombosis in 40 patients who had noncardiac surgery within 6 weeks of BMS implantation. In five of the seven cases antiplatelet therapy was stopped preoperatively (30). In a study by Sharma et al. thienopyridine therapy was discontinued within 90 days of BMS placement (31). In a study of 192 patients undergoing major noncardiac surgery within 2 years of placement of either BMSs or drug-eluting stents (DESs), patients who had surgery within 1 to 6 months after placement (n = 17) and continued dual antiplatelet therapy (aspirin plus a thienopyridine) through the perioperative period had no major cardiac events. In those who discontinued antiplatelet therapies (n = 13), 30.7% suffered a major event. For those who underwent late surgery (unclear if aspirin was continued or not), only 1 of 162 had a major cardiac event. In this study there was no difference in cardiovascular events between BMSs and DESs. There was also no difference in the incidence of transfusion between those on dual therapy and those who had antiplatelet drugs withheld (32).

In February of 2007, the ACC/AHA in conjunction with the Society for Cardiovascular Angiography and Interventions (SCAI), the American College of Surgeons (ACS), the American Dental Association (ADA), and the American College of Physicians (ACP), published an advisory statement regarding the premature discontinuation of dual antiplatelet therapy after coronary stents (33). It recommended that strong consideration be given to the placement of BMSs in patients likely to undergo surgery within 12 months and that elective surgery be deferred for 1 year in patients with DESs who would be at high risk for perioperative bleeding if dual antiplatelet therapy were continued. For patients with a DES who need surgical procedures within 12 months of stent placement and in whom discontinuation of thienopyridine therapy is absolutely necessary, it is advised that aspirin be continued and thienopyridine therapy restarted as soon as possible. There is limited evidence regarding how soon after either DES or BMS placement surgery can safely be conducted if dual therapy can be continued. A certain period of time is required for the stent to settle and there is also concern regarding smooth muscle proliferation in response to the endothelial injury during placement.

PHARMACOLOGIC INTERVENTIONS

Beta Blockers

Beta blockers protect the heart by improving myocardial oxygen balance by slowing the HR and reducing contractility. Decreasing the HR not only improves diastolic coronary filling, but also decreases myocardial oxygen consumption. Beta blockers may stabilize coronary plaques by decreasing shear forces and through an anti-inflammatory effect. Stability lowers the incidence of atherosclerotic plaque rupture or fissuring. In ischemia-induced arrhythmias, beta blockers have a membrane stabilizing effect. Finally, beta blockers can cause a shift in the balance of metabolism to glucose from free fatty acids, which could improve efficiency of the muscle energy (34).

The first randomized controlled trial of perioperative beta blockade was published in 1996 by Dennis Mangano and the Multicenter Study of Perioperative Ischemia Research Group (McSPI group) (35). In this study 200 patients who needed major noncardiac surgery and had either a history of CAD or two or more risk factors for CAD were randomized to receive placebo or atenolol on the day of surgery and for 7 days or until hospital discharge. There was no statistically significant difference in outcome during the 7-day perioperative period between the atenolol and placebo groups; however, during the first 6 to 8 months after the study there were 12 cardiac events in the control group compared to none in the atenolol group. The results remained significant to the end of the study period, with a 15% reduction in 2-year, event-free survival. In a secondary analysis, Wallace et al. found a 30% to 50% reduction in perioperative ischemia (36).

The strongest evidence for perioperative beta blockers to date comes from the Dutch Echocardiographic Cardiac Risk Evaluation Applying Stress Echocardiography (DECREASE) trial from Poldermans et al. (37). Patients with one or more risk factors underwent DSE. Those with a positive DSE result were randomized to placebo or perioperative bisoprolol. Excluded were patients with extensive WMAs or strong evidence of left main or three-vessel CAD and patients with asthma or taking beta blocker therapy. Bisoprolol, initiated on average 37 days and at least 1 week preoperatively, was continued for 30 days postoperatively. From 1,351 patients screened, 112 patients were enrolled. The 30-day cardiac mortality decreased from 17% in the control group to 3.4% in the study group and nonfatal MI decreased from 17% to 0%.

The subsequent literature is less encouraging. The Perioperative Beta-Blockade for Patients Undergoing Infra-renal Vascular Surgery (POBBLE) trial enrolled 103 patients who were randomized to placebo or metoprolol, typically the night before surgery, and for 7 days postoperatively (38). Patients were excluded if they had a history of MI within 2 years of surgery or angina with a positive stress test. There was no statistically significant difference in 30-day cardiovascular morbidity and mortality. Symptomatic bradycardia and hypotension were higher in the study group, with an increased requirement of inotropic support. The Metoprolol after Vascular Surgery (MaVS) trial studied 496 patients who had major vascular surgery of which 297 patients had an RCRI of 1 (1 point given for undergoing vascular surgery) and 47 patients had an RCRI of ≥3 (39). Patients were randomized to placebo or metoprolol 2 hours preoperatively and then postoperatively for up to 5 days. In patients with an RCRI of <2 there was no statistically significant difference in 30-day cardiovascular outcome. In those with an RCRI of ≥3, the incidence of 30-day complications was higher in the metoprolol group, 7 of 19 versus 4 of 28, although the number of events was too small for significance. There was a significantly higher incidence of need for treatment of bradycardia and hypotension in the metoprolol group. The Diabetic Postoperative Mortality and Morbidity (DIPOM) trial included 921 diabetic patients >40 years of age who needed major nonvascular surgery lasting >1 hour. Patients were excluded if they had indications for outpatient beta blocker treatment, which was not otherwise specified. Metoprolol or placebo was given the night before surgery and continued for 7 days or until hospital discharge. There was no statistically significant difference in cardiovascular outcome over the 18-month follow-up (40).

Lindenauer et al. published a retrospective cohort study conducted by searching a database used by 329 participating hospitals for quality assessment (41). A total of 119,454 patients were given beta blockers perioperatively, defined as the administration of beta blockers within the first or second day of hospitalization. There was no effect on in-hospital mortality when evaluated for the entire cohort (2.3% vs. 2.4%). For patients with an RCRI score ≥3, beta blockers were protective; patients with an RCRI score of 1 had no mortality benefit. For those with an RCRI of 0, in-hospital mortality increased with the use of perioperative beta blockade.

A recent systematic review and meta-analysis was published in 2007 by Wiesbauer et al. (42), who found 70 trials that met their inclusion criteria. Perioperative beta blockers in noncardiac surgery decreased the incidence of myocardial ischemia but did not significantly reduce the incidence of PMI, arrhythmias, length of hospital stay, or mortality.

The literature regarding perioperative beta blockade is far from conclusive, but beta blockers are a part of optimal medical therapy for perioperative cardiac protection. The critical questions are to whom should they be administered, when, and for how long? Whether different beta blockers are superior should be determined. Recent studies suggest that beta blockers may not be effective if HR is not well controlled or if patients are at low risk.

There are several considerations regarding the optimal protocol for perioperative beta blockade. Feringa et al. studied 272 vascular surgery patients and their beta blocker doses (43). In multivariate analysis, higher beta blocker doses were significantly associated with a lower incidence of myocardial ischemia, troponin T release, and long-term mortality. Higher HR during ECG monitoring was significantly associated with an increased incidence of myocardial ischemia, troponin T release, and long-term mortality. The authors suggested that controlling HR <70 bpm was ideal. There is also some evidence to suggest that long-acting agents are superior because of a lower incidence of plasma level troughs. A longer preoperative administration period allows better titration with less under- and overdosing. When Redelmeier et al. reviewed 37,151 patients who had received atenolol or metoprolol before surgery, they found that 1,038 patients experienced an MI or died. The rate was significantly lower for patients given atenolol than for those given metoprolol (2.5% vs. 3.2%, p <0.001). The decreased risk with atenolol persisted after adjustment for measured demographic, medical, and surgical factors. The authors concluded that the metoprolol group did not have as low a perioperative cardiac risk as patients given atenolol, because of possible acute withdrawal after missed atenolol doses. This supported the use of longer-acting agents with tight HR control (44).

In 2006, the ACC/AHA updated its recommendations for perioperative beta blockade (45). The current Focused Update to the ACC/AHA Guidelines on perioperative beta blockade advocates that perioperative beta blockade is a class I indication (conditions for which there is evidence for and/or general agreement that the procedure or treatment is beneficial, useful, and effective) to be used in patients previously taking beta blockers and those with a positive stress test who need major vascular surgery (Table 3.8). The use of these agents in those with a history of CAD but without documented ongoing ischemia or undergoing less invasive procedures is a class II recommendation (conditions for which there is conflicting evidence and/or a divergence of opinion about the usefulness/efficacy of a procedure or treatment but the weight of evidence/opinion is in favor of usefulness/efficacy). Previous contraindications (e.g., chronic obstructive pulmonary disease [COPD] and stable CHF) are only relative contraindications and beta blockers are well tolerated in these patients.

Antiplatelet Agents

Chronic aspirin therapy for both primary and secondary prevention of atherosclerotic disease is now extremely common. The U.S. Preventative Services Task Force recommends aspirin for primary prevention in patients considered at increased risk for the

Table 3.8. Recommendation for perioperative beta blockade

Surgical Procedure	No Clinical Risk Factors	One or More Clinical Risk Factors	CHD or High Cardiac Risk
Vascular	Class IIb Level of evidence: B	Class IIb Level of evidence: B	Patients found to have myocardial ischemia on preoperative testing Class I Level of evidence: B[a] Class IIa Level of evidence: B[b]
High-/Intermediate-risk	[c]	Class IIb Level of evidence: C	Class IIa Level of evidence: B
Low-risk	[c]	[c]	[c]

[a]Applies to patients found to have coronary ischemia on preoperative testing.
[b]Applies to patients found to have coronary heart disease.
[c]Indicates insufficient data. See text for further discussion.
CHD = coronary heart disease.
Class I: Conditions for which there is evidence for and/or general agreement that the procedure/therapy is useful and effective.
Class II: Conditions for which there is conflicting evidence and/or a divergence of opinion about the usefulness/efficacy of performing the procedure/therapy.
Class IIa: Weight of evidence/opinion is in favor of usefulness/efficacy.
Class IIb: Usefulness/efficacy is less well established by evidence/opinion.
Class III: Conditions for which there is evidence and/or general agreement that the procedure/therapy is not useful/effective and in some cases may be harmful.
From Fleisher LA, Beckman JA, Brown KA, et al. ACC/AHA 2007 guidelines on perioperative cardiovascular evaluation and care for noncardiac surgery: A report of the American College of Cardiology/American Heart Association Task Force on Practice Guidelines (writing committee to Revise the 2002 Guidelines on Perioperative Cardiovascular Evaluation for Noncardiac Surgery). *J Am Coll Cardiol* 2007;50:e159–241.

development of CAD. The AHA/ACC Guidelines for Secondary Prevention for Patients with Coronary and Other Atherosclerotic Vascular Disease recommend indefinite aspirin therapy with 75 to 162 mg (46). Traditionally aspirin was withheld for at least 5 days before elective surgery to decrease the risk of perioperative bleeding. Recently, as the protective role of antiplatelet therapy has been better appreciated, the practice of aspirin withdrawal preoperatively has been questioned. Case reports of cardiovascular events after the cessation of aspirin preoperatively and experimental data suggest a rebound increase in platelet activity with acute cessation after chronic therapy. A meta-analysis evaluating the perioperative cardiovascular risks of discontinuing aspirin versus the risk of perioperative bleeding complications from its continuation was published in 2005 (47). Retrospective investigations showed that aspirin withdrawal preceded up to 10.2% of all acute cardiovascular events. Acute coronary events occurred 8.5 ± 3.6 days after aspirin withdrawal. In 41 studies (10 randomized) with 14,981 patients that evaluated perioperative bleeding in patients taking aspirin, incidence of bleeding complications increased in patients taking aspirin by a factor of 1.5, but severity of bleeding did not increase, except in intracranial surgery and perhaps transurethral resection of the prostate. In 2002, the French Society of Anesthesiology and Intensive Care published a consensus statement regarding aspirin taken perioperatively (48). Aspirin increased bleeding moderately but without an increased need for transfusion. The statement cautioned against the practice of aspirin cessation, particularly in vascular surgical patients, because of the risk of cardiovascular events. Finally, if aspirin discontinuation is felt to be necessary, doses should be resumed as soon as possible, preferably within 6 hours of surgery. The American College of Chest Physicians has recommended preoperative aspirin therapy for patients who need carotid endarterectomy and prosthetic femoral-popliteal bypass (49).

The literature is limited regarding the perioperative use of other antiplatelet medications such as the thienopyridines, clopidogrel and ticlopidine, or glycoprotein IIb/IIIa inhibitors. Concern about bleeding has led most practitioners to advise patients to discontinue or avoid these medications before most surgeries. Other than in cardiac surgery, however, there is no evidence to prove an increased incidence of major bleeding complications in noncardiac surgery. There is some evidence to suggest that surgery, even vascular surgery in a patient taking thienopyridines, can be performed safely. Except for protection against stent thrombosis, there is no evidence to support the superiority of thienopyridines over aspirin alone for the prevention of perioperative cardiac events.

Statins

Statins have anti-inflammatory actions that can stabilize coronary plaque. Statin drugs enhance the production of nitric oxide, which improves endothelial function and inhibits platelet aggregation. They have also been shown to decrease the proliferation of smooth muscle in response to injury and scavenge oxygen free radicals.

Hindler et al. recently published a meta-analysis of eight studies of noncardiac surgery (50). The use of preoperative statin therapy was associated with a 4.4% absolute reduction in perioperative mortality (from 6.1% to 1.7%). There was no statistically significant improvement in the one study of nonvascular surgery.

The efficacy of acute statin therapy compared to chronic has not been extensively studied. Durazzo et al. randomized 100 patients who needed vascular surgery to receive atorvastatin or placebo for 45 days preoperatively, irrespective of serum cholesterol levels (51). Cardiac complications decreased significantly 6 months after surgery in the treated group, 8% versus 26%. In this small number of patients the results of acute short-term therapy were effective.

Although the protective effects of statins appear impressive, their use is not without complication. Muscle symptoms such as cramps or myalgias occur, but in general, at a rate similar to that with placebo. Minor elevations of creatine kinase (CK) are not uncommon. More serious side effects such as hepatotoxicity, myositis, and rhabdomyolysis have been reported. The mechanism of these side effects is unclear. In the reported cases of postoperative rhabdomyolysis, possible precipitating factors included prolonged immobility, unusual patient positioning, and prolonged use of statins (52,53). The AHA Clinical Advisory on the Use and Safety of Statins advised that statins be withheld in patients who have major surgery (54).

In an effort to clarify the risk of statin use in patients who have major vascular surgery, Schouten et al. screened 981 consecutive patients (55). A total of 182 patients were on chronic therapy and another 44 had statin therapy initiated 31 to 52 days before surgery because preoperative tests showed elevated serum cholesterol. Muscle complaints were noted and CK levels were checked preoperatively and then on postoperative days 1, 3, and 7. Patients taking statins had a slight increase in their baseline CK versus nonusers (75 vs. 46 U/dL) but remained within the normal range. No patients complained of muscle weakness or muscle pain during the perioperative period. There was no statistically significant difference in postoperative CK levels between users and nonusers or between acute and chronic statin users. There is growing concern regarding the risks associated with acute discontinuation of statins. In one study of patients who had acute coronary syndromes, mortality increased by sevenfold in patients who stopped statin therapy abruptly (56). Acute withdrawal of therapy led to increased oxidative stress and endothelial dysfunction in mice (57).

Statin therapy is effective as a cardioprotective tool perioperatively. The risk of rhabdomyolysis in patients who continue therapy in the perioperative period appears small, and the associated risk of acute withdrawal may very well be higher. Acute therapy was safe in the Schouten study, which had a small number of patients. The current ACC/AHA guidelines advocate continuing statins as a Class I recommendation.

Nitroglycerin

Nitroglycerin has been a mainstay of anti-ischemic therapy, but its value during the perioperative period is controversial. Two randomized clinical trials have focused on nitroglycerin and high-risk noncardiac surgery patients, and no benefit was seen in a meta-analysis (58). Many of the effects of nitroglycerin are mimicked by anesthetic agents. These effects minimize the potential beneficial effects of nitroglycerin and potentially lead to profound hypotension. The evidence does not support the routine prophylactic use of nitroglycerin.

α_2-Adrenergic Agonists

α_2-Adrenergic agonists have been used as adjuvants to anesthetic management. Ellis et al. (59) randomly assigned high-risk patients who had noncardiac surgery to receive either clonidine or a placebo. Incidence of intraoperative but not postoperative ischemia decreased significantly with clonidine. Stuhmeier et al. randomly assigned patients who had elective vascular surgery to receive either an α_2-adrenergic agonist or a placebo (60). Incidence of perioperative myocardial ischemia was reduced significantly with fewer nonfatal MIs in the group who received the α_2-adrenergic agonist. Wallace et al. randomized 190 patients and demonstrated that perioperative administration of clonidine for 4 days to patients at risk for CAD significantly reduces the incidence of perioperative myocardial ischemia and postoperative death (61). Clonidine may be useful for the management of postoperative hypertension because it is available in oral and transdermal formulations. Clonidine stimulates central α_2 receptors and thereby decreases sympathetic outflow to the vasculature, producing vasodilation and lowering BP. It is particularly appropriate for the patient taking clonidine preoperatively to continue this drug to avoid the clonidine withdrawal syndrome. Abrupt cessation of clonidine can lead to a withdrawal syndrome characterized by rebound hyperactivity of the central autonomic and sympathetic nervous systems. Patients have symptoms similar to symptoms of a pheochromocytoma or severe hypertension with marked agitation. Levels of noradrenaline, adrenaline, and total and free 3-methoxy-4-hydrophenylglycol, indices of sympathetic hyperactivity, are very high. Clonidine should not be used in patients with high-grade conduction disturbances.

Perioperative administration of mivazerol, an intravenous α_2-adrenergic agonist, was associated with a significantly reduced incidence of myocardial ischemia with no difference in cardiac events. A large-scale trial of mivazerol is being analyzed, the results of which should provide important data for management of high-risk patients.

Calcium Channel Antagonists

The calcium channel blockers may be useful in the management of postoperative hypertension. These agents lower BP by reducing afterload but may produce reflex tachycardia; this condition is particularly true with the use of dihydropyridine compounds such as nifedipine. A meta-analysis was unable to demonstrate benefits of the use of these agents in noncardiac surgery (58).

Intra-Aortic Balloon Counterpulsation

In high-risk patients with unstable angina or severe CAD, an intra-aortic balloon counterpulsation device has been placed before induction of anesthesia. In several small case series, perioperative morbidity and mortality were low (62,63). Because the use of an intra-aortic balloon counterpulsation is associated with risks and requires additional skills for placement and knowledge to manage, the physician must determine if the benefits outweigh these risks.

REFERENCES

1. Eagle KA, Berger PB, Calkins H, et al. ACC/AHA guideline update for perioperative cardiovascular evaluation for noncardiac surgery-executive summary: a report of the American College of Cardiology/American Heart Association Task Force on Practice Guidelines (committee to update the 1996 Guidelines on

Perioperative Cardiovascular Evaluation for Noncardiac Surgery). *J Am Coll Cardiol*. 2002;39:542–553.

1A. Fleisher LA, Beckman JA, Brown KA, et al. ACC/AHA 2007 guidelines on perioperative cardiovascular evaluation and care for noncardiac surgery: A report of the American College of Cardiology/American Heart Association Task Force on Practice Guidelines (Writing Committee to Revise the 2002 Guidelines on Perioperative Cardiovascular Evaluation for Noncardiac Surgery). *J Am Coll Cardiol* 2007;50:e159–241.

2. Mangano DT, Browner WS, Hollenberg M, et al. Association of perioperative myocardial ischemia with cardiac morbidity and mortality in men undergoing noncardiac surgery. *N Engl J Med*. 1990;323:1781–1788.

3. Landesberg G, Mosseri M, Zahger D, et al. Myocardial infarction after vascular surgery: the role of prolonged stress-induced, ST depression-type ischemia. *J Am Coll Cardiol*. 2001;37:1839–1845.

4. Landesberg G. The pathophysiology of perioperative myocardial infarction: facts and perspectives. *J Cardiothorac Vasc Anesth*. 2003;17:90–100.

5. Dawood MM, Gutpa DK, Southern J, et al. Pathology of fatal perioperative myocardial infarction: implications regarding pathophysiology and prevention. *Int J Cardiol*. 1996;57:37–44.

6. Cohen MC, Aretz TH. Histological analysis of coronary artery lesions in fatal postoperative myocardial infarction. *Cardiovasc Pathol*. 1999;8:133–139.

7. Naghavi M, Libby P, Falk E, et al. From vulnerable plaque to vulnerable patient: a call for new definitions and risk assessment strategies: part II. *Circulation*. 2003;108:1772–1778.

8. Keats AS. The ASA Classification of physical status-a recapitulation. *Anesthesiology*. 1978;49:233.

9. Goldman L, Caldera DL, Nussbaum SR, et al. Multifactorial index of cardiac risk in noncardiac surgical procedures. *N Engl J Med*. 1977;297:845–850.

10. Detsky A, Abrams H, McLaughlin J, et al. Predicting cardiac complications in patients undergoing non-cardiac surgery. *J Gen Intern Med*. 1986;1:211–219.

11. Eagle KA, Coley CM, Newell JB, et al. Combining clinical and thallium data optimizes preoperative assessment of cardiac risk before major vascular surgery. *Ann Int Med*. 1989;110:859–866.

12. Lee TH, Marcantonio ER, Mangione CM, et al. Derivation and prospective validation of a simple index for prediction of cardiac risk of major noncardiac surgery. *Circulation*. 1999;100:1043–1049.

13. Shah KB, Kleinman BS, Sami H, et al. Reevaluation of perioperative myocardial infarction in patients with prior myocardial infarction undergoing noncardiac operations. *Anesth Analg*. 1990;71:231–235.

14. Tarhan S, Moffitt EA, Taylor WF, et al. Myocardial infarction after general anesthesia. *JAMA*. 1972;220:1451–1454.

15. Hertzer NR, Bevan EG, Young JR, et al. Coronary artery disease in peripheral vascular patients: a classification of 1000 coronary angiograms and results of surgical management. *Ann Surg*. 1984;199:223–233.

16. Paul SD, Eagle KA, Kuntz KM, et al. Concordance of preoperative clinical risk with angiographic severity of coronary artery disease in patients undergoing vascular surgery. *Circulation.* 1996;94:1561–1566.

17. Mangano DT, London MJ, Tubau JF, et al. Dipyridamole thallium-201 scintigraphy as a preoperative screening test. A reexamination of its predictive potential. Study of Perioperative Ischemia Research Group. *Circulation.* 1991;84:493–502.

18. Baron JF, Mundler O, Bertrand M, et al. Dipyridamole-thallium scintigraphy and gated radionuclide angiography to assess cardiac risk before abdominal aortic surgery. *N Engl J Med.* 1994; 330:663–669.

19. L'Italien GJ, Paul SD, Hendel RC, et al. Development and validation of a Bayesian model for perioperative cardiac risk assessment in a cohort of 1,081 vascular surgical candidates. *J Am Coll Cardiol.* 1996;27:779–786.

20. Poldermans D, Arnese M, Fioretti PM, et al. Improved cardiac risk stratification in major vascular surgery with dobutamine-atropine stress echocardiography. *J Am Coll Cardiol.* 1995; 26:648–653.

21. Froehlich JB, Karavite D, Russman PL, et al. American College of Cardiology/American Heart Association preoperative assessment guidelines reduce resource utilization before aortic surgery. *J Vasc Surg.* 2002;36:758–763.

22. Reilly DF, McNeely MJ, Doerner D, et al. Self-reported exercise tolerance and the risk of serious perioperative complications. *Arch Intern Med.* 1999;159:2185–2192.

23. Poldermans D, Bax JJ, Schouten O, et al. Should major vascular surgery be delayed because of preoperative cardiac testing in intermediate-risk patients receiving beta-blocker therapy with tight heart rate control? *J Am Coll Cardiol.* 2006;48:964–969.

24. Falcone RA, Nass C, Jermyn R, et al. The value of preoperative pharmacologic stress testing before vascular surgery using ACC/AHA guidelines: a prospective, randomized trial. *J Cardiothorac Vasc Anesth.* 2003;17:694–698.

25. McFalls EO, Ward HB, Moritz TE, et al. Coronary-artery revascularization before elective major vascular surgery. *N Engl J Med.* 2004;351:2795–2804.

26. Fleisher LA, Rosenbaum SH, Nelson AH, et al. Preoperative dipyridamole thallium imaging and Holter monitoring as a predictor of perioperative cardiac events and long tem outcome. *Anesthesiology.* 1995;83:906–917.

27. Beattie WS, Abdelnaem E, Wijeysundera DN, et al. A meta-analytic comparison of preoperative stress echocardiography and nuclear scintigraphy imaging. *Anesth Analg.* 2006;102:8–16.

28. Ward HB, Kelly RF, Thottapurathu L, et al. Coronary artery bypass grafting is superior to percutaneous coronary intervention in prevention of perioperative myocardial infarctions during subsequent vascular surgery. *Ann Thorac Surg.* 2006;82: 795–800.

29. Landesberg G, Berlatzky Y, Bocher M, et al. A clinical survival score predicts the likelihood to benefit from preoperative thallium scanning and coronary revascularization before major vascular surgery. *Eur Heart J.* 2007;28:533–539.

30. Kaluza GL, Joseph J, Lee JR, et al. Catastrophic outcomes of noncardiac surgery soon after coronary stenting. *J Am Coll Cardiol.* 2000;35:1288–1294.

31. Sharma AK, Ajani AE, Hamwi SM, et al. Major noncardiac surgery following coronary stenting: when is it safe to operate? *Catheter Cardiovasc Interv.* 2004;63:141–145.

32. Schouten O, van Domburg RT, Bax JJ, et al. Noncardiac surgery after coronary stenting: early surgery and interruption of antiplatelet therapy are associated with an increase in major adverse cardiac events. *J Am Coll Cardiol.* 2007;49:122–124.

33. Grines CL, Bonow RO, Casey DE Jr, et al. Prevention of premature discontinuation of dual antiplatelet therapy in patients with coronary artery stents: a science advisory from the American Heart Association, American College of Cardiology, Society for Cardiovascular Angiography and Interventions, American College of Surgeons, and American Dental Association, with representation from the American College of Physicians. *J Am Coll Cardiol.* 2007;49:734–739.

34. Schouten O, Bax JJ, Dunkelgrun M, et al. Pro: beta-blockers are indicated for patients at risk for cardiac complications undergoing noncardiac surgery. *Anesth Analg.* 2007;104:8–10.

35. Mangano DT, Layug EL, Wallace A, et al. Effect of atenolol on mortality and cardiovascular morbidity after noncardiac surgery. Multicenter Study of Perioperative Ischemia Research Group. *N Engl J Med.* 1996;335:1713–1720.

36. Wallace A, Layug B, Tateo I, et al. Prophylactic atenolol reduces postoperative myocardial ischemia. McSPI Research Group. *Anesthesiology.* 1998;88:7–17.

37. Poldermans D, Boersma E, Bax JJ, et al. The effect of bisoprolol on perioperative mortality and myocardial infarction in high-risk patients undergoing vascular surgery. Dutch Echocardiographic Cardiac Risk Evaluation Applying Stress Echocardiography Study Group. *N Engl J Med.* 1999;341:1789–1794.

38. Brady AR, Gibbs JS, Greenhalgh RM, et al. Perioperative betablockade (POBBLE) for patients undergoing infrarenal vascular surgery: results of a randomized double-blind controlled trial. *J Vasc Surg.* 2005;41:602–609.

39. Yang H, Raymer K, Butler R, et al. The effects of perioperative beta-blockade: results of the Metoprolol after Vascular Surgery (MaVS) study, a randomized controlled trial. *Am Heart J.* 2006;152:983–990.

40. Juul AB, Wetterslev J, Gluud C, et al. Effect of perioperative beta blockade in patients with diabetes undergoing major noncardiac surgery: randomised placebo controlled, blinded multicentre trial. *BMJ.* 2006;332:1482.

41. Lindenauer PK, Pekow P, Wang K, et al. Perioperative betablocker therapy and mortality after major noncardiac surgery. *N Engl J Med.* 2005;353:349–361.

42. Wiesbauer F, Schlager O, Domanovits H, et al. Perioperative beta-blockers for preventing surgery-related mortality and morbidity: a systematic review and meta-analysis. *Anesth Analg.* 2007;104:27–41.

43. Feringa HH, Bax JJ, Boersma E, et al. High-dose beta-blockers and tight heart rate control reduce myocardial ischemia and

troponin T release in vascular surgery patients. *Circulation*. 2006;114(1 Suppl):1344–1349.

44. Redelmeier D, Scales D, Kopp A. Beta blockers for elective surgery in elderly patients: population based, retrospective cohort study. *BMJ*. 2005;331:932.

45. Fleisher LA, Beckman JA, Brown KA, et al. ACC/AHA 2006 guideline update on perioperative cardiovascular evaluation for noncardiac surgery: focused update on perioperative beta-blocker therapy: a report of the American College of Cardiology/American Heart Association Task Force on Practice Guidelines (writing committee to update the 2002 Guidelines on Perioperative Cardiovascular Evaluation for Noncardiac Surgery): developed in collaboration with the American Society of Echocardiography, American Society of Nuclear Cardiology, Heart Rhythm Society, Society of Cardiovascular Anesthesiologists, Society for Cardiovascular Angiography and Interventions, and Society for Vascular Medicine and Biology. *Circulation*. 2006;113:2662–2674.

46. Smith SC Jr, Allen J, Blair SN, et al. AHA/ACC guidelines for secondary prevention for patients with coronary and other atherosclerotic vascular disease: 2006 update: endorsed by the National Heart, Lung, and Blood Institute. *Circulation*. 2006; 113:2363–2372.

47. Burger W, Chemnitius JM, Kneissl GD, et al. Low-dose aspirin for secondary cardiovascular prevention—cardiovascular risks after its perioperative withdrawal versus bleeding risks with its continuation—review and meta-analysis. *J Intern Med*. 2005; 257:399–414.

48. Samama CM, Bastien O, Forestier F, et al. Antiplatelet agents in the perioperative period: expert recommendations of the French Society of Anesthesiology and Intensive Care (SFAR) 2001–summary statement. *Can J Anaesth*. 2002;49:S26–35.

49. Clagett GP, Sobel M, Jackson MR, et al. Antithrombotic therapy in peripheral arterial occlusive disease: the Seventh ACCP Conference on Antithrombotic and Thrombolytic Therapy. *Chest*. 2004;126(Suppl):609S–626S.

50. Hindler K, Shaw AD, Samuels J, et al. Improved postoperative outcomes associated with preoperative statin therapy. *Anesthesiology*. 2006;105:1260–1272.

51. Durazzo AE, Machado FS, Ikeoka DT, et al. Reduction in cardiovascular events after vascular surgery with atorvastatin: a randomized trial. *J Vasc Surg*. 2004;39:967–975.

52. Kersten JR, Fleisher LA. Statins: the next advance in cardioprotection? *Anesthesiology*. 2006;105:1079–1080.

53. Forestier F, Breton Y, Bonnet E, et al. Severe rhabdomyolysis after laparoscopic surgery for adenocarcinoma of the rectum in two patients treated with statins. *Anesthesiology*. 2002;97:1019–1021.

54. Pasternak RC, Smith SC Jr, Bairey-Merz CN, et al. ACC/AHA/NHLBI Clinical Advisory on the Use and Safety of Statins. *Circulation*. 2002;106:1024–1028.

55. Schouten O, Kertai MD, Bax JJ, et al. Safety of perioperative statin use in high-risk patients undergoing major vascular surgery. *Am J Cardiol*. 2005;95:658–660.

56. Heeschen C, Hamm CW, Laufs U, et al. Withdrawal of statins increases event rates in patients with acute coronary syndromes. *Circulation*. 2002;105:1446–1452.
57. Vecchione C, Brandes RP. Withdrawal of 3-hydroxy-3-methylglutaryl coenzyme A reductase inhibitors elicits oxidative stress and induces endothelial dysfunction in mice. *Circ Res*. 2002;91:173–179.
58. Stevens RD, Burri H, Tramer MR. Pharmacologic myocardial protection in patients undergoing noncardiac surgery: a quantitative systematic review. *Anesth Analg*. 2003;97:623–633.
59. Ellis JE, Drijvers G, Pedlow S, et al. Premedication with oral and transdermal clonidine provides safe and efficacious postoperative sympatholysis. *Anesth Analg*. 1994;79:1133–1140.
60. Stuhmeier KD, Mainzer B, Cierpka J, et al. Small, oral dose of clonidine reduces the incidence of intraoperative myocardial ischemia in patients having vascular surgery. *Anesthesiology*. 1996;85:706–712.
61. Wallace AW, Galindez D, Salahieh A, et al. Effect of clonidine on cardiovascular morbidity and mortality after noncardiac surgery. *Anesthesiology*. 2004;101:284–293.
62. Siu SC, Kowalchuk GJ, Welty FK, et al. Intra-aortic balloon counterpulsation support in the high-risk cardiac patient undergoing urgent noncardiac surgery. *Chest*. 1991;99:1342–1345.
63. Shayani V, Watson WC, Mansour MA, et al. Intra-aortic balloon counterpulsation in patients with severe cardiac dysfunction undergoing abdominal operations. *Arch Surg*. 1998;133:632–635.

4

Nonischemic Heart Disease and Vascular Disease

Ann T. Tong and Marc A. Rozner

Preoperative evaluation identifies patients who might need further assessment or treatment of comorbid conditions. A significant number of patients undergoing surgery have cardiac disease. In some patients, cardiac conditions are discovered during preoperative evaluation, and treatment can be lifesaving. Often, preoperative evaluation leads to a modification of the anesthetic plan to optimize postoperative outcomes. This chapter provides a comprehensive review of hypertension, nonischemic cardiomyopathy, valvular heart disease, rhythm disturbances, pacemakers, implantable cardioverter defibrillators (ICDs), carotid bruits, peripheral arterial disease, and the transplanted heart. The final section discusses preoperative drug management. This chapter excludes ischemic heart disease, which is covered in Chapter 3.

HYPERTENSION

Systemic arterial hypertension (Table 4.1) is common, and its prevalence increases with age. According to the Joint National Committee for the Prevention, Detection, Evaluation, and Treatment of High Blood Pressure Report (JNC 7), hypertension affects approximately 50 million individuals in the United States and approximately 1 billion worldwide (1). In only 34% of patients with known hypertension is it adequately controlled, and 30% of patients are unaware that they have hypertension. The relationship between blood pressure (BP) and cardiovascular disease (CVD) is continuous and independent of other risk factors. High BP increases the risk of myocardial infarction (MI), heart failure (HF), stroke, and kidney disease. For individuals between 40 and 70 years old, each increment in systolic and diastolic BP of 20 and 10 mm Hg, respectively, doubles the risk of lifetime CVD. The preoperative evaluation is a unique opportunity to identify patients with hypertension and initiate or arrange appropriate therapy.

The patient with hypertension is evaluated so that the information obtained will aid in perioperative management. For example, patients with hypertension have a higher incidence of silent ischemia than the general population (2), but the presence of hypertension is not a predictor of increased postoperative complications. Left ventricular hypertrophy (LVH) increases the risk of coronary artery disease (CAD) and perioperative myocardial ischemia, but regression of left ventricular (LV) mass requires many months of antihypertensive therapy.

Table 4.1. Classification and management of hypertension in adults

Category	Systolic (mm Hg)	Diastolic (mm Hg)	Lifestyle Modification	Pharmacologic Therapy Indicated
Normal	<120	<80	Encourage	
Prehypertension	120–139	80–89	Yes	High-risk patients with risk factors for CVD
Stage 1 hypertension	140–159	90–99	Yes	Yes
Stage 2 hypertension	>160	>100	Yes	Yes

CVD, cardiovascular disease.
Adapted from the Seven Report of the Joint National Committee on Detection, Evaluation, and Treatment of High Blood Pressure (JNC 7) (1)

Table 4.2. Cardiovascular risk factors

Major risk factors
Hypertension
Cigarette smoking
Obesity (body mass index >30)
Physical inactivity
Dyslipidemia
Diabetes mellitus
Age (>55 yr for men, >65 yr for women)
Family history of premature cardiovascular disease (men <55 yr, women <65 yr)

Target organ damage
Heart
    Left ventricular hypertrophy
    Angina or prior myocardial infarction
    Prior coronary revascularization
    Heart failure
Stroke or transient ischemic attack
Chronic kidney disease
Peripheral arterial disease
Retinopathy

Chobanian AV, Bakris GL, Black HR, et al. The Seventh Report of the Joint National Committee on Prevention, Detection, Evaluation, and Treatment of High Blood Pressure: the JNC 7 report. *JAMA.* 2003;289:2560–2572.

History and Physical Examination

In the initial evaluation of patients with a history of hypertension:

- Identify other cardiovascular risk factors that may affect prognosis and treatment (Table 4.2).
- Assess the presence of target organ damage and CVD.
- Identify the causes of hypertension (Table 4.3).

The physical examination focuses on verification of BP in both arms, auscultation for the presence of bruit (carotid, abdominal, femoral), palpation of the thyroid gland, and verification of the

Table 4.3. Causes of hypertension

Sleep apnea
Chronic kidney disease
Renovascular disease
Coarctation of the aorta
Primary aldosteronism
Cushing syndrome
Chronic steroid use
Pheochromocytoma
Thyroid or parathyroid disease
Drug induced or drug related

presence of rales/crackles in lungs. The presence of murmurs, heart sounds S_3 and S_4, and peripheral edema guides selection of other cardiac testing.

Laboratory Testing

Serum electrolytes, blood urea nitrogen (BUN), creatinine, and calcium are part of the initial evaluation of hypertension. Patients with suspected renal insufficiency or poorly controlled hypertension should have these tests done preoperatively. Electrolytes need to be obtained in a patient on diuretics or potassium-sparing drugs (e.g., angiotensin-converting enzyme inhibitors [ACEIs] or aldosterone antagonists). A urinalysis may identify renal insufficiency.

Cardiac Testing

Electrocardiography (ECG) can identify LVH, left atrial (LA) abnormality, or a prior MI. Reasonable physicians continue to debate the need for a preoperative ECG in an asymptomatic patient with limited CVD risk, since abnormalities are not predictive of major postoperative events in a general surgical population, even in the elderly (3). However, in a hypertensive patient with significant CVD risk factors or having high-risk surgery, the presence of LVH or ST-segment depression on an ECG predicts adverse cardiac events. It is reasonable to obtain a preoperative ECG in these patients. If a significant ECG abnormality (multiple Q waves, LVH with strain, widespread low-voltage QRS, or widespread ST-segment elevation or depression) is found, transthoracic echocardiography (TTE) may be indicated to assess LVH, diastolic dysfunction, wall motion abnormality, or valvular disease.

Preoperative Preparation and Anesthetic Implication

For patients with controlled hypertension, the main issues include the need for stress testing and administration of their usual antihypertensive drugs on the day of surgery. Preoperative stress testing is discussed in Chapter 3.

There seems to be no argument regarding the continuation of beta blockers, clonidine, and calcium channel blockers into the perioperative environment. The continuation of diuretics can necessitate a urinary catheter, produce unwanted volume contraction, or predispose to electrolyte abnormalities. There remains debate about continuation of ACEIs and angiotensin receptor antagonists (ARBs), since these agents have been shown to produce postinduction hypotension (4), sometimes profound and refractory to conventional therapy (5). It is our practice to hold these drugs on the day of surgery, since many anesthetic agents lower BP. Other centers hold them only for patients with well-controlled BP, those having major surgery with significant fluid shifts and/or blood loss, or those taking multiple antihypertensives. See the section on Preoperative Management of Drug Therapy.

Patients identified during a preoperative evaluation prior to the day of surgery with untreated, poorly treated, or uncontrolled hypertension should be started on antihypertensive therapy appropriate to their comorbid diseases and the interval to surgery. For patients seen 1 to 2 days prior to surgery, some providers will initiate calcium channel blockade (e.g., amlodipine 5 to 10 mg daily, including the day of surgery) to reduce exaggerated BP responses in these patients. The institution of diuretics, which have the best long-term outcomes for antihypertensive therapy (6), often requires weeks to achieve the desired effect.

The primary issue for a patient who presents on the day of surgery with poorly controlled or uncontrolled hypertension (systolic BP >220 mm Hg and/or diastolic >110 mm Hg) is the need for further preoperative management prior to induction of anesthesia. Traditionally, surgery for these patients has been delayed to allow further treatment. However, a meta-analysis of this topic and reviewed in the American College of Cardiology/ American Heart Association (ACC/AHA) Perioperative Guidelines (7) clearly shows that delaying surgery to initiate treatment does not improve outcome in the patient *without* end-organ damage (8). In fact, across many studies, none of the patients with "uncontrolled systemic hypertension" sustained a major perioperative cardiac event. These patients demonstrate perioperative hemodynamic lability and exaggerated response to surgical stimuli, but this response does not seem to lead to cardiac complications in the absence of severe CAD. Thus, although these patients might have increased perioperative complexity, delaying their surgery provides no benefit and can increase their overall cost of medical care (9). Therefore, treatment of BP on the day of surgery, titrated to prevent significant hypotension (especially with anesthetic induction), as well as the ability to manage the patient's hypertension and other comorbid diseases throughout the perioperative period, appears sufficient in most cases. In their recent review of the literature, Hanada et al. concluded: "In order to minimize the risk of cardiovascular complications, achieving hemodynamic stability is more important than the absolute target values of intraoperative blood pressure control" (10).

The issue of perioperative beta blockade arises in these patients. Many experts now believe that initiation of beta blocker therapy (atenolol, metoprolol, or bisoprolol) in the clinic or on the day of surgery will reduce the incidence of perioperative cardiac events (11,12), and guidelines have been issued (13). Care should be taken to ensure continuation of these drugs throughout the perioperative period.

Nevertheless, some cases are found in which delay of surgery may be warranted based on the preoperative BP. A hypertensive crisis, defined as evidence of ongoing end-organ damage with severely elevated BP, requires treatment as a medical emergency. With symptoms of new headache or visual disturbances, the patient might be at risk for a cerebral hemorrhage, and treatment before the induction of anesthesia is warranted. Similarly, elevated BP of an episodic nature, particularly when associated with intermittent headaches or palpitations, raises the possibility of a pheochromocytoma, and elective cases should be delayed to permit further investigation.

HEART FAILURE AND CARDIOMYOPATHY

Heart failure (HF) remains a common problem in the United States, affecting >5 million individuals (2% of the population), with 550,000 new cases diagnosed annually. The prevalence increases with age; HF affects 1% of individuals between the ages of 50 and 59 years, and >10% of individuals >80 years old (14). Although mortality from coronary heart disease (CHD) and hypertension has declined significantly in the past 40 years, overall mortality in patients diagnosed with HF has remained the same. Patients with compensated HF (history of HF exacerbations, but without jugular venous distention [JVD], crackles, and S_3) have a 5% to 7% incidence of cardiac complications, whereas those with decompensated HF have a 20% to 30% incidence of cardiac complications.

Ischemic heart disease and hypertension remain the most common causes of HF. Other etiologies include valvular diseases, hypertrophic cardiomyopathies (HCMs), restrictive or infiltrative conditions (sarcoidosis, hemochromatosis, amyloidosis), myocarditis, arrhythmogenic right ventricular (RV) cardiomyopathy, HIV, metabolic conditions (hyper-/hypothyroidism), toxicity (alcohol, cocaine, chemotherapy, radiation), peripartum disorders, and muscular dystrophies. In some patients, the cause cannot be identified (idiopathic HF).

Patients with HF undergo myocardial remodeling (LVH, chamber dilation, and interstitial fibrosis) and demonstrate disturbed hormonal, cytokine, and neural regulatory function. HF can be asymptomatic or cause fatigue, dyspnea, and fluid retention. Most published studies of HF evaluate patients with systolic dysfunction. In one study of patients who had surgery and an S_3 gallop and JVD, 20% experienced cardiac death and 14% experienced serious cardiac complications (18).

HF may be systolic (decreased LV ejection fraction [LVEF], abnormal contraction), diastolic (elevated filling pressures and abnormal relaxation but normal LVEF), or both. Diastolic HF (also called HF with preserved LV systolic function) accounts for as many as 40% of HF cases (16). Patients with diastolic HF have elevated LV filling pressures secondary to a stiff noncompliant ventricle, but near normal LV systolic function. Unlike systolic HF, for which there is substantial evidence-based medicine derived from multiple large-scale randomized trials, treatment of diastolic HF remains empiric and is based mostly on anecdotal information.

In the past, assessment of LV diastolic function required invasive hemodynamic and/or angiographic measurement, performed during a cardiac catheterization. Doppler echocardiographic assessments of LV filling patterns, yielding reliable and useful measures of diastolic performance and LV hemodynamics, have become available. Patients can now be classified into those with normal filling pressures and diastolic function; those with mild abnormalities of impaired relaxation; and those with more severe abnormalities reflective of a restrictive filling pattern and elevated LA pressure (17). The significance of such measurements is well established in patients with chronic HF in whom Doppler filling parameters independently convey information about symptoms, exercise limitation, and prognosis, as well as response to therapy (18).

Patients with diastolic HF poorly tolerate rapid fluid administration, which can result in pulmonary edema. Tachycardia,

Table 4.4. New York Heart Association classification of dyspnea

Class	Description
I	Dyspnea with more than ordinary activity (e.g., prolonged exertion at work or recreation)
II	Dyspnea with ordinary activity (e.g., climbing stairs rapidly or more than one flight of stairs at normal pace, walking uphill, walking more than two blocks)
III	Marked limitation of ordinary physical activity (e.g., dyspnea walking one to two blocks, climbing one flight of stairs, "comfortable at rest")
IV	Inability to carry out any physical activity without dyspnea, short of breath at rest

which shortens the diastolic filling period, can be problematic. Atrial fibrillation (AF), with the loss of atrial contribution, especially with a rapid ventricular response, can produce significant hemodynamic compromise.

History and Physical Examination

History and physical examination help confirm the diagnosis and determine the physiologic state and functional status of the patient. Functional status is classified using the New York Heart Association (NYHA) classification (Table 4.4). Similarly, the new staging system (Table 4.5) is used to emphasize the role of risk factors in the development of HF.

Most patients with HF complain of dyspnea. Other symptoms include paroxysmal nocturnal dyspnea, orthopnea, fatigue, generalized weakness, chest pain, and nonproductive nocturnal cough. Because pulmonary, renal, or hepatic diseases can cause similar symptoms, symptoms alone cannot reliably be used to predict the severity of cardiac dysfunction or prognosis (19). Table 4.6 shows common physical findings of HF. Determining the cause(s) and precipitating factor(s) of HF provides insight into appropriate testing and therapy, and any patient with untreated or newly discovered HF should be referred for additional evaluation and treatment before surgery unless emergent surgery is needed.

Diagnostic Testing

Table 4.7 shows useful diagnostic tests for patients with HF. The diagnosis requires objective evidence of cardiac dysfunction at rest. LVEF is best assessed by TTE, although radionuclide angiography or contrast ventriculography have been used. TTE also provides information on diastolic function, wall motion abnormalities, LVH, valvular abnormalities, and cardiac hemodynamics, thus making it the test of choice. A normal echocardiogram rules out significant HF.

LVEF has been studied as a predictor of short- and long-term prognosis in patients who undergo noncardiac surgery.

Table 4.5.   Stages of heart failure

At Risk for Heart Failure		Heart Failure	
Stage A: No structural heart disease No symptoms of HF	Stage B: Structural disease No signs or symptoms of HF	Stage C: Structural disease Prior or current symptoms of HF	Stage D: Refractory HF
Presence of hypertension, atherosclerotic disease, diabetes, metabolic syndrome, cardiotoxins, family history of HF	History of MI, LV remodeling (LVH, low LVEF), asymptomatic valvular disease	Presence of dyspnea, fatigue, reduced exercise tolerance	Presence of symptoms at rest

HF, heart failure; LV, left ventricular; LVEF, left ventricular ejection fraction; LVH, left ventricular hypertrophy; MI, myocardial infarction.
Adapted from Hunt SA, ACC/AHA Task Force on Practice Guidelines. ACC/AHA 2005 guideline update for the diagnosis and management of chronic heart failure in the adult: a report of the American College of Cardiology/American Heart Association Task Force on Practice Guidelines (writing committee to update the 2001 Guidelines for the Evaluation and Management of Heart Failure). *J Am Coll Cardiol.* 2005;46:e1–82. Available at: http://content.onlinejacc.org/cgi/reprint/46/6/e1.

According to the ACC guidelines, the greatest risk of perioperative ischemic events is believed to be in patients with a resting LVEF <35%, but this finding has not been a consistent predictor (6). In fact, a meta-analysis shows that preoperative LVEF determination adds little value, if any, to preoperative risk stratification (20).

Natriuretic peptide levels are now routinely used to distinguish dyspnea from pulmonary causes from HF, especially in the setting of clinical uncertainty. B-type natriuretic peptide (BNP) is a 32-amino-acid peptide released predominantly from the ventricles

Table 4.6.   Common physical findings in heart failure patients

Resting tachycardia
Pulmonary basilar crackles
Peripheral/dependent edema
S_3 gallop
Jugular venous distention
Hepatojugular reflex
Laterally displaced apical pulse
Unexplained weight gain
Oliguria

Table 4.7. Diagnostic testing for heart failure

Test	Findings
ECG	A normal ECG suggests that the diagnosis of chronic HF should be carefully reviewed. The negative predictive value of a normal ECG to exclude LV systolic dysfunction exceeds 90%.
Chest radiography	Chest radiography should be part of the initial diagnostic workup in HF. It has predictive value only in the context of typical signs and symptoms and an abnormal ECG.
Laboratory tests	Routine evaluation includes complete blood count, serum electrolytes, creatinine, glucose, hepatic enzymes, and urinalysis. Some experts also recommend thyroid function tests as well as serum ferritin and transferrin saturation levels. In acute exacerbations exclude acute myocardial infarction by myocardial specific enzyme analysis.
Natriuretic peptides	Plasma concentrations of certain natriuretic peptides can be helpful in the diagnostic process. These peptides may be most useful clinically as a "rule out" test because of their consistent and high negative predictive values.
Echocardiography	Objective evidence of cardiac dysfunction at rest is necessary for the diagnosis of HF. Echocardiography is the preferred method.
Pulmonary function	Lung function measurements are of little value in diagnosing chronic HF. They might be useful in excluding respiratory causes of breathlessness.
Holter monitoring	Conventional Holter monitoring is of no value in the diagnosis of chronic HF, although it may detect and quantify the nature, frequency, and duration of atrial and ventricular arrhythmias that could be causing or exacerbating symptoms of HF.
Exercise testing	In clinical practice, exercise testing is of limited value for the diagnosis of HF. A normal maximal exercise test in a patient not receiving treatment for HF excludes HF as a diagnosis. Exercise testing in chronic HF may be useful for prognostic stratification.
Additional noninvasive tests	When echocardiography at rest has not provided enough information or in severe or refractory chronic HF or in patients with coronary artery disease, further noninvasive imaging may include stress testing (echocardiography, nuclear cardiology) or cardiac magnetic resonance imaging.
Invasive investigation	Invasive investigation is generally not required to establish the presence of chronic HF but may be important in elucidating the cause in individual patients (e.g., endomyocardial biopsy) or to obtain prognostic information.

ECG, electrocardiogram; HF, heart failure; LV, left ventricular.
Adapted from Remme WJ, Swedberg K. Comprehensive guidelines for the diagnosis and treatment of chronic heart failure. Task force for the diagnosis and treatment of chronic heart failure of the European Society of Cardiology. *Eur J Heart Fail.* 2002;4:11–22.

in response to volume and pressure overload. In the BNP Multinational Study, which evaluated patients with dyspnea in an emergency department, a BNP level of >100 pg/mL had a diagnostic accuracy for HF of 83.4% (21). Overall, BNP levels had similar positive and negative predictive values for both systolic and diastolic HF (22). Patients with more severe dyspnea, prior MI, and higher heart rates (HRs) were more likely to have higher BNP levels and systolic HF. Other disease entities such as MI, pulmonary embolus, severe sepsis, renal failure, and hypothyroidism can elevate BNP, and BNP level may be <100 pg/mL in appropriately treated patients with compensated HF or obesity.

Elevated levels of N-terminal pro-BNP preoperatively are strongly associated with mortality and major adverse cardiac events in patients having major vascular surgery (23). Elevated BNP levels predict increased rates of cardiac events (cardiac death, nonfatal MI, pulmonary edema, and ventricular tachycardia) in patients who have noncardiac surgery (24).

Treatment

Medical management includes ACEIs or ARBs, beta blockers, diuretics, digoxin, hydralazine, nitrates, anticoagulants, and aldosterone inhibitors (25). Invasive management includes implantation of a cardiac generator with multisite ventricular pacing (see below). Multiple clinical trials have shown ACEIs and beta blockers provide survival benefits, and beneficial effects appear shortly after starting therapy (26). Diuretics improve symptoms, but have not been studied in a survival trial. Digoxin may be used in patients who remain symptomatic despite ACEIs, beta blockers, and diuretics. Aldosterone antagonists (spironolactone and eplerenone) provide additional survival benefits in patients with severe symptomatic HF or those with a previous MI. Hydralazine and nitrates may be used in patients intolerant of ACEIs or ARBs or who have significant renal dysfunction; they also have incremental survival benefits in the African American population (27). Short-acting calcium channel antagonists are contraindicated in systolic HF. They depress LV function, worsen symptoms, increase neurohormone levels, and increase the risk of death. Their role in the treatment of HF with preserved LV systolic function is uncertain.

Preoperative Preparation and Anesthetic Implication

Surgery should be delayed for patients with decompensated HF, if possible, until their condition and treatment have been optimized. Consensus guidelines for the management of acute decompensated HF divide patients by the adequacy of their cardiac output (28). Patients with low cardiac output require inotropes, which should be continued perioperatively if surgery cannot be delayed. At present, there is no agreement regarding how long after an episode of decompensated HF to delay elective surgery. Patients with decompensated HF might benefit from invasive hemodynamic monitoring to guide therapy; however, the use of pulmonary artery catheters or central venous pressure monitoring remains controversial (29,30). In one review of preoperative hemodynamic optimization, only patients in the highest-risk group benefited and only when supranormal values for oxygen delivery were achieved (31). The medical management of HF before an elective surgical procedure may require adjustment of medications on an outpatient basis or an admission to a hospital. HF remains a complex and chronic disease often requiring coordination among anesthesiologists and consultants for optimal perioperative outcomes.

Patients with acute volume overload likely require intravenous diuretics. In the absence of hypotension, IV vasodilators (nitroglycerin, nitroprusside, or nesiritide) may be added to diuretic therapy for rapid improvement of congestive symptoms. Nesiritide, a peptide identical to human BNP, reduces LV filling pressure and systemic and pulmonary vascular resistance and increases cardiac output (32). Potential side effects include hypotension similar to that with nitroglycerin and worsening renal function at higher doses. In patients who had cardiac surgery, nesiritide had a favorable effect on urine output and renal function when preoperative serum creatinine was elevated (33). The *routine* use of IV inotropic agents such as dobutamine and milrinone is generally not indicated, except in cases of severely depressed cardiac output in an inpatient setting.

See the section on Preoperative Management of Drug Therapy for recommendations for the day of surgery.

HYPERTROPHIC OBSTRUCTIVE CARDIOMYOPATHY

Although infrequent, hypertrophic obstructive cardiomyopathy (HCM) can increase the risk of hemodynamic compromise in the perioperative period. Patients typically have marked degrees of LVH, reduced ventricular compliance, hyperdynamic LV systolic function, and systolic anterior motion of the mitral valve (MV) with or without a dynamic pressure gradient in the subaortic area.

A history of cardiac symptoms, especially chest pain, dyspnea, and syncope, should be carefully determined. The systolic murmur of the condition is characteristic, and auscultation during passive leg elevation or with the patient changing from the standing to the squatting position typically demonstrates a decrease in the intensity of the murmur. The Valsalva maneuver increases the intensity of the murmur. TTE is useful for evaluation. A retrospective evaluation of 35 patients with documented HCM who had undergone noncardiac surgery demonstrated a high rate of perioperative HF but no cardiac deaths (34). Therefore, an appropriate course is to proceed to surgery while avoiding hypovolemia.

VALVULAR HEART DISEASE

Differentiating a functional from a structural heart murmur remains paramount, and often difficult, in the preoperative evaluation of a patient for noncardiac surgery. Most functional murmurs are from turbulent blood flow across the aortic or the pulmonary outflow tracts. The murmur begins after S_1 with ejection of blood from the ventricle. As the flow increases, the murmur intensity increases, and as the flow decreases, the intensity declines, which gives a crescendo-decrescendo sound to the murmur. This benign murmur is caused by high outflow states (e.g., anemia, hyperthyroidism, pregnancy, exercise), ejection into a dilated vessel

Table 4.8. Grading of murmur intensity

Grade	Description
I	Barely audible
II	Easily audible
III	Intermediate
IV	Murmur accompanied by a thrill
V	Loudest murmur requiring stethoscope + thrill
VI	Murmur heard without a stethoscope + thrill

beyond the valve, or increased transmission of sound through a thin chest wall. In an otherwise healthy patient, the following rarely represents a hemodynamically significant cardiac lesion: A soft systolic ejection murmur of low grade (Table 4.8) loudest at the left sternal border with normal S_1 and S_2, no JVD, normal arterial pulse contour, and no cardiac enlargement. Certain conditions, though, indicate the need for a more extensive evaluation for valvular disease, such as a history of anorectic drug use (dexfenfluramine, fenfluramine, phentermine), rheumatic fever, elderly patients (because of a higher incidence of aortic stenosis [AS]), diastolic murmurs, or abnormal pulse contours.

Murmurs from structural causes may be systolic, diastolic, or continuous, as with a patent ductus arteriosus (PDA). Description of the loudness of the murmur includes assigning a grade of I to VI (Table 4.8). The intensity of the murmurs is determined by the degree of stenosis, the cardiac output, and the amount of turbulent blood flow. Severe stenosis and a low cardiac output frequently results in less turbulent flow. Frequently, the loudest murmurs correlate with minimal lesions, whereas a severe valvular stenosis may be associated with soft murmurs.

With all forms of valvular disease, the presence of pre-existing HF confirmed by preoperative physical examination is associated with a 20% risk of its worsening in the perioperative period. The only exception is AS, which by itself is an independent risk factor for developing HF postoperatively, even without HF preoperatively (15). The location of the loudest sound along with the direction of radiation helps to identify the cardiac structure from which the murmur originates (Table 4.9). A systolic murmur from AS is loudest in the right second intercostal space and radiates to the carotid arteries, whereas a systolic murmur from mitral regurgitation (MR) is best heard at the apex and radiates to the left axilla and base of the heart. Often, determining the origin of a murmur is difficult. In these situations, specific maneuvers that alter the cardiac hemodynamics help to identify the origin and significance of the murmur. For example:

- Deep inspiration augments venous return and accentuates murmurs in the right heart (e.g., tricuspid regurgitation).
- The Valsalva maneuver decreases right and left ventricular filling and reduces the intensity of most murmurs except those associated with HCM and mitral valve prolapse (MVP), in which the murmur is paradoxically accentuated with Valsalva's maneuver.

Table 4.9. Characteristics of pathologic murmurs

Condition	Location	Timing	Description	Severity
Mitral stenosis	Apex	Middiastolic	Opening snap; low-pitched rumble radiates to the axilla	Intensity correlates poorly but duration correlates well
Mitral regurgitation	Apex	Holosystolic	High pitched, blowing; loud S_3 radiates to the axilla	Significant if loud with S_3 gallop
Mitral valve prolapse	Apex	Late systolic	Crescendo, midsystolic click	Decreased end-diastolic volume or increased contractility increases the intensity and duration of the murmur
Aortic stenosis	Second right and left parasternal interspaces	Midsystolic	Crescendo-decrescendo diamond, radiates to the carotids; S_3 and S_4 if significant	Contour of diamond parallels the instantaneous pressure gradient; as long as cardiac output is maintained, excellent correlation between intensity, length, and severity
Aortic insufficiency	Third and fourth parasternal interspace; if loudest at the right, consider aortic root	Holodiastolic	Decrescendo, blowing, high pitched, radiates to the carotids; Austin-Flint rumble at the apex	
Hypertrophic cardiomyopathy	Apex, lower left sternal edge	Midsystolic	Reversed or single S_2 and S_4; Valsalva maneuver increases intensity	Decreased diastolic volume or increased contractility increases intensity of the murmur

Adapted from Eisen N, Reich DL. The patient with valvular heart disease. *Probl Anesth.* 1997;9:157.

- Standing reduces LV volume and accentuates murmurs of HCM and MVP.
- Squatting increases venous return and systemic arterial resistance and thus afterload. This maneuver increases most murmurs except those murmurs of HCM and MVP.
- Sustained hand-grip exercise increases systemic arterial BP and HR, often accentuating murmurs of MR, aortic insufficiency (AI), and mitral stenosis (MS), but diminishing murmurs of AS and HCM.
- Amyl nitrate inhalation decreases afterload, thereby increasing the intensity of murmurs associated with valvular stenosis while diminishing those of AI and MR.

Evaluation of a murmur likely to be hemodynamically significant and related to structural heart disease requires TTE. Often, the patient will have undergone previous TTE evaluation, and effort should be expended to obtain the results to avoid duplication.

Because each of the valvular lesions has different implications for perioperative management and the risk of surgery in a patient with significant AS is extremely high, evaluation to define the extent of valvular insufficiency, stenotic area, and flow gradient is necessary. Occasionally, invasive tests must be performed, despite thorough evaluation with a history, physical examination, and noninvasive tests. For example, evidence of MR and papillary muscle dysfunction suggests the presence of ischemic heart disease, so additional testing with stress or cardiac catheterization may be needed.

MITRAL STENOSIS

MS, which is most commonly associated with rheumatic heart disease, is more frequently found in women than men. Symptoms of MS manifest 10 to 20 years after the acute disease (Table 4.10). MS is often associated with MR. It is an isolated lesion in approximately 20% of patients.

Symptoms of MS result from increased LA pressure and reduced cardiac output. The elevated LA pressure mimics symptoms of LV failure, even though LV contractility is normal. Pulmonary hypertension frequently develops, and right ventricular (RV) function may be compromised.

Physical findings include a diastolic rumble best heard in the apex following an opening snap. S_1 is loud, and the presence of a loud P_2 suggests pulmonary hypertension (Table 4.9). RV overload represents severe disease and produces an RV lift, JVD, ascites, hepatomegaly, and peripheral edema.

TTE or cardiac catheterization may be useful to define the severity of disease. The normal adult MV has an area of 4 to 6 cm². Stenosis is mild when the MV area is 1.5 to 2.5 cm² and moderate when the area is 1.1 to 1.5 cm². MS is critical when the area is 0.6 to 1.0 cm² and the resting mean transvalvular gradient is >10 mm Hg. MS and a dilated LA are associated with a greater frequency of AF, which also promotes clot formation.

Increases in HR reduce LV filling across a stenotic MV and increase the transmitral pressure gradient. Tachycardia in the perioperative period can produce patient complaints. Beta

Table 4.10. Vascular abnormalities, cardiac symptoms and their relationship to prognosis

Condition	Symptom Onset	Symptom	Prognosis
Mitral stenosis	Symptoms usual with valve area <1.5 cm²	Dyspnea, PND, orthopnea, fatigue, chest pain, palpitations, hemoptysis, hoarseness, AF, embolic phenomena, RVF (ascites, peripheral edema)	20% die within 1 yr of developing symptoms; NYHA class I, 85% 10-yr survival; NYHA class II, 50% 10-yr survival; NYHA class III, 20% 10-yr survival; NYHA class IV, 0% 5-yr survival
Mitral regurgitation			
Acute	Immediate	HF, fatigue, dyspnea, AF	Critical
Chronic	Usually asymptomatic for many years	HF, dyspnea, AF, fatigue	Well tolerated for many years
Aortic stenosis	Symptoms usual with valve area <1 cm², 15% die suddenly without previous symptoms	Angina with exertion; nitroglycerin syncope; syncope with exertion; HF	Asymptomatic, severe AS 1 yr survival 67% 2 yr survival 56% 5 yr survival 38%
Aortic insufficiency			
Acute	Immediate	HF	Critical
Chronic	Symptomatic for many years	Dyspnea, fatigue	Well tolerated for years; 50% of patients with severe AI live 10 yr; once symptoms develop, they progress rapidly; patients with palpitations have an average 5 yr survival

AF, atrial fibrillation; HF, heart failure; NYHA, New York Heart Association; PND, paroxysmal nocturnal dyspnea; RVF, right ventricular failure.
Adapted from Eisen N, Reich DL. The patient with valvular heart disease. *Probl Anesth.* 1997;9:157, and Varadarajan P, Kapoor N, Bansal RC, et al. Clinical profile and natural history of 453 nonsurgically managed patients with severe aortic stenosis. *Ann Thorac Surg* 2006;82:2111.

blockers may be used to reduce HR to maximize hemodynamic conditions. Antiarrhythmic agents may prevent AF in patients in whom this arrhythmia is likely, such as those with frequent premature atrial contractions. The development of AF indicates the need for anticoagulation therapy to prevent thrombus formation. Unrecognized MS must be included in the differential diagnosis of pulmonary edema in the perioperative period.

MITRAL REGURGITATION

MR is found more frequently than MS and can be acute or chronic. It develops from leaflet pathology (MVP, rheumatic heart disease, infective endocarditis, collagen vascular diseases), subvalvular pathology (papillary muscle dysfunction, rupture of chordae tendineae), or annular dilation (LV dilation secondary to CAD or cardiomyopathy). The most common cause of MR in the United States is MVP.

The presentation of MR is more gradual than that of any other valvular lesion. Symptoms usually appear only in the late stages with onset of LV dysfunction. Patients complain of fatigue, weight loss, and weakness consistent with low cardiac output. Associated symptoms of RV failure may be seen (Table 4.10).

Chronic MR often results in eccentric cardiac hypertrophy, and cardiac enlargement is observed on physical examination. On auscultation, a holosystolic murmur is heard in the apical area with radiation to the axilla or base of the heart. An S_3 may be present from either HF or rapid filling of the LV by the large volume of blood in the LA (Table 4.9).

No single test exists to quantify the severity of MR. TTE can provide a semiquantitative measure as well as calculated regurgitant fraction through the use of Doppler hemodynamics. Transesophageal echocardiography (TEE) might be needed, especially in cases of an eccentric jet. Left ventriculography provides additional but imperfect estimates of severity, since patients usually have a large LV end-diastolic volume without a change in LV end-diastolic pressure because of increased compliance.

In severe MR, LV function may be reduced, LA and pulmonary vascular pressures are elevated, and AF may be present. MR is not likely to cause abrupt clinical deterioration in the perioperative period, unless other valvular lesions (e.g., AS) or LV dysfunction is present. In the one series, MR was a significant univariate correlate of perioperative cardiac morbidity and postoperative mortality, but the predictive value did not persist after control for other criteria of heart disease in a multivariate analysis.

MITRAL VALVE PROLAPSE

MVP, also known as *floppy valve syndrome* and *systolic click-murmur syndrome*, is a common but highly variable syndrome, most often found in women 15 to 30 years of age. Patients generally remain asymptomatic but occasionally progress to severe and symptomatic MR. They may complain of atypical chest pain, lightheadedness, palpitations, and syncope. Men with MVP who are >55 years of age have the highest incidence of infectious and hemodynamic complications.

Preoperative evaluation focuses on differentiating between patients with purely functional disease and those with significant degeneration of the MV and hemodynamically significant MR. The most common finding is a mid- or late nonejection systolic click with or without a crescendo-decrescendo systolic murmur (Table 4.9). TTE is useful to identify either thickening or a systolic displacement of the MV leaflet into the LA; patients with these findings are at risk of developing severe MR or infective endocarditis.

Management of asymptomatic patients consists of reassurance. Presence of MVP or an isolated click uncomplicated by other symptoms does not warrant cardiologic evaluation. Many patients with MVP take beta blockers for palpitations and atypical pain, and these medications should be continued perioperatively. Appropriate treatment of other complications (symptomatic arrhythmia, symptomatic or severe MR, transient ischemic attacks) is warranted.

AORTIC SCLEROSIS AND STENOSIS

Aortic sclerosis is present in approximately 25% of adults >65 years of age and is a risk factor for CAD similar to classic risk factors (age, gender, hypertension, smoking, cholesterol level, diabetes) (35). Aortic sclerosis is associated with adverse clinical outcome: A 50% increased risk of MI and cardiovascular death compared with patients with a normal aortic valve (AV) (36). Sclerosis can progress to AS.

AS usually starts decades before the onset of symptoms. It is an idiopathic disease resulting from degeneration and calcification of the aortic leaflets present in older patients. This active disease process involves lipid accumulation, inflammation, and calcification, with many similarities to atherosclerosis. Stenosis is more likely to develop in patients who have a congenitally bicuspid aortic valve. Although rheumatic heart disease may cause AS, it is less common than MS and always occurs with MV disease. The severity of AS is based on the aortic jet velocity, the mean transvalvular pressure gradient, and the valve area (Table 4.11). The transvalvular gradient will be lower with LV dysfunction.

TTE evaluation should be performed for any patient with known AS and changing symptoms and signs. Patients with asymptomatic AS should undergo TTE follow-up yearly for severe AS, every 1–2 years for moderate AS, and every 3–5 years for mild AS (37).

Table 4.11. Severity of aortic stenosis

Grade	Aortic Jet Velocity (m/sec)	Mean Transvalvular Pressure Gradient (mm Hg)	Aortic Valve Area (cm^2)
Mild	<3	<25	≥1.5
Moderate	3–4	25–40	1.0–1.5
Severe	4–4.5	40–50	0.7–1.0
Critical	>4.5	>50	<0.7

The classic symptoms of AS are angina, syncope, and HF. The average time from onset of symptoms to death is 2 years with HF, 3 years with syncope, and 5 years with angina. Because of the frequently fatal nature of this lesion (80% of patients who die have had symptoms for <4 years) and the propensity of AS to cause sudden unexpected death (presumably from arrhythmias) in 10% of patients, surgical intervention is recommended for patients with symptomatic and hemodynamically significant AS.

The most common physical finding in AS is a systolic murmur, best heard over the right second intercostal space with radiation to the neck. In the mild version, the murmur peaks early in systole and often produces a thrill. In the severe version, the murmur peaks late in systole and becomes softer as cardiac output diminishes. The carotid upstroke has a diminished amplitude and slow rise (*parvus et tardus*) in severe AS. S_2 may be paradoxically split because of a delay in LV emptying (Table 4.9).

Angina may be from concomitant CAD, but more often results from a supply:demand mismatch with normal coronaries. The increase in LV transmural pressure decreases supply, and the demand is increased by the increase in afterload and myocardial hypertrophy. Patients with AS and angina should undergo cardiac catheterization to rule out CAD. HF can be a result of systolic dysfunction (increased afterload and decreased contractility), diastolic dysfunction (increased LV wall thickness and collagen deposition), or both (Table 4.10).

The presence of moderate to severe AS increases the risk associated with noncardiac surgery, and the ACC/AHA guidelines for perioperative cardiac evaluation recommend that elective noncardiac surgery be postponed or canceled until AV replacement (AVR) or valvuloplasty is performed in patients with severe, symptomatic AS (6). Studies have shown, however, that noncardiac surgery with appropriate monitoring can be performed safely in selected patients with severe AS.

Since the Goldman study showing that AS is an independent risk factor for postoperative morbidity, awareness of the intraoperative risk has heightened (15). Improvements in anesthetic techniques have resulted in a favorable perioperative outcome in patients with severe AS who undergo noncardiac surgery. Use of aggressive intraoperative monitoring and avoidance of adverse hemodynamic changes likely have helped to achieve this improvement. Patients with severe AS may benefit from intra-arterial BP and central venous pressure monitoring, pulmonary artery catheterization, and TEE. Almost all operations requiring central neuraxial or general anesthesia in patients with severe AS require intra-arterial BP monitoring. Other invasive monitoring (pulmonary artery catheterization, TEE) may be indicated, depending on the severity of the surgery and the potential for significant fluid shifts or hemodynamic perturbations. Intraoperative TEE can provide valuable information about valvular and myocardial anatomy and function that can facilitate anesthetic management.

AORTIC INSUFFICIENCY

AI results from any condition that prohibits adequate diastolic opposition of the AV leaflets such as abnormalities of the AV leaflets, the aortic root, or both. Valvular pathology includes rheumatic heart disease (which may lead to a fibrous, calcified AV), infective endocarditis, trauma, a bicuspid AV (which may result in AI or a combination of AS/AI), myxomatous proliferation of the AV, and collagen vascular diseases. Causes of aortic root dilation include cystic medial necrosis of the aorta (Marfan syndrome), age-related degeneration, dissection, hypertension, ankylosing spondylitis, osteogenesis imperfecta, syphilitic aortitis, and collagen vascular diseases. AI can be acute (trauma, aortic dissection) or chronic. Acute AI, characterized by a sudden onset of pulmonary edema and hypotension, should be considered a surgical emergency. If physical examination and TTE show evidence of early closure of the MV and HF, then the patient benefits most from AVR.

Patients with isolated, chronic AI typically rarely experience abrupt deterioration abruptly in the perioperative period. In chronic AI, LV volume overload causes LV dilation and eccentric hypertrophy. The enlarged LV produces a large stroke volume that is ejected into the aorta. The large stroke volume causes systolic hypertension, but the regurgitant blood flow into the LV during diastole produces a low diastolic pressure. The net effect is a widened pulse pressure.

The murmur of AI is typically a high-pitched, blowing diastolic murmur after S_2, best heard over the left sternal border and accentuated when the patient leans forward. A diastolic rumble (Austin Flint murmur), best heard over the cardiac apex, results from the impinging of the aortic jet on the MV (causing it to vibrate) and simultaneous filling of the LV from the LA during diastole (Table 4.9). Peripheral signs of the hyperdynamic circulation are the Corrigan or water-hammer pulse (bounding full carotid pulse with a rapid downstroke), the Musset sign (head bobbing), pistol shot sounds over the femoral artery, and the Duroziez sign (to and fro murmur after application of gentle pressure over the femoral artery).

History and Physical Examination

The history and physical examination guide further investigation. One should attempt to determine from the patient or records whether the murmur is new. The *absence* of such a history does not establish that the murmur is indeed new. AS is more common in males and MVP is more common in females.

A history of syncope associated with a murmur suggests AS, HCM (history of multiple syncopal events), or thromboemboli from a dilated LA caused by MV disease. Syncope can also result from conduction abnormalities, often with structural disease of the MV. Complaints of chest pain or discomfort may indicate the presence of critical AS, HCM, or MR with pulmonary congestion. Dyspnea on exertion may be caused by AS, HCM, or pulmonary congestion from MV disease. A family history of premature sudden death, syncope, and murmur can be important clues for the diagnosis of HCM.

The physical examination focuses on findings associated with the presumed valvular stenotic lesion. For example, in the patient with AS, evaluation of the carotid pulse contour and timing can help determine the severity of the stenosis.

Rales in the patient with MR or MS suggest LA volume overload.

Diagnostic Testing

The surface ECG can provide important clues in the evaluation of murmurs. LVH can be from AI or AS; LA enlargement may be from MV disease; and right atrial (RA) enlargement may be from tricuspid valve disease. A chest radiograph can provide information regarding the cardiac silhouette and pulmonary vasculature. TTE has proven to be the best noninvasive test to evaluate a murmur, and any patient with LVH on ECG and a systolic murmur should undergo TTE evaluation. TTE allows determination of both the severity of the valvular disease and the possible resultant systolic dysfunction and pulmonary hypertension. Other noninvasive tests for evaluating valvular disease include radionuclide ventriculography, fluoroscopy, and magnetic resonance imaging (MRI). Occasionally, TEE may be needed to determine the severity of the valvular lesion.

BALLOON VALVULOPLASTY BEFORE NONCARDIAC SURGERY

Although the long-term outcome for patients who undergo aortic balloon valvuloplasty is generally poor because of restenosis, this procedure may be used for palliation when AVR cannot be performed due to serious comorbid conditions. The considerable procedure-related morbidity and mortality must be carefully considered before recommending this procedure to lower the risk of noncardiac surgery.

Balloon aortic valvuloplasty often decreases the severity of AS, but does not alter the natural history of AS. Balloon valvuloplasty often results in symptomatic improvement; however, the post-valvuloplasty valve area is usually <1.0 cm^2, the major periprocedural complication rate is $\sim5\%$, and the 6-month restenosis rate is high (38). Fatal cardiac arrest has been reported in 3%, but the procedural mortality may be even higher. In a report of 492 patients who underwent balloon aortic valvuloplasty, 4.9% died within the first 24 hours after the procedure and 7.5% died during the hospitalization. Acute catastrophic complications, including ventricular perforation, acute severe AI, cerebrovascular accident, and limb amputation, have been reported in 6% of patients (39).

A study presented at the 2007 Society of Cardiovascular Angiography and Interventions meeting showed that percutaneous AVR with an investigational device may be an option for high-risk patients (40). In 17 patients from 64 to 90 years of age with severe AS (AV area <0.6 cm^2) who had percutaneous AVR, only one patient died in the hospital. The 30-day postprocedure mean AV area was 1.4 cm^2, the mean LVEF was 56%, and NYHA clinical class improved by one grade. Five of the patients who died of other causes had satisfactory valve function at autopsy.

In contrast to aortic valvuloplasty, mitral balloon valvuloplasty is often a reasonable alternative to MV surgery. Results have been favorable, especially in younger patients with MS who do not have severe MV leaflet thickening or significant subvalvular fibrosis and calcification.

PROSTHETIC HEART VALVES

More than 60,000 patients undergo cardiac valve replacement each year in the United States. Issues important in the perioperative period include managing long-term anticoagulation therapy, reducing the risk of infective endocarditis (see Chapter 17), preventing valve thrombosis, and ruling out significant valve-related hemolysis.

Although mechanical prosthetic valves have greater durability than bioprosthetic valves, they are more thrombogenic. The risk of valve thrombosis is greatest in patients with caged-ball prosthetic valves (Starr-Edwards). Single tilting-disk prosthetic valves (Björk-Shiley, Medtronic-Hall, Omnicarbon) have an intermediate risk of valve thrombosis, and bileaflet tilting-disk prostheses (St. Jude Medical, CarboMedics, Edwards Duromedics) pose the lowest risk among the mechanical valves. Bioprosthetic valves available in the United States are porcine heterograft (Carpentier-Edwards, Hancock), pericardial (Carpentier-Edwards), and stentless valves.

The management of warfarin anticoagulation therapy in the perioperative period remains the most difficult aspect of care for patients with mechanical prosthetic valves. The risk of discontinuing anticoagulants must be weighed against the benefit of a reduced likelihood of perioperative bleeding. See Chapters 7 and 17 for specific recommendations.

CONDUCTION BLOCKS

First-degree atrioventricular block exists when the PR interval is >0.20 seconds at a HR of 50 to 100 beats per minute (bpm). First-degree block usually represents a benign abnormality and rarely results in significant impairment. Progression to complete heart block (CHB), while rare, has been reported during spinal anesthesia (41).

Two types of second-degree block have been described. The more benign, Mobitz type I block (Wenckebach block), usually results from atrioventricular nodal delay. As seen in Figure 4.1, the PR interval progressively prolongs until a beat is finally blocked, after which the cycle begins again. Rarely progressing to CHB, Mobitz type I block can be abolished by the use of vagolytic agents like atropine sulfate. Mobitz type II block is the result of infranodal block and can progress to CHB. As seen in Figure 4.2, atrioventricular conduction is interrupted, manifested as a

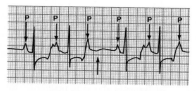

Figure 4.1. An electrocardiogram recorded from a patient with Mobitz type I block. There is progressive elongation of the PR interval until a P wave is completely blocked and a ventricular beat is dropped.

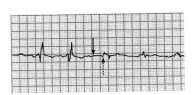

Figure 4.2. An electrocardiogram recorded from a patient with a Mobitz type II block that occurs without progressive elongation of the PR interval. This patient has a pacemaker that is tracking his atrial rhythm.

blocked beat without progression of the PR interval. Pacemaker placement is routinely recommended for patients with Mobitz type II block.

In third-degree (complete) heart block (Fig. 4.3), all atrial beats are blocked and the ventricles, if depolarizing, are driven by a pacemaker distal to the site of the block. Acquired permanent CHB (i.e., not part of an acute coronary syndrome or active myocardial ischemia) always requires permanent pacemaker placement.

Finally, intraventricular conduction delays (IVCDs) or left bundle hemiblocks could suggest underlying CAD or simply reflect fibrosis of the conduction system (Lenègre disease in younger patients, Lev disease in older patients). Complete left bundle branch block (LBBB; Fig. 4.4) or right bundle branch block (RBBB; Fig. 4.5) can be normal variants or represent CAD. In an early Framingham report, the presence of BBB was not associated with the development of new CHD (42).

According to Eriksson et al., ischemic heart disease and BBB often coexist, but their etiologies may not be the same (43). Several studies have found an increased mortality among patients with BBB and concomitant cardiovascular disease. In large numbers of patients from multiple study populations who have been followed longitudinally, the presence of LBBB, but not RBBB, has been associated with a lifelong increased risk of cardiovascular disease, including MI, HF, and death (43–45).

Many physicians believe that a new LBBB is pathognomonic for cardiac disease. A detailed history documenting the absence

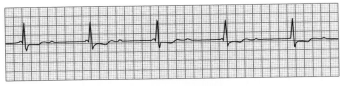

Figure 4.3. Electrocardiogram showing probable third-degree heart block (HB). The atrial rate is 75 bpm. The ventricular rate is 38 bpm. Although this is likely a true third-degree HB, the possibility of 2:1 second-degree block cannot be ruled out, with a profound first-degree HB present (800 msec PR interval).

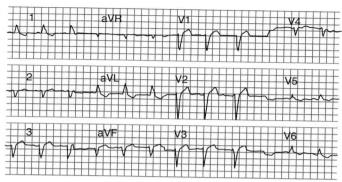

Figure 4.4. Electrocardiogram showing left bundle branch block.

of CAD risk factors (male gender, advancing age, family history, poor functional tolerance, hypertension, diabetes, hypercholesterolemia, or smoking) and symptomatology (chest pain, dyspnea with activity, palpitations, diaphoresis, or syncope) probably eliminates the need for an ischemic workup. An old ECG with a similar pattern provides the best evidence for stability, and a discussion with the patient about the condition might prevent a future unnecessary workup. Patients with new LBBB should undergo TTE evaluation to determine LV systolic function. RBBB can be associated with ischemic heart or lung disease, or arise independently. A history of palpitations or syncope should prompt an arrhythmia investigation, since 1% to 4% of patients with BBB progress to high-grade atrioventricular block per year, requiring pacemaker implantation (43).

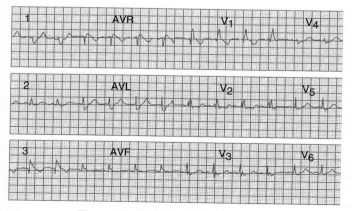

Figure 4.5. Right bundle branch block.

In general, indications for use of a temporary pacemaker during the perioperative period are the same as those for a permanent pacemaker. The patient with an IVCD and normal LVEF rarely will require any pacing. The presence of a complete LBBB increases the probability of developing CHB during insertion of a pulmonary artery (PA) catheter. Numerous strategies have been advocated for the insertion of the PA catheter, including the use of external pacing devices in case CHB develops. Use of a pacing PA catheter may be considered, but frequently the block develops during flotation, and adequate ventricular capture cannot be obtained in this situation. Removal of the PA catheter frequently restores normal rhythm. Based on a study of 39 patients, perioperative progression to CHB in patients with IVCD or hemiblock would be unlikely (46).

SUPRAVENTRICULAR TACHYCARDIAS

The underlying mechanism of supraventricular tachycardia (SVT) is either re-entry or ectopic atrial foci (e.g., ectopic atrial tachycardia or AF). In a re-entry SVT, the mechanism involves dissociation of the conduction tissue into two pathways, one of which exhibits unidirectional block and the other prolonged conduction. An atrial impulse is conducted antegrade to the ventricle over the slowly conducting pathway, as the other has a unidirectional block. The impulse then re-enters the atrial tissue in a retrograde fashion over the pathway that has a unidirectional block. Meanwhile, the pathway with the prolonged conduction has time to regain responsiveness, and the same impulse can be conducted antegrade over this pathway. Once initiated, the re-entry cycle becomes self-perpetuating, resulting in SVT. The re-entry mechanism has been demonstrated in the sinoatrial (SA) and atrioventricular nodes, in the His-Purkinje system, and over accessory pathways such as in Wolff-Parkinson-White (WPW) syndrome. WPW represents a special situation, since the impulse can be conducted both retrograde and antegrade via the bundle of Kent (see below). Sometimes, a concealed bypass tract is present in which the impulse is conducted only in retrograde fashion and the atrioventricular node serves as the antegrade conductor.

Occasionally, SVT of re-entrant origin can be terminated by vagal maneuvers (carotid sinus massage, Valsalva maneuver), which alter atrioventricular conduction. Pharmacologic interventions for re-entry SVT include adenosine, beta blockers, calcium channel blockers, and digoxin. Nonpharmacologic interventions include atrial overdrive pacing (atrial pacing at a rate higher than the SVT with abrupt termination, resulting in resumption of sinus rhythm). SVT because of a concealed bypass tract can be treated by ablation of the tract. Patients with SVT and hemodynamic compromise are treated with synchronized countershock beginning at 50 joules (J) with stepwise increases to 360 J (with an older, monophasic discharge defibrillator) or 25 J increasing to 200 J (for biphasic discharge defibrillators).

SVT may result from rapidly firing ectopic atrial foci with rapid conduction over the atrioventricular node rather than a re-entrant pathway. Various degrees of atrioventricular block may be present resulting in a slower ventricular rate. Vagal

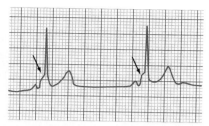

Figure 4.6. Electrocardiogram of a patient with Wolff-Parkinson-White syndrome. Note the delta wave (arrow).

maneuvers are not effective in terminating SVT in this situation because the mechanism does not involve re-entry.

In the WPW syndrome, anomalous atrial to ventricular conduction is over an accessory pathway. Conduction across this bypass tract results in a short PR interval (<0.12 seconds) and an initial slurring (delta wave) during the inscription of the QRS complex, and may be associated with a wide QRS complex (Fig. 4.6).

The accessory pathway in patients with WPW syndrome is capable of bidirectional conduction, which may culminate in a re-entrant SVT without atrioventricular nodal involvement. As discussed below, in patients with AF who also have WPW syndrome, conduction over an accessory pathway results in a rapid ventricular rate or ventricular fibrillation (VF) and abrupt hemodynamic compromise. Atrioventricular nodal blocking agents (beta blockers, calcium channel blockers, and digoxin) are used with extreme caution in patients who have WPW syndrome and SVT because these drugs may shorten the refractory period in the accessory pathways, which can increase the ventricular rate and precipitate VF. Cardioversion is indicated for hemodynamic compromise. Procainamide or lidocaine increases the refractory period of the slows accessory pathway and slows conduction. Radiofrequency catheter or surgical ablation of the accessory pathway offers a permanent cure in patients with WPW syndrome and SVT.

ATRIAL FIBRILLATION

Patients with AF (Fig. 4.7) may have one of the following patterns, often progressing over time: Intermittent (paroxysmal), persistent (can be cardioverted), or permanent (resistant to cardioversion).

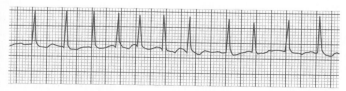

Figure 4.7. Electrocardiogram showing atrial fibrillation.

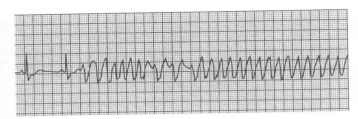

Figure 4.8. Electrocardiogram (ECG) demonstrating atrial fibrillation with conduction over an aberrant pathway in a patient with Wolff-Parkinson-White syndrome. The ventricular response exceeds 300 bpm in some portions of the ECG, and the rhythm is irregularly irregular, which is characteristic of atrial fibrillation.

Some patients with AF who have undergone successful conversion to sinus rhythm with electrical or pharmacologic cardioversion are maintained on antiarrhythmic drugs. These drugs should be continued in the perioperative period if the AF is adequately controlled. Ventricular rate control, an important aspect of AF care, can be achieved either pharmacologically (digoxin, beta blockers, calcium channel blockers) or by nonpharmacologic methods (catheter ablation, placement of a permanent pacemaker). These drugs should be continued in the perioperative period.

Two groups of patients with AF need further, and sometimes immediate, intervention. The first group has an inappropriately fast ventricular response (>180 bpm). Atrioventricular conduction may be across accessory pathways, such as occurs in the WPW syndrome (Fig. 4.8). Elective surgery in patients with ventricular rates >100 bpm, or who have rapid-fire salvos, should be delayed until the rate is controlled.

The second group has inappropriately slow ventricular rates (<90 bpm) without treatment with atrioventricular nodal blocking agents. These patients may have underlying atrioventricular nodal disease, and slow conduction may be a manifestation of sick sinus syndrome (SSS).

The patient with AF represents a unique challenge because of the risk of thromboembolism. Patients may be taking warfarin or aspirin, depending on their thrombotic risk. Stroke may be a devastating complication of an embolic phenomenon, and the goal must be to balance the risk of stroke against the risk of bleeding if anticoagulation is continued. A complete management guide has been published by the ACC/AHA (47). See the section Anticoagulant and Antiplatelet Drugs in Chapters 7 and 17 for recommendations.

VENTRICULAR ARRHYTHMIAS

Patients with ventricular premature beats (VPBs) (Fig. 4.9) during preoperative testing present a dilemma regarding further cardiac evaluation. VPBs are differentiated from atrial premature contractions (APCs) by their origin. VPBs originate in the ventricle and are identified by a wide QRS complex (>0.12 seconds)

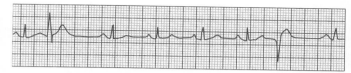

Figure 4.9. Electrocardiogram showing multifocal premature ventricular complexes.

because of abnormal ventricular depolarization and repolarization. An APC originates in the atrium, resulting in a P wave and an unchanged QRS complex. VPB can be classified and graded according to the morphology, frequency, and other characteristics proposed by Lown (Table 4.12).

The Lown classification has limitations for stratifying the risk of sudden cardiac arrest. For example, both couplets and ventricular tachycardia (VT) are better indicators of sudden cardiac arrest than R-on-T VPBs. A clinically useful classification has been developed that is based on the nature of the arrhythmia, underlying heart disease, and the potential for sudden cardiac arrest. Contributing factors such as hypokalemia, hypomagnesemia, acidosis, alkalosis, endocrine abnormalities, and drug toxicities are ruled out. Myocardial ischemia and LV systolic dysfunction are considered. Based on these factors, patients with VPB may be classified as follows:

Benign: Patients with ventricular arrhythmias (e.g., single VPB) but without structural heart disease or hemodynamic compromise are at no risk for sudden cardiac arrest or future major arrhythmic events.

Potentially lethal: Patients with >30 VPB/hour or nonsustained VT without hemodynamic compromise usually have underlying structural heart disease. They are at moderate to high risk for sudden cardiac arrest or a major arrhythmic event. Even in apparently healthy individuals >55 years of age there is an increased cardiac event rate (MI, death) compared to similar

Table 4.12. Lown's grading of ventricular premature beats (VPBs)

Grade	Description
1	Uniform VPB <30/h
2	Uniform VPB >30/h
3	Multiform VPB
4a	Couplets (two consecutive VPBs)
4b	Ventricular tachycardia (three or more consecutive VPBs)
5	R-on-T VPB (potential to progress to ventricular tachycardia)

R-on-T: A premature ventricular complex in the electrocardiogram interrupting the T wave of the preceding beat.

patients with <30 VPBs/hour (48). Some might benefit from the placement of an ICD (49).

Lethal: Patients with lethal ventricular arrhythmias (sustained VT, VF, syncope, hemodynamic compromise) usually have underlying structural heart disease and reduced LVEF. Many are at very high risk for sudden cardiac arrest. Most of these patients benefit from the placement of an ICD (49).

Patients with benign VPBs need no further cardiac evaluation, and treatment is primarily to relieve symptoms. Patients with potentially lethal or lethal arrhythmias, however, should have further cardiac evaluation (TTE, electrophysiologic [EP] testing, signal-averaged ECG, cardiac catheterization) and pharmacologic treatment (antiarrhythmic agents) or nonpharmacologic intervention (ablation, ICD). Many patients with a history of arrhythmia and sudden cardiac arrest benefit from an ICD, a topic that is addressed later in this chapter. When patients are taking antiarrhythmic agents, the class of medication and potential intraoperative medications that can be used should be understood (see Antiarrhythmic Drugs). Patients with VPBs and heart disease should have electrolyte levels and an ECG evaluated preoperatively.

SICK SINUS SYNDROME

Patients with SSS can be asymptomatic but often have syncope or palpitations. In SSS, the automaticity of the sinus node is diminished, and inappropriate sinus bradycardia is often associated with varying degrees of SA block or even sinus arrest. Frequently, the bradycardia is punctuated with SVT (bradycardia-tachycardia syndrome). Figure 4.10 presents ECGs recorded over several days in a patient with SSS.

Patients with SSS can be difficult to manage intraoperatively because of their inability to respond with appropriate ventricular rates to the stress of surgery and anesthesia or their propensity

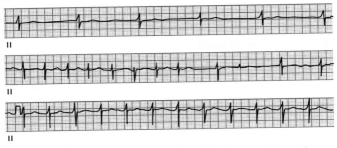

Figure 4.10. Different electrocardiographic patterns observed over a 2- to 3-week period in a patient with bradycardia-tachycardia syndrome. The electrocardiogram (ECG) in the first panel shows sinus arrest with a junctional rhythm of 50 bpm. The ECG in the middle panel (recorded 5 days later) shows atrial fibrillation. The ECG in the bottom panel (recorded 12 days later) shows supraventricular tachycardia at a rate of 130 bpm.

to develop tachyarrhythmias. Moreover, the already diminished automaticity of the SA node may be depressed further by anesthetic and vagotonic agents. These patients should be monitored carefully and may require transvenous pacing. Although pacing is the treatment of choice for symptomatic bradycardia, it is less predictable in suppressing SVT. Patients with SVT may benefit from the use atrioventricular nodal blocking agents (digoxin, beta blockers, calcium channel blockers), in addition to pacemaker placement.

PACEMAKERS

More than 2 million individuals in the United States have permanent cardiac pacemakers. Identifying the manufacturer of the pacemaker allows quick access to expert advice and assistance (from the manufacturer) if issues arise. Perioperative management of these devices is generally based on expert opinion, because no established evidence-based guidelines have been published.

Pacemakers are designated with a five-letter code, although frequently only the first three or four are used. The first three letters describe the basic antibradycardia functions, the fourth describes "rate modulation," and the fifth describes pacemakers with multisite atrial and/or ventricular pacing (50). See Table 4.13 for pacemaker classification.

Preoperatively, the indication for the pacemaker placement as well as the pacemaker manufacturer should be identified. The status of and treatment for HF, CAD, valvular heart disease, arrhythmias, and concomitant diseases like hypertension and diabetes should be known and optimized. On physical examination, the location of the pulse generator should be determined. Occasionally, the pulse generator may become mobile and loose as a result of external manipulation by the patient (Twiddler syndrome).

Pacemaker function is tested preoperatively (and, generally, postoperatively) by comprehensive evaluation using a programmer (51). If preoperative interrogation of the device cannot be performed in a timely manner, a preoperative chest radiograph should be reviewed for pacemaker identification code, number of wires, continuity of wires, and identification of the device as a pacemaker or ICD. In general, patients should be monitored postoperatively until a comprehensive evaluation of the pacemaker is completed.

Electrocautery with monopolar and, rarely, bipolar systems may interfere with pacemakers by causing oversensing. Coagulation electrocautery is more likely to cause problems than is cutting cautery (52). If monopolar electrocautery must be used, the tool should be kept at least 4 to 6 inches from the pacemaker to minimize interference. The current return pad should be placed so that the current does not cross the generator, the lead system, or the chest. Ventricular oversensing (most common) will "convince" the pacemaker that ventricular systoles are present, so ventricular pacing will be inhibited. Atrial oversensing in a dual chamber mode (i.e., DDD) can lead to increased ventricular pacing rates as the pacemaker attempts to "track" this atrial activity.

Table 4.13. Generic pacemaker code

Position I	Position II	Position III	Position IV	Position V
Chambers paced	Chambers sensed	Response to sensing	Programmability	Multisite pacing
O = None	**O** = None	**O** = None	**O** = None	**O** = None
A = Atrium	**A** = Atrium	**I** = Inhibited	**R** = Rate Modulation	**A** = Atrium
V = Ventricle	**V** = Ventricle	**T** = Triggered		**V** = Ventricle
D = Dual (A + V)	**D** = Dual (A + V)	**D** = Dual (T + I)		**D** = Dual (A + V)

From Bernstein AD, Daubert JC, Fletcher RD, et al. The revised NASPE/BPEG generic code for antibradycardia, adaptive-rate, and multisite pacing. North American Society of Pacing and Electrophysiology/British Pacing and Electrophysiology Group. *Pacing Clin Electrophysiol.* 2002;25:260–264.

Rate modulation, an important component of many pacemakers, is designed for the chronotropically incompetent heart. Atrial chronotropic incompetence is defined as the inability to exceed 70% of maximum predicted HR for a given level of metabolic demand or inability to reach a HR of 100 bpm during exercise. Rate-adaptive pacemakers have been designed to increase pacing at the onset of exercise and decrease the rate with rest. Many pacemakers detect mechanical forces such as direct pressure on the generator or vibrations from body movements. Some pacemakers with minute ventilation sensors use chest wall electrical impedance, which varies during the respiratory cycle, to detect "exercise." All sensors can be fooled (e.g., by mechanical ventilation, vibration, and chest "prepping"). Specifically, with minute ventilation sensing devices, connection to an ECG monitor or the use of monopolar electrocautery can result in a paced tachycardia, leading to inappropriate pharmacologic or electrical therapy (53). As a result, most experts and the 2002 ACC/AHA guidelines recommend disabling rate modulation while the patient has a risk of exposure to electromagnetic interference (EMI), which can occur in the preoperative area, the operating and recovery rooms, and intensive care units (54,55).

A pacemaker can be programmed to an asynchronous mode to avoid interference problems. However, asynchronous pacing can cause R-on-T phenomena and precipitate an undesirable tachyarrhythmia (e.g., VT) (56). In cases of emergent surgery or situations in which the pacemaker is not able to be interrogated, a magnet can be placed over the pacemaker while recording the ECG to evaluate the magnet and function of the pacemaker. Not all pacemakers respond to magnet placement with asynchronous pacing. Prophylaxis for infective endocarditis is not recommended for patients with permanent pacemakers.

IMPLANTABLE CARDIOVERTER DEFIBRILLATORS

The preoperative evaluation of the patient with an ICD should focus on indication for the device, because ICDs are implanted for known arrhythmias or prophylaxis against arrhythmogenic potential. Nearly all of these patients have significant cardiomyopathy and systolic HF, often from CAD. As with pacemakers, identifying the manufacturer of the ICD allows quick access to expert advice and assistance from the company if issues arise. If the type of ICD is unknown, a chest radiograph might reveal the manufacturer's logo.

Currently, nearly every ICD can provide complex antibradycardia pacing with rate responsiveness, antitachycardia pacing, and low-energy cardioversion in addition to shock. Since antitachycardia pacing is generally painless, many patients do not know that they have received therapy for a VT until the ICD is interrogated with a programmer.

Because there are multiple causes of inhibition or triggering intraoperatively, most experts recommend disabling antitachycardia therapy during any case in which EMI is expected (51). The ICD can misinterpret electrocautery as an arrhythmia and discharge inappropriately. In certain cases and with certain ICDs magnet placement may be appropriate but only after consultation with an ICD expert. The generic comment "just put a magnet on it" is inappropriate until after the ICD is comprehensively checked. Some devices from Guidant or CPI permanently disable antitachyarrhythmic therapy after magnet placement for >30 seconds (57). In fact, many ICDs (from Guidant, CPI, St. Jude Medical, or Pacesetter) can be programmed to ignore a magnet altogether, and no ICD will change to asynchronous brady-pacing with magnet placement. Currently, Guidant recommends disabling the magnet sensor permanently in many ICDs owing to a magnet switch problem (58). If the magnet sensor has been disabled, it will no longer respond to magnet placement. If patient movement during the procedure is a concern, the ICD should be disabled to shock therapy even if no EMI is expected since shocks can arise from unexpected arrhythmias or lead problems. Placement of a central line also requires the disabling of shock therapy, since the guidewire might touch the lead and precipitate a shock, which could injure the patient or damage the ICD (59).

Current expert recommendations include a preoperative ICD interrogation. For emergency cases, placement of a magnet might be the only option while assistance is en route. At the completion of surgery, the ICD should be evaluated and reactivated. Therefore, elective surgery on a patient with an ICD may not be appropriate in all locations if facilities to evaluate the device are not available. A patient with disabled antitachycardia therapy must be monitored electrocardiographically until the ICD is checked and re-enabled. If the ICD was checked preoperatively, and no EMI, rhythm disturbance, or reprogramming took place, then the ICD need not be retested. Caution must be observed if a magnet is placed on an ICD manufactured by Guidant (formerly CPI), because some of these ICDs can have antitachycardia therapy permanently disabled by >30 seconds of magnet placement (57). Contacting the patient's electrophysiologist preoperatively remains the best course of action.

PERIPHERAL ARTERIAL DISEASE

Peripheral arterial disease (PAD), formerly called peripheral vascular disease, refers to arterial occlusive or aneurysmal disease in the aorta or major arterial trunks supplying the brain, visceral organs, and limbs. The etiology of this process can be acquired (smoking, hypertension, diabetes, hyperlipidemia) or an inborn metabolic disorder (Marfan and Ehlers-Danlos syndromes). The incidence of PAD increases with age, and generally affects men more than women to at least age 75 years (60).

Clinical manifestations of PAD contribute to acute and chronic illnesses that are associated with decreased functional capacity, impaired quality of life, and increased risk of premature death. Because the underlying pathophysiology of PAD results from altered structure and function of the arterial system, patients with PAD often have renal, cardiac, and cerebrovascular disease (61).

History, Physical Examination, and Testing

In patients with PAD, the history elicits comorbidities likely to increase the risk of perioperative problems, such as poor functional reserve, CAD, prior stroke or transient ischemic attack (TIA), diabetes, or renal insufficiency. The physical examination focuses on the signs of significant treatable diseases as well as any cardiac findings that would suggest cardiac dysfunction. The peripheral pulses are evaluated and documented. A recent ECG is obtained preoperatively. Obtaining a creatinine level is important because these patients may have renal insufficiency and may receive radiocontrast dye during vascular procedures. See Chapter 8 for a detailed discussion of this topic.

Recommendations

Administration of beta blockers, especially in high-risk populations, leads to decreases in perioperative cardiac morbidity and mortality. In fact, in recent guidelines, perioperative beta blockade has been recommended with level 1 or 2 evidence for nearly every high-risk surgery patient (13). Care must be taken to ensure continued administration of beta blockers during the postoperative period. Clonidine might be a useful substitute for the patient with contraindications to beta blockade (62). The ACC/AHA has published guidelines for these higher-risk patients, which include immediate smoking cessation; appropriate treatment of hypertension, dyslipidemia, and diabetes; and institution of beta blockers and antiplatelet therapy (aspirin or clopidogrel but not warfarin) (63).

Control and optimization of concomitant diseases (hypertension, CAD, diabetes) should be considered perioperatively. The diagnostic evaluation and treatment (whether percutaneous or surgical) of cerebrovascular disease or CAD to treat asymptomatic disease in PAD patients could needlessly delay surgery. Even though 60% to 80% of PAD patients will have significant CAD (64), individuals with low to moderate cardiovascular risk factors who can tolerate administration of beta blockers will not benefit from an extensive investigation to reduce cardiac risk (65). When 510 patients with known, stable CAD were randomly allocated to coronary artery revascularization or medical management with beta blockers, statin, and aspirin before elective surgery for either an expanding abdominal aortic aneurysm or severe symptoms of PAD, no short- or long-term benefit accrued to those who had revascularization. Vascular surgery was significantly delayed in that group compared to the medical management group (54 days vs. 18 days from randomization) resulting in more deaths before surgery (10 vs. 1) (66). Even in patients with high-risk coronary artery anatomy with extensive exercise-induced ischemia on stress testing, preoperative revascularization produced no benefit in survival or myocardial infarction reduction, although only 101 patients were studied (67). Additionally, the recent statement from the ACC/AHA regarding the need to continue aspirin and thienopyridine antiplatelet therapy for at least 30 days after a bare-metal coronary artery stent or for a year after a drug-eluting stent placement could lead to considerable delay of vascular surgery (68).

CAROTID BRUIT

The presence of an asymptomatic carotid bruit is not correlated with the severity of underlying carotid stenosis or the risk of perioperative stroke (69). It does, however, signal an increased risk of stroke, but does not correlate with the location or mechanism of the stroke. The majority of strokes in patients undergoing cardiac surgery, including those with carotid stenosis, are embolic and are either contralateral to the affected carotid artery or bilateral (70). The Asymptomatic Carotid Atherosclerosis Study found decreased cerebrovascular morbidity and overall mortality after surgery for asymptomatic carotid stenosis of $\geq 60\%$ as measured by diameter reduction, provided that good-risk patients underwent surgery by a surgeon whose record of surgical mortality and morbidity was $<3\%$ (71).

Patients who have a symptomatic carotid bruit and a history of TIAs, lacunar strokes, nondisabling cortical stroke in the territories supplied by the internal carotid artery, or ophthalmic TIAs should be evaluated for carotid artery disease because their risk of perioperative stroke is high (70). Patients with symptomatic carotid stenosis within the previous 6 months benefit from carotid revascularization before undergoing cardiac or major vascular surgery (72). The North American Symptomatic Carotid Endarterectomy Study revealed a clear benefit of carotid endarterectomy for stroke prevention in patients with high-grade stenosis of $\geq 70\%$ who had a nondisabling stroke or TIA in the previous 6 months (73). Carotid endarterectomy is acceptable but not proven treatment for patients with a TIA or a nondisabling stroke in the previous 6 months and a stenosis of 50% to 69%. Carotid endarterectomy is of uncertain benefit in patients who have experienced a TIA or mild nondisabling stroke and have stenosis of $<50\%$.

History and Physical Examination

For patients with a carotid bruit, a detailed history elicits symptoms of TIAs (amaurosis fugax, tingling, numbness or weakness of the face and/or extremities) or CVAs; a careful neurologic examination documents any abnormal findings, and a complete cardiovascular examination confirms the presence of associated cardiovascular disease. This examination assesses for bruits in other vessels (abdominal, renal, femoral) and for heart sounds S_3 and S_4 or murmurs.

Diagnostic Testing

Carotid Doppler ultrasound is $>95\%$ sensitive for hemodynamically significant stenosis. A cerebral angiogram, the gold-standard test, carries a risk of stroke or death of 0.5% to 1.2%. Magnetic resonance angiography (MRA) complements carotid ultrasound because of high specificity and sensitivity but is more costly and less widely available. Transcranial Doppler ultrasonography, which does not directly evaluate the degree of carotid stenosis, is often used in conjunction with carotid ultrasonography to assess the intracranial circulation and hemodynamic significance of the carotid stenosis. All patients with symptomatic carotid stenosis should undergo noncontrast brain computed tomography (CT) or MRI to rule out silent infarcts. Other tests to rule out associated CVD include ECG, TTE, and stress testing if clinically indicated by history or abnormal results on cardiac tests.

Routine evaluation of an asymptomatic carotid bruit before noncardiac surgery is controversial. If the patient is scheduled for major surgery with anticipation of significant blood loss or fluid shifts, evaluation should be considered. Some patients with hemodynamically significant, high-grade, asymptomatic carotid stenosis, especially bilateral stenoses, may benefit from carotid revascularization before elective surgery. An asymptomatic carotid bruit also should be evaluated if the patient has symptoms of angina; a history of significant CAD, severe PAD, prior carotid endarterectomy, or contralateral carotid artery occlusion; or the presence of other risk factors for perioperative stroke (age >70 years, female, hypertension, diabetes, renal insufficiency, smoking, COPD, HF, LVEF <40%, AF, or atherosclerosis of the ascending aorta).

THE PATIENT WITH A TRANSPLANTED HEART

In the patient with a transplanted heart, preoperative evaluation focuses on the functional status of the transplanted heart. Usually, the transplanted heart lacks autonomic reflexes and will not produce pain with ischemia. Patients with a transplanted heart undergo periodic evaluation for the presence of CAD via coronary angiography or stress testing and for myocardial function via TTE or multiple-gated acquisition scan (MUGA). The most recent results should be documented.

A transplanted heart has decreased ventricular compliance and is preload dependent. Patients demonstrate chronotropic incompetence to exercise, anemia, and trauma, because the donor SA node is denervated and does not have direct autonomic regulation. As a result, they have 50% to 70% of the exercise capacity of healthy individuals of the same gender and age. After a heart transplant, the ECG might show two sets of P waves, one from the original SA node, which has autonomic regulation but is blocked by the suture line, and the other from the donor heart, which drives the HR (Fig. 4.11).

The patient with a heart transplant is evaluated for evidence of rejection, especially in the first 3 months when the incidence is highest. Low cardiac output and dysrhythmias may be caused by rejection and are evaluated by TTE and ECG. Endomyocardial biopsy may be needed to confirm rejection, which could require high-dose immunosuppressive therapy.

Immunosuppressive therapy should be continued in the perioperative period. Although immunosuppressants are given in

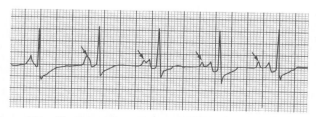

Figure 4.11. Electrocardiogram demonstrating two sets of P waves in a patient with a heart transplant. The P waves indicated by the arrows are from the recipient sinus node. The P waves preceding the QRS complex are from the donor heart.

combination to minimize dose-related toxicity of individual agents, significant adverse effects are still associated with their use. Glucocorticoids can cause adrenal suppression, glucose intolerance, and hypertension; thus, preoperative evaluation should include a glucose level and consideration of perioperative stress doses of steroids (see Chapter 17). Patients on azathioprine might have myelosuppression, including leukopenia, anemia, and thrombocytopenia, so a complete blood count (CBC) with platelets is warranted. Some patients can develop pancreatitis, hepatitis, and hepatic veno-occlusive disease, which require liver and pancreatic testing. Cyclosporine is a nephrotoxic agent and can cause renal dysfunction, electrolyte abnormalities, hypertension, hyperlipidemia, and diabetes. Tacrolimus has similar side effects to cyclosporine. Sirolimus can cause hyperlipidemia, thrombocytopenia, neutropenia, and anemia. Immunosuppressed patients are at a greater risk of opportunistic infections and should have minimal exposure to sources of nosocomial infection (e.g., central and intravascular catheters, mechanical ventilators).

PREOPERATIVE MANAGEMENT OF DRUG THERAPY

To provide an optimal anesthetic and optimal control of adverse hemodynamic perturbations, one must understand a patient's pre-existing drug therapy. Review of limited data suggests that it is safe to continue the vast majority of drugs until the time of surgery, especially in cases in which withdrawal could lead to adverse hemodynamic changes.

α_1-Adrenergic Antagonist Drugs

The α_1-adrenergic antagonist drugs, including prazosin, terazosin, doxazosin, and tamsulosin, are used to control hypertension and benign prostatic hyperplasia. No significant studies have been conducted of the perioperative use of these drugs. These drugs can cause tachycardia through unopposed β-adrenergic activity and hypotension is possible, especially in a volume-depleted patient. However, especially in the case of prazosin, which leaves the prejunctional α_2 receptors intact, the tachycardia is blunted through negative feedback. Most providers continue these drugs throughout the perioperative period, although there are some reports of refractory hypotension (74), especially when these drugs are given with other antihypertensives or in the presence of a neuroaxial block (75).

α_2-Adrenergic Agonist Drugs

The α_2-adrenergic agonists control BP by a centrally mediated stimulation of α_2 receptors, which decreases sympathetic outflow. This class of drugs includes clonidine, methyldopa, guanabenz, and guanfacine. Withdrawal from these drugs may result in rebound hypertension. If the patient is taking an oral medication, methyldopa administered parenterally or clonidine administered via a transdermal patch can be substituted. α_2 Agonists decrease anesthetic requirements and decrease the hemodynamic lability in hypertensive patients. Clonidine decreases analgesic requirements and anxiety and provides sedation. Other possible benefits include attenuation of opiate withdrawal and decreased postoperative shivering, both of which may have adverse hemodynamic effects and precipitate or worsen ischemic heart disease. Most providers continue these drugs throughout the perioperative period.

Angiotensin-converting Enzyme Inhibitors, Angiotensin II Receptor Antagonists, and Renin Antagonists

ACEIs include benazepril, captopril, enalapril, enalaprilat (IV), fosinopril, lisinopril, moexipril, perindopril, quinapril, ramipril, spirapril (not in the United States), and trandolapril. Angiotensin II receptor antagonists include candesartan, eprosartan, irbesartan, losartan, olmesartan, telmisartan, and valsartan. Recently approved is aliskiren, the first direct renin-inhibiting agent. These drugs are indicated for hypertension, HF (afterload reduction, cardiac remodeling), post-MI to improve survival, and diabetic nephropathy. Although no contraindications exist to continuing these drugs perioperatively when patients have been taking them chronically, administering them on the morning of surgery might cause profound, refractory hypotension (4,5). Patients taking these drugs are more sensitive to hypovolemia. ACEIs can cause hyperkalemia. Electrolytes and creatinine level should be obtained preoperatively. It is our practice to hold these drugs on the day of surgery, since many anesthetic agents lower BP. Other centers hold them only for patients with well-controlled BP, those having major surgery with significant fluid shifts and/or blood loss, or those on multiple antihypertensive drugs.

Antiarrhythmic Drugs

Most antiarrhythmic drugs should be continued through the perioperative period. Some of the class I antiarrhythmic drugs like quinidine and procainamide can potentiate the inhalational agents and cause myocardial depression. Class I antiarrhythmics can promote arrhythmias (torsades de pointes), and preoperative evaluation should include an ECG to measure the QT interval. The QT interval represents the duration of ventricular systole and is measured from the beginning of the QRS complex to the end of the T wave. The normal QT interval, corrected for HR (QTc), is usually <0.425 seconds. QTc is calculated by dividing the QT interval by the square root of the R-R interval.

Some inhalational agents decrease liver biotransformation of drugs. Because most of the antiarrhythmic drugs are metabolized in the liver, consideration should be given to reducing the dosages of these drugs. Long-term use of amiodarone can cause serious adverse effects. Patients should undergo evaluation every 4 to 6 months to detect pulmonary toxicity via pulmonary function tests and chest radiography and thyroid dysfunction by measurement of the thyroid profile. Concomitant use of amiodarone with warfarin can potentiate the anticoagulant effect. Amiodarone, a myocardial depressant with a half-life of 30 days, can increase the serum concentration of digoxin, quinidine, and procainamide. It can cause bradycardia (atropine resistant), atrioventricular block, and severe hypotension. Planning for surgery should include preparation for pacing and cardiac support.

Beta Blockers

Beta blockers are commonly used to treat cardiac diseases, especially CAD, hypertension, SVT, and HCM. These drugs are continued throughout the perioperative period. Their withdrawal can lead to hypertension, tachycardia, and recurrence of tachyarrhythmias or worsen or precipitate ischemia by altering the oxygen supply:demand balance. Giving beta blockers in combination with calcium channel blockers or class I antiarrhythmic drugs (quinidine, procainamide, disopyramide) carries a risk of prolonging atrioventricular conduction, resulting in complete heart block. Beta blockers decrease hepatic blood flow and can prolong the effects of drugs metabolized by the liver. Beta blockers should be continued throughout the perioperative period.

Calcium Channel Blockers

Calcium channel blockers (CCBs) commonly used to treat hypertension include amlodipine, felodipine, nifedipine, and nicardipine. They are also used for SVT (verapamil, diltiazem) and ischemic heart disease, especially vasospastic angina. Most experts recommend continuation of these drugs in the perioperative period, although high doses might precipitate hypotension. CCBs do not have the same rebound effects from withdrawal as do beta blockers. The safety of using short-acting CCBs in patients with CAD is controversial.

CCBs might potentiate nondepolarizing neuromuscular blocking agents. Verapamil and diltiazem potentiate the depression of cardiac contractility and atrioventricular conduction block by the volatile anesthetics. Some of the newer agents (e.g., amlodipine) have less negative inotropic effect. Nifedipine can potentiate the vasodilatory effect of volatile agents. Verapamil or diltiazem, combined with beta blockers, can lead to complete heart block. Most providers continue these drugs throughout the perioperative period.

Digoxin

Digoxin is used for both cardiomyopathy and AF. Patients taking digoxin long term continue taking it perioperatively. Digoxin has a narrow therapeutic window, with normal therapeutic levels between 1 and 1.5 ng/mL. Patients at risk for toxicity include those with hypovolemia, electrolyte abnormalities, renal failure, or hypothyroidism; those who are elderly; and those taking other drugs such as diuretics, antiarrhythmics, or agents that block the atrioventricular node. Serum potassium levels may fluctuate in patients who take diuretics or are critically ill, predisposing to digoxin toxicity. Any dysrhythmia with digoxin should be considered a manifestation of digoxin toxicity. Paroxysmal atrial tachycardia (PAT) with 2:1 atrioventricular block is pathognomonic of digoxin toxicity (Fig. 4.12).

Other side effects of digoxin toxicity include VPBs, bigeminy, junctional tachycardia, second-degree atrioventricular block, VT, nausea, anorexia, vomiting, diarrhea, altered mental status, agitation, lethargy, scotoma, and altered perception of colors. Preoperative prophylactic loading dose administration of digoxin to

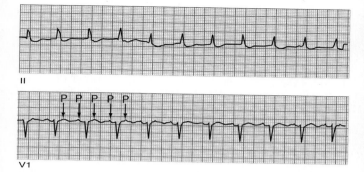

Figure 4.12. Electrocardiogram demonstrating paroxysmal atrial tachycardia with 2:1 block in a patient with digoxin toxicity. Atrial rate is 200 bpm, and ventricular rate is 100 bpm.

patients with diminished cardiac reserve to prevent AF remains controversial. All patients on digoxin should have evidence of stable digoxin level, electrolytes, and renal function. Most providers continue digoxin throughout the perioperative period.

Diuretics

The major categories of diuretics include loop diuretics (furosemide, bumetanide, torsemide), thiazides (hydrochlorothiazide), osmotic diuretics (mannitol), related sulfonamide compounds (indapamide), and potassium-sparing diuretics (spironolactone, eplerenone). Volume depletion and hypokalemia may predispose patients to dysrhythmias. Patients taking diuretics may experience hyponatremia, hypomagnesemia, hypocalcemia, and hyperglycemia. Diuretics are generally discontinued or taken in reduced doses preoperatively to avoid hypovolemia, prerenal azotemia, and intraoperative hypotension. The continuation of diuretics may necessitate a urinary catheter, produce unwanted volume contraction, or predispose to electrolyte abnormalities. Many providers withhold diuretics on the day of surgery until after the surgery is complete. Intravenous diuretics can always be administered if necessary during surgery. Electrolytes should be obtained preoperatively.

REFERENCES

1. Chobanian AV, Bakris GL, Black HR, et al. The Seventh Report of the Joint National Committee on Prevention, Detection, Evaluation, and Treatment of High Blood Pressure: the JNC 7 report. *JAMA.* 2003;289:2560–2572.
2. Boon D, Piek JJ, van Montfrans GA. Silent ischaemia and hypertension. *J Hypertens.* 2000;18:1355–1364.
3. Liu LL, Dzankic S, Leung JM. Preoperative electrocardiogram abnormalities do not predict postoperative cardiac complications in geriatric surgical patients. *J Am Geriatr Soc.* 2002;50:1186–1191.

4. Comfere T, Sprung J, Kumar MM, et al. Angiotensin system inhibitors in a general surgical population. *Anesth Analg.* 2005;100:636–644.

5. Bertrand M, Godet G, Meersschaert K, et al. Should the angiotensin II antagonists be discontinued before surgery? *Anesth Analg.* 2001;92:26–30.

6. ALLHAT Officers and Coordinators for the ALLHAT Collaborative Research Group. Major outcomes in high-risk hypertensive patients randomized to angiotensin-converting enzyme inhibitor or calcium channel blocker vs diuretic: the Antihypertensive and Lipid-Lowering Treatment to Prevent Heart Attack Trial (ALLHAT). *JAMA.* 2002;288:2981–2997.

7. Fleisher LA, Beckman JA, Brown KA, et al. ACC/AHA guidelines for perioperative cardiovascular evaluation and care for noncardiac surgery. *J Am Coll Cardiol.* 2007;50:e159–241. Available at: http://www.acc.org. Accessed September 28, 2007.

8. Howell SJ, Sear JW, Foex P. Hypertension, hypertensive heart disease and perioperative cardiac risk. *Br J Anaesth.* 2004;92: 570–583.

9. Weksler N, Klein M, Szendro G, et al. The dilemma of immediate preoperative hypertension: to treat and operate, or to postpone surgery? *J Clin Anesth.* 2003;15:179–183.

10. Hanada S, Kawakami H, Goto T, et al. Hypertension and anesthesia. *Curr Opin Anaesthesiol.* 2006;19:315–319.

11. Mangano DT, Layug EL, Wallace A, et al. Effect of atenolol on mortality and cardiovascular morbidity after noncardiac surgery. Multicenter Study of Perioperative Ischemia Research Group. *N Engl J Med.* 1996;335:1713–1720.

12. Poldermans D, Boersma E, Bax JJ, et al. The effect of bisoprolol on perioperative mortality and myocardial infarction in high-risk patients undergoing vascular surgery. Dutch Echocardiographic Cardiac Risk Evaluation Applying Stress Echocardiography Study Group. *N Engl J Med.* 1999;341: 1789–1794.

13. Fleisher LA, Beckman JA, Brown KA, et al. ACC/AHA 2006 guideline update on Perioperative Cardiovascular Evaluation for Noncardiac Surgery: focused update on Perioperative Beta-blocker Therapy—a report of the American College of Cardiology/American Heart Association Task Force on Practice Guidelines (writing committee to update the 2002 Guidelines on Perioperative Cardiovascular Evaluation for Noncardiac Surgery). *Anesth Analg.* 2007;104:15–26.

14. Thom T, Haase N, Rosamond W, et al. Heart disease and stroke statistics—2006 update: a report from the American Heart Association Statistics Committee and Stroke Statistics Subcommittee. *Circulation.* 2006;113:e85–151.

15. Goldman L, Caldera DL, Nussbaum SR, et al. Multifactorial index of cardiac risk in noncardiac surgical procedures. *N Engl J Med.* 1977;297:845–850.

16. Vasan RS, Benjamin EJ, Levy D. Prevalence, clinical features and prognosis of diastolic heart failure: an epidemiologic perspective. *J Am Coll Cardiol.* 1995;26:1565–1574.

17. Rakowski H, Appleton C, Chan KL, et al. Canadian consensus recommendations for the measurement and reporting of diastolic dysfunction by echocardiography: from the Investigators of

Consensus on Diastolic Dysfunction by Echocardiography. *J Am Soc Echocardiogr*. 1996;9:736–760.

18. Traversi E, Pozzoli M, Cioffi G, et al. Mitral flow velocity changes after 6 months of optimized therapy provide important hemodynamic and prognostic information in patients with chronic heart failure. *Am Heart J*. 1996;132:809–819.

19. Remme WJ, Swedberg K. Comprehensive guidelines for the diagnosis and treatment of chronic heart failure. Task force for the diagnosis and treatment of chronic heart failure of the European Society of Cardiology. *Eur J Heart Fail*. 2002;4:11–22.

20. Karkos CD, Baguneid MS, Triposkiadis F, et al. Routine measurement of radioisotope left ventricular ejection fraction prior to vascular surgery: is it worthwhile? *Eur J Vasc Endovasc Surg*. 2004;27:227–238.

21. McCullough PA, Nowak RM, McCord J, et al. B-type natriuretic peptide and clinical judgment in emergency diagnosis of heart failure: analysis from Breathing Not Properly (BNP) Multinational Study. *Circulation*. 2002;106:416–422.

22. Maisel AS, McCord J, Nowak RM, et al. Bedside B-Type natriuretic peptide in the emergency diagnosis of heart failure with reduced or preserved ejection fraction. Results from the Breathing Not Properly Multinational Study. *J Am Coll Cardiol*. 2003;41:2010–2017.

23. Feringa HH, Schouten O, Dunkelgrun M, et al. Plasma N-terminal pro-B-type natriuretic peptide as long-term prognostic marker after major vascular surgery. *Heart*. 2007;93:226–231.

24. Dernellis J, Panaretou M. Assessment of cardiac risk before noncardiac surgery: brain natriuretic peptide in 1590 patients. *Heart*. 2006;92:1645–1650.

25. Hunt SA, ACC/AHA Task Force on Practice Guidelines. ACC/AHA 2005 guideline update for the diagnosis and management of chronic heart failure in the adult: a report of the American College of Cardiology/American Heart Association Task Force on Practice Guidelines (writing committee to update the 2001 Guidelines for the Evaluation and Management of Heart Failure). *J Am Coll Cardiol*. 2005;46:e1–82. Available at: http://content.onlinejacc.org/cgi/reprint/46/6/e1.

26. Krum H, Roecker EB, Mohacsi P, et al. Effects of initiating carvedilol in patients with severe chronic heart failure: results from the COPERNICUS Study. *JAMA*. 2003;289:712–718.

27. Taylor AL, Ziesche S, Yancy C, et al. Combination of isosorbide dinitrate and hydralazine in blacks with heart failure. *N Engl J Med*. 2004;351:2049–2057.

28. Didomenico RJ, Park HY, Southworth MR, et al. Guidelines for acute decompensated heart failure treatment. *Ann Pharmacother*. 2004;38:649–660.

29. Sandham JD, Hull RD, Brant RF, et al. A randomized, controlled trial of the use of pulmonary-artery catheters in high-risk surgical patients. *N Engl J Med*. 2003;348:5–14.

30. Connors AF Jr, Speroff T, Dawson NV, et al. The effectiveness of right heart catheterization in the initial care of critically ill patients. SUPPORT Investigators. *JAMA*. 1996;276:889–897.

31. Davies SJ, Wilson RJ. Preoperative optimization of the high-risk surgical patient. *Br J Anaesth*. 2004;93:121–128.

32. Butler J, Emerman C, Peacock WF, et al. The efficacy and safety of B-type natriuretic peptide (nesiritide) in patients with renal insufficiency and acutely decompensated congestive heart failure. *Nephrol Dial Transplant*. 2004;19:391–399.

33. Beaver TM, Winterstein AG, Shuster JJ, et al. Effectiveness of nesiritide on dialysis or all-cause mortality in patients undergoing cardiothoracic surgery. *Clin Cardiol*. 2006;29:18–24.

34. Thompson RC, Liberthson RR, Lowenstein E. Perioperative anesthetic risk of noncardiac surgery in hypertrophic obstructive cardiomyopathy. *JAMA*. 1985;254:2419–2421.

35. Stewart BF, Siscovick D, Lind BK, et al. Clinical factors associated with calcific aortic valve disease. Cardiovascular Health Study. *J Am Coll Cardiol*. 1997;29:630–634.

36. Otto CM, Lind BK, Kitzman DW, et al. Association of aortic-valve sclerosis with cardiovascular mortality and morbidity in the elderly. *N Engl J Med*. 1999;341:142–147.

37. American College of Cardiology/American Heart Association Task Force on Practice Guidelines, Society of Cardiovascular Anesthesiologists, Society for Cardiovascular Angiography and Interventions, et al. ACC/AHA 2006 guidelines for the management of patients with valvular heart disease: a report of the American College of Cardiology/American Heart Association Task Force on Practice Guidelines (writing committee to revise the 1998 Guidelines for the Management of Patients With Valvular Heart Disease): developed in collaboration with the Society of Cardiovascular Anesthesiologists: endorsed by the Society for Cardiovascular Angiography and Interventions and the Society of Thoracic Surgeons. *Circulation*. 2006;114:e84–e231.

38. Dauterman KW, Michaels AD, Ports TA. Is there any indication for aortic valvuloplasty in the elderly? *Am J Geriatric Cardiol*. 2003;12:190–196.

39. Holmes DR Jr, Nishimura RA, Reeder GS. In-hospital mortality after balloon aortic valvuloplasty: frequency and associated factors. *J Am Coll Cardiol*. 1991;17:189–192.

40. Asgar AW, Berry C, Marcheix B, et al. Percutaneous aortic valve replacement with the 18 FR and 21 FR Corevalve revalving system. Society for Cardiovascular Angiography and Interventions 30th Annual Scientific Sessions, May 25, 2007.

41. Bernards CM, Hymas NJ. Progression of first degree heart block to high-grade second degree block during spinal anaesthesia. *Can J Anaesth*. 1992;39:173–175.

42. Kreger BE, Anderson KM, Levy D. QRS interval fails to predict coronary disease incidence. The Framingham Study. *Arch Intern Med*. 1991;15:1365–1368.

43. Eriksson P, Wilhelmsen L, Rosengren A. Bundle-branch block in middle-aged men: risk of complications and death over 28 years. The Primary Prevention Study in Goteborg, Sweden. *Eur Heart J*. 2005;26:2300–2306.

44. Dhingra R, Pencina MJ, Wang TJ, et al. Electrocardiographic QRS duration and the risk of congestive heart failure: the Framingham Heart Study. *Hypertension*. 2006;47:861–867.

45. Fahy GJ, Pinski SL, Miller DP, et al. Natural history of isolated bundle branch block. *Am J Cardiol*. 1996;77:1185–1190.

46. Gauss A, Hubner C, Meierhenrich R, et al. Perioperative transcutaneous pacemaker in patients with chronic bifascicular block or left bundle branch block and additional first-degree atrioventricular block. *Acta Anaesthesiol Scand.* 1999;43:731–736.

47. Fuster V, Ryden LE, Cannom DS, et al. ACC/AHA/ESC 2006 Guidelines for the Management of Patients with Atrial Fibrillation: a report of the American College of Cardiology/American Heart Association Task Force on Practice Guidelines and the European Society of Cardiology Committee for Practice Guidelines (writing committee to revise the 2001 Guidelines for the Management of Patients With Atrial Fibrillation): developed in collaboration with the European Heart Rhythm Association and the Heart Rhythm Society. *Circulation.* 2006;114:e257–e354.

48. Sajadieh A, Nielsen OW, Rasmussen V, et al. Ventricular arrhythmias and risk of death and acute myocardial infarction in apparently healthy subjects of age ≥55 years. *Am J Cardiol.* 2006;97:1351–1357.

49. Buxton AE, Lee KL, Fisher JD, et al. A randomized study of the prevention of sudden death in patients with coronary artery disease. Multicenter Unsustained Tachycardia Trial Investigators. *N Engl J Med.* 1999;341:1882–1890.

50. Bernstein AD, Daubert JC, Fletcher RD, et al. The revised NASPE/BPEG generic code for antibradycardia, adaptive-rate, and multisite pacing. North American Society of Pacing and Electrophysiology/British Pacing and Electrophysiology Group. *Pacing Clin Electrophysiol.* 2002;25:260–264.

51. American Society of Anesthesiologists Task Force on Perioperative Management of Patients with Cardiac Rhythm Management Devices. Practice advisory for the perioperative management of patients with cardiac rhythm management devices: pacemakers and implantable cardioverter-defibrillators: a report by the American Society of Anesthesiologists Task Force on Perioperative Management of Patients with Cardiac Rhythm Management Devices. *Anesthesiology.* 2005;103:186–198.

52. Rozner MA. Review of electrical interference in implanted cardiac devices. *Pacing Clin Electrophysiol.* 2003;26(4 Pt 1):923–925.

53. Lau W, Corcoran SJ, Mond HG. Pacemaker tachycardia in a minute ventilation rate-adaptive pacemaker induced by electrocardiographic monitoring. *Pacing Clin Electrophysiol.* 2006;29:438–440.

54. Levine PA. Response to "rate-adaptive cardiac pacing: implications of environmental noise during craniotomy." *Anesthesiology.* 1997;87:1261.

55. Madsen GM, Andersen C. Pacemaker-induced tachycardia during general anaesthesia: a case report. *Br J Anaesth.* 1989;63:360–361.

56. Preisman S, Cheng DC. Life-threatening ventricular dysrhythmias with inadvertent asynchronous temporary pacing after cardiac surgery. *Anesthesiology.* 1999;91:880–883.

57. Rasmussen MJ, Friedman PA, Hammill SC, et al. Unintentional deactivation of implantable cardioverter-defibrillators in health care settings. *Mayo Clin Proc.* 2002;77:855–859.

58. Guidant. Urgent medical device safety information and corrective action (Contak Renewal [3,4,RF] ICD [magnet switch]).

June 23, 2005. Available at: http://www.guidant.com/physician_communications/RENEWAL3_RENEWAL4.pdf. Accessed January 1, 2007.

59. Varma N, Cunningham D, Falk R. Central venous access resulting in selective failure of ICD defibrillation capacity. *Pacing Clin Electrophysiol*. 2001;24:394–395.

60. Criqui MH, Fronek A, Barrett-Connor E, et al. The prevalence of peripheral arterial disease in a defined population. *Circulation*. 1985;71:510–515.

61. Ness J, Aronow WS. Prevalence of coexistence of coronary artery disease, ischemic stroke, and peripheral arterial disease in older persons, mean age 80 years, in an academic hospital-based geriatrics practice. *J Am Geriatr Soc*. 1999;47:1255–1256.

62. Wallace AW, Galindez D, Salahieh A, et al. Effect of clonidine on cardiovascular morbidity and mortality after noncardiac surgery. *Anesthesiology*. 2004;101:284–293.

63. Hirsch AT, Haskal ZJ, Hertzer NR, et al. ACC/AHA 2005 guidelines for the management of patients with peripheral arterial disease (lower extremity, renal, mesenteric, and abdominal aortic): executive summary. A collaborative report from the American Association for Vascular Surgery/Society for Vascular Surgery, Society for Cardiovascular Angiography and Interventions, Society for Vascular Medicine and Biology, Society of Interventional Radiology, and the ACC/AHA Task Force on Practice Guidelines (writing committee to develop Guidelines for the Management of Patients With Peripheral Arterial Disease) endorsed by the American Association of Cardiovascular and Pulmonary Rehabilitation; National Heart, Lung, and Blood Institute; Society for Vascular Nursing; TransAtlantic Inter-Society Consensus; and Vascular Disease Foundation. *J Am Coll Cardiol*. 2006;47:1239–1312. Available at: http://www.acc.org/qualityandscience/clinical/guidelines/pad/index.pdf.

64. Mendelson G, Aronow WS, Ahn C. Prevalence of coronary artery disease, atherothrombotic brain infarction, and peripheral arterial disease: associated risk factors in older Hispanics in an academic hospital-based geriatrics practice. *J Am Geriatr Soc*. 1998;46:481–483.

65. Boersma E, Poldermans D, Bax JJ, et al. Predictors of cardiac events after major vascular surgery: role of clinical characteristics, dobutamine echocardiography, and beta-blocker therapy. *JAMA*. 2001;285:1865–1873.

66. McFalls EO, Ward HB, Moritz TE, et al. Coronary-artery revascularization before elective major vascular surgery. *N Engl J Med*. 2004;351:2795–2804.

67. Poldermans D, Schouten O, Vidakovic R, et al. A clinical randomized trial to evaluate the safety of a noninvasive approach in high-risk patients undergoing major vascular surgery: the DECREASE-V Pilot Study. *J Am Coll Cardiol*. 2007;49:1763–1769.

68. Grines CL, Bonow RO, Casey DE Jr, et al. Prevention of premature discontinuation of dual antiplatelet therapy in patients with coronary artery stents: a science advisory from the American Heart Association, American College of Cardiology, Society for Cardiovascular Angiography and Interventions, American

College of Surgeons, and American Dental Association, with representation from the American College of Physicians. *J Am Coll Cardiol.* 2007;49:734–739.

69. Mackey AE, Abrahamowicz M, Langlois Y, et al. Outcome of asymptomatic patients with carotid disease. Asymptomatic Cervical Bruit Study Group. *Neurology.* 1997;48:896–903.

70. Naylor AR, Mehta Z, Rothwell PM, et al. Carotid artery disease and stroke during coronary artery bypass: a critical review of the literature. *Eur J Vasc Endovasc Surg.* 2002;23:283–294.

71. Endarterectomy for asymptomatic carotid artery stenosis. Executive Committee for the Asymptomatic Carotid Atherosclerosis Study. *JAMA.* 1995;273:1421–1428.

72. Chaturvedi S, Bruno A, Feasby T, et al. Carotid endarterectomy—an evidence-based review: report of the Therapeutics and Technology Assessment Subcommittee of the American Academy of Neurology. *Neurology.* 2005;65:794–801.

73. Beneficial effect of carotid endarterectomy in symptomatic patients with high-grade carotid stenosis. North American Symptomatic Carotid Endarterectomy Trial Collaborators. *N Engl J Med.* 1991;325:445–453.

74. Gregoretti S. Intraoperative hypotension in a patient treated with terazosin, a new alpha-adrenergic receptor antagonist. *J Clin Anesth.* 1994;6:170–171.

75. Lydiatt CA, Fee MP, Hill GE. Severe hypotension during epidural anesthesia in a prazosin-treated patient. *Anesth Analg.* 1993; 76:1152–1153.

76. Eisen N, Reich DL. The patient with valvular heart disease. *Probl Anesth.* 1997;9:157.

Pulmonary Diseases

Evans R. Fernández Pérez, Ognjen Gajic,
Juraj Sprung, and David O. Warner

The aim of this chapter is to provide a framework for the preoperative evaluation of patients with lung diseases. Anesthesiologists should know when to request a consult for these patients and whether the ordering of expensive tests is irrelevant or unnecessary. This chapter first outlines the pertinent history, physical findings, diagnostic testing algorithms, and management of patients with common lung diseases, including asthma, cystic fibrosis (CF), and chronic obstructive pulmonary disease (COPD). We also discuss methods for evaluating patients with dyspnea or a history of tobacco use. We consider how to optimize medical management (when to use corticosteroids or intensify bronchodilator regimens) and how to identify high-risk surgical patients. A brief discussion of lung volume reduction surgery and lung transplantation is also included.

ASTHMA

Asthma is a chronic inflammatory airway disease produced by cellular and chemical mediators. The underlying cause of airway inflammation is unknown. Its consequences include bronchial smooth muscle hypertrophy and hyperplasia, microvascular leakage leading to bronchial wall edema, increased mucus production, and activation of airway neurons. In asthmatics the bronchi become hyperresponsive to a variety of stimuli and the airway wall is remodeled. The hallmark of asthma is airway obstruction characterized by wheezing, shortness of breath, chest tightness, and cough. In most severe cases air entry is diminished ("silent chest") and pulsus paradoxus is prominent. These symptoms are usually associated with widespread and variable airflow limitation that is partially reversible either spontaneously or with treatment. Bronchoconstriction can be precipitated by unknown triggers or allergen exposure; irritants such as fumes or cigarette smoke; viral infection; medications; and instrumentation of the larynx, trachea, and airways (1,2). Not all patients who wheeze have asthma and not all patients who have asthma wheeze. The differential diagnoses include COPD, vocal cord dysfunction, respiratory irritants from gastroesophageal reflux disease (GERD), congestive heart failure (CHF; "cardiac asthma"), allergic bronchopulmonary aspergillosis, drug-induced bronchospasm, cystic fibrosis, bronchiolitis obliterans, hypersensitivity pneumonitis, airway obstruction, and α_1-antitrypsin deficiency. Spirometry is the initial preferred diagnostic tool. A normal spirometry, however, does not exclude asthma. Patients with suspected asthma and normal spirometry can benefit from an inhalational challenge with methacholine or by response to asthma therapy. The National Asthma Education and Prevention Program (1) has

Table 5.1. Asthma classifications by severity

Classification	Symptoms	Lung Function
Step 1: Mild intermittent	• Daytime two or fewer times per week • Nighttime two or fewer times per month • Brief exacerbations • Asymptomatic between exacerbations • Intensity of exacerbations varies	• PEF variability <20% • FEV_1 ≥80% • PEF ≥80%
Step 2: Mild persistent	• Daytime more than two times per week but less than one time per day • Nighttime more than two times per month • Exacerbations may affect activity	• PEF variability 20%–30% • FEV_1 ≥80% • PEF ≥80%
Step 3: Moderate persistent	• Daytime symptoms daily • Nighttime symptoms more than one time per week • Exacerbations affect activity • Exacerbations two or more times per week • Exacerbations last days • Daily use of inhaled short-acting β_2-agonists	• PEF variability >30% • FEV_1 >60% but <80% • PEF >60% but <80%
Step 4: Severe persistent	• Daytime symptoms continual • Nighttime symptoms frequent • Symptoms limit physical activity • Exacerbations frequent	• PEF variability >30% • FEV_1 ≤60% • PEF ≤60%

FEV_1, forced expiratory volume in 1 second; PEF, peak expiratory flow.
Adapted from the National Asthma Education and Prevention Program. *NIH*. 1997;97–4051.

classified asthma into four levels of severity to guide therapy (Tables 5.1 and 5.2). The classification is based on both the severity and frequency of symptoms.

CHRONIC OBSTRUCTIVE PULMONARY DISEASE

COPD is characterized by chronic airflow limitation that is not fully reversible. Airflow limitation is usually progressive and associated with lung inflammation. It can be caused by noxious particles or gases from cigarette smoke or occupations (e.g., coal miners, grain handlers, and cement or cotton workers), environmental pollutants, and host factors (e.g., genetic causes such as α_1-antitrypsin deficiency; childhood illnesses such as low birth

Table 5.2. Asthma management according to level of severity

Quick relief for all patients	Bronchodilator as needed for symptoms. Intensity of treatment will depend upon severity of exacerbation.
	– Preferred treatment: Short-acting inhaled β_2-agonists by nebulizer or face mask and space/holding chamber
	– Alternative treatment: Oral β_2-agonist
	With viral respiratory infection
	– Bronchodilator every 4–6 hours up to 24 hours; in general, repeat no more than once every 6 weeks
	– Consider systemic corticosteroid if exacerbation is severe or patient has history of previous severe exacerbations
	Use of short-acting β_2-agonists more than two times a week in intermittent asthma (daily, or increasing use in persistent asthma) may indicate the need to initiate (increase) long-term-control therapy.
Mild intermittent	No daily medication needed
Mild persistent	Preferred treatment:
	– Low-dose inhaled corticosteroid (with nebulizer, MDI with holding chamber or with face mask)
	Alternative treatment:
	– Cromolyn (nebulizer is preferred or MDI with holding chamber)
	OR
	– Leukotriene receptor antagonist

Moderate persistent

Preferred treatment:
– Low-dose inhaled corticosteroids and long-acting inhaled β_2-agonists

OR

– Medium-dose inhaled corticosteroids

Alternative treatment:
– Low-dose inhaled corticosteroids and either leukotriene receptor antagonist or theophylline

If needed (particularly in patients with recurring severe exacerbations):

Preferred treatment:
– Medium-dose inhaled corticosteroids and long-acting inhaled β_2-agonists

Alternative treatment:
– Medium-dose inhaled corticosteroids and either leukotriene receptor antagonist or theophylline

Severe persistent

Preferred treatment:
– High-dose inhaled corticosteroids

AND

– Long-acting inhaled β_2-agonists

AND, if needed,

– Corticosteroid tablets or syrup long term (2 mg/kg/day, generally do not exceed 60 mg/day). Try to reduce systemic corticosteroids and maintain control with high-dose inhaled corticosteroids.

MDI, metered dose inhaler.
Reproduced from National Asthma Education and Prevention Program. Expert panel report: Guidelines for the Diagnosis and Management of Asthma Update on Selected Topics—2002. *J Allergy Clin Immunol.* 2002;110(5 Suppl):S141–219.

weight, respiratory infections, and childhood asthma). Inflammation eventually alters lung parenchyma and pulmonary vasculature (3).

COPD includes chronic bronchitis and emphysema. Differential diagnoses include asthma, CHF, bronchiectasis, tuberculosis, obliterative bronchiolitis, and diffuse panbronchiolitis (4).

Emphysema is defined by the American Thoracic Society and European Respiratory Society (ATS/ERS) as "a condition of the lung characterized by abnormal permanent enlargement of the airspaces distal to terminal bronchioles, accompanied by destruction of their walls, and without obvious fibrosis" (3). The destruction is defined as "non-uniformity in the pattern of respiratory airspace enlargement so that the orderly appearance of the acinus and its components is disturbed and may be lost." The pathogenesis of emphysema in smokers is not well known and may be the result of inherited or acquired proteolytic activity against extracellular matrix proteins in the lungs. Damage to elastic fibers leads to alveolar wall enlargement, and septal destruction appears to be the critical event (5). Diffusing lung capacity measured with carbon monoxide (DL_{CO}) decreases and lung parenchymal density appears reduced on chest radiography or computed tomography (CT).

Three main morphologic patterns of emphysema are recognized: (a) proximal acinar emphysema that involves the upper lung zones (centrilobular emphysema, typical of COPD, and dust-related emphysema such as coal worker pneumoconiosis); (b) panacinar emphysema that commonly involves the lower lung zones (e.g., α_1-antitrypsin deficiency); and (c) distal acinar or paraseptal emphysema, the least common form, as an isolated lesion or in combination with other forms.

Chronic bronchitis is bronchitis that is experienced on most days for at least 3 months of a year for at least 2 successive years or recurrent excessive bronchial mucus secretion (not attributed to other diseases such as bronchiectasis) that severely impairs expiratory flow rates (3). In chronic bronchitis, the mucous glands enlarge from hyperplasia and hypertrophy of cells as well as airway inflammation (5).

Clinical Aspects

The patient with COPD usually experiences dyspnea, chronic cough, wheezing, and sputum production that worsens after a viral respiratory infection (1). Diaphragmatic excursion and dynamic hyperinflation decrease and the anterior-posterior chest diameter increases, limiting exercise. Advanced disease may produce signs of hypoxia (polycythemia, cyanosis, clubbing), hypercarbia (asterixis), and wasting. Table 5.3 summarizes the stages and medical management of COPD as defined by the National Heart Lung and Blood Institute/World Health Organization global initiative (4). Pulmonary symptoms may vary considerably in a given patient over time. While there is no universally accepted definition for the acute exacerbation of COPD, the ATS and ERS guidelines define an exacerbation as an increase in the patient's daily symptoms of dyspnea, cough, or sputum beyond normal day-to-day variability and severe enough to require a change in management.

Table 5.3 Stages and therapy at each stage of chronic obstructive pulmonary disease

New	0: At Risk	I: Mild	II: Moderate	III: Severe	IV: Very Severe
Characteristics	• Chronic symptoms • Exposure to risk factors • Normal spirometry	• FEV_1/FVC <70% • FEV_1 ≥80% • With or without symptoms	• FEV_1/FVC <70% • 50% ≤FEV_1 <80% • With or without symptoms	• FEV_1/FVC <70% • 30% ≤FEV_1 <50% • With or without symptoms	• FEV_1/FVC <70% • FEV_1 <30% or FEV_1 <50% predicted plus chronic respiratory failure
	Avoidance of risk factor(s); influenza vaccination				
		Add short-acting bronchodilator when needed			
			Add regular treatment with one or more long-acting bronchodilators *Add* rehabilitation		
				Add inhaled glucocorticosteroids if repeated exacerbations	
					Add long-term oxygen if chronic respiratory failure *Consider* surgical treatments

FEV_1, forced expiratory volume in 1 second; FVC, forced vital capacity.
Classification based on postbronchodilator response. Respiratory failure is defined as arterial partial pressure of oxygen <60 mm Hg with or without arterial partial pressure of CO_2 >50 mm Hg while breathing air at sea level.
Reproduced from Fabbri L, Pauwels RA, Hurd SS. Global strategy for the diagnosis, management, and prevention of chronic obstructive pulmonary disease: GOLD executive summary updated 2003. *COPD.* 2004;1:105–141.

Spirometry is the primary diagnostic tool, with findings typically including a reduced forced expiratory volume in 1 second (FEV_1) and normal to increased lung capacity. Spirometry, however, does not provide a complete assessment of disease severity. For example, in a cohort study, the body mass index, airflow obstruction (predicted FEV_1), dyspnea (score on the Modified Medical Research Council dyspnea scale; Table 5.4), and 6-minute walk distance for exercise tolerance were combined in a multidimensional 10-point scale on which higher scores indicated a higher risk of death. This index better predicted all-cause and respiratory mortality in patients with COPD compared with the FEV_1 alone, which itself had little predictive value (6).

Surgical Treatment of Chronic Obstructive Pulmonary Disorder

Lung volume reduction surgery (LVRS) and lung transplantation are two surgical options for patients with advanced COPD. LVRS may be useful as a primary therapy for patients with COPD or a bridge to lung transplantation. The National Emphysema Therapy Trial, a multicenter randomized controlled clinical trial

Table 5.4 Modified dyspnea scale of the Medical Research Council

Grade	Description
1	Not troubled by breathlessness except with strenuous exercise
2	Troubled by shortness of breath when hurrying on the level or walking up a slight hill
3	Walks slower than people of the same age on the level because of breathlessness or has to stop for breath when walking at own pace on the level
4	Stops for breath after walking approximately 100 yards or after a few minutes on the level
5	Too breathless to leave the house or breathless when dressing or undressing

Reproduced from Mahler DA, Weinberg DH, Wells CK, et al. The measurement of dyspnea: Contents, interobserver agreement, and physiologic correlates of two new clinical indexes. *Chest.* 1984;85:751–758.

comparing medical therapy versus medical therapy plus LVRS, showed that a subset of patients with upper lobe–predominant emphysema and low maximal workload after rehabilitation had lower mortality and better exercise capacity and health status compared to that achieved by intense medical management (7). At the same time, the study showed that patients with an FEV_1 <20% of predicted value and either homogenously distributed emphysema or severely impaired gas exchange should not undergo surgery (7). LVRS enhances ventilatory function by improving vital capacity (increasing lung compliance, decreasing chest wall elastic recoil, enhancing diaphragmatic function) and ventilation-perfusion matching (8).

Lung transplantation is a treatment, not a cure, for a variety of end-stage lung diseases. COPD is the most common indication for lung transplantation (United Network for Organ Sharing online database; www.unos.org). In selected patients with advanced COPD and limited life expectancy, lung transplantation improves pulmonary function, exercise capacity, and quality of life. As the number of transplants continues to increase and survival improves, patients with complications related to the transplanted lung(s) as well as lung transplant patients with unrelated disorders undergo procedures more frequently (9). The 1-, 5- and 10-year survival in patients with emphysema after lung transplant is approximately 80%, 50%, and 35%, respectively (10).

POST LUNG TRANSPLANT PATIENT

Risk assessment and strategies to reduce perioperative pulmonary complications of post lung transplant patients should focus on graft function, risk of infection, and adverse effects of immunosuppression (Table 5.5) (11). The time, type (e.g., single or double lung), and indication for the transplant and the type and level of immunosuppression are determined. A pulmonologist

Table 5.5   Side effects of immunosuppressives with a direct impact on anesthetic and perioperative management

	CyA	Tacr	Aza	Ster	MMF	ATG	OKT3
Anemia	−	−	+	−	+	−	−
Leucopenia	−	−	+	−	+	+	+
Thrombocytopenia	−	−	+	−	+	−	−
Hypertension	++	+	−	+	−	−	−
Diabetes	+	++	−	++	−	−	−
Neurotoxicity	+	+	−	+	−	−	−
Renal insufficiency	+	++	−	−	−	−	−
Anaphylaxis	−	−	−	−	−	+	+
Fever	−	−	−	−	−	+	+

ATG = anti-thymocyte globuin, Aza = azathioprine, CyA = cyclosporine A, MMF = mycophenolate mofetil, OKT3 = monoclonal antibodies directed against CD-3 antigen of the surface of human T-lymphocytes, Ster = steroids, Tacr = tacrolimus (FK506).
Reproduced from Kostopanagiotou G, Smyrniotis V, Arkadopoulos N, et al. Anesthetic and perioperative management of adult transplant recipients in nontransplant surgery. *Anesth Analg.* 1999;89:613–622.

specializing in transplantation should be consulted. A complete blood count (CBC) to monitor leukocyte and platelet levels and a creatinine level are needed if patients are taking cyclosporine or tacrolimus. If a patient has respiratory symptoms (e.g., dyspnea), a chest radiograph and spirometry are indicated. Routine surveillance bronchoscopy to detect asymptomatic rejection or infection and pulmonary function tests (PFTs) to detect graft complications are often recommended.

CYSTIC FIBROSIS

CF is an autosomal recessive, chronic, progressive, multisystem disease. The incidence varies widely among ethnic groups. According to the American Lung Association, approximately 30,000 Americans have CF and approximately 1,000 new cases are diagnosed each year. CF is the most common lethal hereditary genetic disease in Caucasians. It is caused by abnormalities in a membrane chloride channel protein (encoded by the CF transmembrane conductance regulator gene) that alters chloride transport and water flux across the apical surface of epithelial cells. More than 1,000 mutations have been identified.

The diagnosis is established by the finding of elevated sweat chloride concentration (>60 mEq/L) plus at least one of the following: Chronic airway disease (typically bronchiolitis with airway obstruction and/or bronchiectasis), exocrine pancreatic insufficiency (most frequent extrapulmonary manifestation), or a history of CF diagnosed in a parent, sibling, or first cousin. The most common clinical manifestations and treatment options are outlined in Table 5.6.

Table 5.6 Clinical manifestations and management of patients with cystic fibrosis

Involved Systems	Management
Respiratory • Bronchiectasis • Sinusitis • Reactive airway disease • Hemoptysis • Allergic bronchopulmonary aspergillosis • Recurrent pneumonia • Pneumothorax	• Airway clearance (e.g., chest physiotherapy) • Inhaled and systemic antimicrobials • Inhaled and systemic steroids • Mucolytic agents (e.g., DNA-se) • Bronchodilators • Bronchial artery embolization • Lung transplant
Gastrointestinal • Meconium ileus • Small bowel obstruction • Rectal prolapse	• Osmotic enteral solutions • Hydration • Surgical correction
Endocrine • Diabetes mellitus • Pancreatitis • Fat and fat-soluble vitamin malabsorption	• Insulin administration • Bisphosphonates • Pancreatic enzyme replacement • Vitamin supplementation • Nutritional support
Hepatobiliary • Biliary cirrhosis • Portal hypertension • Cholelithiasis	• Ursodeoxycholic acid • Available therapies for portal hypertension and the complications of liver cirrhosis
Genitourinary • Obstructive azoospermia (bilateral absence of the vas deferens)	• Artificial insemination and genetic counseling

RESTRICTIVE LUNG DISEASE

Restrictive lung disorders are characterized by a reduction in total lung capacity (TLC). The FEV_1 and forced vital capacity (FVC) are reduced proportionally and the FEV_1:FVC ratio is usually normal or increased.

The etiology of restrictive lung disease may be pulmonary or extrapulmonary. Pulmonary causes include, but are not limited to, idiopathic interstitial pneumonia, secondary interstitial lung disease (e.g., connective tissue or drug induced), lung resection, atelectasis, pneumonia, and advanced pneumoconiosis. The interstitial diseases comprise a large part of this category and are characterized by fibrosis, inflammation, or both. Extrapulmonary restrictive disorders are divided into those involving the chest wall (e.g., kyphoscoliosis, ankylosing spondylitis, pregnancy), the respiratory muscles (e.g., diaphragmatic paralysis, myasthenia gravis, polymyositis), or the pleural cavity (e.g., pleural effusion, pneumothorax, fibrothorax, cardiomegaly).

If maximum voluntary ventilation is reduced, the cause may be neuromuscular weakness, or poor cooperation or coordination during testing. The preoperative management assesses muscle strength, with particular attention to respiratory function. The maximum inspiratory and expiratory pressures are sensitive but not specific in detecting neuromuscular weakness. Appropriate medical therapy for the patient's restrictive lung disease prior to an elective procedure is essential. Consultation with a pulmonary specialist is recommended.

DYSPNEA

Dyspnea is the most common symptom in patients with cardiopulmonary disease. A consensus statement of the ATS defined dyspnea as the "subjective experience of breathing discomfort that consists of qualitatively distinct sensations that vary in intensity" (12). The experience derives from interactions among multiple physiologic, psychological, social, and environmental factors and may induce secondary physiologic and behavioral responses (12). Dyspnea is associated with conditions in which the respiratory drive is increased or the respiratory system is subject to an increased mechanical load.

The sensation of dyspnea seems to originate with the activation of sensory systems involved with respiration. Sensory information is, in turn, relayed to higher brain centers where central processing of respiratory-related signals and contextual, cognitive, and behavioral influences shape the ultimate expression of the evoked sensation (12). Dyspnea is a complex symptom and cannot be linked conclusively with a specific pathophysiologic mechanism. Possible mechanisms of dyspnea in selected conditions are outlined in Figure 5.1.

The assessment of dyspnea is a critical part of the preoperative evaluation. The evaluation method tries to standardize symptoms by history and physical examination and by initial and subsequent diagnostic testing (Fig. 5.1).

History and Physical Examination

Dyspnea is either acute or chronic. The most common causes of acute dyspnea are COPD, asthma, and CHF. Two thirds of patients with chronic dyspnea (longer than 1 month) have asthma, COPD, interstitial lung diseases, and/or cardiomyopathy (13). Dyspnea may be intermittent (e.g., asthma), recurrent (e.g., CHF), or persistent (e.g., patients with COPD and/or interstitial lung disease) and may be influenced by position. Dyspnea when the patient is in the right or left lateral decubitus position is called trepopnea. It may signify unilateral lung disease, such as pleural effusion or obstruction of the proximal tracheobronchial tree. When the patient lies with the affected lung down, gravitational forces increase perfusion of a dependent lung that cannot ventilate well. Orthopnea, or dyspnea on recumbency, typically occurs at night in patients with left ventricular (LV) dysfunction, obstructive sleep apnea (OSA), GERD, or asthma. Platypnea is dyspnea that worsens in the upright position. It is called platypnea-orthodeoxia, when arterial oxygen desaturation is caused by right to left intracardiac shunts (14), intrapulmonary shunts (15), liver disease (16), or pulmonary resection (17).

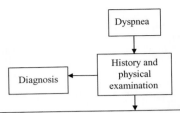

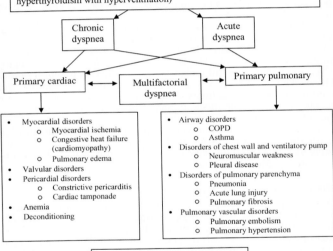

Dyspnea

History and physical examination

Diagnosis

Initial diagnostic tests*

Suspected cardiac etiology: Chest radiograph (e.g., pulmonary edema, cardiomegaly), ECG (arrhythmias, MI), echocardiogram (e.g. evaluation of ventricular function in heart failure), BNP (e.g., >400 pg/mL in CHF)

Suspected pulmonary etiology: Chest radiograph (e.g., pneumonia, pneumothorax), ABG (e.g., hypoxemic/hypercarbic respiratory failure), spirometry (e.g., reduced expiratory flows in COPD/asthma)

Multifactorial/miscellaneous etiology: CBC (e.g., anemia), creatinine (e.g., renal failure), electrolytes (e.g., hyponatremia in hypervolemia), TFTs (e.g., hyperthyroidism with hyperventilation)

Chronic dyspnea

Acute dyspnea

Primary cardiac

Multifactorial dyspnea

Primary pulmonary

- Myocardial disorders
  - Myocardial ischemia
  - Congestive heat failure (cardiomyopathy)
  - Pulmonary edema
- Valvular disorders
- Pericardial disorders
  - Constrictive pericarditis
  - Cardiac tamponade
- Anemia
- Deconditioning

- Airway disorders
  - COPD
  - Asthma
- Disorders of chest wall and ventilatory pump
  - Neuromuscular weakness
  - Pleural disease
- Disorders of pulmonary parenchyma
  - Pneumonia
  - Acute lung injury
  - Pulmonary fibrosis
- Pulmonary vascular disorders
  - Pulmonary embolism
  - Pulmonary hypertension

Unrevealing cause of dyspnea: consider cardiopulmonary exercise testing (Fig. 5.2)

*After a history and examination are obtained, diagnostic tests are based on pretest disease probability or likelihood that a patient has a given condition. The sensitivity and specificity of the test and the prevalence of disease in the population are important. In addition, clinical guidelines (e.g., clinical prediction rules) can guide the clinician.

Patients with various cardiopulmonary diseases use different words or phrases to describe their sensation of dyspnea (18,19). A detailed medical history should list precipitating factors, severity (Table 5.4), timing, positional factors, and associated features. Physical findings associated with dyspnea may provide diagnostic clues: Distended jugular veins (heart failure), carotid bruits (coronary artery disease), cyanosis (hypoxemia), tachypnea (rapid shallow breathing in a patient with neuromuscular disease), pulsus paradoxus (in a patient with acute severe COPD and/or asthma exacerbation), increased pulmonic component of the second heart sound (pulmonary hypertension), displacement of the maximal cardiac impulse toward the xiphoid process (ventricular hypertrophy in a patient with heart failure), or hyperresonance to percussion, prolonged expiration, and wheezing (COPD or asthma).

Diagnostic Testing

After the history and physical examination are complete, specific preoperative diagnostic testing in patients with dyspnea should be tailored according to cardiac risk factors and/or underlying respiratory diseases. For example, if the cause of dyspnea seems to be cardiovascular, noninvasive cardiac testing (electrocardiogram [ECG], transthoracic echocardiogram, stress testing) and even coronary angiography may be warranted before surgery. Natriuretic peptide levels have proved valuable in the initial differentiation of acute dyspnea caused by CHF from noncardiogenic causes. The N-terminal fragment (NT-proBNP) at cut points of >450 pg/mL for patients <50 years of age and >900 pg/mL for patients ≥50 years of age is highly sensitive and specific for the diagnosis of acute CHF (20). An NT-proBNP level <300 pg/mL has a negative predictive value of 99% for ruling out acute CHF (20). A chest radiograph is important in the initial evaluation of patients with dyspnea, but the absence of abnormal findings does not rule out significant cardiopulmonary disease. PFTs and CT of the chest may provide evidence of emphysema or diffuse interstitial lung disease not otherwise seen on chest films.

CBC, thyroid function testing, and ventilation/perfusion (V/Q) scanning or CT angiogram are useful to identify conditions that can contribute to dyspnea such as anemia, hyperthyroidism, and pulmonary thromboembolism, respectively. For patients with unexplained dyspnea and for whom initial test results are nondiagnostic, cardiopulmonary exercise testing (CPET) is a useful tool for differentiating among cardiac or pulmonary from other causes such as neuromuscular disorders, hematopoietic disorders,

←

Figure 5.1. Algorithm for dyspnea. Only some initial tests are described in the algorithm. Parallel testing (e.g., multiple tests at once) increases sensitivity (i.e., disease is less likely to be missed; desirable in life-threatening situations). Serial testing increases specificity (e.g., evaluating a patient with stable chronic dyspnea). ABG, arterial blood gases; BNP, Brain natriuretic peptide; CBC, complete blood count; CHF, congestive heart failure; COPD, chronic obstructive pulmonary disease; ECG, electrocardiogram; MI, myocardial ischemia; TFTs: thyroid function tests.

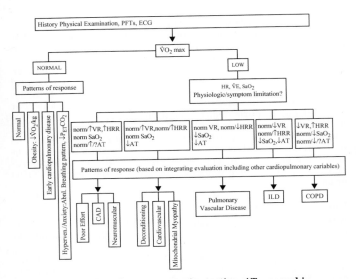

Figure 5.2. Cardiopulmonary exercise testing. AT, anaerobic threshold; CAD, coronary artery disease; COPD, chronic obstructive pulmonary disease; ECG, electrocardiogram; HR, heart rate; HRR, heart rate reserve; ILD, interstitial lung disease; $P_{ET}CO_2$, expired carbon dioxide; PFTs, pulmonary function tests; SaO_2, arterial oxygen saturation; $\dot{V}E$, ventilation; $\dot{V}O_2$, oxygen consumption; $\dot{V}O_2$ max, maximum oxygen consumption; VR, ventilatory reserve. Reproduced from ATS/ACCP statement on cardiopulmonary exercise testing. *Am J Respir Crit Care Med.* **2003;167(2):211–277.**

psychological factors (e.g., anxiety syndromes), or deconditioning (e.g., obesity) (21). According to the ATS/ERS, "the CPET provides a global assessment of the integrative exercise responses which are not adequately reflected through the measurement of individual organ system function. This relatively noninvasive, dynamic physiologic testing permits the evaluation of both submaximal and peak exercise responses, provides the physician with relevant information for clinical decision making" (21). Results from CPET may direct subsequent diagnostic testing to target the suspected organ system or help in limiting further testing (Fig. 5.2) (21).

SMOKING

Smoking leads to mucous gland enlargement and goblet cell hyperplasia, hypersecretion of mucus, disruption of mucociliary clearance, and impairment of local lung defenses (e.g., antiproteases), and can contribute to an increased risk for bacterial infection, small airway inflammation and remodeling, and bronchial reactivity (22). The FEV_1 normally declines by approximately 25 to 30 mL/year in nonsmokers, but this decline is accelerated in smokers and might be as high as 100 mL/year in those with COPD who continue to smoke (23–25). Smoking cessation does not dramatically improve the FEV_1 but rather slows the further decline rate to near that of nonsmokers (26). Patients who smoke are at risk for both pulmonary and nonpulmonary perioperative complications (22,27,28). Abstinence from smoking reduces risk; it appears that several weeks of abstinence is necessary for maximal benefit, parallel to the time required for improvements in pulmonary function (29–32). There is no firm evidence to support earlier conclusions that brief abstinence actually increases the rate of pulmonary complications (28,33). Nonetheless, the longer the duration of preoperative abstinence is, the better. At least 8 weeks of abstinence is required for maximal benefit, consistent with the time needed for the lung to recover from chronic smoke exposure (22,28).

PREOPERATIVE RISK ASSESSMENT FOR POSTOPERATIVE PULMONARY COMPLICATIONS

Postoperative pulmonary complications, which are defined rather broadly and inconsistently in the literature, depend on the type and extent of surgery and patient preoperative function and comorbidities (e.g., CHF). Common complications are atelectasis, retention of tracheobronchial secretions, pneumonia, hypoxemia, pulmonary embolism, respiratory failure with prolonged requirement for mechanical ventilation, and postoperative acute lung injury. Pulmonary complications have been reported in 5% to 10% of the general surgical population and in up to 22% of preoperatively identified high-risk patients (34–36).

As more and more patients with pre-existing pulmonary conditions or other risk factors undergo surgery, pulmonary complications will continue to be an important perioperative consideration. Through medical history, physical examination, and selected diagnostic tests, perioperative pulmonary risk can be assessed accurately to guide treatment and to reduce postoperative risk. A recently validated multifactorial risk index model for identifying patients at risk for developing postoperative respiratory failure may be a useful tool for guiding perioperative respiratory care (36a).

Both pulmonary and nonpulmonary (37) factors add to the risks of anesthesia and surgery. Age, obesity, smoking history, type and anatomic location of the anticipated surgical procedure, type and duration of surgery, and coexisting disease (pulmonary and nonpulmonary) can influence perioperative risks (1,27,34,38). Table 5.7 summarizes the strength of the evidence for the association of patient, procedure, and laboratory test results with postoperative pulmonary complications (39).

Age

Age is an independent risk factor for perioperative pulmonary complications, especially for patients >65 years (39,40). For patients 70 years of age or older, the unadjusted postoperative pulmonary complication estimates range from 4% to 45%, with a median rate of 15% (39). Risk increases with the higher prevalence of coexisting nonpulmonary diseases (37) and the effects of aging on the respiratory system: Loss of elastic lung recoil, greater prevalence of functional airway closure, gradual decrease of the maximal expiratory flow, and impaired protective airway reflexes (27). Age alone, however, is not a contraindication to surgery. Other considerations are functional status and comorbid conditions.

Table 5.7　Summary strength of the evidence for the association of patient, procedure, and laboratory factors with postoperative pulmonary complications

Factor	Strength of Recommendation[a]	Odds Ratio
Potential patient-related risk factor		
Advanced age	A	2.09–3.04
ASA class ≥II	A	2.55–4.87
CHF	A	2.93
Functionally dependent	A	1.65–2.51
CORD	A	1.79
Weight loss	B	1.62
Impaired sensorium	B	1.39
Cigarette use	B	1.26
Alcohol use	B	1.21
Abnormal findings on chest examination	B	NA
Diabetes	C	
Obesity	D	
Asthma	D	
Obstructive sleep apnea	I	
Corticosteroid use	I	
HIV Infection	I	
Arrhythmia	I	
Poor exercise capacity	I	
Potential procedure-related risk factor		
Aortic aneurysm repair	A	6.90
Thoracic surgery	A	4.24
Abdominal surgery	A	3.01
Upper abdominal surgery	A	2.91
Neurosurgery	A	2.53
Prolonged surgery	A	2.26
Head and neck surgery	A	2.21
Emergency surgery	A	2.21
Vascular surgery	A	2.10
General anesthesia	A	1.83
Perioperative transfusion	B	1.47
Hip surgery	D	
Gynecologic or urologic surgery	D	
Esophageal surgery	I	
Laboratory tests		
Albumin level <35 g/L	A	2.53
Chest radiography	B	4.81
BUN level >7.5 mmol/L (>21 mg/dL)	B	Na
Spirometry	I	

ASA, American Society of Anesthesiologists; BUN, blood urea nitrogen; CHF, congestive heart failure; COPD, chronic obstructive pulmonary disease; NA, not available.
[a] Strength of recommendations: A, good evidence to support the particular risk; B, at least fair evidence to support the particular risk; C, at least fair evidence to suggest that the particular factor is not a risk factor; D, good evidence to suggest that the particular factor is not a risk; I, insufficient evidence to determine whether the factor increases risk, and evidence is lacking, is of poor quality, or is conflicting. Reproduced from Smetana GW, Lawrence VA, Cornell JE, American College of Physicians. Preoperative pulmonary risk stratification for noncardiothoracic surgery: systematic review for the American College of Physicians. *Ann Intern Med.* 2006;144:581–595.

Obesity

Obesity has been associated with restrictive pulmonary physiology and decreased expiratory reserve volume and functional residual capacity (e.g., loss of lung volume from atelectasis). Tidal breathing below closing volume, especially when the patient is supine, may lead to intrapulmonary shunting and hypoxemia. Nonetheless, most studies have not shown that an increased body mass index increases risk (40). Obesity is a risk factor for OSA, which makes airway management difficult, increasing complications in the immediate postoperative period. In a retrospective study of patients with OSA who had hip or knee replacement, patients with a diagnosis of OSA had more adverse postoperative outcomes than a group of matched control patients. The rate of postoperative pulmonary complications was not significantly different between the two groups.

Cigarette Smoking

The incidence of perioperative pulmonary complications increases in direct proportion to smoking above a threshold of 10 pack-years (27,38). The available data suggest a modest increase in the risk for postoperative pulmonary complications among current smokers (40).

Type of Surgery and Anesthesia

The incidence of pulmonary complications also is influenced by the surgical site and type of surgical procedure. In general, those close to the diaphragm carry the highest risk. Patients who undergo open aortic and emergency surgeries are at the highest risk for postoperative pulmonary complications (39). The risk of pulmonary complications is increased approximately threefold after a thoracotomy (and increases again after resection of lung tissue) or after nonlaparoscopic upper abdominal surgery (38). After nonabdominal, nonthoracic surgical procedures, risk of pulmonary complications is usually low (27,38).

The incidence of pulmonary complications may be influenced by the type and duration of anesthesia (27,38). The duration of anesthesia is associated with risk of pulmonary complications, recovery room stay, and intensive care unit admission (34). Because longer anesthetics are required for more extensive surgical procedures, this may reflect surgical acuity rather than an effect of anesthesia per se. There are no convincing data to suggest that pulmonary outcomes differ between general and regional anesthetic techniques; therefore, risk for pulmonary complications should not determine anesthetic choice (41). The same is true when regional analgesia is used to provide postoperative analgesia. Although some meta-analyses have suggested a benefit of regional anesthesia, methodologic limitations of the studies preclude such conclusions (42). Despite the fact that general anesthesia appears to be a risk factor on a basis of adjusted observational data (Table 5.7) (39), systematic review of randomized controlled trials have not consistently reported an effect of the type of anesthesia on postoperative pulmonary complications rates (41). Therefore, as supported by the best randomized trials, there is no evidence that regional analgesia improves pulmonary risk (41). Regional techniques may pose challenges to the patients with pulmonary disease. Unintentionally high neuraxial level or blockade of the phrenic nerve during inter-scalene brachial plexus blocks may cause intercostal respiratory muscles or diaphragmatic paralysis, which may be deleterious for patients with reduced ventilatory reserve (i.e., COPD).

Comorbid Conditions and Exercise Capacity

Measures of general health status, such as the American Society of Anesthesiologists (ASA) physical status score and pre-existing pulmonary disease, are important for determining risks for postoperative pulmonary complications. COPD and asthma are significant risk factors, especially if poorly controlled. Patients with abnormal findings on lung examination such as crackles, wheezes, and decreased breath sounds are at increased risk for pulmonary complications after abdominal surgery (43). Other factors that may influence pulmonary complications include the severity and stability of pulmonary disorders (e.g., a recent increase in productive cough or poorly controlled asthma with wheezing) as well as nonpulmonary factors (e.g., spontaneous or provocable myocardial ischemia) (34,37,38).

Functional dependence and decreased exercise capacity increase the risk of postoperative pulmonary and cardiac complications. Exercise is impaired if the patient cannot walk four blocks on level ground or climb two flights of stairs without symptoms. The most common underlying causes of poor exercise capacity are cardiac limitation and deconditioning. If capacity is limited by problems of gas exchange or respiratory reserve, the risk of adverse pulmonary events after surgery may be high.

DIAGNOSTIC TESTING TO ASSESS RISK

Laboratory tests and imaging studies must be individualized to the complexity of the clinical situation. Studies have not shown consistent benefit from any specific test or imaging study, although many tests are routinely ordered or even required by institutional policy. The literature does not support ordering "routine" preoperative tests unless required to answer a specific question about a patient's condition. Diagnostic testing is selective according to patient risk factors and risk of surgery (Table 5.8). Preoperative spirometry, arterial blood gases, and chest radiography should not be used routinely for predicting risk of postoperative pulmonary complications (40). Specific testing may be necessary for surgical planning for patients scheduled for lung resection. For example, the risk of postoperative respiratory insufficiency or death is greater in patients undergoing a pneumonectomy with a preoperative FEV_1 <2 L or 50% of predicted, a maximal voluntary ventilation <50% predicted, or a DL_{CO} of the lung <60% predicted (3). Thus, patients scheduled for lung resection should generally undergo spirometry, and for selected patients, lung DL_{CO} should be determined (44).

If patients anticipating lung resection surgery have preoperative abnormalities in FEV_1 or DL_{CO}, it is essential to estimate the likely postresection pulmonary reserve. The amount of residual lung function after lung resection can be estimated by using

Table 5.8   Recommendations for preoperative diagnostic tests

Test	Consider Performing if
Electrocardiogram	Signs or symptoms of cardiac or severe pulmonary disease (angina, cor pulmonale, etc.)
Coagulation studies	Use of anticoagulants (because of prior pulmonary embolism, deep venous thrombosis, atrial fibrillation, etc.) or a history or coagulation abnormalities
Hemoglobin level	Polycythemia (chronic hypoxemia)
Pulse oximetry/arterial blood gases	Cyanosis or oxygen dependency
Serum electrolytes	Use of digoxin, diuretics, angiotensin receptor antagonists, or steroids
Serum creatinine concentration	Therapy with potentially nephrotoxic medications such as cyclosporine
Chest radiography	Signs or symptoms of cardiopulmonary disease
Spirometry	Presence of dyspnea
	Patient will undergo lung resection
	Presence of significant pulmonary symptoms or disease

From Smetana GW, Lawrence VA, Cornell JE, American College of Physicians. Preoperative pulmonary risk stratification for noncardiothoracic surgery: systematic review for the American College of Physicians. *Ann Intern Med.* 2006;144:581–595.

radionuclide quantitative lung scanning coupled with spirometry. The FEV_1 from spirometry is obtained and is the only other value needed in this calculation. Residual FEV_1 is predicted by multiplying the FEV_1 by the percentage of radioactive counts from the nonoperative lung or lung region according to the following equation (45):

Predicted postoperative FEV_1

$$= FEV_1 \times \frac{\text{Radioactive counts in nonoperative lung}}{\text{Radioactive counts from both lungs}}$$

A calculated predicted postoperative FEV_1 of at least 0.8 L (27) or >40% of the predicted normal value suggests that the patient has sufficient lung tissue to tolerate the procedure (38). A predicted postoperative FEV_1 or DL_{CO} <40% indicates an increased risk for perioperative complications. CPET should be performed in these patients to further define the perioperative risks before surgery. Risk for perioperative complications can generally be stratified by calculation of maximal oxygen consumption ($\dot{V}O_2$ max). Patients with preoperative $\dot{V}O_2$ max >20 mL/kg/minute are not at increased risk of complications or death; a $\dot{V}O_2$ max <15 mL/kg/minute indicates an increased risk of perioperative complications; and patients with a $\dot{V}O_2$ max <10 mL/kg/minute have a very high risk for postoperative complications (45). Alternative types of exercise testing include stair climbing and the 6-minute walk (45–47). Although often not performed in a standardized manner, stair climbing can predict $\dot{V}O_2$ max. In general terms, patients who can climb five flights of stairs have a $\dot{V}O_2$ max >20 mL/kg/minute. Conversely, patients who cannot climb one flight of stairs have a $\dot{V}O_2$ max <10 mL/kg/minute. Oxyhemoglobin desaturation during an exercise test has been associated with an increased risk for perioperative complications (47). Table 5.8 has suggestions for preoperative testing for patients with pulmonary disease.

PREOPERATIVE RECOMMENDATIONS TO PREVENT POSTOPERATIVE PULMONARY COMPLICATIONS

A comprehensive medical assessment (37) should be performed to treat underlying lung disease. Consultation with a pulmonologist may be helpful for patients with severe lung disease or those awaiting lung transplantation, pneumonectomy, or lung volume reduction. Standard preventive strategies are always appropriate, regardless of the risk assessment. These strategies are smoking cessation (32) before planned surgery and training in incentive spirometry or intermittent positive pressure breathing to reduce the risk of postoperative atelectasis (3). One study demonstrated that preoperative intensive inspiratory muscle training reduced the incidence of postoperative pulmonary complications and duration of postoperative hospitalization in patients at high risk for developing a pulmonary complication after coronary artery bypass graft surgery. Figure 5.3 summarizes the recommendations for identification of patients at risk for perioperative pulmonary complications and gives suggestions for prophylactic measures to decrease the risks.

For patients at high risk for postoperative pulmonary complications, more aggressive preventive strategies are added to the standard strategies. Additional measures include the following (Tables 5.2 and 5.3):

- Lung disease should be controlled preoperatively (e.g., bronchodilator therapy and, if needed, oral prednisone before elective surgery may reduce complications in a patient with moderate to severe persistent asthma). Measures to control active infection (e.g. antibiotics) can reduce the incidence and severity of perioperative pulmonary complications (38).
- Measures aimed to prevent deep venous thrombosis (DVT) and pulmonary embolism (PE) are important for all major operations, especially for orthopedic operations, in which the incidence of thrombosis may be as high as 60% (48–50). Heparin prophylaxis can help to reduce the incidence of DVT and death in high-risk patients. Prevention of DVT in the lower extremities inevitably reduces the frequency of PE. Populations at risk (e.g., neuro- or orthopedic surgery, a history of PE or DVT) must be identified so that safe and efficient prophylactic antithrombotic measures can be used. The American College of Chest Physicians' Seventh Consensus Conference on Antithrombotic Therapy has published guidelines, which are reviewed in Chapter 7 (51).

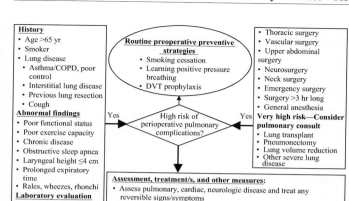

Figure 5.3.   Preoperative evaluation of patients with pulmonary disease: Risk assessment, treatments, and other measures aimed at risk reduction.

- Atelectasis and hypoxemia often develop in the perioperative period (52). Incentive spirometry and other lung expansion strategies are beneficial. The use of continuous positive airway pressure (CPAP) may reduce pulmonary complications in patients at risk for hypoxemia after extubation and reduce the incidence of tracheal reintubations (53). Patients who use CPAP should be instructed to bring their devices to the hospital on the day of surgery. Preparation may facilitate earlier extubation or prevent reintubation (54).

- Elective procedures should be delayed for patients with acute exacerbations of COPD or asthma. There are no data on how long after an acute exacerbation the patient remains at risk.

- Corticosteroids may be administered in "stress doses" for those whose hypopituitary-adrenal axis (HPA) is suppressed from recent prolonged corticosteroid therapy. Long-term (months to years) administration of >5 mg of prednisone daily increases the risk of HPA suppression (55). Patients who have received >20 mg/day of prednisone or its equivalent for >3 weeks may require supplementation (Table 5.9) (see Chapters 6 and 17 for more details). Adults who have received only inhaled corticosteroids rarely need systemic corticosteroids in the perioperative period to prevent adrenal insufficiency (56). Corticosteroids may be used to improve preoperative pulmonary function, but there is no evidence that routine parenteral corticosteroids are necessary for all patients with reactive airway disease.

CONCLUSION

The goal of preoperative assessment is to identify patients with pre-existing pathologies or predisposing factors that increase the risk for postoperative pulmonary complications. A detailed

Table 5.9   Perioperative corticosteroid administration in adrenal insufficiency

Type of Surgery	Corticosteroid Treatment
Major (i.e., cardiopulmonary bypass)	Hydrocortisone 100 mg IV every 8 hours ×3 doses, with dose 1 before surgery; then hydrocortisone 50 mg IV every 8 hours ×3 doses; then hydrocortisone 25 mg IV every 8 hours ×3 doses; then resume usual outpatient dose
Moderate (i.e., open cholecystectomy, lower extremity revascularization)	Hydrocortisone 50 mg IV every 8 hours ×3 doses; then hydrocortisone 25 mg IV every 8 hours ×3 doses; then resume usual outpatient dose
Minor (i.e., inguinal herniorrhaphy)	Take usual oral dose preoperatively; double first postoperative dose (optional); then resume usual outpatient dose

From Salem M, Tainsh RE Jr, Bromberg J, et al. Perioperative glucocorticoid coverage. A reassessment 42 years after emergence of a problem. *Ann Surg.* 1994;219:416–425.

preoperative history and physical examination are paramount for risk stratification. In addition to perioperative management, preventive efforts should be focused on optimizing the patient's medical condition preoperatively to minimize postoperative pulmonary complications. When estimating risk, consider both patient- and procedure-related risk factors that may affect the postoperative course. Preoperative diagnostic tests should be ordered based on the clinical characteristics of each patient; routine testing is not justified. Finally, key preoperative interventions should be considered such as smoking cessation, incentive spirometry and deep breathing exercises, intensive inspiratory muscle training, and optimization of respiratory, nutritional, and cardiac status in patients with lung disease, all of which effectively help prevent postoperative pulmonary complications.

REFERENCES

1. National Asthma Education and Prevention Program. Expert Panel Report: Guidelines for the Diagnosis and Management of Asthma Update on Selected Topics–2002. *J Allergy Clin Immunol.* 2002;110:S141–219.
2. Folkerts G, Busse WW, Nijkamp FP, et al. Virus-induced airway hyperresponsiveness and asthma. *Am J Respir Crit Care Med.* 1998;157:1708–1720.
3. Celli BR, MacNee W. Standards for the diagnosis and treatment of patients with COPD: a summary of the ATS/ERS position paper. *Eur Respir J.* 2004;23:932–946.
4. Fabbri L, Pauwels RA, Hurd SS. Gold Scientific Committee. Global strategy for the diagnosis, management, and prevention

of chronic obstructive pulmonary disease: GOLD executive summary updated 2003. *COPD*. 2004;1:105–141.

5. Repine JE, Bast A, Lankhorst I. Oxidative stress in chronic obstructive pulmonary disease. Oxidative Stress Study Group. *Am J Respir Crit Care Med*. 1997;156:341–357.

6. Celli BR, Cote CG, Marin J, et al. The body-mass index, airflow obstruction, dyspnea, and exercise capacity index in chronic obstructive pulmonary disease. *N Engl J Med*. 2004;350:1005–1012.

7. Fishman A, Martinez F, Naunheim K, et al. A randomized trial comparing lung-volume-reduction surgery with medical therapy for severe emphysema. *N Engl J Med*. 2003;348:2059–2073.

8. Utz JP, Hubmayr RD, Deschamps C. Lung volume reduction surgery for emphysema: out on a limb without a NETT. *Mayo Clin Proc*. 1998;73:552–566.

9. Trulock EP. Lung transplantation. *Am J Respir Crit Care Med*. 1997;155:789–818.

10. Trulock EP, Edwards LB, Taylor DO, et al. The Registry of the International Society for Heart and Lung Transplantation: twentieth official Adult Lung and Heart-Lung Transplant Report—2003. *J Heart Lung Transplant*. 2003;22:625–635.

11. Kostopanagiotou G, Smyrniotis V, Arkadopoulos N, et al. Anesthetic and perioperative management of adult transplant recipients in nontransplant surgery. *Anesth Analg*. 1999;89:613–622.

12. Dyspnea. Mechanisms, assessment, and management: a consensus statement. American Thoracic Society. *Am J Respir Crit Care Med*. 1999;159:321–340.

13. Pratter MR, Curley FJ, Dubois J, et al. Cause and evaluation of chronic dyspnea in a pulmonary disease clinic. *Arch Intern Med*. 1989;149:2277–2282.

14. Wranne B, Tolagen K. Platypnoea after pneumonectomy caused by a combination of intracardiac right-to-left shunt and hypovolaemia. Relief of symptoms on restitution of blood volume. *Scand J Thorac Cardiovasc Surg*. 1978;12:129–131.

15. Robin ED, Laman D, Horn BR, et al. Platypnea related to orthodeoxia caused by true vascular lung shunts. *N Engl J Med*. 1976;294:941–943.

16. Santiago SM Jr, Dalton JW Jr. Platypnea and hypoxemia in Laennec's cirrhosis of the liver. *South Med J*. 1977;70:510–512.

17. Begin R. Platypnea after pneumonectomy. *N Engl J Med*. 1975;293:342–343.

18. Simon PM, Schwartzstein RM, Weiss JW, et al. Distinguishable types of dyspnea in patients with shortness of breath. *Am Rev Respir Dis*. 1990;142:1009–1014.

19. Scano G, Stendardi L, Grazzini M. Understanding dyspnoea by its language. *Eur Respir J*. 2005;25:380–385.

20. Januzzi JL Jr, Camargo CA, Anwaruddin S, et al. The N-terminal Pro-BNP investigation of dyspnea in the emergency department (PRIDE) study. *Am J Cardiol*. 2005;95:948–954.

21. American Thoracic Society, American College of Chest Physicians. ATS/ACCP statement on cardiopulmonary exercise testing. *Am J Respir Crit Care Med*. 2003;167:211–277.

22. Egan TD, Wong KC. Perioperative smoking cessation and anesthesia: a review. *J Clin Anesth*. 1992;4:63–72.

23. Cooper CB. Assessment of pulmonary function in COPD. *Semin Respir Crit Care Med*. 2005;26:246–252.

24. Fletcher C, Peto R. The natural history of chronic airflow obstruction. *BMJ*. 1977;1:1645–1648.

25. Sandford AJ, Chagani T, Weir TD, et al. Susceptibility genes for rapid decline of lung function in the lung health study. *Am J Respir Crit Care Med*. 2001;163:469–473.

26. Scanlon PD, Connett JE, Waller LA, et al. Smoking cessation and lung function in mild-to-moderate chronic obstructive pulmonary disease. The Lung Health Study. *Am J Respir Crit Care Med*. 2000;161:381–390.

27. Okeson GC. Pulmonary dysfunction and surgical risk. How to assess and minimize the hazards. *Postgrad Med*. 1983;74:75–83.

28. Warner DO. Perioperative abstinence from cigarettes: physiologic and clinical consequences. *Anesthesiology*. 2006;104:356–367.

29. Bluman LG, Mosca L, Newman N, et al. Preoperative smoking habits and postoperative pulmonary complications. *Chest*. 1998;113:883–889.

30. Kotani N, Kushikata T, Hashimoto H, et al. Recovery of intraoperative microbicidal and inflammatory functions of alveolar immune cells after a tobacco smoke-free period. *Anesthesiology*. 2001;94:999–1006.

31. Moores LK. Smoking and postoperative pulmonary complications. An evidence-based review of the recent literature. *Clin Chest Med*. 2000;21:139–146.

32. Warner MA, Offord KP, Warner ME, et al. Role of preoperative cessation of smoking and other factors in postoperative pulmonary complications: a blinded prospective study of coronary artery bypass patients. *Mayo Clin Proc*. 1989;64:609–616.

33. Barrera R, Shi W, Amar D, et al. Smoking and timing of cessation: impact on pulmonary complications after thoracotomy. *Chest*. 2005;127:1977–1983.

34. Wong DH, Weber EC, Schell MJ, et al. Factors associated with postoperative pulmonary complications in patients with severe chronic obstructive pulmonary disease. *Anesth Analg*. 1995;80:276–284.

35. McAlister FA, Bertsch K, Man J, et al. Incidence of and risk factors for pulmonary complications after nonthoracic surgery. *Am J Respir Crit Care Med*. 2005;171:514–517.

36. McAlister FA, Khan NA, Straus SE, et al. Accuracy of the preoperative assessment in predicting pulmonary risk after nonthoracic surgery. *Am J Respir Crit Care Med*. 2003;167:741–744.

36a. Johnson RG, Arozullah AM, Neumayer L, et al. Multivariable predictors of postoperative respiratory failure after general and vascular surgery: Results from the patient safety in surgery study. *J Am Coll Surg*. 2007;204(6):1188–1198.

37. Merli GJ, Weitz HH. Approaching the surgical patient. Role of the medical consultant. *Clin Chest Med*. 1993;14:205–210.

38. Mohr DN, Lavender RC. Preoperative pulmonary evaluation. Identifying patients at increased risk for complications. *Postgrad Med*. 1996;100:241–251.

39. Smetana GW, Lawrence VA, Cornell JE, American College of Physicians. Preoperative pulmonary risk stratification for

noncardiothoracic surgery: systematic review for the American College of Physicians. *Ann Intern Med*. 2006;144:581–595.

40. Qaseem A, Snow V, Fitterman N, et al. Risk assessment for and strategies to reduce perioperative pulmonary complications for patients undergoing noncardiothoracic surgery: a guideline from the American College of Physicians. *Ann Intern Med*. 2006;144:575–580.

41. Lawrence VA, Cornell JE, Smetana GW. Strategies to reduce postoperative pulmonary complications after noncardiothoracic surgery: systematic review for the American College of Physicians. *Ann Intern Med*. 2006;144:596–608.

42. Rodgers A, Walker N, Schug S, et al. Reduction of postoperative mortality and morbidity with epidural or spinal anaesthesia: results from overview of randomised trials. *BMJ*. 2000;321:1493.

43. Lawrence VA, Dhanda R, Hilsenbeck SG, et al. Risk of pulmonary complications after elective abdominal surgery. *Chest*. 1996;110:744–750.

44. Schuurmans MM, Diacon AH, Bolliger CT. Functional evaluation before lung resection. *Clin Chest Med*. 2002;23:159–172.

45. Wyser C, Stulz P, Soler M, et al. Prospective evaluation of an algorithm for the functional assessment of lung resection candidates. *Am J Respir Crit Care Med*. 1999;159:1450–1456.

46. Datta D, Lahiri B. Preoperative evaluation of patients undergoing lung resection surgery. *Chest*. 2003;123:2096–2103.

47. Beckles MA, Spiro SG, Colice GL, et al. The physiologic evaluation of patients with lung cancer being considered for resectional surgery. *Chest*. 2003;123:105S–114S.

48. Haas S. Prevention of venous thromboembolism: recommendations based on the International Consensus and the American College of Chest Physicians Sixth Consensus Conference on Anti-thrombotic Therapy. *Clin Appl Thromb Hemost*. 2001;7:171–177.

49. Clagett GP, Anderson FA Jr, Geerts W, et al. Prevention of venous thromboembolism. *Chest*. 1998;114:531S–560S.

50. Geerts W, Ray JG, Colwell CW, et al. Prevention of venous thromboembolism. *Chest*. 2005;128:3775–3776.

51. Geerts WH, Pineo GF, Heit JA, et al. Prevention of venous thromboembolism: the Seventh ACCP Conference on Antithrombotic and Thrombolytic Therapy. *Chest*. 2004;126:338S–400S.

52. Brooks-Brunn JA. Postoperative atelectasis and pneumonia. *Heart Lung*. 1995;24:94–115.

53. Squadrone V, Coha M, Cerutti E, et al. Continuous positive airway pressure for treatment of postoperative hypoxemia: a randomized controlled trial. *JAMA*. 2005;293:589–595.

54. Bohner H, Kindgen-Milles D, Grust A, et al. Prophylactic nasal continuous positive airway pressure after major vascular surgery: results of a prospective randomized trial. *Langenbecks Arch Surg*. 2002;387:21–26.

55. Bromberg JS, Alfrey EJ, Barker CF, et al. Adrenal suppression and steroid supplementation in renal transplant recipients. *Transplantation*. 1991;51:385–390.

56. Goldmann DR. Surgery in patients with endocrine dysfunction. *Med Clin North Am*. 1987;71:499–509.

Endocrine and Metabolic Disorders

Vivek K. Moitra and BobbieJean Sweitzer

Anesthesiologists face several preoperative challenges when patients with endocrine disorders need surgery. Patients may present with an endocrinopathy requiring surgery, or more commonly, have an endocrine abnormality that complicates surgical and anesthetic management. Physiologic perturbations during the perioperative period may precipitate an endocrine crisis. To anticipate and prevent complications from an endocrine disorder, underlying conditions should be thoroughly evaluated before surgery. One endocrine disorder often occurs in concert with another to produce recognized syndromes of endocrinopathies such as multiple endocrine neoplasia (MEN) syndrome (Table 6.1). This chapter reviews the preoperative assessment and management of patients with endocrine disorders.

DIABETES MELLITUS

Diabetes mellitus (DM) is a disorder characterized by abnormal carbohydrate metabolism, which causes hyperglycemia. Hyperglycemia impairs vasodilation and induces a chronic proinflammatory, prothrombotic, and proatherogenic state leading to vascular complications (1). Although DM potentially affects all tissues, atherosclerotic vascular, renal, and nervous system effects such as peripheral vascular disease (PVD), renal insufficiency, and cerebrovascular disease are of greatest relevance to the anesthesiologist. Diabetics commonly have autonomic dysfunction, which manifests as orthostatic hypotension, loss of beat-to-beat heart rate variability, and delayed gastric emptying.

According to recent recommendations by the American Diabetes Association and the World Health Organization, DM is classified by the underlying disease etiology (i.e., type 1 vs. type 2) rather than by age of onset (i.e., juvenile-onset vs. adult-onset DM) or treatment modality (i.e., insulin-dependent vs. non–insulin-dependent DM) (2) (Table 6.2).

The insulin deficiency in type 1 DM is the result of autoimmune-mediated destruction of pancreatic beta cells. Patients depend on exogenous insulin to regulate metabolism. Onset of type 1 DM is at a younger age than onset of type 2 DM, and sensitivity to insulin is normal. Lack of insulin may precipitate diabetic ketoacidosis, a complex and potentially life-threatening metabolic derangement. Some patients with longstanding type 1 DM in tight control have repeated episodes of asymptomatic hypoglycemia and failure of counterregulatory mechanisms that result in hypoglycemic unawareness, even when blood glucose levels are dangerously low. In contrast, the peripheral insulin resistance of type 2 DM is often coupled with a failure to secrete insulin because of pancreatic beta cell dysfunction. Weight gain and abdominal or

Table 6.1. Characteristics of multiple endocrine neoplasia (MEN) syndromes

MEN Type 1 (Werner Syndrome)	MEN Type IIa (Sipple Syndrome)	MEN Type IIb (also known as MEN Type III)
Neoplastic tissue Parathyroid adenoma Pituitary adenoma Pancreatic islet cell Carcinoid (rare) Meningioma (rare) Lipoma (rare)	**Neoplastic tissue** Medullary thyroid carcinoma Pheochromocytoma Parathyroid adenoma **Other features** Cutaneous lichen amyloidosis (rare) Hirschsprung disease (rare)	**Neoplastic tissue** Medullary thyroid carcinoma Pheochromocytoma Mucosal neuroma Intestinal gan- glioneuromatosis **Other features** Skeletal deformities/ marfanoid habitus

visceral fat, independent of body mass index, are associated with an increased risk of developing type 2 DM (3).

Patients with DM may not experience classic cardiac chest pain but rather may be prone to "silent" myocardial ischemia. A diagnosis of DM has the same predictive value for a peri-operative cardiovascular event as a history of ischemic heart disease, compensated or prior heart failure, renal insufficiency, and cerebrovascular disease (4,5). Patients with DM but without previous MI carry the same level of risk for coronary events as nondiabetic patients with previous MI (6). In fact, patients with DM are considered risk equivalents for coronary artery disease (CAD), mandating intensive antiatherosclerotic therapy (7).

An elevated blood glucose is often a result of the stress response, and its presence can provide the practitioner with insight into the severity of a patient's illness. Hyperglycemia has emerged as a marker of outcome in diverse settings including MI, stroke, and trauma (8). Preoperatively, it is critical to distinguish between hyperglycemia as a marker of acute illness and its potential as a reversible, treatable, and independent variable of outcome.

Table 6.2. Classification of diabetes mellitus by disease etiology

Classification	Disease Etiology	Description
Type 1	Insulin deficiency	Autoimmune destruction of pancreatic beta cells
Type 2	Insulin resistance	Peripheral insulin resistance often coupled with a failure to secrete insulin

Currently, the American Diabetes Association recommends a target HbA1c of <7% for patients with type 2 DM. HbA1c, or glycosylated hemoglobin, is a measure of long-term glucose control, typically the past 3 months. Lower levels of HbA1c are associated with reduced microvascular and neuropathic complications. An elevated HbA1c is associated with a greater risk of cardiovascular events, an increase in postoperative infectious complications, and an increase in gastric fluid volumes (9–11).

With poor glycemic control, serum and tissue proteins are glycosylated, and abnormal collagen is deposited in connective tissues and joints. Consequently, diabetics with a history of chronic hyperglycemia may develop stiff joint syndrome, reducing joint mobility (cervical, atlanto-occipital) and contributing to a difficult laryngoscopy. Although the risk of limited joint mobility increases as HbA1c values increase, currently no data show that poor glycemic control predicts a difficult airway (12).

Patients with DM are prone to skin lesions from infection or ischemia. Peripheral neuropathy with pre-existing sensory deficits may complicate attempts to assess the adequacy of a regional anesthetic. Diabetics have an increased incidence of renal dysfunction, delayed gastric emptying due to gastropathy, retinopathy, erectile dysfunction, and cerebrovascular disease manifesting as transient ischemic attacks (TIAs), stroke, or vascular dementia.

Diabetics often have complex medicine regimens, and insulin prescriptions are a common source of error. Use of sulfonylurea agents with very long half-lives (e.g., chlorpropamide) is associated with hypoglycemia in the fasting patient. The use of metformin, an insulin sensitizer, is associated with lactic acidosis. However, this is rare in the absence of hepatic or renal dysfunction. In the past, varying opinions suggested discontinuing metformin for up to 48 hours before surgery. However, there are very little data supporting this recommendation. Several newer oral agents (acarbose, pioglitazone) used as single-agent therapy do not carry a risk of hypoglycemia in the fasting patient.

Interview, History, and Physical Examination

Patients are questioned about symptoms of CAD (chest discomfort, shortness of breath with exertion). The absence of chest pain is not reassuring in diabetics who may have "silent" ischemia. See Chapter 3 for a more detailed discussion of the history and physical examination in patients with known or suspected CAD. In addition, symptoms of diabetic autonomic neuropathy (orthostatic hypotension, spastic bladder, early satiety, heartburn, vomiting after meals), peripheral neuropathy, TIAs, or stroke should be noted. Renal insufficiency from diabetic nephropathy and claudication secondary to PVD are elicited. Patients with type 1 DM are questioned about ketoacidosis; those with type 2, about hyperglycemic, hyperosmolar coma. The frequency, severity, and symptoms of hypoglycemic episodes are established. A history of neck and joint immobility and previous difficult intubation should be documented.

Table 6.3. Preoperative evaluation of the patient with diabetes

Cardiovascular	Myocardial ischemia (may be silent), other risk factors for coronary artery disease (see Chapter 3)
	Blood pressure, heart rate, orthostatic hypotension, peripheral pulses
Neurologic	History of stroke, peripheral neuropathy, autonomic dysfunction
	Motor, sensory neurologic examination
Gastrointestinal	Gastroparesis, gastroesophageal reflux
Renal	Renal function, diuretic and/or dialysis dependence
	Volume status, skin turgor, mucous membranes, neck veins
Endocrine	Glucose control, history of diabetic ketoacidosis or hyperosmolar coma, presence of other endocrine disorders (Table 6.1)
HEENT	History of difficult intubation, complete airway evaluation including assessment of neck mobility

HEENT, head, eyes, ears, nose, and throat.

The characteristics of organ systems in patients with DM are in Table 6.3. Patients with PVD often exhibit discrepancies in blood pressure (BP) at different sites of measurement. BP in both arms should be compared. Orthostatic measurements should be performed. Orthostatic changes (a decrease in systolic BP of at least 20 mmHg or a decrease in diastolic pressure of at least 10 mmHg within 3 minutes of standing) occur with autonomic dysfunction.

Examination of peripheral pulses (presence or absence, quality, bruits) provides information about vascular pathology and information for planning invasive monitoring cannulation sites. Because of positioning considerations during surgery, the location of skin lesions should be documented. Motor and sensory deficits should be noted.

Diagnostic Testing

Recommendations for diagnostic tests appear in Table 6.4.

A single morning glucose value or even multiple readings taken only after an overnight fast do not adequately reflect a diabetic patient's long-term glucose control. An estimation of glycemic control can be obtained through an examination of blood glucoses at different times of the day over a course of weeks or an HbA1c. An ECG is useful in identifying the presence of ischemic heart disease and establishing a baseline for comparison. Further stress testing may be necessary in symptomatic and asymptomatic patients who may have "silent ischemia" (see Chapter 3). Stress imaging can be useful in diabetic patients who may not have

Table 6.4.   Diagnostic tests for patients with diabetes mellitus

Test	Rationale
Electrocardiogram	Provides information about ischemic cardiac disease and serves as a baseline for comparison should hemodynamic complications develop
Electrolyte panel	Provides information about volume, osmolarity, and acid–base status
Blood glucose	Provides information about glucose control and serves as a marker of illness
HbA1C	Provides information about long-term glucose control and associated complications
Specialized testing (see Chapter 3 for cardiac testing)	Provides information about coronary artery disease in patients who may have asymptomatic disease

angina during an exercise stress test (13). A creatinine level is necessary to evaluate renal function in diabetic patients.

Implications for Perioperative and Anesthetic Management

The anesthesiologist should know which type of insulin the patient is taking (Table 6.5). In order to simplify perioperative glucose control, the anesthesiologist should consider discontinuing all oral agents on the day of surgery (DOS) and use insulin therapy for glucose management.

Physicians should consider preadmitting patients prone to diabetic ketoacidosis (those with type 1 DM) or patients known to be particularly susceptible to hypoglycemia. The medical regimen is designed in consultation with the patient's primary care physician or endocrinologist. Because type 1 diabetics do not produce insulin, they must take insulin on the DOS even when they are fasting or normoglycemic to avoid ketoacidosis. The following suggestions are recommended for patients with DM scheduled for surgery:

- Surgery for patients with DM (especially type 1) should be scheduled as the first case of the day.
- Pre-, intra-, and postoperative blood glucose levels should be determined.
- Up until the DOS continue all insulin regimens as scheduled.
- Type 1 diabetics take a small amount (usually one third to one half) of their usual morning long-acting insulin (e.g., lente or NPH) on the DOS.
- Type 2 diabetics take none or up to half the dose of long-acting or combination (70/30 preparations) insulins on the DOS.
- Patients with an insulin pump continue only their basal rate on the DOS.

Table 6.5. Types of insulin and perioperative management

Type of Insulin	Onset	Peak	Duration	Perioperative Management
Rapid acting				
Humalog/Lispro	15–30 min	30–90 min	3–5 hr	Omit on the DOS
Novolog/Aspart	10–20 min	40–50 min	3–5 hr	Omit on the DOS
Apidra/Glulisine	20–30 min	30–90 min	1–2.5 hr	Omit on the DOS
Short acting				
Regular (R) Humulin or Novolin	30 min–1 hr	2–5 hr	5–8 hr	Omit on the DOS For patients on an insulin pump: Continue basal rate on the DOS
Intermediate acting				
NPH (N)	1–2 hr	4–12 hr	18–24 hr	Half or none on DOS
Lente (L)	1–2.5 hr	3–10 hr	18–24 hr	Half or none on DOS
Long acting				
Ultralente (U)	30 min–3 hr	10–20 hr	20–36 hr	Half or none on DOS
Glargine/Lantus	1.5 hr	No peak; insulin delivered steadily	20–24 hr	Half or none on DOS
Levemir or detemir	1–2 hr	6–8 hr	Up to 24 hr	Half or none on DOS
Premixed				
Humulin 70/30	30 min	2–4 hr	14–24 hr	Half or none on DOS
Novolin 70/30	30 min	2–12 hr	Up to 24 hr	Half or none on DOS
Novolog 70/30	10–20 min	1–4 hr	Up to 24 hr	Half or none on DOS
Humulin 50/50	30 min	2–5 hr	18–24 hr	Half or none on DOS
Humalog mix 75/25	15 min	30 min–2 hr	16–20 hr	Half or none on DOS

DOS, day of surgery.
Adapted from http://diabetes.webmd.com/diabetes.types.insulin. Accessed October 7, 2007.

- Discontinue all rapid- and short-acting insulins on the DOS (unless administered via pump).
- Long-acting sulfonylureas such as chlorpropamide may be discontinued several days before surgery, especially if prolonged fasting is anticipated.
- Shorter-acting oral agents should be discontinued on the DOS.
- Metformin should be discontinued on the DOS.
- Metformin should not be restarted if there is a risk of renal and/or hepatic failure. This is especially a concern after the administration of radiographic contrast.

THYROID DISORDERS

Thyroid hormones regulate metabolism and have numerous systemic effects. The physiologic effects of thyroid hormone include a general increase in most of the body's metabolic processes. Synergistic actions of thyroid hormone and catecholamines stimulate the cardiovascular system with elevated heart rate, blood pressure, and cardiac output. Thyroid-stimulating hormone (TSH) is secreted by the anterior pituitary gland and stimulates the synthesis and secretion of triiodothyronine (T3) and thyroxine (T4) by the thyroid gland. TSH, in turn, is regulated by two mechanisms. First, T3 and T4, through negative feedback, inhibit TSH secretion by suppressing the release of the hypothalamic hormone, thyrotropin-releasing hormone (TRH). Second, TSH concentration is regulated directly by TRH.

In general, successful treatment of overt thyroid dysfunction has been associated with an improvement in survival. Some studies have suggested that patients with mild to moderate thyroid disease are not at a greater risk of major perioperative complications (14,15). In contrast, with severe thyroid dysfunction, surgery and stress can precipitate myxedema coma or thyroid storm (16,17). Myxedema coma can be life threatening and is characterized by profound lethargy or coma and often occurs with hypothermia. Hypothyroidism can coexist with occult adrenal insufficiency. Thyroid storm is a state of cardiovascular or nervous system decompensation in a patient with severe hyperthyroidism after a destabilizing event such as surgery, MI, stroke, infection, or trauma. Symptoms include fever out of proportion to any evidence of infection; tachydysrhythmia, often resistant to pharmacologic therapy; cardiovascular collapse with hypotension; dehydration from fever, perspiration, or diarrhea; and alterations in mental status.

In hypothyroidism, hyponatremia may occur from the inability to suppress secretion of antidiuretic hormone (ADH).

Interview, History, and Physical Examination

Preoperative evaluation may uncover a history of an adequately or inadequately treated thyroid disorder. The history should include the cause of the condition (inflammatory, postsurgical, pituitary insufficiency); the treatment prescribed and any changes in the regimen; and systemic symptoms of the thyroid disorder. Investigation of symptoms such as tachycardia, tremors, palpitations, cold intolerance, fatigue, lethargy, weight gain, and constipation is useful to determine if a patient is euthyroid (Table 6.6).

Table 6.6.   Preoperative evaluation of the patient with a thyroid disorder

Hyperthyroidism	
General	Hyperkinesis, warm moist skin, carpal tunnel syndrome, tremor
Cardiovascular	Palpitations, tachycardia, atrial fibrillation, systolic hypertension
Neurologic	Fatigue, weakness, nervousness, tremor, proximal muscle weakness
Gastrointestinal	Changes in appetite or bowel movement frequency, weight loss despite increased appetite
Endocrine	Increased perspiration, irregular menses
HEENT	Stare, lid lag, eyelid retraction, chemosis, proptosis, localized myxedema (Graves disease), tracheal deviation, goiter, dysphagia, chronic cough, dyspnea, orthopnea, hoarseness
Hypothyroidism	
General	Slow movements, slow speech, dry sallow skin, nonpitting edema (myxedema), cold intolerance
Cardiovascular	Bradycardia, diastolic hypertension, low-voltage electrocardiogram, enlarged cardiac silhouette on chest radiograph
Pulmonary	Hypoventilation
Neurologic	Fatigue, sleepiness, depression, paresthesias, delayed relaxation of deep tendon reflexes
Gastrointestinal	Weight gain, constipation
Endocrine	Irregular menses, menorrhagia
HEENT	Periorbital edema, enlarged tongue, tracheal deviation, goiter, dysphagia, chronic cough, dyspnea, orthopnea, hoarseness

HEENT, head, eyes, ears, nose, and throat.

Physical findings associated with hypo- or hyperthyroidism should be noted during the preoperative evaluation (Table 6.6). A thorough evaluation of the head and neck is essential to identify airway compromise (e.g., a deviated or narrowed trachea, enlarged tongue, vocal cord paresis) or the presence of intraoral thyroid tissue (the "lingual thyroid"), which may complicate laryngoscopy and intubation. Patients with Graves ophthalmopathy may exhibit proptosis with or without conjunctival edema (chemosis), enhancing the risk for ocular injury under general anesthesia.

Diagnostic Testing

Preoperative diagnostic tests for patients with thyroid disorders are listed in Table 6.7.

Although the prevalence of thyroid disorders remains high, there is little evidence to support the routine screening of asymptomatic patients without risk factors for thyroid disease.

Table 6.7.   Diagnostic tests for patients with a thyroid disorder

Test	Rationale
Chest radiograph, ultrasound, computed tomography, or magnetic resonance imaging	Evaluate airway abnormalities
Electrocardiogram	Rhythm disturbances such as tachycardia, atrial fibrillation, and low-voltage QRS
Echocardiogram	Evaluate ventricular function and presence of pericardial effusion
Electrolyte panel	Evaluate abnormal electrolytes, particularly sodium
Thyroid function tests	Assess thyroid function and adequacy of treatment

TSH levels can be used to monitor thyroid function. Relying on the TSH alone can be misleading if patients have been treated recently for thyrotoxicosis or have pituitary disease, nonthyroidal illness, or thyroid hormone resistance. Because numerous drugs and systemic pathologies affect the degree of protein binding, measurement of total thyroid hormone concentrations has been largely replaced by measurement of free hormone concentrations (free T3 and free T4). Thyroid function tests may be less useful in a variety of circumstances such as nonthyroidal illness, previously known as "euthyroid sick syndrome"; subclinical hyperthyroidism (abnormal TSH levels with normal free T3 and free T4); alterations in protein binding; and administration of medications such as dopamine, amiodarone, and glucocorticoids. Under these conditions, clinical, metabolic, and end-organ measures (i.e., ECG and electrolyte levels) may be helpful in the assessment of thyroid function.

Implications for Perioperative and Anesthetic Management

For patients with thyroid disorders:

- Elective surgery should be postponed until patients are euthyroid.
- An endocrinology consult is needed for noneuthyroid patients who require urgent or emergent surgery.
- Hyperthyroid patients requiring urgent surgery are often treated with beta blockers, iodine, antithyroid medications, and glucocorticoids.
- Hyperthyroid patients should take antithyroid medications (e.g., propylthiouracil [PTU] and methimazole, which have short half-lives, 6 to 8 hours) on the DOS.
- Intravascular volume may be depleted in hyperthyroid patients.
- Hyperthyroid patients are at risk for thyroid storm perioperatively.
- Because T4 has a half-life of 7 to 10 days, hypothyroid patients can miss several days of T4 without adverse consequences.

- Hypothyroid patients may have a decreased cardiac output from decreased heart rate and myocardial contractility.
- Patients with severe hypothyroidism may have an impaired respiratory response to hypoxia and hypercapnia (18).

DISORDERS OF CALCIUM METABOLISM

Understanding calcium homeostasis is essential to appreciating the anesthetic risks of patients with hypocalcemia and hypercalcemia. Parathyroid hormone (PTH) regulates extracellular calcium concentration through action on the bone, kidney, and intestine. PTH secretion is activated by hypocalcemia and elevated phosphorous levels. The net effect of PTH is to increase extracellular calcium. An excess or deficiency of calcium can disrupt coagulation, neurotransmitter and hormone secretion, neuromuscular excitability, muscle contraction, hormone action, and enzyme function.

Hypocalcemia

Common causes of hypocalcemia are listed in Table 6.8. Patients with rhabdomyolysis, pancreatitis, sepsis, burns, fat embolism syndrome, recent massive transfusion, hypoalbuminemia, hypomagnesemia, or renal insufficiency are at risk for hypocalcemia. Chronic hypocalcemia may have few clinical signs or symptoms, whereas rapidly developing hypocalcemia may have impressive clinical effects. The most common setting for symptomatic hypocalcemia is within 12 to 24 hours after surgery, particularly after total or subtotal thyroidectomy or four-gland parathyroid exploration or removal.

Longstanding hypocalcemia with hyperphosphatemia and PTH deficiency is associated with calcification of the basal ganglia with extrapyramidal signs. Hypocalcemia can cause neuromuscular irritability, arrhythmias, congestive heart failure (decreased myocardial contractility), and hypotension. Acute, severe hypocalcemia (total serum calcium levels <7.5 mg/dL, normal albumin) is a medical emergency associated with death from laryngeal spasm or grand mal seizures.

Interview, History, and Physical Examination

The recommendations for history and physical examination are found in Table 6.8. Symptoms of hypocalcemia may include perioral or acral paresthesias and spontaneous tetany. Neuronal irritability can be detected by tapping the facial nerve below the zygoma. In hypocalcemic patients, this results in ipsilateral contractions of the facial muscle with twitching of the corner of the mouth (Chvostek sign). Carpal spasm of the hand (Trousseau sign) can be elicited by 3 minutes of occlusive pressure with a blood pressure cuff. Cataracts and deposits of calcium are seen in the lens.

Diagnostic Testing

Diagnostic tests are listed in Table 6.9.

Hypocalcemia can cause cardiac conduction disturbances. ECG abnormalities include prolonged QT intervals and marked QRS and ST changes. These changes can mimic changes associated

Table 6.8. Preoperative evaluation of patients with calcium disorders

Hypercalcemia

Etiology	Endocrine: Hyperparathyroidism, hyperthyroidism, multiple endocrine neoplasia syndromes, acromegaly, pheochromocytoma, adrenal insufficiency Malignancy: Solid tumors: Breast, lung, pancreas, kidneys, ovary; Hematologic cancers: Myeloma, lymphosarcoma, adult T-cell lymphoma, Burkitt lymphoma (rare) Granulomatous disease: Sarcoidosis, histoplasmosis, coccidioidomycosis, tuberculosis Drugs: Theophylline, lithium, thiazides, vitamin D, calcium-containing antacids, vitamin A Other: AIDS, renal diseases, familial genetic causes, immobilization, osteopenia, osteoporosis
Cardiovascular	Hypertension, electrocardiogram conduction changes, digitalis toxicity, shortened QT interval
Neurologic	Weakness, atrophy, fatigue, seizures, memory loss, lethargy, psychosis, disorientation, hyporeflexia, airway protection
Gastrointestinal	Nausea, vomiting, anorexia, abdominal pain, constipation, pancreatitis, peptic ulcers, dehydration
Renal	Polyuria, nephrolithiasis, oliguric failure (late), volume status (skin turgor, mucous membranes, neck veins)

Hypocalcemia

Etiology	Endocrine: Hypoparathyroidism pseudohypoparathyroidism Drugs: Contrast media containing ethylene diamine tetraacetate (EDTA), loop diuretics, anticonvulsants Electrolytes: Hyperphosphatemia, phosphate therapy, hypomagnesemia Gastrointestinal: Liver failure, intestinal malabsorption, pancreatitis Other: Hemosiderosis, amyloidosis, renal failure, rhabdomyolysis, chemotherapy or tumor lysis, vitamin D deficiency, lack of sun exposure, dietary deficiency, hypoalbuminemia, osteoblastic metastases, critical illness, alkalosis, burns, toxic shock, fat embolism, massive transfusion (citrate intoxication)
Cardiovascular	Symptoms of congestive heart failure, dyspnea, peripheral edema, hypotension, dysrhythmia, catecholamine resistance
Neurologic	Paresthesias (acral, perioral), spontaneous tetany, seizure, weakness, Chvostek sign, Trousseau sign, extrapyramidal signs, muscle spasms, carpal/pedal spasm, altered mental status, seizures
HEENT	Cataracts, history of laryngeal spasm, stridor, apnea

HEENT, head, eyes, ears, nose, and throat. AIDS = acquired immunodeficiency syndrome.

Table 6.9.   Diagnostic tests for patients with calcium disorders

Test	Rationale
Electrocardiogram	For QT interval and ST changes
Electrolyte panel	Calcium, phosphorous, magnesium,
Creatinine	and albumin levels

with an acute MI or conduction abnormalities. Ventricular dysrhythmia is a rare complication of hypocalcemia.

Evaluation of calcium status is typically determined by measuring total serum calcium and albumin levels. A rough correction for protein-binding abnormalities can be made by assuming a change in total calcium of 0.8 mg/dL (0.2 mmol/L) for every 1 mg/dL change in albumin from 4.0 mg/dL. Ionized calcium levels are a more accurate indicator of calcium activity than serum calcium and albumin. For patients with an unknown etiology of hypocalcemia, a creatinine level should be ordered to evaluate renal function. An elevated serum phosphorus level with normal renal function supports the diagnosis of hypoparathyroidism. Phosphorous and magnesium levels should be evaluated in hypocalcemic patients.

Implications for Perioperative and Anesthetic Management

For patients with hypocalcemia:

- Patients with chronic hypocalcemia should take their calcium and vitamin D supplements before surgery.
- Acute hypocalcemia may cause neurologic or cardiovascular dysfunction.
- Treatment of acute hypocalcemia is with intravenous elemental calcium with close monitoring of serum calcium levels every 2 hours.

Hypercalcemia

Hypercalcemia can be categorized as either parathyroid dependent or non–parathyroid dependent. Disorders of the parathyroid gland that result in hypercalcemia include primary and tertiary hyperparathyroidism, familial hypocalciuric hypercalcemia, and lithium-induced hypercalcemia. Primary hyperparathyroidism occurs in the setting of inappropriate or autonomous secretion of PTH from the parathyroid glands. Secondary hyperparathyroidism often occurs in the setting of chronic renal failure when there is glandular hyperplasia from continuous stimulation from hyperphosphatemia and hypocalcemia. Eventually these glands may enlarge and become autonomous resulting in an oversecretion of PTH causing hypercalcemia (tertiary hyperparathyroidism). Hypercalcemia of malignancy is usually associated with destructive bone lesions or secretion of a PTH-like tumor peptide (PTH-RP). Hypercalcemia from parathyroid disease is associated with bone loss and osteoporosis. Multiple non–parathyroid-dependent hypercalcemic conditions exist (Table 6.8).

Interview, History, and Physical Examination

Signs and symptoms of hypercalcemia include cognitive deficits ranging from minimal memory loss to coma, constipation, excess stomach acid secretion, ulcer symptoms, polyuria, and renal stones. Once hypercalcemia is confirmed, use of potentiating medications should be considered. These include calcium-containing antacids; hydrochlorothiazide diuretics, which reduce renal calcium excretion; and lithium, which causes four-gland parathyroid hyperplasia. A malignancy should be considered.

Hypercalcemia often has no physical signs. The patient should be assessed for hypertension, hyporeflexia, and muscle weakness or atrophy. The patient's ability to protect the airway should be assessed if mental status is depressed. There may be evidence of volume depletion from anorexia, pancreatitis, renal tubular dysfunction, or vomiting.

Diagnostic Testing

Diagnostic tests are listed in Table 6.9.

Patients with primary hyperparathyroidism or hypercalcemia may exhibit T-wave abnormalities, ST-segment depressions, or shortening of the QT interval (19).

Implications for Perioperative and Anesthetic Management

For patients with calcium disorders:

- Mild to moderate hypercalcemia (total calcium <12 mg/dL) generally does not require specific treatment.
- Moderate hypercalcemia (total calcium 12 to 14 mg/dL) can be treated with saline hydration, oral administration of furosemide, and adequate salt and water intake.
- Severe hypercalcemia (total calcium >14 mg/dL) is life threatening and is treated with saline, diuretics, bisphosphonates, calcitonin, mithramycin, and glucocorticoids.
- Hypercalcemia enhances digitalis toxicity.

PITUITARY-ADRENAL CONDITIONS

Corticotropin-releasing hormone (CRH) from the hypothalamus regulates the production of adrenocorticotropic hormone (ACTH) by the anterior pituitary gland. ACTH controls the production of the glucocorticoid cortisol from the adrenal cortex. Cortisol production is essential for stress responses, hemodynamic stability, and temperature regulation. The average basal adrenal cortisol secretion is 30 mg/day. During maximal stress, adrenal cortisol output may increase 10-fold, up to 300 mg/day. A key feature of hypothalamic-pituitary-adrenal (HPA) physiology is negative feedback suppression of pituitary ACTH release by high levels of endogenous or exogenous glucocorticoids. Long-term glucocorticoid therapy is common for asthma, rheumatoid arthritis, and other inflammatory conditions, and for immune suppression in transplant patients. Thus, many patients are at risk for suppression of their endogenous HPA axis. The adrenal cortex produces a second steroid hormone, aldosterone, that is under the control of potassium levels and the renin-angiotensin system. Aldosterone increases the reabsorption of sodium from the renal distal tubule and the excretion of potassium. This hormone is central to normal fluid and electrolyte balance. Primary adrenal insufficiency (hemorrhage, tumor, infection) results in loss of both aldosterone and cortisol. Aldosterone secretion is preserved in secondary adrenal insufficiency from exogenous steroid therapy. Abnormalities in the HPA system are most commonly encountered in patients undergoing long-term treatment with glucocorticoids for medical conditions.

Adrenal Hormone Excess

In Cushing disease, a pituitary tumor producing ACTH leads to elevated glucocorticoid production. With ectopic ACTH or CRH production from lung tumors or other neoplasms and primary adrenal neoplasms, glucocorticoid oversecretion is possible. Mineralocorticoid excess may result from adrenal aldosteronoma or hyperplasia. Excess mineralocorticoids make the body retain sodium and water. Cushing syndrome is the clinical manifestation of excessive corticosteroid levels. It can be caused by ACTH hypersecretion (Cushing disease) or prolonged high-dose therapeutic glucocorticoid administration. Major manifestations of hypercorticalism relevant to anesthesia are hypertension, obesity, myopathy, and glucose intolerance or frank diabetes mellitus.

Adrenal Insufficiency

Adrenal insufficiency follows suppression of the HPA axis or destruction of the adrenal or the pituitary gland. Primary adrenal insufficiency is uncommon and associated with autoimmune adrenalitis, tuberculosis, and HIV. Some HIV patients have a peripheral resistance to glucocorticoids and up to 20% of patients with advanced AIDS have adrenal insufficiency (20). The most common cause of adrenal insufficiency is iatrogenic. In patients who take >20 mg/day of prednisone or its equivalent for >3 weeks, the HPA axis is suppressed. The HPA axis is not suppressed in patients who take <5 mg/day of prednisone or its equivalent. If 5 to 20 mg/day of prednisone or its equivalent is taken for >3 weeks, the HPA axis may or may not be suppressed. An intact HPA responds to the stress of surgery, trauma, and infection by increasing adrenal output of glucocorticoids. Glucocorticoids modify the effect of catecholamines on vascular tone. Hypotension refractory to vasopressor therapy and fluid resuscitation has been described in septic and elderly patients who are unable to mount an adequate stress response during illness (21,22).

Interview, History, and Physical Examination

The duration and dosage of steroid therapy should be recorded.

Signs and symptoms of hypercortisolemia include proximal muscle weakness; early fatigue; hypertension; emotional lability; abnormal central fat deposition, especially in the face, between the scapulae ("buffalo hump"), and in the abdomen; bruising; cutaneous striae; osteoporosis; acne; and virilization in women. Symptoms of CAD, diabetes mellitus, and osteoporosis should be investigated.

The examination of the patient with HPA system disorders should include recording of vital signs, particularly the blood pressure with orthostatic signs (Table 6.10). Evaluation of muscle

Table 6.10.   Preoperative evaluation of patients with hypothalamic-pituitary-adrenal disorders

General	Body habitus
Cardiovascular	Blood pressure, orthostatic hypotension, hypertension
Neurologic	Myopathy, weakness
Endocrine	Steroid use (dose, duration), presence of multiple endocrine disorders
Dermatologic	Skin integrity
HEENT	Oral thrush

HEENT, head, eyes, ears, nose, and throat.

wasting and proximal myopathy should be performed. An assessment of skin and connective tissue integrity aids in planning regional anesthesia and vascular access. Evaluation of the oropharynx may reveal oral thrush, which is common in patients treated with steroids and may complicate airway management. Postponement of elective procedures may be indicated while the infection is treated.

Diagnostic Testing

The diagnostic tests suggested for these patients appear in Table 6.11. Measurements of electrolyte and glucose levels are indicated because they can be abnormal in HPA disorders. Although patients with Cushing syndrome may have a history of bruising, coagulation studies and a platelet count should be normal. Because patients with HPA disorders may have electrolyte abnormalities, hypertension, and/or CAD, an ECG is indicated.

Implications for Perioperative and Anesthetic Management

For patients with HPA disorders:

- Electrolyte and glucose abnormalities are common in disorders of the HPA axis.
- Coexisting myopathy should be recognized because of the possibility of increased sensitivity to muscle relaxants and respiratory insufficiency postoperatively.
- Adrenal insufficiency can be associated with vasodilation and hypotension refractory to vasopressor therapy and fluid resuscitation.

Table 6.11.   Diagnostic tests for patients with a hypothalamic-pituitary-adrenal disorder

Test	Rationale
Blood glucose	Hyperglycemia in patients with glucocorticoid excess
Electrocardiogram	Assess for ventricular hypertrophy or coronary artery disease
Electrolyte panel	Electrolyte abnormalities are common

- Hypovolemia should be anticipated in patients with adrenal insufficiency.
- Patients continue their glucocorticoid or mineralocorticoid replacement therapy and antihypertensive and cardiac regimens on the DOS.
- Steroid supplementation is advisable for major procedures in patients with Cushing syndrome or in patient's taking >20 mg/day of prednisone or its equivalent.
- The risk of adrenal insufficiency remains for up to 1 year after the cessation of high-dose steroid therapy.

See Chapter 17 for a detailed discussion of perioperative steroid replacement recommendations.

OTHER PITUITARY GLAND DISORDERS

In addition to ACTH, the anterior pituitary gland secretes several other trophic hormones. Acromegaly associated with excess growth hormone is of principal concern for the anesthesiologist. Excessive growth hormone secretion stimulates overgrowth of skin, connective tissue, cartilage, bone, and viscera. Characteristic findings of soft tissue overgrowth include an enlarged jaw (macrognathia) and excessive size of hands and feet. Neuropathies secondary to entrapment of nerves may occur. Pharyngeal and laryngeal soft tissue overgrowth and macroglossia lead to obstructive sleep apnea (OSA), although many acromegalics also have a central sleep apnea etiology. The acromegalic patient may have abnormal facies, an enlarged nose and tongue, and a hypertrophic epiglottis. Tongue enlargement and soft tissue hypertrophy in the hypopharynx may complicate mask ventilation, laryngoscopy, and intubation. Acromegalics have an increased incidence of hypertension, left ventricular hypertrophy (LVH), diastolic dysfunction, and valvular abnormalities. Acromegalic patients are prone to CAD and CHF. Acromegalics may complain of symptoms secondary to pituitary enlargement (i.e., headaches and visual impairment). There is an increased incidence of diabetes mellitus with acromegaly. Although the thyroid gland is normal, secondary hypothyroidism due to pituitary dysfunction may occur in acromegalics.

The posterior pituitary gland secretes ADH, also known as *vasopressin*. This peptide hormone controls the excretion of water by the kidney. In diabetes insipidus (DI), dilute urine formation is copious (>1 L/hour) because of ADH deficiency, with the potential for hypernatremia and depletion of intravascular volume. This condition may be seen after head injury or pituitary surgery.

Interview, History, and Physical Examination

BP measurement is important because of the common occurrence of hypertension. These patients need to be evaluated for heart disease (CHF, CAD). Evaluation of the airway is important for the patient with acromegaly. Acromegalics need to be questioned about the diagnosis of or symptoms consistent with OSA (snoring, daytime somnolence). A complete neurologic examination including visual fields and documentation of any sensory or motor deficits is important. The presence or absence of the signs and symptoms of thyroid dysfunction should be documented (see the thyroid section of this chapter). Patients with DI are examined specifically to estimate volume status (orthostatic signs; see the DM section of this chapter for description of orthostatic BP determination). Medications, especially the use of the synthetic ADH analog desmopressin acetate in patients with diabetes insipidus, should be documented.

Diagnostic Testing

Glycemic control should be evaluated. An ECG is indicated. Sodium levels should be determined in patients with DI. Thyroid function tests (TFTs) should be done since the signs and symptoms of hypothyroidism are nonspecific. If OSA or CHF is present or suspected, an echocardiogram is indicated.

Implications for Perioperative and Anesthetic Management

- Acromegalic patients should be alerted to the possibility of intubation while awake.
- Advanced planning for difficult airway management to ensure equipment and personnel are available is important.
- Patients with DI continue their hormone therapy.
- Desmopressin acetate (a chemically modified vasopressin) can be administered by injection (intravenously or subcutaneously), endotracheal tube insufflation, nasal spray, or mouth.
- Volume status and sodium levels are the principal concern in DI.

CARCINOID TUMORS

Carcinoid tumors are rare neuroendocrine tumors, which typically arise from the gastrointestinal (GI) tract but may be found in the bronchi or pancreas. Mediators released from carcinoid tumors in the GI tract enter the portal venous circulation and are metabolized by the liver before they reach the systemic circulation. Carcinoid syndrome is the constellation of signs and symptoms (flushing, diarrhea, telangiectasias, and bronchospasm) that occurs when the circulation of vasoactive mediators such as serotonin, tachykinins, histamine, kallikrein, and prostaglandins bypass liver metabolism (23). Flushing can be accompanied by tachycardia or supraventricular arrhythmias.

The release of serotonin has been implicated in the development of carcinoid heart disease, which is characterized by endocardial fibrosis of right-sided heart valves resulting in tricuspid regurgitation and pulmonic stenosis (23). Signs of right-sided CHF such as peripheral edema and hepatomegaly may occur. Gastrointestinal pathology or the avid uptake of tryptophan (the precursor for serotonin) by tumor cells can lead to malnutrition. Carcinoid syndrome is more likely to be present in metastatic GI tumors or primary tumors outside of the GI tract. Carcinoid tumors are associated with MEN type 1, and the presence or absence of parathyroid, pancreatic, and pituitary disease should be identified preoperatively (Table 6.1).

Interview, History, and Physical Examination

The symptoms of carcinoid syndrome (Table 6.12) should be elicited. In the majority of patients (95%) the features of carcinoid syndrome are absent; instead, patients experience gastrointestinal symptoms such as nausea, bleeding, or abdominal pain.

Table 6.12. Preoperative evaluation of patients with carcinoid tumors

Cardiovascular	Palpitations, dizziness, orthostatic symptoms, tricuspid and pulmonary murmurs, hypertension, orthostatic hypotension, right-sided heart failure, peripheral edema, enlarged liver, jugular venous distension
Gastrointestinal	Abdominal pain, nausea, malnutrition, gastrointestinal bleeding, diarrhea
Pulmonary	Wheezing
Dermatologic	Flushing, erythema, telangiectasias, mucous membranes, skin turgor

A history of frequent or protracted bouts of diarrhea suggests the possibility of fluid and electrolyte abnormalities. The patient's nutritional status should be assessed. The patient should be questioned about a history of shortness of breath, chest pain, and functional status. A history of lower extremity swelling and right upper quadrant pain should be sought.

An estimation of the preoperative fluid status can be through assessment of vital signs and any orthostatic changes (see the diabetes section of this chapter). Because bronchospasm is a component of the carcinoid syndrome, a lung examination is essential. The chest examination includes auscultation for cardiac murmurs, S_3 or S_4, and rales. Jugular venous distension (JVD), peripheral edema, and hepatomegaly should be noted.

Diagnostic Testing

Suggestions for preoperative diagnostic tests are given in Table 6.13. Although urinary 5-HIAA levels do not predict the

Table 6.13. Diagnostic tests for patients with established carcinoid tumors

Test	Rationale
Electrocardiogram	Assess dysrhythmias
Echocardiogram	Evaluate right-sided heart dysfunction and valvular abnormalities
Electrolyte panel	Abnormalities are common because of dehydration, diarrhea, and malnutrition
Prealbumin	Assessment of severity of illness and malnutrition
Imaging studies (computerized tomography, magnetic resonance imaging, radionucleotide scans, chest radiograph, bronchoscopy)	Identify location of tumor

physiologic response to surgical manipulation, the presence of elevated urinary 5-HIAA levels and carcinoid heart disease may increase perioperative morbidity and mortality (24). The anesthesiologist determines the location of the tumor through evaluation of radionucleotide or computerized tomography (CT) scans, magnetic resonance imaging (MRI), and bronchoscopy. An echocardiogram and ECG are necessary to evaluate for the presence of carcinoid heart disease and supraventricular arrhythmias.

Implications for Perioperative and Anesthetic Management

- Identify the location of the tumor and the presence of carcinoid syndrome.
- Be alert for intravascular volume depletion and electrolyte abnormalities.

Specific perioperative pharmacotherapy includes H_1 and H_2 histamine receptor blockers, ketanserin (serotonin receptor antagonist), droperidol, phenylephrine, and octreotide acetate.

PHEOCHROMOCYTOMA

Pheochromocytomas are catecholamine-secreting tumors composed of chromaffin tissue derived from the embryonic neural crest (25). The presenting feature of pheochromocytoma is typically severe, sustained, or paroxysmal hypertension, which may be accompanied by headache, palpitations, pallor, feelings of apprehension, and excessive diaphoresis. In resection of a pheochromocytoma, manipulation of the tumor releases catecholamines, causing significant hemodynamic perturbations that may result in morbidity and mortality. An excess of catecholamines can cause hyperglycemia and renal vasoconstriction, compromising renal perfusion and function. Myocardial dysfunction occurs from catecholamine-induced hypertrophic cardiomyopathy, angina, MI, CHF, hypertension, or dysrhythmias. In resection of a pheochromocytoma, manipulation of the tumor releases catecholamines, causing significant hemodynamic perturbations that may result in morbidity and mortality. Marked hemodynamic fluctuations are also possible after tumor removal (26). A multidisciplinary team including the anesthesiologist, an endocrinologist, and the surgeon should be involved in preoperative preparation.

Interview, History, and Physical Examination

Table 6.14 summarizes the important history and focus of examination for patients with pheochromocytoma. Heart rate and BP need to be assessed with orthostatic changes (see the diabetes section of this chapter). Symptoms of chest pain and shortness of breath should be sought. Auscultation of the heart for murmurs and arrhythmias and the lungs for rales is important. JVD, hepatomegaly, and peripheral edema should be noted. Simple palpation of a pheochromocytoma may precipitate a hypertensive crisis, so careful examination of the abdomen is important. The presence of other associated endocrinopathies should be investigated (Table 6.1).

Table 6.14. **Preoperative evaluation of patients with pheochromocytoma**

Cardiovascular	Palpitations, tachycardia, diaphoresis, pallor, angina, history of myocardial infarction, dyspnea, orthopnea, hypertension, heart rate, congestive heart failure (S_3 or S_4 gallop, jugular venous distention, pulmonary crackles), intravascular volume depletion (orthostatic hypotension, dry mucous membranes, poor skin turgor)
Neurologic	Headache, diaphoresis, feelings of apprehension
Gastrointestinal	Abdominal pain, nausea, malnutrition, gastrointestinal bleeding, diarrhea, palpation may precipitate a crisis

Diagnostic Testing

Table 6.15 summarizes the diagnostic tests for patients with a pheochromocytoma. The preoperative ECG of patients with a pheochromocytoma may show prolonged corrected Q-T (QTc) intervals and high QRS amplitudes reflecting ventricular hypertrophy (27). ST-segment and T-wave changes may suggest ischemia. Echocardiography is useful to detect cardiac dysfunction. The chest radiograph rules out pulmonary edema or cardiomegaly in patients with signs and symptoms of pulmonary edema or CHF. Electrolyte levels, blood urea nitrogen, creatinine, and glucose values are obtained.

Implications for Perioperative and Anesthetic Management

- A low dose of phenoxybenzamine (i.e., 10 mg twice daily) can be initiated in the outpatient setting and can be increased by 10-mg increments over the course of 10 to 14 days.
- Patients are encouraged to measure their BP in the sitting and standing position twice daily during adjustment of alpha blockade therapy.

Table 6.15. **Diagnostic tests for patients with pheochromocytoma**

Test	Rationale
Electrocardiogram	Assess heart rate, rhythm, conduction abnormalities, myocardial ischemia, ventricular hypertrophy
Echocardiogram	Evaluate ventricular function
Chest radiograph	Pulmonary edema, cardiomegaly
Electrolyte panel	Assess renal function
Blood glucose	Hyperglycemia as a monitor of stress
Complete blood count	Hematocrit to establish baseline level and monitor replacement

- Clinical endpoints for alpha blockade dosing include orthostasis, stable BP control, and elimination of symptoms.
- Published criteria for adequate α-adrenergic blockade include a BP <160/90 mmHg, orthostatic hypotension, resolution of ST-segment abnormalities, and infrequent premature ventricular contractions (28).
- Initiating beta blockade without adequately establishing alpha blockade may worsen hypertension through unopposed vasoconstriction.
- Despite the use of α- and β-adrenergic blockade, patients may still manifest significant intraoperative hemodynamic lability (26).
- Large tumors, prolonged anesthesia, and elevated urinary metabolites are associated with adverse perioperative events.
- Hemodynamic lability and arrhythmias are common.

Part of the improvement in perioperative outcomes for patients undergoing pheochromocytoma resection has been attributed to adequate α- and β-adrenergic blockade (25,26). These therapies may prevent the catecholamine surges associated with intraoperative tumor manipulation. Preoperative α- and β-adrenergic blockade can improve cardiac function (29,30).

PORPHYRIAS

The porphyrias are a collection of conditions resulting from abnormal biosynthesis of heme. Genetic defects in key enzymes lead to the accumulation of heme precursors. The porphyrias are classified by the location of the enzyme defect (hepatic or erythropoietic) or by the presence of acute symptoms (Table 6.16). Three of the subtypes—acute intermittent porphyria (AIP), variegate porphyria (VP), and hereditary coproporphyria (HCP)—have been called *inducible porphyrias* because they are associated with the precipitation of crises by anesthetic agents.

Patients with porphyrias can have photosensitivity, especially with sun exposure; abdominal pain; peripheral neuropathies; or mental disturbances. Autonomic instability and motor dysfunction may occur. Abnormalities in the cranial nerve or motor examination may suggest impending respiratory failure and an increased risk of aspiration (31,32). Some of the neurologic motor defects may take months or years to resolve. Abdominal pain is usually not proportional to clinical findings and is thought to stem from autonomic neuropathy and alternating areas of spastic and relaxed bowel (32).

Interview, History, and Physical Examination

In patients complaining of abdominal pain, nausea, and vomiting, certain associated symptoms such as confusion, anxiety, peripheral neuropathies, and red-purple urine should prompt the clinician to investigate the possibility of an undiagnosed porphyria (31). The subtype of porphyria should be characterized and clinical manifestations such as photosensitivity and neurologic abnormalities should be documented. Triggering agents should be identified.

There is no evidence of peritonitis on abdominal examination. Skin lesions should be noted.

Table 6.16.   Classification of human porphyrias

Type	Presentation	Photosensitivity	Neurovisceral Manifestations
Hepatic porphyrias			
ALA dehydratase deficiency (plumboporphyria)	Acute	−	+
Acute intermittent porphyria	Acute/inducible	−	+
Hereditary coproporphyria	Acute/inducible	+	+
Variegate porphyria	Acute/inducible	+	+
Porphyria cutanea tarda	Nonacute	+	−
Erythropoietic porphyrias			
Congenital erythropoietic porphyria	Nonacute	+	−
Erythropoietic protoporphyria	Nonacute	+	−

+ indicates yes; − indicates no.

Table 6.17. Preoperative evaluation of patients with porphyrias

Cardiovascular	Dizziness, tachycardia, blood pressure, orthostatic hypotension
Neurologic	Mental status changes, anxiety, confusion, peripheral neuropathies, cranial nerve dysfunction (bulbar symptoms), sensory and motor examination
Gastrointestinal	Abdominal pain, nausea, vomiting, abdominal examination
Dermatologic	Photosensitivity, excessive sweating, skin lesions from sun exposure, hypertrichosis
Reproductive	Pregnancy

The preoperative examination and diagnostic tests for patients with porphyrias are summarized in Tables 6.17 and 6.18.

Diagnostic Testing

Laboratory determinations include measurement of electrolyte levels. In patients who are dehydrated, blood urea nitrogen and creatinine levels are ordered to evaluate for prerenal azotemia. Porphyria exacerbations may be more frequent during pregnancy, and a pregnancy test to uncover the possibility of pregnancy should be considered.

Implications for Perioperative and Anesthetic Management

- Identify and avoid common triggering agents (Table 6.19).
- The presence of skin lesions affects positioning and choice of regional anesthesia.
- Patients are often hypovolemic and have electrolyte abnormalities in the setting of an acute attack.
- Dehydration, stress, and surgery can precipitate an attack.

Identifying anesthetic agents that trigger porphyria has been difficult, because attacks may also be caused by stress and surgery. General anesthesia can mask an acute attack of porphyria. Medicolegal concerns, however, may deter the clinician

Table 6.18. Diagnostic tests for patients with porphyria

Test	Rationale
Electrolyte panel, magnesium	Hyponatremia, hypokalemia, hypomagnesemia, and renal dysfunction possible with dehydration
Blood urea nitrogen/creatinine	Prerenal azotemia in patients at risk for intravascular volume depletion
Pregnancy test	Pregnancy has been associated with acute attacks
Electrocardiogram	Assessment of electrolyte abnormalities

Table 6.19. Common perioperative drugs implicated in precipitating attacks of porphyria

Avoid	Use With Caution
Aminophylline	Angiotensin-converting enzyme inhibitors
Amiodarone	Calcium channel blockers
Antibiotics	Dantrolene
Barbiturates	Diclofenac
Cannabis	Fluconazole
Carbamazepine	H_2 blockers
Chloramphenicol	Hydralazine
Clindamycin	Ketorolac
Clonidine	Macrolides
Dapsone	Metoclopramide
Doxycycline	Metronidazole
Ergots	Midazolam
Etomidate	Nitroprusside
Pentazocine	Odansetron
Phenytoin	Proton pump inhibitors
Sulphonamide	Pyridostigmine
Valproic acid	Quinolones
	Rifampicin
	Tetracyclines
	Theophylline

This list is not complete and is not intended as a substitute for clinical judgment. Unlisted drugs cannot be assumed to be safe. A more detailed listing of drug information and porphyrias can be found at http://www.porphyria.uct.ac.za. Accessed October 7, 2007.

from administering a regional anesthetic in patients at risk for neurologic complications of the underlying disease.

ACKNOWLEDGEMENT

The authors acknowledge and appreciate the contributions to the previous edition of this chapter by Stephanie L. Lee, M.D., Robert A. Peterfreund, M.D., and Mark Dershwitz, M.D. The authors thank Jerome Klafta, M.D., for his helpful discussion in the preparation of the section on pheochromocytomas. In addition, the authors thank Sally Kozlik for her invaluable editorial assistance.

REFERENCES

1. Beckman JA, Creager MA, Libby P. Diabetes and atherosclerosis. *JAMA.* 2002;287:2570–2581.
2. Report of the expert committee on the diagnosis and classification of diabetes mellitus. *Diabetes Care.* 2003;26(Suppl 1):S5–20.
3. Koh-Banerjee P, Wang Y, Hu FB, et al. Changes in body weight and body fat distribution as risk factors for clinical diabetes in US men. *Am J Epidemiol.* 2004;159:1150–1159.
4. Fleisher LA, Beckman JA, Brown KA, et al. ACC/AHA guidelines on perioperative cardiovascular evaluation and care for

noncardiac surgery. *J Am Coll Cardiol*. 2007;50:e159–241. www. acc.org. Accessed September 28, 2007.

5. Lee TH, Marcantonio ER, Mangione CM, et al. Derivation and prospective validation of a simple index for prediction of cardiac risk of major noncardiac surgery. *Circulation*. 1999;100:1043–1049.

6. Haffner SM, Lehto S, Ronnemaa T, et al. Mortality from coronary artery disease in subjects with type 2 diabetes and in nondiabetic subjects with and without prior myocardial infarction. *N Engl J Med*. 1998;339:229–234.

7. Executive Summary of the Third Report of the National Cholesterol Education Program (NCEP) expert panel on detection, evaluation, and treatment of high blood cholesterol in adults (Adult Treatment Panel III). *JAMA*. 2001;285:2486–2497.

8. Smiley DD, Umpierrez GE. Perioperative glucose control in the diabetic or nondiabetic patient. *South Med J*. 2006;99:580–589.

9. Selvin E, Marinopoulos S, Berkenblit G, et al. Meta-analysis: glycosylated hemoglobin and cardiovascular disease in diabetes mellitus. *Ann Intern Med*. 2004;141:421–431.

10. Dronge AS, Perkal MF, Kancir S, et al. Long-term glycemic control and postoperative infectious complications. *Arch Surg*. 2006;141:375–380.

11. Jellish WS, Kartha V, Fluder E, et al. Effect of metoclopramide on gastric fluid volumes in diabetic patients who have fasted before elective surgery. *Anesthesiology*. 2005;102:904–909.

12. Silverstein JH, Gordon G, Pollock BH, et al. Long-term glycemic control influences the onset of limited joint mobility in type 1 diabetes. *J Pediatr*. 1998;132:944–947.

13. Albers AR, Krichavsky MZ, Balady GJ. Stress testing in patients with diabetes mellitus. *Circulation*. 2006;113:583–592.

14. Ladenson PW, Levin AA, Ridgway EC, et al. Complications of surgery in hypothyroid patients. *Am J Med*. 1984;77:261–266.

15. Weinberg AD, Brennan MD, Gorman CA. Outcome of anesthesia and surgery in hypothyroid patients. *Arch Intern Med*. 1983;143:893.

16. Abbott TR. Anaesthesia in untreated myxoedema. *Br J Anaesth*. 1967;39:510–514.

17. Kim JM, Hackman L. Anesthesia for untreated hypothyroidism: report of three cases. *Anesth Analg*. 1977;56:299–302.

18. Ladenson PW, Goldenheim PD, Ridgeway EC. Prediction and reversal of blunted ventilatory responsiveness in patients with hypothyroidism. *Am J Med*. 1988;84:877–882.

19. Lind L, Ljunghall S. Pre-operative evaluation of risk factors for complications in patients with primary hyperparathyroidism. *Eur J Clin Invest*. 1995;25:955–958.

20. Piédrola G, Casado JL, López I, et al. Clinical features of adrenal insufficiency in patients with acquired immune deficiency syndrome. *Clin Endocrinol*. 1996;45:97–101.

21. Annane D, Briegel J, Sprung CL, et al. Corticosteroid insufficiency in acutely ill patients. *N Engl J Med*. 2003;348:2157–2159.

22. Rivers EP, Gaspari M, Abi Saad G. Adrenal insufficiency in high-risk surgical ICU patients. *Chest*. 2001;119:889–896.

23. Graham GW, Unger BP, Coursin DB. Perioperative management of selective endocrine disorders. *Int Anesthesiol Clin*. 2000;38:31–67.

24. Kinney MA, Warner ME, Nagorney DM, et al. Perianesthetic risks and outcomes of abdominal surgery for metastatic carcinoid tumours. *Br J Anaesth*. 2001;87:447–452.
25. Kinney MAO, Narr BJ, Warner MA. Perioperative management of pheochromocytoma. *J Cardiothorac Vasc Anesth*. 2002;16:359–369.
26. Kinney MA, Warner ME, van Heerden JA, et al. Perianesthetic risks and outcomes of pheochromocytoma and paraganglioma resection. *Anesth Analg*. 2000;91:1118–1123.
27. Stenstrom G, Swedberg K. QRS amplitudes, QTc intervals and ECG abnormalities in pheochromocytoma patients before, during, and after treatment. *Acta Med Scand*. 1988;224:231–235.
28. Roizen MF, Schreider BD, Hassan SZ. Anesthesia for patients with pheochromocytoma. *Anesthesiol Clin North Am*. 1987;5:269–275.
29. Lam JB, Shub C, Sheps SG. Reversible dilation of hypertrophied left ventricle in pheochromocytoma: serial two-dimensional echocardiographic observations. *Am Heart J*. 1985;109:613–615.
30. Nanda AS, Feldman A, Liang CS. Acute reversal of pheochromocytoma-induced catecholamine cardiomyopathy. *Clin Cardiol*. 1995;18:421–423.
31. Jensen NF, Fiddler DS, Striepe V. Anesthetic considerations in porphyrias. *Anesth Analg*. 1995;80:591–599.
32. James MFM, Hift RJ. Porphyrias. *Br J Anaesth*. 2000;85:143–153.

Hematologic Issues

Ajay Kumar and Amir K. Jaffer

Preoperative hematologic disorders are commonly encountered by the clinician performing the preoperative evaluation. Without recognition and management, they can lead to excessive bleeding or thrombosis, which can affect the patient's morbidity and mortality perioperatively. Each patient's risk of bleeding and thrombosis is determined by finding any established or undiagnosed underlying medical condition that might predispose the patient to such an increased risk. Sometimes a pre-established condition poses a challenge to the clinician. The condition may be related to the need for surgery or an unrelated chronic disease.

ANEMIA

Anemic individuals have less than the normal number of red blood cells (from underproduction, increased loss, or destruction) or less than the normal quantity of hemoglobin (Hgb) in the blood, thereby decreasing the blood's oxygen-carrying capacity. The World Health Organization has designated <13 g/dL as the cutoff value for adult men and <12 g/dL for nonpregnant women.

Anemia is the most common hematologic diagnosis among surgical patients preoperatively. Anemia is either related to the condition prompting the surgery (e.g., cancer, gastrointestinal or genitourinary bleeding, metorrhagia) or underlying medical conditions (e.g., sickle cell disease, rheumatoid arthritis, metorrhagia). The estimates of perioperative anemia prevalence vary widely, from 5% in geriatric women with hip fractures to 75.8% in patients with Duke's stage D colon cancer (1).

The prevalence of perioperative anemia varies because of differences in the definition of anemia, the types of surgeries studied, and patients' comorbidities. Preoperative anemia is associated with morbidity and mortality after surgery because blood transfusion requirements are increased as is the risk of postoperative infection (2,3). Therefore, it is prudent to delay major elective surgery and improve the patient's medical condition when preoperative anemia is discovered (Fig. 7.1).

History and Physical Examination

All patients are asked about a history of anemia during the preoperative evaluation. Patients with known anemia are questioned about the onset, previous Hgb values, symptoms, and management. Patients without an established history are asked about the following symptoms and their time of onset and duration:

- Palpitations and tachycardia, which might suggest underlying cardiovascular decompensation
- Fatigue, angina, and dyspnea, which might suggest tissue hypoxia

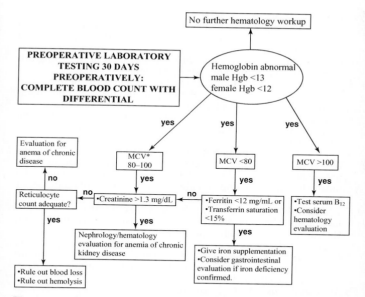

Figure 7.1. Preoperative anemia. MCV, mean corpuscular volume. (From Goodnough LT, Shander A, Spivak JL, et al. Detection, evaluation, and management of anemia in the elective surgical patient. *Anesth Analg.* 2005;101:1858–1861.)

- Bone pain, which might suggest an underlying myeloproliferative disorder or cancer
- History of blood transfusions, which might explain the circumstances surrounding previous blood loss
- Skin should be examined for pallor and petechiae
- Enlarged lymph nodes and hepatosplenomegaly, which may suggest disorders often associated with anemia

Diagnostic Tests

All patients scheduled for major elective surgery should have Hgb levels measured within 30 days of surgery. If anemia discovered preoperatively is unrelated to the condition for which surgery is to be performed, the surgery is delayed (2). The evaluation focuses on the cause for the anemia. The initial evaluation includes a complete blood count (CBC), peripheral smear, and corrected reticulocyte count, which will determine whether anemia is hyperproliferative from loss or destruction of red blood cells (RBCs) or hypoproliferative from a decrease in marrow production (e.g., anemia of chronic disease). The mean corpuscular volume (MCV) (Fig. 7.1) can help determine the etiology of anemia but additional tests (2) such as the following may be necessary:

- Iron (Fe) and total iron binding capacity (TIBC) or transferrin. Fe and TIBC are low with anemia from chronic disease. Fe is low and TIBC is high with iron deficiency anemia. Patients >50 years of age usually need a gastrointestinal (GI) workup with upper endoscopy (EGD) and colonoscopy. Subsequent repletion with iron such as ferrous sulfate 325 mg orally may be needed two or three times daily.

- Ferritin. Ferritin levels of <30 ng/mL in men and <10 ng/mL in women suggest iron deficiency anemia.
- Serum B_{12} and RBC folate levels. Low levels of B_{12} or folate can lead to macrocytic anemia. Patients need vitamin supplementation to correct the underlying anemia.
- Hemoccult testing is necessary to document blood loss from the GI tract, but false-positive and -negative results are common with this test.
- Type and screen (T&S) provide information about the patient's blood type and the presence of red cell antibodies. If the antibody screen is positive, additional tests are performed to identify the antibodies present and to rule out other clinically significant antibodies to red cell antigens. These tests may be completed within a few hours or may take days if sent out to a reference laboratory. Completion time and blood availability depends on the number of antibodies present, antibody reactivity, and frequency of the corresponding antigen in the donor population. Once clinically significant antibodies are identified, national standards require the blood bank to provide antigen-negative, crossmatch-compatible units for transfusion.
- Type and cross (T&C) is an order for a T&S plus a request for a specified number of RBC units. Depending on the results of the T&S, units may be readily available (no clinically significant antibodies identified) or may require special screening for antigen-negative units (when clinically significant antibodies are identified).

We recommend comprehensive, multifaceted blood conservation to achieve optimal outcomes for elective noncardiac surgery (Fig. 7.2). This method starts with identifying the cause of anemia

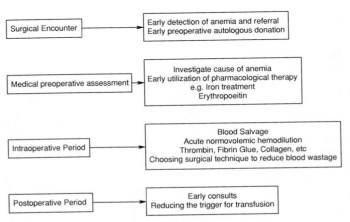

Figure 7.2. Multifaceted approach to perioperative blood conservation.

and treating it before surgery. Erythropoietin-α may be a preoperative option for anemia of chronic disease in patients with Hgb <13 g/dL for noncardiac, nonvascular surgery such as major joint replacement. Intraoperatively several blood salvage techniques are also available for blood conservation (Fig. 7.2).

ASSESSMENT OF BLEEDING RISK

To determine the preoperative risk of bleeding, questions (4) are asked regarding the following:

- Excessive bruising
- Bleeding after brushing teeth
- Nose bleeds
- Prolonged bleeding after cuts
- Severe prolonged menstrual periods
- History of occult or frank blood loss through the GI or genitourinary tract
- Excessive bleeding after dental extraction, surgery, or childbirth
- History of hemophilia or a coinherited familial hematologic disorder
- Personal history of liver disease, renal failure, hypersplenism, or hematologic or collagen vascular disease
- Current or recent use of medications that may interfere with hemostasis

The physical examination focuses on signs of petechiae, purpura, hematomas, jaundice, and cirrhosis, which alert the clinician that postoperative bleeding may be an issue.

For patients who do not have risk factors such as coagulopathy, history of liver disease, malabsorption, malnutrition, trauma, or hemorrhage, the overall risk of postoperative hemorrhage and death is extremely low. In high-risk patients (i.e., patients with one of the above criteria), the risk of postoperative hemorrhage is 10-fold higher, but the risk of death is still extremely low (4).

The prothrombin time (PT), activated partial thromboplastin time (aPTT), and platelet counts are highly reproducible and automated. These tests were not designed to determine the risk of perioperative bleeding, but rather to detect factor deficiencies. In general, the PT and aPTT do not predict postoperative hemorrhage. The platelet count, however, may be useful. It can be low in certain diseases such as cirrhosis or be normal but dysfunctional in patients with end-stage renal disease (ESRD). Routine testing of PT, aPTT, and platelet count is not recommended or cost effective without findings on history or physical examination of bleeding or thrombosis.

An elevated aPTT can be the result of a *hyper-* or a *hypo*coagulable state. A common cause of a prolonged aPTT is exposure of the patient to heparin and can be determined from the patient history. A prolonged aPTT can result from factor deficiencies or inhibitors, or circulating anticoagulants. A mixing study, where blood from the patient with the prolonged aPTT is combined with blood from a patient with normal coagulation, can further aid in diagnosis. Circulating anticoagulants or factor inhibitors do not allow the correction of aPTT during mixing studies; deficiencies will be supplied by the normal blood and the aPTT will correct. Lupus anticoagulants and antiphospholipid antibodies do not cause bleeding but increase the risk for arterial or venous thrombotic events. Factor VIII inhibitors can cause life-threatening hemorrhage perioperatively. Laboratory analysis is usually diagnostic for anticardiolipin antibodies and anti-β_2 glycoprotein-1 antibodies. The dilute Russell viper venom time is the most sensitive for lupus anticoagulants. Factor VIII inhibitors take 2 to 3 hours and lupus anticoagulant and antiphospholipid antibodies work much more rapidly during mixing studies. In summary, risk for postoperative bleeding is better correlated with positive history and physical examination than with screening tests. Patients with isolated elevated aPTT need a repeat aPTT. Then mixing studies are performed followed by measurement of ristocetin cofactor activity and von Willebrand factor (vWF) antigen levels.

The result of the bleeding time test is technician dependent and affected by drugs the patient may be taking. It correlates poorly with postoperative bleeding. There is no role for ordering a bleeding time perioperatively and many institutions no longer perform this test.

SICKLE CELL ANEMIA

Sickle cell anemia or sickle cell disease (SCD) is usually a chronic, well-compensated hemolytic anemia with an appropriate reticulocytosis. Vaso-occlusive phenomena and hemolysis are the clinical hallmarks of SCD, an inherited disorder caused by homozygosity for the abnormal Hgb, hemoglobin S (HgbS). Vaso-occlusion results in recurrent painful episodes and a variety of serious organ system complications that can lead to lifelong disabilities or early death. The disorder is most severe in patients with SCD (homozygosity for HgbS), of intermediate severity in hemoglobin SC disease (HgbSC, combined heterozygosity for hemoglobins S and C), and generally benign in those with sickle cell trait (heterozygosity for HgbS).

Patients with SCD are generally considered at risk for perioperative complications even without known cardiopulmonary disease. These problems may arise from perioperative hypoxia, hypoperfusion, and acidosis, which cause erythrocytes to sickle, thus precipitating vaso-occlusion and organ dysfunction.

Although an optimal level of Hgb is not known, perioperative transfusion has been utilized routinely during intermediate- and high-risk surgery in these patients. The Cooperative Study of Sickle Cell Disease observed 3,765 patients with a mean follow-up of 5.3 ± 2.0 years. It concluded that surgery was safe in patients with SCD and preoperative transfusion was beneficial for all surgical risk levels, although in most patients who had low-risk surgery and did not receive blood transfusions, complication rates were low (5).

When two regimens were compared in 604 surgical procedures in patients with SCD, a conservative transfusion regimen (correcting anemia to 10 g/dL and decreasing HgbS to about 60%) was as effective as an aggressive regimen (reducing HgbS to 30% or less) in preventing perioperative complications. The conservative approach resulted in half as many transfusion-associated complications. The recommendation from the study was that all patients with SCD who need major surgery be prepared in advance with transfusion to correct their anemia to an Hgb of approximately 10 g/dL and HgbS to approximately 60% (6).

GLUCOSE-6-PHOSPHATE DEHYDROGENASE DEFICIENCY

Glucose-6-phosphate dehydrogenase (G6PD) deficiency is an X-linked inherited disease. Hemolysis results after exposure to infections, drugs, and certain substances (antipyretics, sulfanil-amides, nitrates, antimalarials) that produce peroxide and cause oxidation of Hgb and RBC membranes and lead to Heinz body formation. The severity of hemolysis depends on the amount of the offending agent and enzymatic activity in the patient. During surgery, hypoxia, sustained mechanical ventilation, and need for blood and blood products increase the risk for hemolysis. Autoantibody-coated erythrocytes rapidly undergo destruction in the reticuloendothelial system in autoimmune hemolytic anemia. This destruction leads to severe hemolysis. This disease, a Coombs (+) hemolytic anemia, responds well to steroids. Steroid drugs should be instituted until signs of hemolysis disappear. In patients with sustained hemolysis despite steroid therapy, splenectomy is advocated. Normothermia is maintained because hypothermia is a known trigger for hemolysis. In the postoperative period, patients are monitored for hemolysis with regular Hgb and haptoglobin levels. Patients with ongoing postoperative hemolysis should receive steroids (7).

HEMOPHILIA

Hemophilias are a group of inherited coagulation disorders including those with deficiencies of factors VIII and IX. Factor VIII deficiency (hemophilia A) and factor IX deficiency (hemophilia B or Christmas disease) are X-linked recessive diseases. They exhibit a range of clinical severity that correlates well with assayed factor levels. Patients with hemophilia have a prolonged aPTT and a normal PT. Even mild trauma experienced in daily life makes them bleed. Bleeding deep in the tissues is often severe enough to require urgent fasciotomy of extremities or craniotomy for a rapidly expanding hematoma. Recurrent hemarthrosis may require corrective or palliative procedures because of destructive changes in joints. Approximately 50% of operations in hemophiliacs are orthopedic (8).

Hemophilia A occurs almost exclusively in males. The incidence of hemophilia A is 1 in 10,000, and it accounts for 85% of patients with hemophilia. The severity of the bleeding varies from kindred to kindred, but within a given family relatives are likely to be affected similarly. The severity of bleeding relates directly to the degree of factor VIII deficiency.

The fragility of the hemophilic clot, which may undergo premature fibrinolysis causing rebleeding, delayed wound healing, and thus impaired outcome, is a challenge to surgical intervention in the hemophilic patient. Ideally a hematologist should be involved in the perioperative care and preparation of such patients prior to surgery. Surgical preparation includes detailed coagulation tests along with blood typing as outlined in Table 7.1. A detailed factor replacement plan needs to be in place before surgery based on the

Table 7.1. Required preoperative testing in a hemophiliac

- Platelet count
- Platelet aggregation with agonists
- Activated partial thromboplastin time
- Prothrombin time
- Factor levels
- Inhibitor testing
- Fibrinogen
- Factor response recording

response to recovery time. The program should include the dosing schedule during the rehabilitation period. Factors VIII and IX levels should be closely monitored from postoperative day 1 and maintained at 75% to 100% for 72 hours after surgery and at 50% until healing is complete, which usually takes about 2 weeks. Recombinant or purified factor concentrates are infused and peak and trough levels are monitored to modify the doses as needed. It is estimated that each unit of factor concentrate increases the factor levels by 2% per kilogram. Intramuscular injections are avoided in hemophiliacs to prevent hematoma formation. Venous thromboembolism (VTE) prophylaxis may be offered to hemophiliacs if their factors are adequately replaced (8).

VON WILLEBRAND DISEASE

von Willebrand disease is caused by qualitative and quantitative deficiencies in factor VIII. Factor VIII and the vWF circulate as a complex. The disease has autosomal dominant (types 1, 2A, and 2B) and recessive (type 3) modes of inheritance and affects both genders (Table 7.2). In the majority of cases, vWD is identified as a result of bleeding episodes in childhood. Use of aspirin in vWD markedly increases hemostatic defects. Clinically significant vWD is almost always associated with a prolonged aPTT but a normal PT. Mild cases may have a normal aPTT. Levels of vWF increase during acute reactions, which can mask the laboratory diagnosis. If the patient experiences only mild bleeding and frequent bruising, this deficiency may be unsuspected (4,9,10).

A von Willebrand panel includes a test for ristocetin cofactor (a functional assay for vWF, the presence of which leads to platelet aggregation when the antibiotic ristocetin is added), a test for vWF antigen (an immunologic test), and a factor VIII activity level. Many forms of vWD exist because of quantitative and qualitative differences in the vWF produced (Table 7.2). The distinction of various subtypes is essential for determining appropriate therapy.

Desmopressin (desmopressin acetate, or 1-desamino-8-D-arginine vasopressin [DDAVP]) is useful in patients with hemophilia A and vWD type 1. Desmopressin increases endothelial cell release of factor VIII, vWF, and plasminogen activator. An intravenous dose of 0.3 μg/kg in 50 mL of saline can produce a prompt threefold to fourfold increase in vWF activity. Desmopressin should be given slowly (over 15 to 30 minutes) to avoid

Table 7.2.   Types of von Willebrand disease

Type	Characteristics	Treatment
1	80% of cases; quantitative defect	Desmopressin[a]
2A	Abnormal multimer pattern; quantitative and qualitative defect	Desmopressin[a]
2B	Rare; abnormal multimer pattern; quantitative and qualitative defect; autosomal dominant	Desmopressin[a] may produce thrombocytopenia
2M	Qualitative defect; normal multimer pattern	Desmopressin[a]
2N	Qualitative defect; vWF levels are normal; only factor VIII is reduced	Desmopressin[a] effect may be too short lived
3	Rare; low to nondetectable levels of vWF	Desmopressin[a] usually not effective

vWF, von Willebrand factor.
[a]Desmopressin acetate (DDAVP). With type 2B or when desmopressin acetate is not effective, vWF-containing factor VIII concentrates or cryoprecipitate may be used instead.

hypotension, flushing, tachycardia, and headache. The goal is to raise vWF to 80 to 100 U/dL, replace abnormal vWF, and raise levels of factor VIII. Administration of desmopressin results in considerable variation in vWF levels. The response pattern in individual patients can be determined by infusing desmopressin and following the change in factor VIII and vWF. A nasal spray of desmopressin delivering a dose of 150 μg into each nostril may be useful in patients with vWD. Desmopressin probably should not be used more frequently than every 48 hours because depletion of endothelial stores may cause tachyphylaxis. Epsilon-aminocaproic acid (4 g orally every 4 hours) or tranexamic acid (1.5 g orally every 8 hours) should be given to counteract the release of plasminogen activator by desmopressin (4,9,10).

If cryoprecipitate is infused, then the response is monitored by measuring a ristocetin cofactor activity level. The goal is to increase the ristocetin cofactor activity level to more than 50%. Treatment is repeated every 12 hours until clinical bleeding is controlled. Many factor VIII concentrates do not provide effective therapy for vWD because they do not contain vWF. Humate-P has been approved by the U.S. Food and Drug Administration for use in patients with vWD (4,9,10).

Administration of desmopressin may be dangerous for patients with type 2B vWD because an increase in abnormal vWF may cause increased binding to platelets, resulting in removal of platelets and thrombocytopenia. Abnormal vWF can be replaced with normal vWF using cryoprecipitate or factor VIII concentrates that contain vWF. The fibrinolytic inhibitor epsilon-aminocaproic acid may be used, especially in circumstances in which local fibrinolysis can be expected, such as dental extraction (9,10).

THROMBOCYTOPENIA

Thrombocytopenia is defined as a platelet count of <150,000/mm^3. Thrombocytopenia from inherited disorders generally defines the bleeding symptoms, but this cause is rare. The causes of thrombocytopenia include decreased production, sequestration, or increased destruction of platelets (Table 7.3).

Table 7.3. Causes of thrombocytopenia

Decreased production
Congenital
  Bernard-Soulier syndrome (loss of glycoprotein 1b)
  Alport syndrome
  May-Hegglin anomaly
  Wiskott-Aldrich syndrome

Acquired
  Bone marrow infiltration
    Metastatic cancers
    Myelofibrosis
  Ineffective thrombopoiesis
    Folate, B$_{12}$, or iron deficiency
    Myelodysplastic syndrome

Increased destruction
Idiopathic
Drugs
  Immune mechanism
    For example, penicillin, digitalis derivatives, sulfa
      compounds, quinine, quinidine phenytoin, heparin,
      ampicillin
  Nonimmune mechanism
    For example, ticlopidine, mitomycin, cisplatin,
      cyclosporine

Drugs that alter platelet function
    For example, nonsteroidal anti-inflammatory agents,
      β-lactam antibiotics, heparin, isoniazid, penicillin,
      aminoglycosides

Autoimmune
  Chronic lymphocytic leukemia
  Systemic lupus erythematosus
  Thyroid disease
  Hypogammaglobulinemia
  Antiphospholipid syndrome
  Posttransfusion purpura
  Sepsis

Nonimmune
  Preeclampsia
  Hemolytic-uremic syndrome
  Thrombotic thrombocytopenic purpura
  Cardiopulmonary bypass
  Disseminated intravascular coagulation

In otherwise healthy patients, pseudothrombocytopenia from platelet agglutination caused by ethylenediaminetetraacetic acid (EDTA) should always be ruled out. EDTA is a chelating agent that is widely used to sequester di- and trivalent metal ions in blood collection tubes when CBC is determined. The workup for thrombocytopenia includes a peripheral smear examination (Fig. 7.3). A preoperative finding of thrombocytopenia is investigated and corrected because it poses a risk of bleeding inversely related to the platelet count. Surgery can generally proceed when levels are >50,000/mm^3 as long as platelets are supplemented as needed. In general, neuroaxial blockade is contraindicated at levels <100,000/mm^3. For a given platelet count, the risk of bleeding increases when anemia, fever, infection, or a platelet function defect (e.g., use of aspirin or nonsteroidal anti-inflammatory drugs [NSAIDs]) coexist. In consumptive disorders caused by drugs, discontinuation of the drug should lead to a normal platelet count within 5 to 10 days. If thrombocytopenia is caused by disseminated intravascular coagulation (DIC), treatment should be directed at the underlying disease (11).

Idiopathic (autoimmune) thrombocytopenic purpura (ITP) in adults is usually a chronic disorder of insidious onset. It is characterized by a reduced platelet count, increased peripheral destruction of platelets, and augmented platelet production. Autoantibodies, which are produced against platelets and possibly against megakaryocytes, lead to the phagocytic destruction of platelets. The diagnosis of ITP is based solely on clinical criteria because platelet antibody studies and bone marrow aspiration are of uncertain value. The history, physical examination, and peripheral blood smear can exclude most alternatives (11).

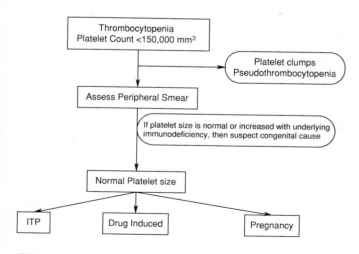

ITP = idiopathic thrombocytopenic purpura

Figure 7.3. Algorithm for investigation of isolated thrombocytopenia in a healthy person. ITP, idiopathic thrombocytopenic purpura.

The treatment of chronic ITP is supportive, not curative, and is directed toward the inactivation or removal of the major site of platelet destruction and antiplatelet antibody production, the spleen. Corticosteroids prevent sequestration of antibody-coated platelets by the spleen and probably impair antibody production. Gamma globulin or platelet transfusions are used in urgent situations.

Thrombocytopenia in the presence of heparin should raise concerns for heparin-induced thrombocytopenia (HIT), which usually occurs within 5 to 10 days after initiation of heparin. Approximately 30% of cases occur within 24 hours after initiation of heparin. This condition is often referred to as rapid-onset HIT. Patients who experience rapid-onset HIT usually have had exposure to heparin within the previous 30 days. Some of the associated complications include arterial thromboses, deep venous thrombosis (DVT), pulmonary emboli (PE), cerebral sinus thrombosis, and thromboses of arteriovenous (AV) fistulas. Arterial thrombosis seems more common in patients with cardiovascular disease such as stroke, myocardial infarction (MI), and cardiac thromboses. The overall risk of HIT depends on the type of heparin and patient characteristics. It can be catastrophic if undiagnosed or untreated; up to 30% of patients die. An additional 10% to 20% of patients will require an amputation. Half of all patients with HIT will have a thrombosis in 30 days. Treatment of HIT is immediate discontinuation of heparin. Alternative anticoagulants include the heparinoid drug danaparoid sodium, as well as direct thrombin inhibitors such as lepirudin and argatroban. Low-molecular-weight heparin (LMWH) use is contraindicated if HIT is suspected (12,13).

THROMBOCYTOSIS

Thrombocytosis, defined as a platelet count of $>500,000/mm^3$, may be physiologic (exercise, parturition, epinephrine), primary (a myeloproliferative disorder with increased platelet production independent of normal regulatory control), or secondary (associated with iron deficiency or neoplastic, chronic inflammatory, and postoperative states). The platelet count usually returns to normal with treatment of the underlying disorder. Patients with polycythemia vera or essential thrombocythemia (primary thrombocytosis) (5,6) have an increased risk of thrombotic or bleeding events, respectively. The risk of thrombosis and hemorrhage seems to be increased in older patients and those with prior thrombotic or hemorrhagic events. Use of aspirin may worsen the hemorrhagic tendency. No specific platelet count is predictive of hemorrhage or thrombosis. The most common sites of hemorrhage are mucosal surfaces; the most common thrombotic events are mesenteric and deep vein thromboses; PE; and cerebral, coronary, and peripheral arterial occlusions. Secondary thrombocytosis rarely leads to platelet count $>1,000,000/mm^3$, and the cause may be obvious from the history, physical examination, or radiologic or blood testing. Treatment of the underlying disorder usually returns the platelet count to normal. Thromboembolic events are rare in patients with secondary thrombocytosis or chronic myelogenous leukemia. Plateletpheresis has been used (e.g., in serious hemorrhage or thrombosis; before an emergency operation); however, it is rarely necessary. Because the half-life of platelets is 7 days, medical therapy with hydroxyurea and anagrelide does not provide an immediate effect.

THROMBOPHILIAS

Pathogenesis for VTE is multifactorial, often involving acquired or environmental risk factors as well as genetic predisposition. These risk factors can be a circulatory (stasis), an endothelial (vessel wall injury), or a hypercoagulable state (changes in composition of blood). Hypercoagulability, which can be inherited or acquired, is sometimes called thrombophilia. Routine preoperative screening for hypercoagulability in the asymptomatic individual is not useful (4); however, in the setting of a previously experienced VTE and known thrombophilia (such as factor V Leiden, prothrombin gene mutation, protein C or protein S deficiency), patients receive aggressive pharmacologic prophylaxis with either unfractionated heparin (UFH) 5,000 U SC three times daily, LMWH such as enoxaparin 40 mg SC once daily or dalteparin SC 5,000 U once daily, or fondaparinux 2.5 mg SC once daily (14). If patients will undergo major surgery, extended prophylaxis for 4 weeks can be entertained. Patients with history of antiphospholipid antibodies taking long-term therapy will need bridging therapy with UFH or LMWH as discussed in a subsequent section.

PREVENTION OF VENOUS THROMBOEMBOLISM

During the routine preoperative evaluation, the risk of postoperative VTE should be estimated using both *patient- and surgery-specific* factors. The most recent guidelines of the American College of Chest Physicians (ACCP) stratify patients based on both factors (14). Their four risk categories for postoperative VTE are as follows:

Low risk: Patients who need minor surgery, are <40 years old, and have no additional risk factors for VTE

Moderate risk: Patients who need minor surgery and have additional risk factors, or need major surgery, are 40 to 60 years old, and have no additional risk factors

High risk: Patients >60 years of age who need major surgery and have no other risk factors or patients who need major surgery, are 40 to 60 years old, and have additional risk factors

Highest risk: Patients with multiple risk factors who need major surgery, or patients who need surgeries with the highest risk: Hip or knee arthroplasty, hip-fracture surgery, pelvic or abdominal cancer surgery, major trauma surgery, or surgery for spinal cord injury

Risk factors for VTE include advanced age (>40 years), prior VTE, obesity, heart failure, paralysis, cancer, and the presence of a molecular hypercoagulable state (e.g., protein C deficiency, factor V Leiden) (14).

The nonpharmacologic options to prevent VTE include the following:

• Ambulation for all patients as soon as possible after surgery

- Elastic compression stockings for low-risk patients or stockings in combination with pharmacologic measures for higher-risk patients
- Intermittent pneumatic compression devices alone in high-risk surgical patients; the fit must be proper and devices must be maintained on the patient for ~15 hours a day for maximal benefit

These modalities may be used in those patients at high risk for bleeding after major surgery (e.g., after craniotomy or spine surgery). Additionally, they are often used in combination with pharmacologic prophylaxis in the highest-risk patients (14).

The pharmacologic options to prevent VTE include the following:

- **Aspirin,** which inhibits platelet aggregation, is not very effective for prophylaxis against VTE. The ACCP guidelines recommend *against* its use as the single prophylactic agent.
- **Unfractionated heparin**, which inhibits factors II and X, is inexpensive but has a short half-life requiring SC dosing two to three times daily for maximal benefit. The anticoagulant effect can be easily reversed with protamine if needed. Use of UFH carries a significant risk of HIT (~3% in the postoperative setting).
- **Warfarin** (Coumadin) inhibits vitamin K–dependent clotting factors II, VII, IX, and X. It is inexpensive and can be administered orally. It requires monitoring with an international normalized ratio (INR), interacts with multiple drugs and foods, and has a narrow therapeutic index. It takes approximately 5 days to achieve maximal anticoagulant effect; therefore, patients are at increased risk for VTE while the INR is subtherapeutic.
- **Low-molecular-weight heparins** are derived from UFH through a chemical process. They preferentially inhibit factor X more than factor II. They are well absorbed from subcutaneous tissue and can be administered one to two times daily. They are cleared by the kidneys and cause less HIT compared to UFH. Although they cost more than the generic drugs such as UFH and warfarin, they may be more cost effective because less intensive monitoring is required. Enoxaparin (Lovenox) can be used for patients with renal insufficiency with creatinine clearances of <30 mL/minute as long as the patient does not have end-stage renal disease on dialysis by decreasing the recommended dose from 40 mg SC once daily to 30 mg SC once daily.
- **Fondaparinux** (Arixtra) is a synthetic pentasaccharide that inhibits factor X, has a long half-life of 18 hours, and is administered once daily SC. It has a rapid onset of action, but the anticoagulant effect cannot be easily reversed in case of severe bleeding. Cleared by the kidneys, the drug is contraindicated in patients with creatinine clearances <30 mL/minute. It does not cause HIT. It is best to start this drug at least 12 hours after surgery but generally it is started 18 to 24 hours after surgery to minimize the risk of bleeding.

We recommend the use of the ACCP guidelines for VTE prophylaxis. These are outlined in Table 7.4.

Table 7.4. Recommendations for venous thromboembolism prevention for patients according to type of surgery

Type of Surgery	Type of Prophylaxis[a]	Duration
Low-risk general surgery	Early mobilization	Until ambulation or discharge
Moderate-risk general surgery	UFH 5,000 U SC bid or LMWH	Until ambulation or discharge
High-risk general surgery	UFH 5,000 U SC tid or LMWH plus IPC or GCS	Until ambulation or discharge, but up to 28 days in major abdominal or pelvic cancer surgery is preferred
Vascular surgery	UFH 5,000 U SC bid or tid or LMWH	Until ambulation or discharge
Laparoscopic gynecologic surgery >30 min	UFH 5,000 U SC tid or LMWH plus IPC or GCS	Until ambulation or discharge
Major gynecologic surgery	UFH 5,000 U SC tid or LMWH plus IPC or GCS	Until ambulation or discharge
Urologic surgery other than low risk	UFH 5,000 U SC tid or LMWH plus IPC or GCS	Until ambulation or discharge
Major joint arthroplasty (e.g., total knee or hip)	LMWH or warfarin or fondaparinux	At least 10 days; up to 28–35 days is preferred
Hip fracture surgery	Fondaparinux or LMWH or warfarin	At least 10 days and up to 28 days is preferred
Neurosurgery • Extracranial • Intracranial	IPC ± GCS IPC ± GCS; LMWH or UFH can be added if bleeding risk is acceptable	Until ambulation or discharge

[a]LMWH dosing = enoxaparin 40 mg SC qd, dalteparin 5,000 IU SC qd, tinzaparin 75 IU/kg qd, or fondaparinux 2.5 mg SC qd.
bid, twice daily; GCS, graded compression stocking; IPC, intermittent pneumatic compression; LMWH, low-molecular-weight heparin; qd, every day; tid, three times daily; UFH, unfractionated heparin.
Adapted from Geerts WH, Pineo GF, Heit JA, et al. Prevention of venous thromboembolism: the Seventh ACCP Conference on Antithrombotic and Thrombolytic Therapy. *Chest.* 2004;126(3 Suppl):338S–400S.

PERIOPERATIVE MANAGEMENT
OF ANTITHROMBOTIC THERAPY

Aspirin irreversibly inhibits cyclooxygenase-1 (COX-1) by acetylating a serine residue at position 530. The inhibition prevents the conversion of arachidonate to the unstable prostaglandin (PG) intermediate PGH_2, which is converted to thromboxane (Tx) TxA_2, a potent vasoconstrictor and platelet agonist. Aspirin has a half-life of 15 to 20 minutes and irreversibly inhibits platelets, an effect that persists for 7 to 10 days, which approximates platelet lifespan. Therefore, it should be discontinued 7 to 10 days before surgery if the risk of bleeding outweighs the benefits of aspirin administration. Anytime a drug is discontinued before surgery or a procedure, the risks and benefits must be weighed against each other, including the indication for the therapy (15) (Table 7.5).

Ticlopidine and clopidogrel are thienopyridine derivatives that are prodrugs, which must be metabolized in the liver to active metabolites. These irreversibly inactivate the platelet adenosine phosphate (ADP) receptor $P2Y_{12}$, one of the two G-protein–coupled receptors that are expressed on the platelet membrane. The combined action of the receptors is necessary for a full activation and aggregation response to stimulation by ADP. Since both these drugs irreversibly inhibit platelets, they must be interrupted 7 to 10 days before surgery (15) (Table 7.5). Chapter 3 includes a detailed discussion of the risks of discontinuing aspirin and the thienopyridines in patients with recent coronary stent placements.

Dipyridamole, a pyrimidopyrimidine derivative with antiplatelet and vasodilator properties, is often combined with aspirin (200 mg dipyridamole + 25 mg aspirin) in a formulation called Aggrenox. The formulation is indicated for secondary stroke prevention in patients with cerebrovascular disease. Dipyridamole has reversible effects on platelet function and has an elimination half-life of approximately 10 hours. If dipyridamole is combined with aspirin, the combination is discontinued 7 to 10 days before elective surgery to eliminate the antiplatelet effects (15) (Table 7.5).

Nonselective NSAIDs reversibly inhibit platelet cyclooxygenase, affecting platelet function. They affect renal prostaglandin synthesis and can potentially induce renal failure in combination with other drugs and hypotension. However, the COX-2 inhibitors (e.g., celecoxib) have much less effect on platelet function. In vitro studies show no increased risk of bleeding with the COX-2 agents. Therefore, we recommend discontinuing the nonselective agents at least 3 days before surgery and continuing the COX-2–selective NSAIDs. To ensure that there is no residual antiplatelet effect at the time of surgery, the NSAID should be stopped at a time that corresponds to five times its elimination half-life. For NSAIDs with a short half-life (2 to 6 hours, such as ibuprofen, diclofenac, ketoprofen, and indomethacin), treatment should be stopped about 2 days before surgery. For NSAIDs with an intermediate half-life (7 to 15 hours, e.g., naproxen, sulindac, and diflunisal), treatment should be stopped 3 to 4 days before surgery. Finally, for NSAIDs with longer half-lives (e.g., meloxicam, nabumetone, and piroxicam),

Table 7.5. Medication management before surgery

Drug	Mode of Action	Discontinue
Aspirin[a] Ticlopidine and clopidogrel[b]	Inhibits cyclooxygenase-1 and interferes with prostaglandin synthesis Irreversibly inactivate the platelet adenosine phosphate (ADP) receptor $P2Y_{12}$, one of the two G-protein–coupled receptors that are expressed on the platelet membrane. Their combined action is necessary for a full activation and aggregation response to stimulation by ADP.	7 days before surgery 7 days before surgery
Dipyridamole	Inhibits platelet function	
Heparin, unfractionated (UFH)	Inhibition of thrombin requires simultaneous binding of heparin to antithrombin-III (AT-III) through the unique pentasaccharide sequence and binding to thrombin through a minimum of 13 additional saccharide units. Inhibition of factor Xa (Xa) requires binding heparin to AT-III through the unique pentasaccharide without the additional requirements for binding to Xa.	7 days before surgery 4–6 hours before surgery
Warfarin	Depletes vitamin K–dependent factors II, VII, IX, and X and proteins C and S	5 days before surgery[c]
Low-molecular-weight heparin (LMWH)	Like UFH, LMWHs produce their major anticoagulant effect by activating AT. The interaction with AT is mediated by a unique pentasaccharide sequence found on less than one third of LMWH molecules. Since a minimum chain length of 18 saccharides (including the pentasaccharide sequence) is required to form ternary complexes among heparin, AT, and thrombin, only the minority of LMWH species are available to inactivate thrombin. In contrast, all LMWH chains containing the high-affinity pentasaccharide catalyze the inactivation of factor Xa.	24 hours before surgery

[a]The risk of bleeding with continuation of aspirin must be balanced with the risk of thrombosis in patients with vascular disease (see Chapters 3 and 17).
[b]Patients on clopidogrel for drug-eluting stents are advised to have elective surgery delayed if possible for at least 12 months; refer to Chapters 3 and 17 for more details.[17]
[c]Patients with mechanical heart valves, atrial fibrillation and multiple risk factors, or recent or recurrent thromboembolism require bridging with heparin or LMWH.

treatment should be stopped 10 days before surgery (15) (Table 7.5).

Perioperative management of patients taking warfarin is often problematic. Warfarin doses must be discontinued or adjusted to avoid excessive bleeding. If the procedure is minor, warfarin can be continued without alteration in dose (Table 7.6). In most cases, warfarin must be discontinued 5 days before surgery to achieve a preoperative INR <1.5. For neurosurgical procedures, cardiac procedures, and some major noncardiac procedures, an INR <1.2 may be preferred. If the patient is elderly, more time may be required for the INR to drop below 1.5.

If the procedure is emergent, then fresh frozen plasma (FFP) and/or vitamin K is used to lower the INR and reverse the effects of warfarin. FFP works immediately and does not affect anticoagulation with warfarin after the procedure. After FFP administration, the INR is monitored at least every few hours to determine the need for additional treatment, because the effects of FFP will dissipate over a few hours. FFP treatment incurs the risks of blood component transfusion.

Recombinant activated factor VII (NovoSeven) may also be useful for the emergent reversal of the warfarin effect without the

Table 7.6.   Safe procedures for patients taking warfarin (no need to discontinue)

Dental
Restorations
Endodontics
Prosthetics
Uncomplicated extractions
Dental hygiene treatment
Periodontal therapy

Gastrointestinal
Upper endoscopy with or without biopsy
Flexible sigmoidoscopy with or without biopsy
Colonoscopy with or without biopsy
Endoscopic retrograde cholangiopancreatography without
     sphincterotomy
Biliary stent insertion without sphincterotomy
Endoscopic ultrasound without fine-needle aspiration
Push enteroscopy of the small bowel

Electroconvulsive therapy

Ophthalmologic
Cataract extractions
Trabeculectomies

Dermatologic
Mohs skin surgery
Simple excisions and repairs

Orthopedic
Joint aspiration
Soft tissue injections
Minor foot procedures

risks of transfusion; however, data are limited and the drug is very expensive.

Vitamin K can also reverse the effects of warfarin. Reversal usually begins 15 minutes after intravenous administration and peaks in 4 to 8 hours. In the case of surgeries that will be performed within 24 hours, it may be best to administer vitamin K intravenously in small doses of 1 to 2 mg. If surgery is not planned within 24 hours, 1 to 2 mg orally is effective.

When warfarin is discontinued, it can place patients at risk for thromboembolism (TE). Knowing why a patient is taking warfarin helps to individualize perioperative management. There are no randomized clinical trials that identify the patients who should receive bridging therapy; however, there are multiple observational trials. Based on the patient's estimated risk of thromboembolism (Table 7.7), either UFH or LMWH can be used as a "bridge" for anticoagulation during the time warfarin is subtherapeutic.

Table 7.7.   Preoperative risk stratification to determine risk of thromboembolism

High risk: Bridging advised
- Venous or arterial thromboembolism within the preceding 3 mo
- Mechanical heart valve
  - In the mitral position
  - Any position with placement in the preceding 3 mo
  - Older valves (tilting disk, cage-ball)
  - Multiple valves
- History of thromboembolism and known hypercoagulable state
  - Antiphospholipid antibody
  - Homozygous factor V Leiden
  - Multiple genetic defects
  - Protein C or S deficiency
- Acute intracardiac thrombus
- Atrial fibrillation
  - With history of stroke, transient ischemic attack (TIA), or systemic embolism
  - Associated with rheumatic valve disease
  - With mechanical valve
  - With multiple risk factors[a] for stroke

Moderate risk: Bridging on a case-by-case basis
- Newer mechanical aortic valve (bileaflet)
- Atrial fibrillation with single risk factor[a]
- Venous thromboembolism
  - Within the past 3–6 mo
  - Idiopathic

Low risk: Bridging not recommended
- Venous thromboembolism
  - >6 mo ago
  - Heterozygous factor V Leiden
- Atrial fibrillation without risk factors[a]

[a]AF risk factors include congestive heart failure, rheumatic heart disease, prior thromboembolic stroke or TIA, age >75 yr, diabetes, or hypertension.

For patients with a history of VTE, the time from the most recent thrombotic episode is the most important risk factor for recurrence if warfarin is not administered. The risk is highest with VTE within the previous 3 months, and these patients will likely benefit from bridging therapy.

The average annual stroke rate in untreated patients with atrial fibrillation (AF) is 4% to 5%. The estimated annual stroke rates for patients range from 1% to >10% depending on the presence of the following risk factors. Patients with three or more of the risks listed below are at relatively high risk for thromboembolism from AF and would likely benefit from bridging anticoagulation with heparin to minimize the risk of periprocedural thromboembolism:

- Congestive heart failure
- Rheumatic heart disease
- Prior thromboembolic stroke or transient ischemic attack (TIA)
- Age >75 years
- Diabetes
- Hypertension (particularly when poorly controlled)

In patients with mechanical heart valves, the risk of stroke while not taking warfarin is generally higher than that of patients with AF.

Patients with mechanical valves in the mitral position and those with older valve models (e.g., ball-in-cage) or those with more than one mechanical valve have a higher risk of thromboembolism than do those with newer-model valves (e.g., St. Jude) and will likely benefit from bridging therapy.

In general, patients at high and moderate thromboembolic risk should receive perioperative bridging therapy. In general, patients at low thromboembolic risk should not receive bridging therapy. The patient's risk for serious bleeding and the increased risk of bleeding during major surgical procedures must be considered. The surgeon should be involved in the discussion. Patients undergoing major procedures should not resume full-dose bridging therapy until hemostasis is secured. Hemostasis may not be established for 2 to 3 days after surgery.

Either UFH or LMWH can be used for bridging therapy. Use of UFH usually requires at least 2 days of hospitalization before the procedure. Care in the hospital is begun with a bolus of 80 U/kg and a continuous IV infusion of 18 U/kg that is adjusted every 6 hours, with a targeted aPTT level of 60 to 80 seconds. Continuous infusions of UFH should be discontinued at least 4 hours before the procedure or 6 hours before for patients with renal insufficiency.

The predictable pharmacokinetics and the bioavailability of subcutaneous LMWH (e.g., dalteparin 100 IU/kg SC q12h or enoxaparin 1 mg/kg SC q12h) allow its preoperative use in an outpatient setting, saving the costs of hospitalization. The last dose of LMWH should always be about 24 hours before the surgery. Table 7.8 outlines a bridging protocol.

Symptomatic epidural hematomas can develop when a spinal or epidural catheter is inserted into or removed from a patient undergoing anticoagulation therapy; special monitoring both pre- and postoperatively may be needed.

Table 7.8.   Protocol for bridging therapy with low-molecular-weight heparin

Preprocedure protocol
- If INR 2–3, stop warfarin 5 days (four doses) before procedure.
- If INR 3–4.5, stop warfarin 6 days (five doses) before procedure.
- Start LMWH[a] 36 hours after last warfarin dose.
- Give last dose of LMWH 24 hours before procedure.
- Ensure patient is thoroughly educated in self-injection and has been provided with written instructions and contact phone number for questions or problems.
- Confer with surgeon and anesthesiologist regarding planned bridging therapy.
- Check INR on morning of procedure.

Postprocedure protocol
- Restart LMWH[a] approximately 24 hours postprocedure, or consider using a thromboprophylaxis dose of LMWH on postprocedure days 1–3 if patient is at high risk for bleeding.
- Confer with surgeon about the planned start time for anticoagulant therapy.
- Start warfarin at patient's preoperative dose on postoperative day 1.
- Monitor daily INR until patient is discharged and periodically thereafter until INR is therapeutic.
- Confer daily by telephone with pharmacist on discharge.
- Do CBC with platelets on day 3 and 7 of LMWH.
- Discontinue LMWH when INR is 2–3 for 2 consecutive days.

CBC, complete blood count; INR, international normalized ratio; LMWH, low-molecular-weight heparin; UFH, unfractionated heparin.

[a]Enoxaparin 1 mg/kg SC q12h or 1.5 mg/kg SC q24h or dalteparin 120 U/kg q12h or dalteparin 200 U/kg SC q24h. For patients with creatinine clearance <30 mL/minute, consider using UFH or enoxaparin 1 mg/kg SC q24h if full-dose LWMH is desired or use 30 mg SC q24h if prophylactic dose of LMWH is desired.

Jaffer AK, Brotman DJ, Chukurmerijee, N. When patients on warfarin need surgery. *Cleve Clin J Med.* 2003.

SPECIAL CONSIDERATIONS WITH NEURAXIAL BLOCKADE

The American Society of Regional Anesthesia (ASRA) (16) has the following recommendations (available online at www.asra.com) when neuraxial blockade is needed for patients receiving antiplatelet or anticoagulant therapy:

- Neuraxial blockade and indwelling catheters are safe in patients on aspirin.
- NSAIDs alone do not significantly increase the risk of spinal hematoma.
- COX-2 inhibitors do not cause platelet dysfunction and neuraxial anesthesia can be safely performed on patients taking these drugs.
- The actual risk of spinal hematoma with thienopyridine derivatives clopidogrel and ticlopidine and the platelet glycoprotein IIb/IIIa receptor antagonists such as abciximab, eptifibatide,

and tirofiban is unknown. The recommendations are to discontinue clopidogrel for 7 days, ticlopidine for 14 days, abciximab for 24 to 48 hours, and tirofiban and eptifibatide for 4 to 8 hours before performing a neuraxial technique.

- Coadministration of antiplatelet and anticoagulant medications is contraindicated with indwelling epidural catheters. Clopidogrel must be discontinued for 7 days before neuraxial blockade.
- Spinal or epidural anesthesia is performed at least 12 hours after the last thromboprophylaxis dose of LMWH (enoxaparin 40 mg SC daily) or dalteparin (5,000 U units once daily), and at least 24 hours after the last full dose of LMWH (e.g., enoxaparin 1 mg/kg q12h, enoxaparin 1.5 mg/kg q24h, or dalteparin 120 U/kg q12h).
- In general, an epidural catheter should not be removed until 12 hours after the last prophylaxis dose of LMWH.
- The first dose of LMWH should be administered no sooner than 2 hours after catheter removal.
- If a *single daily thromboprophylaxis* dose of LMWH is administered, then indwelling catheters may be maintained postoperatively.
- Concurrent use of *twice-daily or therapeutic* LMWH and an indwelling epidural catheter is not recommended.
- The LMWH dose is delayed for 24 hours if the patient experienced excessive trauma during attempted epidural or spinal anesthesia.
- Neuraxial blocks should not be performed in patients chronically taking warfarin unless the warfarin is stopped and the INR is normal.
- Neuraxial catheters should be removed only when the INR is <1.5.
- For patients receiving an initial dose of warfarin prior to surgery, the INR should be checked if the dose was given >24 hours earlier or a second dose has been administered.
- Herbal drugs, by themselves, do not appear to increase the risk of spinal hematoma with neuraxial anesthesia.
- Newer anticoagulants such as thrombin inhibitors and fondaparinux are unknown risks due to a paucity of data and experience. Avoidance of indwelling catheters is recommended (17).

CONCLUSIONS

The preoperative management of the patient with anemia, platelet disorder, or a risk for thrombosis or bleeding is fairly complex. This chapter provides an evidence-based overview with recommendations to manage these commonly encountered perioperative hematologic conditions.

REFERENCES

1. Shander A, Knight K, Thurer R, et al. Prevalence and outcomes of anemia in surgery: a systematic review of the literature. *Am J Med*. 2004;116(Suppl 7A):58S–69S.
2. Goodnough LT, Shander A, Spivak JL, et al. Detection, evaluation, and management of anemia in the elective surgical patient. *Anesth Analg*. 2005;101:1858–1861.
3. Carson JL, Duff A, Poses RM, et al. Effect of anaemia and cardiovascular disease on surgical mortality and morbidity. *Lancet*. 1996;348:1055–1060.

4. Eckman MH, Erban JK, Singh SK, et al. Screening for the risk for bleeding or thrombosis. *Ann Intern Med*. 2003;138:W15–24.

5. Koshy M, Weiner SJ, Miller ST, et al. Surgery and anesthesia in sickle cell disease. Cooperative Study of Sickle Cell Diseases. *Blood*. 1995;86:3676–3684.

6. Vichinsky EP, Haberkern CM, Neumayr L, et al. A comparison of conservative and aggressive transfusion regimens in the perioperative management of sickle cell disease. The Preoperative Transfusion in Sickle Cell Disease Study Group. *N Engl J Med*. 1995;333:206–213.

7. Gayyed NL, Bouboulis N, Holden MP. Open heart operation in patients suffering from hereditary spherocytosis. *Ann Thorac Surg*. 1993;55:1497–1500.

8. Ingerslev J, Hvid I. Surgery in hemophilia. The general view: patient selection, timing, and preoperative assessment. *Semin Hematol*. 2006;43(Suppl 1):S23–26.

9. Michiels JJ, Gadisseur A, Budde U, et al. Characterization, classification, and treatment of von Willebrand diseases: a critical appraisal of the literature and personal experiences. *Semin Thromb Hemost*. 2005;31:577–601.

10. Mannucci PM. Treatment of von Willebrand's Disease. *N Engl J Med*. 2004;351:683–694.

11. Cines DB, Blanchette VS. Immune thrombocytopenic purpura. *N Engl J Med*. 2002;346:995–1008.

12. Bartholomew JR, Begelman SM, Almahameed A. Heparin-induced thrombocytopenia: principles for early recognition and management. *Cleve Clin J Med*. 2005;(Suppl 1):S31–36.

13. Warkentin TE, Kelton JG. Temporal aspects of heparin-induced thrombocytopenia. *N Engl J Med*. 2001;344:1286–1292.

14. Geerts WH, Pineo GF, Heit JA, et al. Prevention of venous thromboembolism: the Seventh ACCP Conference on Antithrombotic and Thrombolytic Therapy. *Chest*. 2004;126(Suppl):338S–400S.

15. Lecompte T, Hardy JF. Antiplatelet agents and perioperative bleeding. *Can J Anaesth*. 2006;53(Suppl):S103–112.

16. Horlocker TT, Wedel DJ, Benzon H, et al. Regional anesthesia in the anticoagulated patient: defining the risks (the second ASRA Consensus Conference on Neuraxial Anesthesia and Anticoagulation). *Reg Anesth Pain Med*. 2003;28:172–197.

17. Grines CL, Bonow RO, Casey DE Jr, et al. Prevention of premature discontinuation of dual antiplatelet therapy in patients with coronary artery stents: a science advisory from the American Heart Association, American College of Cardiology, Society for Cardiovascular Angiography and Interventions, American College of Surgeons, and American Dental Association, with representation from the American College of Physicians. *Circulation*. 2007;115:813–818.

Renal Disease

Padraig Mahon and George D. Shorten

The term *renal impairment* or *renal disease* encompasses a broad spectrum of disease. This continuum ranges from the asymptomatic patient with mildly elevated serum creatinine to the patient with chronic renal failure (CRF) who is dialysis dependent. The broad spectrum makes management of patients with renal disease during the perioperative period challenging.

In this chapter we review the definitions and classifications of renal disease, prevalence of renal disease in the United States population, pathophysiology, preoperative assessment including investigations, and perioperative risk reduction strategies.

DEFINITIONS
A multitude of terms in the literature refer to different stages of the renal disease continuum, partly because of different nomenclatures used in the United States and Europe. It is important to understand these stages to stratify the perioperative risk (Table 8.1). The following are representative definitions from the literature:

- **Renal impairment:** Blood urea nitrogen (BUN) or serum creatinine level increased by >50% of the pretreatment value, to levels >30 mg/dL or 1.5 mg/dL, respectively (1)
- **Chronic renal (kidney) disease (CKD):** The presence of a marker of kidney damage, such as proteinuria (ratio of >30 mg of albumin to 1 g of creatinine on untimed [spot] urine testing), or a decreased glomerular filtration rate (GFR) for ≥ 3 months (GFR <60 mL/minute^{-1}/1.73 m^{-2})
- **Acute renal failure (ARF):** Abrupt and sustained decrease in renal function resulting in retention of nitrogenous (urea and creatinine) and nonnitrogenous waste products (to qualify for inclusion in this category patients must have a urine output <0.5 mL/kg^{-1}/hour^{-1}) (2)
- **Chronic renal failure:** A GFR <15 mL/minute^{-1}/1.73 m^{-2}, usually accompanied by signs and symptoms of uremia, or the need for initiation of kidney replacement therapy for management of the complications of a decreased GFR
- **End-stage renal disease (ESRD):** Loss of renal function for >3 months (2)

Table 8.1 summarizes a classification system for CKD proposed by the National Kidney Foundation, which stages disease based on GFR (3).

PREVALENCE
More than 20 million adults in the United States have CKD, with millions more at risk (Table 8.1). As incidence of hypertension (responsible for 27%) and diabetes (responsible for 45.5% of ESRD) increases, so too does the prevalence of CKD. The U.S.

Table 8.1.   Stages of chronic kidney disease and prevalence of renal disease in the U.S. population (1988–1998)

Stage	Definition	U.S. Prevalence
1	GFR $\geq$90 mL/min^{-1}/1.73 m^{-2} with evidence of kidney damage[a]	5.9 million
2	GFR = 60–89 mL/min^{-1}/1.73 m^{-2} with evidence of kidney damage[a]	5.3 million
3	GFR = 30–59 mL/min^{-1}/1.73 m^{-2}	7.6 million
4	GFR = 15–29 mL/min^{-1}/1.73 m^{-2}	0.4 million
5	GFR <15 mL/min^{-1}/1.73 m^{-2} or dialysis dependent	0.3 million

GFR, glomerular filtration rate.
[a]Kidney damage defined as pathologic abnormalities or markers of damage, including abnormalities of blood or urine tests or imaging studies.
Adapted from Palevsky MP. Perioperative management of patients with chronic kidney disease or ESRD. *Best Pract Res Clin Anesthesiol.* 2004;18: 129–144; and from National Kidney Foundation, K/DOQI Clinical practice guidelines for chronic kidney disease: evaluation, classification and stratification. *Am J Kidney Dis.* 2002;39(2 suppl 1):S19.

population of dialysis-dependent patients is increasing by 3% to 5% per year. Population-based screening to identify individuals with low GFR is controversial (4). Targeted screening of those with hypertension or diabetes is currently accepted practice. Wider population-based screening, restricted to those with hypertension, diabetes, or age >55 years, can potentially identify 93.2% (95% confidence interval [CI], 92.4% to 94%) of patients with CKD (GFR <60 mL/minute^{-1}/1.73 m^{-2}) (5). In the same Norwegian-based study, 20% of individuals with estimated GFR <30 mL/minute^{-1}/1.73 m^{-2} progressed to ESRD over 8 years of follow-up, compared to 1% to 2% of those with a GFR of 30 to 60 mL/minute^{-1}/1.73 m^{-2}.

CHRONIC KIDNEY DISEASE

Overall perioperative mortality rates in patients with CKD range from 1% to 4%. In patients who undergo cardiac surgery, the estimated mortality rates are greater (10% to 20%). Mortality in dialysis-dependent patients after emergency valve replacement surgery is reported to be 57%. Common causes of mortality in this group include sepsis, bleeding, congestive heart failure (CHF), hypotension, and hyperkalemia.

ACUTE RENAL FAILURE

ARF complicates 2% to 5% of all inpatient admissions. Table 8.2 outlines the causes of in-hospital ARF and associated mortality. Of critically ill patients, 5% to 20% experience an episode of ARF during the course of their illness. ARF occurs in about 19% of patients with moderate sepsis, 23% of those with severe sepsis, and 51% of those with septic shock when blood cultures are positive (6).

Table 8.2. Causes of hospital-acquired acute renal failure: Associated frequency and mortality

Cause	Frequency	Mortality
Decreased renal perfusion	39%	13.6%
Medications	16%	15%
Radiographic contrast media	11%	14%
Surgery	9%	2.8%
Sepsis	6.5%	76%
Post–liver transplant	<5%	28.6%
Post–heart transplant	<5%	35%
Obstruction	<5%	28.6%
Hepatorenal syndrome	<1%	71.4%
Rhabdomyolysis, artifact, glomerulonephritis, nephrectomy, atheroemboli, hypercalcemia, unknown	<1%	

Adapted from Nash OK, Hafeez A, Hou S. Hospital-acquired renal insufficiency. *Am J Kidney Dis.* 2002;3:930–936.

PATHOPHYSIOLOGY

In healthy adults, renal blood flow (RBF) is approximately 1.2 to 1.3 L/minute^{-1} of blood or 20% of cardiac output (7). Blood enters the afferent arteriole and a proportion of plasma is filtered across the glomerular basement membrane and into the proximal tubule for reabsorption and secretion. The filtered component of plasma is referred to as the glomerular filtrate. The GFR in the average 70-kg man is 125 mL/minute^{-1} or approximately 10% of the RBF. Almost all (99%) of this filtrate is normally reabsorbed. In a 24-hour period, the kidneys filter an amount of fluid equal to four times the total body water (TBW) or 60 times the plasma volume (7).

The formation of an adequate glomerular filtration fraction ($^{GFR}/_{RBF}$) depends on RBF and the integrity of the glomerular apparatus, including the capillaries and the basement membrane. RBF is autoregulated between mean arterial pressures of 60 and 150 mm Hg. Autoregulation is prevented by drugs that paralyze smooth muscle. Autoregulation occurs at the level of the afferent arteriole, where nitric oxide (NO) mediates the smooth muscle response to stretch. At low perfusion pressures, angiotensin II constricts the efferent arteriole, thus maintaining filtration pressure across the glomerular membrane. Drugs that interfere with these mediators include nonsteroidal anti-inflammatory drugs (NSAIDs), cyclooxygenase 2 (COX-2) inhibitors, angiotensin-converting enzyme (ACE) inhibitors, and angiotensin II receptor antagonists. These drugs may precipitate renal failure during hypoperfusion. Many patients with existing renal disease who present for surgery will be taking ACE inhibitors. ACE inhibitors are now first-line treatment for the prevention of diabetic nephropathy in diabetic patients. They also confer substantial benefit in patients without diabetes but with advanced renal insufficiency (CKD stage 4; 43% reduction in incidence of ESRD and death at 3.4 years of follow-up) (8). The following help to maintain renal homeostasis:

- Renin angiotensin-aldosterone system
- Angiotensin II
- Antidiuretic hormone (ADH)
- Atrial natriuretic peptide
- Prostaglandins E_2 and I_2 and the kinins

The kidney excretes the end-products of metabolism (urea and acids), retains nutrients (amino acids and glucose), and maintains the volume and composition of body fluids. Disruption of these functions can manifest as the following:

- Nephrotic syndrome
- Acid–base disturbance
- Disorders of potassium homeostasis
- Disorders of sodium homeostasis

The kidney performs a number of secondary functions together with its primary function of excreting end-products of metabolism. Among the secondary functions are the following:

- Erythropoietin production
- Conversion of vitamin D to its active form
- Calcium conservation via the activity of parathyroid hormone (PTH)
- Peptide and protein hormone metabolism (e.g., metabolism of insulin)

Nephrotic Syndrome

The nephrotic syndrome is characterized by heavy urinary protein loss, hypoalbuminemia, and edema. Hypercholesterolemia is almost always present. Urinary protein loss of ≥ 3 to 5 g daily causes hypoalbuminemia. Structural damage to the glomerular basement membrane leads to increased pore size allowing the passage of large molecules. Common causes include diabetic glomerulosclerosis and membranous glomerulopathy.

Acid–Base Disturbance

Normal arterial pH is maintained between 7.38 and 7.42. The normal daily adult diet contains in excess of 70 to 100 mmol of acid. This acid is buffered by intracellular proteins such as hemoglobin and tissue components such as calcium carbonate and calcium phosphate in bone. Most important of all is the bicarbonate-carbonic acid buffer pair generated by the hydration of carbon dioxide (CO_2):

carbonic anhydrase

$$H^+ + HCO_3^- \quad \text{<carbonic anhydrase>} \quad CO_2 + H_2O$$

Acidemia stimulates an increase in ventilation to eliminate CO_2, which limits the decrease in pH. The kidney regenerates the bicarbonate (HCO_3^-) used in the buffering process. The kidney excretes H^+ ions and reabsorbs all filtered HCO_3^- ions, maintaining the plasma HCO_3^- at approximately 25 mEq/L^{-1}. Failure of this mechanism is a common cause of metabolic acidosis, particularly in ARF. Renal tubular acidosis (types 1 to 4) refers to a rare group of genetic diseases (with confusing nomenclature!) in which the renal tubular ability to maintain acid–base balance is impaired.

Disorders of Potassium Homeostasis

Hyperkalemia ($K^+ > 4.9$ mEq/L^{-1}) is caused by diminished excretion due to renal tubular damage or drug interference. The combination of ACE inhibitors with K^+-sparing diuretics (now widely used in the treatment of CHF) in patients with mild renal impairment can precipitate hyperkalemia. NSAIDs, which disrupt prostanoid production, can suppress renin production, resulting in decreased aldosterone levels and hence reduced K^+ excretion. Severe hyperkalemia produces electrocardiogram (ECG) changes including T-wave elevation and can cause sudden death from asystolic arrest. Hyperkalemia causes hyperpolarization of cell membranes, leading to decreased excitability, hypotension, bradycardia, and eventual asystole. Muscle weakness is often the only symptom.

Hypokalemia ($K^+ < 3.3$ mEq/L^{-1}) or K^+ loss via the kidneys is caused by diuretics, mineralocorticoid excess, or renal tubular acidosis. Hypokalemia also results from rapid H^+ ion movement into the extracellular space with K^+ for H^+ ion exchange across cell membranes. Rapid correction of acidosis by hyperventilation or the administration of sodium bicarbonate ($NaHCO_3$) can precipitate hypokalemia. ECG changes include flattened T waves, ST-segment depression, prolonged PR and QT intervals, and atrial and ventricular arrhythmias.

Disorders of Sodium Homeostasis

Intravascular volume is conserved by the action of ADH and aldosterone. Hypovolemia results in ADH release and stimulation of the renin-angiotensin-aldosterone system. ADH is released by the posterior pituitary gland in response to increased osmolality or decreased extracellular volume and increases the permeability of the collecting duct to water. Aldosterone is a mineralocorticoid released by the adrenal cortex in response to angiotensin II. Aldosterone acts on the distal tubule to increase the reabsorption of sodium (Na^+) in exchange for K^+ and H^+.

Hypernatremia ($Na^+ > 144$ mEq/L^{-1}) is most commonly a result of TBW deficit rather than total body Na^+ excess.

Hyponatremia ($Na^+ < 134$ mEq/L^{-1}) is most commonly caused by an excess of TBW rather than a deficit in total body Na^+. In ARF from acute tubular necrosis (ATN), failure to reabsorb Na^+ (primarily a function of the proximal convoluted tubule) can result in excessive Na^+ excretion (>40 mEq/L^{-1}) in the urine.

ETIOLOGY OF CHRONIC RENAL FAILURE

The causes of CRF can be divided into five categories:

1. Congenital and inherited causes
2. Primary and secondary glomerular disease
3. Vascular disease
4. Tubulointerstitial disease
5. Urinary tract obstruction

Table 8.3 lists common causes of renal failure in each of these categories. In many cases, no treatment will reverse the

Table 8.3. Causes of chronic renal failure

Congenital and inherited disease
Polycystic kidney disease
Alport syndrome
Congenital hypoplasia

Glomerular disease
Primary:
  Glomerulonephritides
Secondary:
  Systemic lupus vasculitis
  Diabetic glomerulosclerosis
  Amyloidosis

Vascular disease
Arteriosclerosis
Microscopic polyarteritis
Systemic lupus
Systemic sclerosis with renal involvement

Tubulointerstitial disease
Tubulointerstitial nephritis
Reflux nephropathy
Tuberculosis
Schistosomiasis

Urinary tract obstruction
Urinary calculi
Prostate disease
Retroperitoneal fibrosis
Pelvic mass

underlying cause. Exceptions include removal of obstruction to urinary tract outflow, stenting of a stenosed renal artery, and administering steroids for Goodpasture syndrome and systemic vasculitis.

Diabetes together with poorly controlled hypertension accounts for approximately 70% of cases of CRF. Diabetic nephropathy is caused by renal structural changes. In overt nephropathy, all renal compartments, glomeruli, tubuli, extraglomerular blood vessels, and the interstitium show abnormalities. In essential hypertension one of the earliest renal manifestations is a reduction in total RBF. It is hypothesized that reduced RBF leads to a reduction in pressure and flow in the postglomerular circulation. This reduction may predispose to increased Na^+ reabsorption, which further increases systemic blood pressure (9). Malignant hypertension is accompanied by gross pathologic change and a major disruption in renal function. RBF and GFR are greatly reduced; the renal vasculature may no longer respond to vasodilators (9).

Polycystic kidney disease has an autosomal dominant inheritance in 90% of cases and is the most commonly inherited tubular disorder accounting for 10% of ESRD in the United States.

Extrarenal manifestations include intracranial aneurysms in 10% of patients and mitral valve prolapse in 25% of patients.

ETIOLOGY OF ACUTE RENAL FAILURE

ARF can occur de novo or complicate CKD. The traditional categorization of ARF into prerenal, renal, and postrenal forces the physician to adopt a systematic approach to the patient with ARF (Fig. 8.1). Prerenal causes can often be rapidly corrected. A number of simple tests distinguish prerenal from other causes.

The BUN-to-creatinine (Cr) ratio can be calculated. A ratio >20 favors a prerenal cause, whereas ratios of 10 to 20 occur with renal or postrenal failure. Calculation of the fractional excretion of sodium (FE_{Na}) is useful.

$$FE_{Na} = \frac{P_{Cr}/U_{Cr}}{P_{Na}/U_{Na}}$$

(P_{Cr}, plasma creatinine; U_{Cr}, urine creatinine; P_{Na}, plasma sodium; U_{Na}, urine sodium)

A FE_{Na} <1% is associated with prerenal causes of ARF. A FE_{Na} >1% is most often caused with ATN but may be seen in volume depletion (10% of the time) or in volume depletion with ongoing diuretic therapy (causing salt wasting).

In prerenal ARF, correction of hypovolemia and hypotension is the only means of renal protection. The loop diuretic furosemide is of little use in preventing or treating ARF (10). If the patient remains oliguric (urine output <0.5 mL/kg^{-1}/hour^{-1}) despite normovolemia and adequate mean arterial pressure, the next step is to distinguish between intrinsic pathology and obstructive causes. An ultrasound of the renal tract is indicated to identify changes (enlarged kidneys or dilated ureters) that result from obstruction. Causes of obstruction include ureteric calculi, blood clots, retroperitoneal fibrosis, compressing tumors, and bladder outlet obstruction. Treatment is aimed at decompressing the outflow system and may require nephrostomy, ureteric stenting, or simple catheterization.

When the cause of ARF is not obvious, then intrinsic renal disease such as allergic interstitial nephritis, acute glomerulonephritis, and vasculitis must be considered. These rare causes of ARF require specialist assessment (diagnosis is often made following biopsy) and aggressive treatment.

CLINICAL MEASUREMENT

In healthy individuals GFR remains constant as a result of intrarenal regulatory mechanisms. GFR declines following renal injury or a reduction in RBF. Traditionally, an age-related decline in GFR has been considered "normal." Decreased GFR, however, is an independent predictor of adverse outcome in the elderly population (11).

Measurement or estimation of GFR (eGFR) is necessary to determine renal function. Creatinine clearance (based on the presumption that creatinine production is constant) is a surrogate marker of GFR. Creatinine generation is proportional to muscle mass and is generally greater in men than in women. Individuals of African descent usually have greater serum creatinine concentrations than those of other races. Postoperative conditions (e.g.,

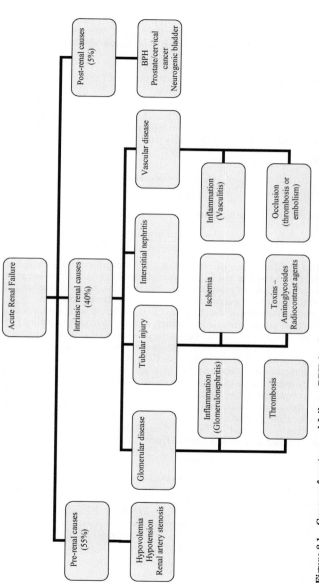

Figure 8.1. Causes of acute renal failure. BPH, benign prostatic hypertrophy. (Adapted from Hilton R. Acute renal failure. *BMJ.* 2006;333:786–789.)

intravascular hemodilution, variable muscle mass, and changes in metabolic rate) complicate the interpretation of serum creatinine measurements (12). GFR can be reduced 50% to 70% without changes in serum creatinine. The classical determination of GFR requires a 24-hour urine collection. Creatinine clearance $(mL/minute^{-1})$ (CC) is estimated by the following formula:

$$CC = U \times V/P \times 100$$

U = urinary creatinine concentration $(mmol/L^{-1})$
V = urine volume (mL)
P = plasma creatinine concentration $(mmol/L^{-1})$

If a 24-hour collection is not feasible, GFR can be estimated from serum creatinine, using the equation from the Modification of Diet in Renal Disease (MDRD) study:

$$eGFR\,(mL/minute/1.73\,m^2)$$
$$= \frac{1.86\,(\text{serum creatinine})^{-1.154} \times (\text{age})^{-0.203}}{(0.742\,\text{if female}) \times (1.210\,\text{if African descent})}$$

Alternatively, the simpler Cockroft-Gault formula may be used:

$$\text{Creatinine clearance} = \frac{(140 - \text{age}) \times \text{wt}\,(kg) \times (0.85\,\text{if female})}{72 \times \text{serum creatinine}\,(mg/dL)}$$

Due to the inclusion of weight in the numerator, as a measure of muscle mass, the equation overestimates creatinine clearance in patients who are edematous or overweight. Online versions of both calculators are available at http://www.nephron.com.

Newer methods of estimating GFR attempt to overcome the reliance on serum creatinine, which is subject to confounding factors. Recently cystatin C, a protein produced at a steady rate by virtually all nucleated cells, has been used to estimate GFR. A 24-hour collection is not required. Cystatin C is not influenced by muscle mass and is identical in men and women. Cystatin C may have an advantage in detecting mildly decreased GFR, whereas serum creatinine may be a better measure at lower levels of GFR. Little data have been published to date regarding its use in the perioperative period.

The tests outlined in Table 8.4 can be used alone or in combination to differentiate prerenal from renal azotemia.

PREANESTHESIA REVIEW

This section outlines the important factors the anesthesiologist should consider preoperatively in the patient with renal disease. A list of potential patient scenarios is presented in Table 8.5.

The early stages of renal failure are often completely asymptomatic despite the accumulation of waste metabolites. Symptoms are common when the BUN exceeds 40 $mmol/L^{-1}$. These symptoms include the following:

• Malaise, loss of energy
• Insomnia
• Pruritus
• Nausea and vomiting
• Symptoms of anemia

Table 8.4. Urine and serum diagnostic indices for differential diagnosis between prerenal and renal azotemia

Measure	Prerenal	Renal
Renal blood flow (mL/min^{-1})	Reduced	Reduced/normal
Urine output $(mL/kg/hr^{-1})$	<0.5	
Creatinine clearance (mL/min^{-1})	Reduced	Reduced
Urine-specific gravity	>1.020	<1.010
Urine osmolality (mOsm/kg)	>500	<350
Urine/plasma osmolality	>1.3	<1.1
Urine sodium (mEq/L)	<20	>40
Urine/plasma urea	>8	<3
Urine/plasma creatinine	>40	<20
Fractional excretion of sodium $(FE_{Na})^a$	<1%	>2%

[a] See page 202 for formula for calculating Fe_{Na}.

- Signs of salt and water retention (i.e., peripheral and pulmonary edema)
- Bone pain from metabolic bone disease
- Paresthesiae and tetany caused by hypocalcemia

In advanced uremia (BUN >50 to 60 mmol/L^{-1}) central nervous system (CNS) symptoms worsen and myoclonic twitching and mental slowing.

Cardiovascular System

Important questions in the cardiac history include the presence of angina and its precipitating factors, a history of myocardial infarction (MI), and exercise tolerance. Exercise capacity, measured as metabolic equivalents (METs), needs to be determined. Complaints of shortness of breath, orthopnea, paroxysmal nocturnal dyspnea, or pedal edema may indicate volume overload. The presence of cardiac risk factors—smoking, diabetes mellitus, obesity, and family history—should be documented in the chart.

Dialysis-dependent renal failure is associated with an increased risk of vascular death. A 25-year-old man with renal

Table 8.5. Clinical spectrum of renal disease

Young, recently diagnosed type 1 diabetic patient
Hypertensive asymptomatic patient with elevated serum creatinine
Overweight type 2 diabetic patient recently diagnosed
Older patient with raised serum creatinine
Chronic renal failure patient, diet and fluid restricted
Peritoneal dialysis patient
Hemodialysis patient
Patient awaiting renal transplant
Patient with functioning graft
Acute renal failure from trauma or rhabdomyolysis
Drug (contrast)-induced acute/chronic renal failure

failure has a >100-fold increased risk of vascular death compared to an age- and sex-matched control. The pathology of the increased vascular morbidity is multifactorial, but important factors include arterial calcification, arterial stiffness, and left ventricular hypertrophy (LVH). Dialysis itself does not appear to accelerate atherosclerosis (13).

Elevated pulmonary artery pressures (PAPs) are found in a high proportion of dialysis patients with an arteriovenous fistula. In a recent study of 42 hemodialysis patients, 20 had pulmonary hypertension (mean PAP, 46; range 36 to 82 mm Hg) (20). Patients with pulmonary hypertension had higher cardiac outputs compared to patients with normal PAP. Temporary closure of the fistula by means of a sphygmomanometer decreased cardiac output and systolic PAP in eight patients (14).

Cardiac autonomic neuropathy manifests as an abnormally elevated resting heart rate (>100 bpm) and lack of heart rate variability during exercise or deep breathing tests (an expiratory:inspiratory ratio [E:I] of >1.17 is abnormal). Systolic dysfunction can result from myocardial fibrosis and calcium overload from secondary hyperparathyroidism. Volume overload from underlying CHF, impaired renal excretion of Na^+ and water, or low oncotic pressure (e.g., in nephrotic kidney disease) can cause pulmonary edema. The clinical characteristics of pericarditis in patients with uremia are similar to those seen in nonuremic patients. Pericarditis is usually painless and occurs in the terminal stages of uremia. Anticoagulants may increase the risk of tamponade in these patients.

Patients undergoing dialysis frequently have elevated serum cardiac troponin T levels. Concentrations of troponin rise during dialysis because of hemoconcentration, which makes it difficult to diagnose acute coronary syndromes. Elevated creatine kinase (CK) levels with a normal Mb fraction are present in at least 30% of patients with CRF. An acute increase in CK following trauma or prolonged immobilization (pressure necrosis) or heroin use is likely caused by rhabdomyolysis. Myoglobinemia and hemoglobinemia predispose to ATN.

Systemic hypertension, if not the cause of renal impairment, is its most common cardiovascular complication, with an incidence >80%. It is not often a feature of Na^+-wasting nephropathies such as polycystic kidney disease or papillary necrosis. Plasma volume expansion from Na^+ and water retention is the most frequent cause of hypertension and may be significantly improved by dialysis. Diastolic dysfunction is associated with LVH from longstanding hypertension. In general, antihypertensive medication should be continued in patients scheduled for surgery.

Hematologic System

Anemia affects 60% to 80% of patients with CRF, reduces quality of life, is associated with increased risk of seizures and hypotensive episodes, and is a risk factor for early death. Maintenance of a hematocrit >30% is associated with decreased mortality in dialysis-dependent patients. However, two recent prospective trials were terminated before completion when a trend was identified toward increased mortality in patients whose hematocrit was maintained >42%, using intravenous iron and recombinant erythropoietin.

Red cell production and survival are decreased in CRF for a variety of reasons:

- Erythropoietin deficiency
- Bone marrow fibrosis from hyperparathyroidism
- Abnormal red cell membranes with greater osmotic fragility

Patients should be asked about erythropoietin/iron treatment and previous transfusion history. The usual dose of erythropoietin is 25 to 50 U/kg^{-1} on alternative days.

Coagulation abnormalities are common in patients on dialysis and those with severe decreases in GFR (<30 mL/minute). Patients with CRF have a tendency toward excessive bleeding in the perioperative period despite normal activated partial thromboplastin time (aPTT), international normalized ratio (INR), and platelet counts. Platelet dysfunction is the primary cause of bleeding. Paradoxically, dialysis-dependent patients have an increased risk of thrombosis that may be associated with the enhanced platelet activation of dialysis (15). Chronic dialysis patients have a twofold increased risk for pulmonary embolism independent of comorbidity (16).

Dialysis-dependent patients are at risk of developing thrombocytopenia from unfractionated heparin used for anticoagulation. There are two distinct syndromes. The first results from heparin-mediated clumping of platelets and affects 10% to 20% of patients. This early decline rarely results in a platelet count <100,000/mm^3. Heparin-induced thrombocytopenia (HIT) is an immunologic phenomenon. Heparin binds to soluble platelet factor 4 (PF 4) and exposes epitopes that then bind IgG, activating them and initiating coagulation. Platelets are consumed in the formation of venous and arterial thrombi.

Recently low-molecular-weight heparins (LMWHs) have been used for anticoagulation during dialysis. Advantages of LMWH are a lesser incidence of HIT, ease of administration, and a longer half-life. LMWH–thrombin complexes are not cleared from blood during dialysis. All LMWH agents used in the United States are metabolized by the liver and eliminated through the kidneys. Some LMWHs appear to have a prolonged half-life in patients with severe CKD or ESRD. Multiple case reports of spontaneous severe hemorrhages have appeared in the literature, particularly in patients with ESRD administered standard doses of enoxaparin. Doses should be adjusted in these patients. In standard doses, tinzaparin does not appear to accumulate to a clinically significant degree in patients with ESRD. Protamine does not fully inactivate LMWH and reversal is unpredictable.

Gastrointestinal System

Liver dysfunction from chronic venous congestion is seen in 5%–10% of patients with severe CRF and volume overload. Viral hepatitis was previously common in dialysis-dependant patients. Fortunately this prevalence has decreased as the need for transfusion in patients with CKD is less with the availability of erythropoietin.

Delayed gastric emptying is common in patients with CRF, particularly in men. The delay appears not to be associated with the presence of gastrointestinal symptoms, underlying renal disease, or *Helicobacter pylori* infection. Diabetic patients with cardiac autonomic neuropathy are more likely to experience delayed gastric emptying than are healthy volunteers. Of 20 patients who underwent peritoneal dialysis, nine had abnormal gastric emptying (solid phase) and four of the nine had delayed liquid emptying (17).

Neurologic System

Uremic neuropathy is a distal, symmetric, mixed motor and sensory polyneuropathy, typically involving the legs more than the arms. Autonomic neuropathy frequently complicates renal failure whether or not caused by diabetes. Cardiovascular autonomic neuropathy is strongly associated with left ventricular hypertrophy in diabetic patients who need hemodialysis.

Electrolytes

Hypocalcemia is common in patients who need dialysis and is managed with calcium and vitamin D supplements. If hypocalcemia is suspected, it is important to ask about paresthesias and cramps. Chvostek sign (contraction of facial muscle after tapping the facial nerve) and Trousseau sign (carpopedal spasm following the application of a tourniquet to the arm for 3 minutes or more) are simple clinical tests that confirm hypocalcemia.

The regulation of plasma phosphate is closely linked to calcium. Phosphate retention owing to reduced renal excretion stimulates production of PTH, which in turn increases reabsorption of calcium from bone. Prolonged hyperparathyroidism results in periarticular and vascular calcification as the calcium phosphate product is deposited. Treatment of chronic hyperphosphatemia is with gut phosphate binders and dialysis.

Hyperkalemia (K^+ >4.9 mEq/L) frequently complicates renal disease. Uncontrollable hyperkalemia is an indication for acute dialysis. Dialysis in the 24 hours before surgery is currently recommended for control of K^+ in the perioperative period in dialysis-dependent patients. Anesthesia should be postponed if possible in patients with K^+ >5.9 mEq/dL^{-1}. The use of suxamethonium causes a transient (10 to 15 minute) increase in plasma K^+ concentration of 0.1 to 0.5 mEq/dL^{-1}. Suxamethonium can be used safely in patients with renal failure (18). In a recent series of 38 patients with moderate hyperkalemia (K^+ $\geq$5.6 mEq/dL^{-1}), none developed dysrhythmias or major morbidity following the administration of suxamethonium (19).

Hypokalemia (K^+ <3.3 mEq/dL^{-1}) occurs in 20% to 30% of patients undergoing continuous ambulatory peritoneal dialysis (CAPD) and requires treatment with diet liberalization or supplementation. Too rapid replacement of K^+ in the perioperative period may cause more problems than hypokalemia itself. Hypokalemia-induced conduction disturbances or diminished contractility should be treated with K^+ replacement given slowly, with continuous ECG monitoring. Chronic hypokalemia (K^+ >2.5 mEq/dL^{-1}) does not cause problems at induction of anesthesia if the patient does not have congestive heart failure or pre-existing arrhythmias and is not taking digitalis.

Hyponatremia (Na^+ <134 mEq/dL^{-1}) can occur in the context of a normal or decreased extracellular volume. The common causes of Na^+ deficiency include vomiting/diarrhea and bowel preparation. Osmotic diuresis from severe uremia, hyperglycemia, or excessive administration of diuretics promotes volume loss with a compensatory increase in ADH, to preserve intravascular volume at the expense of osmolality. Oxytocin and desmopressin (DDAVP) administration can cause hyponatremia with normal extracellular volume. The syndrome of inappropriate antidiuretic hormone (SIADH) classically results in hyponatremia with normal extracellular volume. A rarer cause specific to the CRF population includes excessive water drinking in peritoneal dialysis patients. Symptoms (including confusion, muscle cramps, and lethargy) are attributable to decreased plasma osmolality and do not appear until Na^+ falls below 125 mEq/dL^{-1}. Treatment is slow correction at a rate not exceeding 0.5 to 1/mEq/dL^{-1}/hour^{-1}. The Na^+ deficit can be estimated using the formula:

$$Na^+ deficit = TBW \times (desired\ Na^+ - current\ Na^+)$$

A 70-kg female has a TBW that is approximately 50% of body weight (equal to 35 L). If her current Na^+ is 114 mEq/dL^{-1}, with an ideal minimum level of 130 mEq/dL^{-1}, her total body deficit of Na^+ is approximately 560 mEq. This equates to 3.6 L of normal saline. To correct her deficit at a rate of 0.5 mEq/dL^{-1}/hour^{-1}, the rate of salt administration should be 17.5 mEq Na^+/hour (35 × 0.5 mEq/dL^{-1}/hour^{-1}) or approximately 115 mL/hour of normal saline.

SPECIFIC DOCUMENTATION: THE HISTORY

- The cause of renal failure if known
- The extent of coexisting problems: Diabetes, cardiac and vascular disease, hypertension
- Patient's weight
- Medications
- Previous surgery or anesthesia and any complications (e.g., acute exacerbation of CRF)
- Previous dialysis (temporary or otherwise)
- Vascular access sites

In the Dialysis Patient

- Weight
- Last dialysis session
- Volume of fluid normally removed (Predialysis – postdialysis weight)
- Blood pressure postdialysis
- Electrolytes
- BUN levels predialysis (typically BUN can be expected to fall by 65% following dialysis)
- Daily fluid intake limit
- Amount of urine output (if any) in 24 hours
- Sites of current or old arteriovenous fistulas
- Presence of peritoneal dialysis catheter

In the Transplant Patient

- Weight
- Urine output in 24 hours
- Blood pressure
- Electrolytes
- Position of transplanted kidney(s)
- Native kidneys still in situ?
- Immunosuppressive medications

EXAMINATION

General

- Weight
- Conjunctival/skin pallor
- Ecchymoses

Cardiac

- Peripheral edema
- Jugular venous distension (JVD)
- Pulmonary rales
- Pericardial rub
- Displaced apex beat
- S_3 or S_4 heart sound
- Aortic and pulmonary regurgitation murmurs

Musculoskeletal

- Muscle injury—cause of rhabdomyolysis
- Bone pain secondary renal osteodystrophy
- Spinal pain—possible multiple myeloma in an elderly patient

Vascular

- Pulses
- Site of arteriovenous fistulas/grafts
- Potential intravenous access sites

DIAGNOSTIC TESTING

Patients with advanced renal disease require a complete blood count (CBC) with a platelet count; electrolytes including Na^+, K^+, Ca^{2+}, and Mg^{2+}; and BUN and creatinine levels to be checked. An estimation of creatinine clearance or eGFR is necessary. A coagulation profile is not indicated in the majority of patients with renal impairment unless the patient is taking anticoagulant medications, has an obvious coagulation abnormality with clinical signs, or had dialysis within a few hours before surgery.

For patients on dialysis, these tests are obtained after their last dialysis session or preferably on the day of surgery. In patients who are hypokalemic, serum K^+ is measured on the day of surgery. K^+ measured just before induction of anesthesia is often lower than the value measured 24 to 72 hours previously. Antifactor Xa levels are rarely indicated in patients receiving LMWH. These levels may be useful in specific circumstances when neuroaxial anesthesia is planned and the duration of LMWH is uncertain (e.g., patients with GFR <30 mL/kg/minute^{-1}).

Cardiac Testing

An ECG is indicated for patients with renal disease if the serum creatinine is >2.0 mg/dL^{-1}. This level of creatinine elevation is an American College of Cardiology/American Heart Association (ACC/AHA) risk factor for perioperative cardiac complications. It is equivalent to a prior history of MI or coronary artery disease (CAD) and current angina or diabetes (see Chapter 3).

Severe K$^+$ disturbances result in ECG changes. Hyperkalemia causes peaked T waves and hypokalemia results in flattened T waves and prolonged PR and QT intervals. A pericardial effusion can manifest as low-voltage complexes in all leads. Electrical alternans (varying amplitude of waveform from beat to beat) indicate a large effusion.

Cardiovascular risk factors, the severity of surgery to be undertaken, and the patient's functional capacity determine the need for stress testing. Stress testing should be considered for patients with multiple cardiovascular risk factors who need major surgery (vascular/thoracic) and who have not already been assessed by a cardiologist (see Chapter 3).

Echocardiography is used to evaluate ventricular function and diagnose valvular disease, pericardial effusions, or pulmonary pressures. LVH, which confers an adverse prognosis, is found on echocardiography in 30% to 50% of patients with CKD. Dialysis-dependent patients commonly have aortic valve (AV) and mitral valve (MV) calcification. In a recent case series, valvular changes were present in 64% of patients after a mean of 50 months of dialysis. AV calcification was present in 55% and stenosis in 13% of patients. MV calcification was present in 40% and stenosis in 11% of these patients. AV calcification progresses to stenosis at an accelerated rate in dialysis patients (20). Elevation in the calcium/phosphate product and parathyroid hormone concentrations is the main cause. Valvular abnormalities increase the risk of infective endocarditis in dialysis patients.

Chest Radiograph

In patients with renal disease, a chest radiograph is indicated to confirm a clinical suspicion of pericardial effusion, pulmonary edema, or infection.

PREANESTHETIC PLANNING

The preanesthesia review identifies patients at risk for developing perioperative ARF or worsening of CKD. Patient and surgical risk factors known to precipitate ARF in the perioperative period are shown in Table 8.6.

Euvolemia and perfusion pressure must be maintained. Perioperative fluid deficits from overnight fasting, bowel preparation, diarrhea, and vomiting are corrected before induction of anesthesia. The use of invasive monitoring techniques, including arterial and central venous pressure (CVP) monitoring, may be indicated to guide fluid administration. CVP monitoring guides fluid management during renal transplantation when intraoperative fluid administration is aggressive to maximize early graft function, although the traditional approach of maintaining CVP >15 mm Hg during this procedure has recently been questioned (21). Directed

Table 8.6. Risk factors for the development of perioperative acute renal failure

Patient-Based Factors	Surgical Procedures
Pre-existing renal dysfunction	Cardiopulmonary bypass procedures
Perioperative cardiac dysfunction	Surgery involving aortic cross-clamping
Diabetes	Increased intra-abdominal pressure
Sepsis	Generalized embolization
Hepatic failure	Liver transplantation
Crush injury	Kidney transplantation
Drugs/nephrotoxins	Contrast agents

Adapted from Jarnberg PO. Renal protective strategies in the perioperative period. *Best Pract Res Clin Anaesthesiol.* 2004;18:645–660.

fluid challenges and invasive pressure monitoring during surgery have been shown to decrease duration of hospital stay and morbidity, including cases of renal dysfunction.

If an arteriovenous fistula is likely at some point in the future, then the nondominant arm should be avoided for venous access and central line placement.

Decreased urine output during surgery can be an appropriate tubuloglomerular response to hypovolemia and does not always imply ARF. Urine output during abdominal aortic surgery does not predict postoperative renal failure in patients if normotension and normovolemia are maintained intraoperatively.

Dialysis Patients

Dialysis-dependent patients should have dialysis in the 24 hours before induction of anesthesia to ensure normal K^+ levels and volume status. These patients may have an intravascular fluid deficit after dialysis. Determining the timing of dialysis, how much fluid was removed (e.g., the difference between predialysis and postdialysis weight), and fasting status since dialysis allows some estimation of fluid deficit before induction.

The sites of arteriovenous fistulas or grafts are clearly demarcated preoperatively to prevent inadvertent injury to these structures.

Hyperkalemia

Anesthesia should be postponed if possible in patients with K^+ >5.9 mEq/dL^{-1}. Signs and symptoms of hyperkalemia include muscle weakness and cardiac conduction abnormalities, which become dangerous as K^+ approaches 7 mEq/dL^{-1}. Bradycardia, ventricular fibrillation (VF), and cardiac arrest may result. Patients with chronic hyperkalemia appear to be more resistant to these effects than those with acute hyperkalemia. The use of suxamethonium appears safe in patients with serum K^+ ≤5.6 mEq/dL^{-1}. Major causes of hyperkalemia (plasma K^+ >4.9 mEq/dL^{-1}) include infusion of fresh frozen plasma (FFP), transfusion of old blood, tissue damage, drugs, and hypoxia.

Treatment of hyperkalemia depends on the modalities available to the clinician, the urgency of the situation, and the presence of ECG changes. In a dialysis-dependent patient who needs elective surgery, hyperkalemia should be treated with dialysis. In a patient presenting with ARF who requires urgent surgery, treatment options include the following:

1. If ECG changes are present, administer calcium chloride (CaCl), 0.5 to 1.0 g repeated every 5 minutes if necessary to stabilize the myocardium. Alternatively, give 10 mL 10% calcium gluconate solution slowly.
2. Glucose and insulin shifts K^+ intracellularly. Administer 10 to 15 U of insulin IV with 25 g of glucose (50 mL 50% solution) over 10 to 15 minutes.
3. Inhaled or IV β-agonists (e.g., albuterol or salbutamol) move K^+ intracellularly.
4. Hyperventilation reduces serum K^+ (10 mm Hg decrease in $PaCO_2$ lowers plasma K^+ concentration by 0.5 mEq/dL^{-1}).
5. Administer 50 mEq of $NaHCO_3$ IV over 5 minutes with a repeated dose in 10 to 15 minute as needed.
6. Cation-exchange resins remove K^+ slowly via the gut and are not suitable for acute correction of hyperkalemia but are useful to lower chronic hyperkalemia.

Regional Anesthesia

Renal failure is not a contraindication to regional or neuroaxial anesthesia. Indeed, brachial plexus block is now the anesthetic technique of choice for the construction of forearm arteriovenous fistulas. Each case warrants careful risk–benefit analysis, as no specific recommendations exist in the literature with regard to this population.

KIDNEY TRANSPLANT RECIPIENT

Patients who have a transplanted kidney usually have multisystem disease. Coronary artery disease is common in this population. Hypertension, which may have been present before the transplantation, can also result from immunosuppressive therapy. If the renal allograft is functioning correctly, the serum creatinine will be normal or near normal. GFR and effective RBF will be lower than in individuals without a transplant. Nephrotoxic drugs and NSAIDs should be avoided. Thrombosis of a newly transplanted kidney mediated by acute rejection may require immediate removal of the graft. This population of patients may be acutely unwell with an ongoing systemic inflammatory response resulting in hypotension, vasodilation, hypoperfusion, and metabolic acidosis. Other considerations in a kidney transplant patient include graft site and likely positioning of the patient intraoperatively. Without proper precautions, a prone position for surgery may cause pressure and obstruction of a transplanted kidney in the iliac fossa. Immunosuppressive and antihypertensive medications should be continued perioperatively. If the patient cannot take oral medications postoperatively, a preoperative consultation with the transplant nephrologists may offer other alternatives.

DRUG ADMINISTRATION: PHARMACODYNAMICS AND PHARMACOKINETICS

Table 8.7 outlines the mechanisms of renal toxicity of many commonly used drugs. Special consideration is needed when using NSAIDs in all patients with decreased GFR. Opiates and their metabolites are particularly likely to accumulate in patients with ESRD. Many drugs including antibiotics and some LMWH should be given in reduced doses. Numerous online calculators are available on the following sites: www.globalrph.com/renaldosing2 and www.uphs.upenn.edu/bugdrug/antibiotic_manual/renal.htm.

NSAIDs, selective and nonselective, are strongly associated with renal impairment and precipitation of ARF. Even in healthy individuals with normal renal function NSAIDs decrease creatinine clearance by 18 mL/kg^{-1}/minute^{-1} and K$^+$ excretion by 38 mmol/day on the first postoperative day (22). This transient decrease in renal function is usually benign. Selective COX-2 inhibitors have effects on renal hemodynamics similar to those of nonselective drugs. The U.S. National Kidney Foundation recommends acetaminophen as the analgesic of choice in patients

Table 8.7. Mechanisms of drug-induced renal damage

Mechanism	Drugs
Reduction in renal perfusion through alteration of intrarenal hemodynamics	NSAIDs, ACE inhibitors, cyclosporine, tacrolimus (FK-506), radiocontrast agents, amphotericin B, interleukin-2
Direct tubular toxicity	Aminoglycosides, radiocontrast agents, cisplatin, cyclosporine, tacrolimus, amphotericin B, methotrexate, foscarnet, pentamidine, organic solvents, heavy metals, intravenous immunoglobulin
Heme pigment-induced direct tubular toxicity (rhabdomyolysis)	Cocaine, ethanol, lovastatin
Intratubular obstruction by precipitation of the agent	Acyclovir, sulfonamides, ethylene glycol, chemotherapeutic agents, methotrexate
Allergic interstitial nephritis	Penicillins, cephalosporins, sulfonamides, rifampin, ciprofloxacin, NSAIDs, thiazide diuretics, furosemide, cimetidine, phenytoin, allopurinol
Hemolytic-uremic syndrome	Cyclosporine, tacrolimus, mitomycin, cocaine, quinine, conjugated estrogens

ACE, angiotensin-converting enzyme; NSAIDs, nonsteroidal antiinflammatory drugs.

with underlying kidney disease. A dose of up to 4 g/day is recommended.

The pharmacokinetics of many drugs depends on renal function. Changes in volume of distribution and protein binding affect bioavailability. If salt and water overload or depletion are found in patients with CKD, the changes in volume of distribution affect the concentration of drugs obtained from any fixed dose.

Reduced protein binding from hypoproteinemia or displacement from excess plasma H^+ ions binding to protein sites, which normally bind acidic drugs (such as sulfonamides, penicillin, and salicylates), increases circulating levels of free drug. For drugs with small therapeutic indices, dose regimens should be determined using eGFR. Morphine and meperidine are metabolized in the liver to morphine-6-glucuronide and normeperidine, respectively. Morphine-6-glucuronide has fewer sedative effects than morphine but has a markedly prolonged half-life in patients with CKD not on dialysis (27.1 hours vs. 2.1 hours) than in patients with normal kidney function (23). Normeperidine is less analgesic and has excitatory and convulsant properties and a terminal elimination half-life of 15 to 20 hours in healthy patients and in excess of 40 hours in patients with ARF or CRF.

CONTRAST-INDUCED NEPHROPATHY

Radiocontrast media cause mild transient decreases in GFR in almost all patients. Contrast-induced nephropathy (CIN) is defined as a 25% rise in creatinine above baseline after radiocontrast media have been administered. Diabetic patients and patients with CKD are at highest risk for CIN. The postulated mechanism of renal damage is free radical formation in the renal tubular lumen. Patients requiring dialysis because of CIN have a particularly poor outcome: A 36% in-hospital mortality and a 19% 2-year survival. Transient increases in creatinine are linked to longer hospital and intensive care unit stays.

For patients with CKD (GFR <60 mL/kg^{-1}/minute^{-1}), a CIN-preventative strategy begins in the preoperative period. Figure 8.2 shows a risk prediction diagram developed for patients undergoing percutaneous coronary intervention (PCI). The diagram refers only to PCI, although it may apply to at-risk patients scheduled to receive contrast dye.

Therapeutic strategies aimed at reducing the incidence of CIN are shown in Table 8.8. N-acetylcysteine, an antioxidant, has been studied in the context of CIN. A recent meta-analysis of seven trials (n = 805) demonstrated a 56% reduction in the incidence of CIN in at-risk patients receiving radiocontrast with prior N-acetylcysteine and intravenous hydration versus intravenous hydration alone (24). Perioperative N-acetylcysteine failed to prevent postoperative renal dysfunction in "high-risk" patients undergoing coronary artery bypass grafting (CABG) in a recent Canadian randomized placebo controlled trial (25). The prophylactic administration of N-acetylcysteine to patients with normal renal function is controversial. In a recent study, N-acetylcysteine decreased serum creatinine and increased eGFR, but did not change cystatin C levels in healthy volunteers who received four oral doses (26).

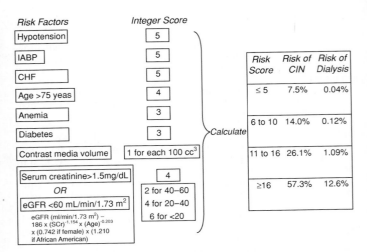

Figure 8.2. Risk prediction diagram for the development of contrast-induced nephropathy and for serious renal failure that requires dialysis after coronary angiography or percutaneous coronary intervention. Anemia, hematocrit <39% for men and <36% for women. CIN, contrast-induced nephropathy; CHF, congestive heart failure functional class III/IV or history of pulmonary edema; eGFR, estimated glomerular filtration rate; hypotension, systolic blood pressure <80 mm Hg for at least 1 hour that requires inotropic support with medications or intra-aortic balloon pump (IABP) within 24 hours of the procedure; SCr, serum creatinine. (Reproduced from Mehran R, Aymong ED, Nikolsky E, et al. A simple risk score for prediction of contrast-induced nephropathy after percutaneous coronary intervention: development and initial validation. *J Am Coll Cardiol.* 2004;44:1393–1399.)

$NaHCO_3$ given before administration of contrast dye is more protective than sodium chloride in animal models of ARF and ischemia. Free radical formation (postulated to cause CIN) is promoted by acidic environments such as those in the renal tubule. Alkalinizing renal tubular fluid with $NaHCO_3$ may reduce injury. A number of small randomized controlled trials support this proposition. The prevailing view is that $NaHCO_3$ may be useful in preventing CIN in high-risk patients.

PHARMACOLOGIC RENOPROTECTIVE STRATEGIES

Multiple interventions have been studied as renoprotective interventions. Unfortunately, most have proved ineffective or have even been shown to increase morbidity and mortality. The most common of these drugs are discussed below.

Dopamine Agonists

In view of its renal vasodilatory and natriuretic effects, dopamine has been extensively studied for renoprotective properties. Low-dose dopamine increases urine output; however, it does not decrease the incidence of sustained renal dysfunction or death in

Table 8.8.   Checklist for contrast-induced nephropathy risk stratification and prevention for patients at risk

1. Calculate eGFR (creatinine clearance) ⟶ high risk if GFR <60 mL/min^{-1}/1.73 m^2.
2. Determine history of or risk of diabetes ⟶ fivefold greater risk with diabetes.
3. Discuss contrast-induced nephropathy risk in informed consent process.
4. Discontinue nonsteroidal anti-inflammatory drugs (NSAIDs) and other renal toxic drugs.
5. Discontinue diuretics the day before and day of procedure.
6. If eGFR <15 mL/min^{-1}/1.73 m^2, obtain nephrology consult to plan for dialysis postprocedure.
7. Hydration with normal saline or sodium bicarbonate 1.5 mL/kg/hour starting 3 hours preprocedure and continuing 6 hours postprocedure.
8. N-acetylcysteine, 600 mg in 30 mL of ginger ale, two doses orally twice a day before and two doses orally twice a day after contrast administration.
9. Iodixanol is the preferred contrast agent for high-risk patients.
10. Limit contrast volume to <100 mL.
11. Ensure urine flow rate is >150 mL/hour after the procedure.
12. Avoid additional contrast dye for 10 days if possible.

eGFR, estimated glomerular filtration rate.
Adapted from McCullough PA, Soman SS. Contrast-induced nephropathy. *Crit Care Clin.* 2005;21:261–280.

patients with sepsis (27). Similarly, dobutamine does not alter RBF, GFR, or urine flow in patients who had vascular surgery. The adverse effects of dopamine include tachyarrhythmias, interpulmonary shunting, tissue necrosis from extravasation, and possible gut ischemia.

Fenoldopam mesylate is a selective dopamine-1-receptor agonist that has been approved for use in hypertensive emergencies (28). Fenoldopam increases renal cortical and medullary blood flow. Human studies involving small numbers of patients reported that fenoldopam possessed renoprotective effects in patients who had cardiopulmonary bypass and infrarenal aneurysm repair. More recent larger studies have failed to show this benefit in patients with early ARF and in cardiac patients postoperatively.

Furosemide, a loop diuretic, blocks reabsorption of Na$^+$ in the thick ascending limb of the loop of Henle. Theoretically furosemide could offer a renoprotective effect by decreasing oxygen and adenosine triphosphate (ATP) consumption because active reabsorption of Na$^+$ is decreased. Unfortunately, this theory is not borne out by clinical trials. A recent meta-analysis of 849 patients failed to identify any benefit of furosemide in the prevention or treatment of ARF (10).

Mannitol is an osmotic diuretic and free radical scavenger. Its use in renal transplant surgery before clamp release is associated with a significant decrease in posttransplant renal failure (29). Apart from the setting of renal transplantation, there is little evidence to support the administration of mannitol for the prevention of perioperative ARF. Mannitol does not prevent ARF after liver transplantation or cardiopulmonary bypass. Administration of mannitol, hydration, and forced alkaline diuresis for the prevention of ARF following crush injuries is widely practiced, but no controlled trials have demonstrated the efficacy of mannitol or alkaline diuresis in patients with rhabdomyolysis.

REFERENCES

1. Sort P, Navasa M, Arroyo V, et al. Effect of intravenous albumin on renal impairment and mortality in patients with cirrhosis and spontaneous bacterial peritonitis. *N Engl J Med*. 1999;341:403–409.
2. Bellomo R, Ronco C, Kellum JA, et al. Acute renal failure definition, outcome measures, animal models, fluid therapy and information technology needs: the Second International Consensus Conference of Acute Dialysis Quality Initiative (ADQI) Group. *Crit Care*. 2004;8:R204–212.
3. National Kidney Foundation, K/DOQI Clinical practice guidelines for chronic kidney disease: evaluation, classification and stratification. *Am J Kidney Dis*. 2002;39 (2 suppl 1):S19.
4. Class CM. Glomerular filtration rate. Screening cannot be recommended on the basis of current knowledge. *BMJ*. 2006;333:1030–1031.
5. Hallan SI, Oien CM, Grootendorst DC, et al. Screening strategies for chronic renal disease in the general population: follow-up of cross sectional health survey. *BMJ*. 2006;333:1047–1050.
6. Schrier RW, Wang W. Acute renal failure and sepsis. *N Eng J Med*. 2004;351:159–169.
7. Ganong WF. Renal function and micturition. In: Ganong WF, ed. *Review of Medical Physiology*. 20th ed. New York: McGraw-Hill; 2001:675–704.
8. Hou FF, Zhang X, Zhang GH, et al. Efficacy and safety of benazepril for advanced chronic renal insufficiency. *N Eng J Med*. 2006;354:131–140.
9. Laragh JH, Blumenfelld JD. Essential hypertension. In: Brenner BM, ed. *Brenner and Rectors's The Kidney*. Vol. 2. Philadelphia: WB Saunders; 2000: 1967–2006.
10. Ho KM, Sheridan DJ. Meta-analysis of frusemide to prevent or treat acute renal failure. *BMJ*. 2006;333:420–423.
11. Kellen M, Aronson A, Roizen MF, et al. Predictive and diagnostic tests of acute renal failure: a review. *Anesth Analg*. 1994;78:134–142.
12. Shiplak MG, Fried LF, Crump C, et al. Cardiovascular disease risk status in elderly patients with renal insufficiency. *Kidney Int*. 2002;62:997–1004.
13. Shoji T, Emoto M, Tabata T, et al. Advanced atherosclerosis in predialysis patients with chronic renal failure. *Kidney Int*. 2002;61:2187–2192.
14. Nakhoul F, Yigla M, Gilman R, et al. The pathogenesis of pulmonary hypertension in haemodialysis patients via arterio-venous access. *Nephrol Dial Transplant*. 2005;20:1686–1692.
15. Kaw D, Malhotra D. Platelet dysfunction and end-stage renal disease. *Semin Dial*. 2006;19:317–322.

16. Tveit DP, Hypolite IO, Hshieh P, et al. Chronic dialysis patients have high risk for pulmonary embolism. *Am J Kidney Dis.* 2002;39:1011–1107.
17. Bird NJ, Streather CP, O'Doherty MJ, et al. Gastric emptying in patients with chronic renal failure on continuous ambulatory peritoneal dialysis. *Nephrol Dial Transplant.* 1994;9:287–290.
18. Thapa S, Brull SJ. Succinylcholine-induced hyperkalemia in patients with renal failure. An old question revisited. *Anesth Analg.* 2000;91:237–241.
19. Schow AJ, Lubarsky DA, Olson RP, Gan TJ. Can succinylcholine be used safely in hyperkalemic patients? *Anesth Analg.* 2002;95:119–122.
20. Umana E, Ahmed W, Alpert MA. Valvular and perivalvular abnormalities in end-stage renal disease. *Am J Med Sci.* 2003;325:237–242.
21. De Gasperi A, Narcisi S, Mazza E, et al. Perioperative fluid management in kidney transplantation: is volume overload still mandatory for graft function? *Transplant Proc.* 2006;38:807–809.
22. Lee A, Cooper MC, Craig JC, et al. Effects of nonsteroidal anti-inflammatory drugs on post operative renal function in normal adults. *Cochrane Database Syst Rev.* 2004;2:CD002765.
23. Hanna MH, D'Costa F, Peat SJ, et al. Morphine-6-glucuronide disposition in renal impairment. *Br J Anaesth.* 1993;7:511–514.
24. Birck R, Krzossok S, Markowetx F, et al. Acetylcysteine for prevention of contrast nephropathy: meta-analysis. *Lancet.* 2003; 362:598–603.
25. Burns KE, Chu MW, Novick RJ. Perioperative N-acetylcysteine to prevent renal dysfunction in high-risk patients undergoing coronary artery bypass surgery: a randomized controlled trial. *JAMA.* 2005;294:342–350.
26. Hoffmann U, Fischereder M, Kruger B, et al. The value of N-acetylcysteine in the prevention of radiocontrast agent-induced nephropathy seems questionable. *J Am Soc Nephrol.* 2004; 15:407–410.
27. Bellomo R, Chapman M, Finfer S, et al. Low dose dopamine in patients with early renal dysfunction: a placebo controlled randomised trial. *Lancet.* 2000;356:2139–2143.
28. Murphy MB, Murray C, Shorten GD. Fenoldopam-a selective peripheral dopamine-receptor agonist for the treatment of severe hypertension. *N Engl J Med.* 2001;345:1548–1557.
29. van Valenberg PL, Hoitsma AJ, Tiggeler RG, et al. Mannitol as an indispensable constituent of an intraoperative hydration protocol in the prevention of acute renal failure after renal cadaveric transplantation. *Transplantation.* 1987;44:784–788.

Hepatobiliary Disease

Susan B. Glick and David B. Glick

The preoperative assessment and management of patients with hepatic and/or biliary disease present many challenges because of the wide-ranging and critical character of the functions performed by the normal liver. This chapter begins with a brief overview of normal liver function followed by a stepwise approach to the preoperative evaluation of the patient without known liver disease. A description of the common diseases that compromise liver function and surgical risk assessment models is then presented. The chapter concludes with a discussion of techniques to minimize operative risk.

LIVER FUNCTION IN HEALTH AND DISEASE

The liver's primary responsibilities—protein synthesis, toxin metabolism, bile production and excretion, and nutrient regulation—make its successful function of paramount importance perioperatively. The liver is divided into acini. The acinus comprises three distinct areas: portal areas from which venous and arterial blood enters the liver through small arteries and veins and bile leaves through bile ducts; sinusoids through which the blood flows to the terminal veins; and hepatocytes, which make up two thirds of the liver's mass. Bile flows from the hepatocytes to the portal areas, that is, in the reverse direction from the flow of blood.

Both the hepatic artery and the portal vein supply the liver with blood. Although the hepatic artery supplies only 20% of the liver's blood, it meets the majority of its oxygen requirements. The portal vein supplies the remaining 80% of the liver's blood. This blood is nutrient rich, having come from the stomach, intestines, pancreas, and spleen.

Liver disease can affect the hepatocytes exclusively, the biliary system exclusively, or both the hepatocytes and the biliary system. Diseases that predominantly damage hepatocytes, known as hepatocellular diseases, include viral hepatitis, alcoholic hepatitis, and autoimmune hepatitis. Diseases that primarily affect the biliary system with bile stasis are known as obstructive diseases. The obstruction may be extrahepatic, also known as obstructive jaundice (e.g., choledocholithiasis and malignant tumors of the bile duct); intrahepatic, also known as cholestatic disease (e.g., primary biliary cirrhosis); or both extrahepatic and intrahepatic (e.g., primary sclerosing cholangitis). Most drug-induced liver disease and some forms of viral hepatitis are both hepatocellular and cholestatic in character.

Diseases of the liver can affect its ability to synthesize proteins, metabolize toxins, produce and excrete bile, and regulate nutrients. Such diseases increase morbidity and mortality in the perioperative setting. The most common causes of perioperative mortality in patients with liver disease are hemorrhage, sepsis, liver failure, and hepatorenal syndrome.

The reasons for hemorrhage are multifactorial. When the liver loses function, it cannot synthesize proteins, including the coagulation factors. Coagulopathy also results from vitamin K deficiency in patients with cholestasis because the inability to secrete bile decreases the absorption of fat-soluble vitamins such as vitamin K. The final contributor to coagulopathy in hepatic disease is thrombocytopenia, found in patients with portal hypertension because of splenic sequestration and the immunologic destruction of platelets.

Ascitic fluid in patients with cirrhosis serves as an ideal culture medium for bacterial pathogens, so there is a constant risk of spontaneous bacterial peritonitis. Cholestasis provides a similarly rich culture medium, frequently resulting in cholangitis. The altered mental status of patients with hepatic encephalopathy increases the risk of aspiration pneumonia. Malnutrition and decreased ability to clear bacterial pathogens may also contribute to the infectious risk.

Hepatic failure is the development of hepatic encephalopathy—a decrease in level of consciousness—in a patient with acute or chronic liver disease. The results of the mental status examination and trail-making test, a paper-and-pencil exercise in which patients are asked to quickly connect 25 numbered circles in order, are abnormal in patients who develop hepatic encephalopathy. Bleeding, infection, and electrolyte disturbances are common precipitants. The serum ammonia level is usually elevated because the liver cannot clear this protein metabolite.

The hepatorenal syndrome is the name given to the renal failure that develops in patients with portal hypertension who have otherwise normally functioning kidneys. It is thought that portal hypertension increases the production of vasodilators in the splanchnic vessels. Splanchnic vasodilation then lowers arterial pressure, which stimulates vasoconstrictors, leading to constriction of the renal vessels and renal compromise.

THE PATIENT WITHOUT KNOWN LIVER DISEASE

The history is used to determine the likelihood that the patient without known liver disease actually has it. To this end, it is important to ask both about symptoms of liver disease and risk factors for hepatic diseases.

History: Symptoms of Liver Disease

Symptoms of liver disease include fatigue, weakness, and malaise. The fatigue is intermittent and often occurs after exertion. Patients awaken feeling rested, but become increasingly tired as the day progresses. Other symptoms include poor appetite and weight loss, generalized abdominal pain, right upper quadrant pain, and bloating. Right upper quadrant pain is caused by stretching or irritation of Glisson's capsule, the well-innervated tissue that covers the liver. Severe right upper quadrant pain may be caused by cholelithiasis/cholecystitis, liver abscess, and occasionally acute hepatitis. Bloating may be due to ascites. Jaundice, dark urine, and pruritus are important symptoms of liver disease. Patients initially notice darkening of the urine, followed by jaundice. The presence of jaundice usually indicates a serum bilirubin level >2.5 mg/dL, a sign that the liver cannot effectively conjugate and excrete bilirubin. Jaundice without darkening of the urine suggests indirect hyperbilirubinemia, found in hemolytic anemia and genetic diseases affecting the conjugation of bilirubin. Pruritus is one of the early manifestations of obstructive liver disease and may affect the patient later in the course of hepatocellular disease.

History: Risk Factors for Liver Disease

Risk factors for liver disease include alcohol use (more than two drinks daily for women and more than three drinks daily for men); sexual activity (men who have sex with men and patients with a lifetime history of multiple sexual partners are at increased risk for hepatitis B); and intravenous drug use (greatest risk factor for hepatitis C). Transfusion history is important; blood transfused before 1986 was not screened for hepatitis B core antibody, and blood transfused before 1992 was not screened for hepatitis C. Tattoos and body piercing increase the risk for hepatitis B. Travel to underdeveloped countries and exposure to children in daycare are risk factors for hepatitis A. Obesity confers risk for nonalcoholic steatohepatosis, which may result in fibrosis. Medications, including prescription medication such as statins, as well as over-the-counter and herbal medications, may cause liver disease. A family history of liver disease, including Wilson disease, hemochromatosis, and α_1-antitrypsin deficiency may increase patients' risk for these disorders. Because both anesthesia and surgery can result in hepatic dysfunction, a history of recent surgery or jaundice following anesthesia are important risk factors.

Physical Examination

The physical examination aims to identify liver disease in the patient without known disease and to classify the severity of liver disease if it is found. On general examination, the patient with advanced liver disease may exhibit muscle wasting and weight loss. The sclerae should be examined in natural light to assess the presence of icterus. Icterus can also be visualized in the membranes under the tongue. The chest should be percussed and auscultated for the presence of pleural effusion. Male patients' breasts may have gynecomastia. The abdomen should be evaluated for hepatomegaly, tenderness over the liver, and splenomegaly. The presence of ascites is suggested by abdominal distension and shifting dullness; however, the physical examination for ascites is unreliable in the presence of small amounts of ascitic fluid. Therefore, when ascites is suspected, ultrasound examination of the abdomen may be necessary to confirm it. Testicular atrophy may be present. Mental status examination may reveal cognitive deficits. The skin should be examined for spider angiomata, usually seen on the arms, face, and upper chest, and characterized by filling from the center of the lesion outward; palmar erythema; and excoriations, suggestive of pruritus from hyperbilirubinemia.

Laboratory Tests

Approximately 1 in 700 patients without known liver disease pre-operatively is found to have liver disease based on laboratory testing (1). Most of these patients do not have advanced disease (2). Therefore, in the absence of a known history of liver disease or a history or physical examination that suggests liver disease, preoperative laboratory testing for liver disease is unnecessary.

Patients with a known history of liver disease and those whose history and/or physical examination suggests liver disease should undergo laboratory testing to confirm the presence and severity of their disease. Serum alanine aminotransferase (ALT) and serum aspartate aminotransferase (AST) measure hepatocyte damage. Bilirubin measures hepatic conjugation and excretion. Alkaline phosphatase measures hepatic excretion. Albumin, prothrombin time (PT), and international normalized ratio (INR) measure protein synthesis.

Should laboratory testing reveal liver disease, additional testing may be required. For example, elevated ALT and AST with a normal alkaline phosphatase suggest hepatocellular damage. Serologic testing for acute hepatitis (hepatitis A IgM antibody, hepatitis B core antibody, hepatitis B surface antigen, and hepatitis C antibody) and chronic hepatitis (hepatitis B surface antigen, hepatitis B surface antibody, and hepatitis C antibody) may be helpful.

Imaging

Should the laboratory testing reveal elevated alkaline phosphatase with relatively normal ALT and AST, imaging of the biliary tract can help determine whether or not the obstruction is extrahepatic. Both abdominal ultrasound and computed tomography (CT) scan may be used to evaluate suspected obstructive jaundice. Either study may reveal dilated biliary ducts. Acute obstruction of the extrahepatic ducts may not be visible by CT or ultrasound and may require magnetic resonance cholangiopancreatography (MRCP) or endoscopic retrograde cholangiopancreatography (ERCP) for diagnosis. MRCP and ERCP are useful for visualizing the biliary tree. CT is helpful for the visualization of hepatic masses; magnetic resonance imaging (MRI) may also be used for this purpose.

Liver Biopsy

While liver biopsy remains the gold standard for the diagnosis of liver disease, current laboratory and imaging studies have decreased the need for this relatively invasive test. Nevertheless, liver biopsy remains important in establishing disease severity.

THE PATIENT WITH KNOWN LIVER DISEASE

The perioperative risk for the patient with known liver disease depends on the type of liver disease, its severity, the planned surgery, and the planned anesthesia.

Type of Liver Disease

Hepatocellular Disease (Acute Hepatitis, Chronic Hepatitis)

Hepatitis is an inflammatory disease of the hepatocytes. Inflammation may be caused by alcohol, viral infection (hepatitis A, hepatitis B, hepatitis C, hepatitis D, and hepatitis E), autoimmune disease, or drug use (both pharmacotherapy and illicit drugs). When hepatocytes are inflamed, they are unable to synthesize proteins, detoxify products of metabolism, regulate nutrient balance, or excrete bile.

Hepatitis A is the most common cause of acute viral hepatitis. It is transmitted by ingestion of contaminated food or water or by contact with an infected person. It is usually self-limited. Hepatitis B causes both acute and chronic hepatitis; it may progress to cirrhosis. The disease is transmitted both sexually and via the bloodstream. Hepatitis C also causes both acute and chronic hepatitis, although the acute phase of the illness is often asymptomatic. It is primarily a blood-borne infection and may progress to cirrhosis. Hepatitis D virus infection does not occur alone but requires coinfection with the hepatitis B virus. Intravenous drug use is the major risk factor for this disease. Hepatitis E virus is uncommon in the United States; it is primarily seen in underdeveloped countries. Like hepatitis A, hepatitis E tends to cause self-limited infections.

Alcoholic hepatitis is associated with chronic, excessive alcohol use (usually five to seven drinks per day for 10 years for men and three to four drinks per day for 10 years for women) and an as yet unexplained genetic predisposition. Among alcoholics, 10% to 20% develop alcoholic hepatitis; this may progress to cirrhosis.

Autoimmune hepatitis is an inflammatory liver disease of unknown etiology. It affects women predominantly, usually those 20 to 40 years old.

Over-the-counter and herbal medications as well as some prescription medications such as acetaminophen, statins, isoniazid, and venlafaxine may cause acute hepatitis.

Acute liver failure, also known as fulminant hepatic failure, is defined as altered mental status (hepatic encephalopathy) and impaired coagulation within 8 weeks of the onset of hepatic disease.

SURGICAL RISK

Acute Hepatitis.   Elective surgery is contraindicated in patients with acute or fulminant viral hepatitis; the mortality rate is 10% to 13% in patients with biopsy-proven viral hepatitis who undergo laparotomy. An additional 11% of patients develop significant complications perioperatively (3).

Elective surgery is also contraindicated in patients with acute alcoholic hepatitis because their mortality rates are 55% to 100% following exploratory laparotomy or portosystemic shunt surgery (4).

Because these results are reported in older studies, it is possible that newer preoperative and intraoperative diagnostic and treatment modalities will lead to better outcomes. In the absence of clear data on this issue, however, it is prudent to delay elective surgery until the acute insult has resolved.

The perioperative risk for patients with drug-induced hepatitis is unknown. Given the high mortality rates for patients with acute viral or alcoholic hepatitis, it seems reasonable to delay elective surgery for patients with drug-induced hepatitis as well.

Chronic Hepatitis. For patients with chronic hepatitis, the extent of hepatic dysfunction predicts operative risk. Patients whose disease is symptomatic or histologically severe have increased risk, especially patients with evidence of end-stage disease such as impaired hepatic synthetic (e.g., prolonged PT or INR or hypoalbuminemia) or excretory function (e.g., hyperbilirubinemia), portal hypertension (e.g., ascites or varices), or bridging or multilobular necrosis on liver biopsy (4,5).

Obstructive Disease

EXTRAHEPATIC OBSTRUCTION/OBSTRUCTIVE JAUNDICE. Extrahepatic obstruction of the bile ducts is often caused by choledocholithiasis (bile duct stones that have either descended from the gallbladder or formed directly inside the bile duct) or from malignancy of the pancreas or biliary tract (often carcinoma of the gallbladder, bile duct, or ampulla of Vater). Patients typically present with jaundice. Patients with choledocholithiasis usually have associated abdominal pain; patients with malignant obstruction may have little or no discomfort.

Surgical Risk. Extrahepatic obstruction increases a patient's risk for perioperative complications including infection (from bacterial colonization of the biliary tree), stress ulcers, disseminated intravascular coagulation, wound dehiscence, and renal failure. The perioperative mortality for these patients ranges from 8% to 28% (6–9).

Predictors of postoperative mortality include preoperative anemia (hematocrit <30%), hyperbilirubinemia (bilirubin >11), and obstruction related to malignant disease. Mortality approaches 60% in patients with all three risk factors; it is 5% in patients without these risk factors (7). Interestingly, preoperative transfusions do not decrease mortality (10).

Azotemia, hypoalbuminemia, and cholangitis are other predictors of mortality. Of patients with obstructive jaundice, 8% experience renal failure postoperatively, usually as a result of acute tubular necrosis (ATN) (11). The reason for renal failure is unclear but may be related to greater absorption of endotoxin. Administering bile salts or lactulose to patients with obstructive jaundice may prevent endotoxemia and the resultant renal vasoconstriction (12,13).

INTRAHEPATIC OBSTRUCTION/CHOLESTASIS. Intrahepatic obstruction of the bile ducts may be caused by primary biliary cirrhosis. Primary biliary cirrhosis is an autoimmune disorder of uncertain etiology found predominantly in women aged 40 to 60 years. Patients often experience fatigue and pruritus, and their antimitochondrial antibodies are usually elevated.

MIXED EXTRAHEPATIC AND INTRAHEPATIC OBSTRUCTION. Primary sclerosing cholangitis causes both extrahepatic and intrahepatic obstruction. Primary sclerosing cholangitis progressively destroys both large and small ducts. Of unknown etiology, it is more frequently found in men than in women, and usually affects patients aged 20 to 30 years. It is associated with inflammatory bowel disease and may progress to cirrhosis.

End-Stage Liver Disease/Cirrhosis

CIRRHOSIS. Cirrhosis represents the end result of many different hepatotoxic processes including alcohol ingestion, viral disease, autoimmune disease, drug use, genetic disorders, cholestasis, and inflammation of the biliary tract. The cirrhotic liver is characterized by fibronodular hyperplasia and bridging fibrosis. Fibronodular hyperplasia represents the liver's attempt to heal itself. Bridging fibrosis is the permanent sequela of hepatocellular destruction.

Functionally, the cirrhotic liver exhibits impaired synthetic function, toxin metabolism, bile production and excretion, nutrient regulation, and portal hypertension. The liver synthesizes almost all of the serum proteins and all coagulation factors except factor VIII. In patients with cirrhotic livers, production of protein, including albumin, is decreased and clotting factors are deficient. Difficulty detoxifying the products of protein metabolism (such as ammonia) results in hepatic encephalopathy. Insufficient excretion of bile causes cholestasis; elevated levels of bilirubin result in jaundice and inability to absorb fat-soluble vitamins such as vitamin K.

Portal hypertension results from the destruction of the hepatic sinusoids by fibronodular hyperplasia and fibrosis. Blood cannot flow easily through the affected hepatic sinusoids, which increases pressure in the splanchnic veins. Portal hypertension results when the pressure in the portal system is at least 5 mmHg higher than the pressure in the inferior vena cava. The small bowel, colon, and spleen become congested. Persistent portal hypertension causes filling of accessory veins especially in the stomach and esophagus. These accessory venous connections between the portal and systemic circuits are known as varices and are the body's attempt to equalize portal and systemic pressures.

Ascites results from portal hypertension together with hypoalbuminemia, increased secretion of antidiuretic hormone (ADH), and retention of sodium by the kidneys.

Cirrhosis also affects the cardiopulmonary system. In patients with advanced liver disease cardiac output increases and systemic vascular resistance decreases. There may also be shunting with decreased tissue perfusion despite the increase in cardiac output.

Ascites and pleural effusions (from portal hypertension) cause atelectasis and restrictive lung disease. Rarely, direct connections form between the portal veins and the pulmonary vessels. This condition, known as hepatopulmonary syndrome, causes hypoxemia from intrapulmonary arteriovenous shunting. Hepatopulmonary syndrome with hypoxemia is a relative contraindication to surgery other than liver transplantation.

Surgical Risk and Risk Prediction Models

Child's Classification.   Child's classification is the best validated way to predict perioperative risk for patients with cirrhosis. Child and Turcotte originally developed a system to predict mortality for patients with liver disease after portocaval shunt surgery (Table 9.1). Their classification included qualitative measures of ascites (none, easily controlled, or poorly controlled), encephalopathy (none, mild, or advanced), and nutritional status (excellent, good, or poor) as well as quantitative measures of bilirubin and albumin. The presence of ascites and the ease with which it is controlled are markers for the degree of portal hypertension and impairment in synthetic function. The presence and severity of encephalopathy measure the liver's ability to detoxify and clear products of metabolism, such as ammonia, which is a byproduct of protein metabolism. Nutritional status, exemplified by muscle wasting, reflects the ability of hepatic synthetic function to keep up with catabolic processes. Bilirubin measures hepatic excretory function, and albumin measures hepatic synthetic function.

Unfortunately, the Child-Turcotte classification has limitations. First, it was never prospectively validated in patients after surgeries other than open portosystemic shunts. Second, subjective assessments of ascites, encephalopathy, and nutritional status made it difficult to apply, especially retrospectively. As a result, Pugh later modified Child and Turcotte's classification system to the Child-Pugh classification system (or, more accurately, the Child-Turcotte-Pugh classification system).

Pugh replaced the assessment of nutritional status with prolongation of the PT, an independent predictor of mortality in the patients he studied who had esophageal transection. He also made the system quantitative by assigning point values to each variable. A total score of 5 to 6 equated to a Child's class A (well-compensated cirrhosis), 7 to 9 to a Child's class B (significant functional compromise), and 10 to 15 to a Child's class C (decompensated cirrhosis). The Child-Turcotte-Pugh classification system is the one most commonly used today; it is now most often referred to as Child's classification (Table 9.2).

The Model for End-Stage Liver Disease.   The model for end-stage liver disease (MELD) is a statistical model developed to predict survival of 3 months or less in patients with cirrhosis following transjugular intrahepatic portosystemic shunting (TIPS). Serum bilirubin, serum creatinine, INR, and etiology of liver disease

Table 9.1.   Child-Turcotte classification

Parameter	A	B	C
Ascites	None	Easily controlled	Poorly controlled
Bilirubin (mg/dL)	<2	2–3	>3
Albumin (g/dL)	>3.5	3.0–3.5	<3.0
Encephalopathy	None	Mild	Advanced
Nutritional status	Excellent	Good	Poor

Table 9.2. Child-Turcotte-Pugh classification

Parameter	Points Assigned		
	1	2	3
Ascites	Absent	Slight	Moderate
Bilirubin (mg/dL)	<2	2–3	>3
Albumin (g/dL)	>3.5	2.8–3.5	<2.8
Prothrombin time			
Seconds over control	<4	4–6	>6
Encephalopathy	None	Grade 1–2	Grade 3–4

(alcoholic, cholestatic, viral hepatitis, or other) were found to be strong predictors of 3-month survival.

$$\text{MELD score} = 3.8\,[\text{Ln serum bilirubin (mg/dL)}] + 11.2\,[\text{Ln INR}]$$
$$+ 9.6\,[\text{Ln serum creatinine (mg/dL)}]$$
$$+ 6.4\,[\times 0 \text{ for alcoholic liver disease,}$$
$$\times 1 \text{ for all other types of liver disease]}$$

Ln = natural logarithm

Ultimately, the etiology of liver disease was excluded from the model because many patients had multiple etiologies of disease. This deletion did not affect the predictive power of the model. This resulted in the modified MELD score, now commonly known simply as the MELD score.

$$\text{The modified MELD score} = 3.8\,[\text{Ln serum bilirubin (mg/dL)}]$$
$$+ 11.2\,[\text{Ln INR}]$$
$$+ 9.6\,[\text{Ln serum creatinine (mg/dL)}]$$
$$+ 6.4$$

Ln = natural logarithm

Because the MELD gives patients a score, rather than placing them in a class (e.g., Child's class A, B or C), it is better able to distinguish disease severity among patients than is Child's classification. MELD is currently used to select patients for transplantation. To prevent overemphasis on renal disease in the risk prediction model, the maximum serum creatinine that can be factored in is 4 (even for patients receiving dialysis). To avoid negative MELD scores (which confer better prognosis than positive scores but are confusing to patients), the minimum level of bilirubin, INR, and serum creatinine is 1. Scores range from 6 to 40 and are reported as the nearest integer; scores >40 are grouped together and treated as 40. Higher scores indicate more severe disease. Online calculators are available to determine the MELD score (e.g., www.unos.org).

Because survival after TIPS is related to underlying liver disease, it was thought that MELD could also be used as a prognostic indicator in patients with a broad range of disease severity expected to undergo a diverse range of surgical procedures. In fact, MELD score was a better predictor of poor outcome than

Child's class in one study of 53 cirrhotic patients who had abdominal surgery (14). In this study, a MELD score ≥14 increased the risk for poor outcome following non–gallbladder-related abdominal surgery and predicted 77% of patients who did poorly postoperatively. Patients whose MELD score was <14 preoperatively generally did well; however, 9% of these patients did poorly.

Patients Who Have Undergone Liver Transplantation

Improved survival rates after liver transplantation (90% at 1 year and 80% at 3 years) suggest that patients with liver transplants will require surgical intervention unrelated to liver disease. Evaluation of the hepatic function of patients with transplanted livers is imperative in the preoperative setting as some primary liver diseases may recur in the transplanted liver (e.g., hepatitis C and autoimmune hepatitis) to cause hepatic dysfunction. Less commonly, chronic rejection may affect hepatic function. The most common nonhepatic complications posttransplantation are hypertension, diabetes, osteoporosis, and renal insufficiency. Immunosuppressive therapy places patients at increased risk for infection.

Type of Surgery

General Principles

Morbidity and mortality are higher following emergency surgery than elective surgery. Perioperative events including hypotension, hepatic ischemia, blood loss, sepsis, and the use of hepatotoxic drugs can worsen liver function. Traction on the abdominal viscera during laparotomy may result in systemic hypotension. Clamping the suprahepatic inferior vena cava or hilar vessels in the operating room may induce hepatic ischemia. Hepatic lobectomy for hepatoma and other extensive procedures can result in significant blood loss. In addition, loss of liver mass in patients who undergo hepatic resection for hepatoma may also worsen liver function. Adhesions seen in patients with prior abdominal surgery can bleed intraoperatively.

Risk Prediction for Patients with Liver Disease Undergoing Surgery Related to Liver Disease

Patients with cirrhosis undergoing TIPS for recurrent variceal bleeding or ascites refractory to medical management whose MELD score is ≥18 have a significantly lower survival rate than patients whose MELD score is 17 or less (15). Following TIPS creation, the 6-month survival rate for patients with a MELD score ≤10 was 100%; for a MELD score of 11 to 17, 75%; for a MELD score of 18 to 24, 61%; and for a MELD score of ≥25, 25%.

Patients with hepatocellular carcinoma undergoing hepatic resection should be carefully evaluated for evidence of underlying liver disease. One retrospective study of 516 patients undergoing hepatic resection for hepatocellular carcinoma found that only 65 of the 516 patients (12.6%) did not have cirrhosis. Of these 65 patients, only eight (12.3%) had a normal liver histologically. Not surprisingly, the survival rate of the patients without cirrhosis was higher than those with cirrhosis (16). Resection of a cirrhotic liver increases morbidity and mortality. Patients with Child's class A cirrhosis generally do well postoperatively. A study of 63 patients with class B and C cirrhosis undergoing resection for hepatocellular carcinoma found that the in-hospital death rate was 14.3% (10.9% for class B and 23.5% for class C); for patients discharged from the hospital, the death rate within 1 month of surgery was 9.5% (6.5% for class B and 17.6% for class C) (17).

The MELD score, which is based on the risk of dying from liver disease within 3 months, is used to prioritize patients for liver transplant surgery. Patients with hepatocellular carcinoma and hepatopulmonary syndrome are afforded additional MELD points to reflect their unmeasured disease severity.

Risk Prediction for Patients with Liver Disease Undergoing Surgery Unrelated to Liver Disease

Either Child's classification or the MELD may be used to predict risk in patients with cirrhosis who have surgery unrelated to liver disease. The Child-Turcotte-Pugh score correlates with perioperative mortality in patients who have abdominal and other nonshunt surgery. In 1984 Garrison et al. evaluated the factors responsible for perioperative morbidity and mortality in 100 cirrhotic patients who underwent abdominal surgery for disease unrelated to cirrhosis. They found that poorly controlled ascites, encephalopathy, elevated bilirubin, prolonged prothrombin time, and decreased albumin, the factors that comprise the Child-Turcotte and Child-Turcotte-Pugh classifications, best predicted morbidity and mortality (18). Emergency surgery was another important predictor of morbidity and mortality.

Of the patients who had undergone emergency surgery, 80% did not survive. Of the patients who survived, 40% had serious complications. The average Child-Turcotte-Pugh score in nonsurviving patients was 2.4 (class A was scored as 1, class B as 2, and class C as 3); the average score of survivors who had complications was 1.6 and of survivors with no complications was 1.25. The need for reoperation, usually resulting from an ascitic leak after surgery, also predicted a high incidence of morbidity and mortality, as did postoperative pulmonary and renal dysfunction (18).

Mansour et al. retrospectively evaluated 92 cirrhotic patients who underwent surgical procedures other than portosystemic shunting (19). Their overall mortality was 26%, 10% for patients of Child's class A, 30% for those of Child's class B, and 82% for those of Child's class C. As in Garrison's study, the need for an emergency procedure increased risk (50% mortality overall, 22% for Child's class A, 38% for Child's class B, and 82% for Child's class C). The most important correlates of mortality were coagulopathy, encephalopathy, ascites, and impaired synthetic and excretory function. Once again, postoperative renal and pulmonary dysfunction were important predictors of poorer outcomes.

The more recent review by Ziser et al. of 733 patients with cirrhosis who had undergone any surgical procedure found that the overall 30-day postoperative mortality rate was 11.6% and complication rate was 30% (20). Risk factors independently associated with mortality included Child's class, ascites, a diagnosis of cirrhosis other than primary biliary cirrhosis, elevated creatinine, chronic obstructive pulmonary disease (COPD), preoperative infection, preoperative upper gastrointestinal bleeding, a high American Society of Anesthesiologists (ASA) physical status score, intraoperative hypotension, and a high surgical severity score (higher scores represent procedures associated with a greater degree of tissue injury).

The evaluation by Northup et al. of nontransplant surgical procedures in patients with cirrhosis including intra-abdominal, musculoskeletal, and cardiovascular procedures found that the MELD score was a significant predictor of 30-day postoperative mortality. A MELD score of 10 was associated with a postoperative mortality of 5%. Using multivariate logistic regression analyses, Northup et al. predicted mortality based on the MELD score. For MELD scores <20, each one-point increase in the MELD score was associated with an approximate 1% increase in mortality; for scores >20, each one-point increase was associated with a 2% increase in mortality (21).

DECREASING THE PERIOPERATIVE RISK

Coagulation Status

Patients with cirrhosis are often coagulopathic. Thrombocytopenia results from splenic sequestration. Production of clotting factors is decreased due to impaired hepatic synthetic function. Cholestasis further hampers clotting factor production by decreasing the ability to absorb the fat-soluble vitamin K. In the absence of overt bleeding, the optimal approach to correction of this coagulopathy is unclear.

In 2005, Caldwell et al. surveyed 95 participants in the Coagulation in Liver Disease symposium to learn about practice variation in assessment of bleeding risk and its prophylactic management in patients with liver disease. Seventy-one percent felt that the INR did not predict risk of postprocedure bleeding. However, 50% would correct the INR preoperatively for a liver biopsy if it were >1.5 and 81% would recommend platelet transfusion prior to liver biopsy for a platelet count <30,000. For placement of an intracranial pressure monitoring device, 55% would correct the INR preoperatively if it were >1.5; 34% would transfuse platelets if the platelet count were ≤50,000 (22).

In the absence of clear data about the prophylactic correction of coagulopathy, correcting the INR to <1.5 and the platelet count to ≥50,000 prior to surgery seems prudent. Vitamin K (10 mg IM, SC, or PO) in the days preceding surgery may improve the INR. This is particularly important for patients who are malnourished or have cholestasis. However, vitamin K will not improve the INR when hepatic synthesis of coagulation factors is impaired. Patients with this problem may require transfusion of fresh frozen plasma immediately prior to the procedure. Platelet transfusions may be necessary to correct the thrombocytopenia.

Renal Status

Because obstructive jaundice increases the risk of renal disease, it is particularly important to avoid additional chemical nephrotoxins, hypovolemia, and other renal hypoperfusion states (e.g., hypotension, heart failure, or sepsis) in the setting of significant hepatic disease. Administering lactulose (30 mL by mouth every 6 hours for 3 days before surgery with the last dose administered within 12 hours of surgery; patients with more than four bowel movements daily on this regimen should have one dose of lactulose held and subsequent doses reduced to 15 mL every 6 hours) or oral bile salts in addition to intravenous fluids the night before surgery reduced postoperative deterioration of renal function (23).

Ascites

Ascites should be controlled preoperatively to reduce the risk of abdominal wound dehiscence and to optimize respiratory function. Sodium (oral and intravenous) should be restricted. Diuretics and therapeutic paracentesis may also help control the patient's ascites. When large-volume paracentesis is required, albumin should be administered simultaneously to decrease the risk of renal dysfunction (24). Aspirated ascitic fluid should be analyzed for spontaneous bacterial peritonitis, which, when present, increases postoperative mortality.

Anemia

While anemia is one of the factors that contribute to high postoperative mortality in patients with obstructive jaundice, correcting the anemia preoperatively is controversial. Some authors feel that this does not improve prognosis (10). Others feel that correcting anemia preoperatively may prevent deterioration in renal function (25).

Encephalopathy

Encephalopathy is commonly precipitated by infection, gastrointestinal bleeding, uremia, hypovolemia, hypoxia, electrolyte imbalances, and sedative use. Patients with encephalopathy should be carefully evaluated for its underlying etiology; when identified, this should be treated aggressively. Lactulose (30 mL by mouth every 6 hours, titrated to two to three bowel movements daily) can be used preoperatively to reduce encephalopathy. Patients who are unable to tolerate lactulose may obtain benefit from oral rifaximin therapy; however, this use is not currently approved by the U.S. Food and Drug Administration.

Nutrition

Optimizing nutritional status by administering supplemental enteral or parenteral feedings is helpful for patients with alcoholic hepatitis and may be beneficial for patients with cirrhosis and malnutrition.

Infection

Patients with obstructive jaundice benefit from the perioperative administration of broad-spectrum antibiotics, a therapy that decreases the frequency of postoperative infections without affecting mortality. Preoperative endoscopic biliary drainage decreases mortality for patients with cholangitis and choledocholithiasis but is ineffective for patients with malignant obstruction of the biliary tract. Transhepatic drainage of the biliary tree is also ineffective in this setting.

Anesthetic Considerations

Many of the characteristics of patients with liver diseases discussed previously in this chapter have direct bearing on the plans and conversations that take place on the day of surgery. These include decisions regarding anesthetic technique and the choice of specific anesthetic agents.

Anesthetic Technique

Because many patients with liver disease have coagulation abnormalities, operations on these patients that would otherwise be performed using neuraxial blocks (spinal or epidural anesthetics) would be inappropriate if the patient's INR on preoperative testing is >1.3 because of the increased risk of epidural hematoma (see Chapter 7). These considerations should be explained to the patient preoperatively.

Choice of Anesthetic Agents

Planning the anesthetic for a patient who has liver disease requires the use of agents that minimize additional damage to the already compromised liver and do not require significant hepatic function for clearance to avoid postoperative complications due to persistence of drugs used intraoperatively. While a complete discussion of the relative merits and liabilities of various agents is beyond the scope of this chapter, a brief outline of the common considerations follows.

Volatile Agents

The degree to which volatile anesthetics are metabolized by the liver mirrors the degree to which they cause hepatotoxicity. Because the liver does not metabolize isoflurane and the newer haloalkanes desflurane and sevoflurane as extensively as halothane or enflurane, the former agents carry a lesser risk of hepatitis. Of all of the volatile anesthetics, halothane has the greatest risk of hepatotoxicity. There are two types of halothane hepatitis. One is minor, seen in 10% to 30% of patients exposed to halothane, and consists of a mild increase in the ALT postoperatively, often accompanied by fever, nausea, and fatigue. The hepatitis resolves spontaneously in 1 to 2 weeks. There are no signs of immune disease in these patients.

The second type of halothane hepatitis is less common, seen in only 1 in 10,000 to 30,000 patients who receive halothane, but is much more serious and can be fatal. This type of halothane hepatitis is autoimmune in nature. The trifluoroacetyl metabolite of halothane is thought to induce the formation of neohepatic antigens, to which patients develop IgG antibodies. The resultant antibody–neoantigen reaction causes hepatitis. Although halothane is now rarely used for adult patients in the United States, patients previously exposed to it may develop cross-sensitivity to other fluorinated volatile anesthetics that have trifluoroacetyl metabolites, including enflurane, isoflurane, and desflurane. Thus, identifying previous episodes of halothane-induced liver injury is an important part of the preoperative workup. Sevoflurane is the anesthetic choice for patients with a history of halothane-induced hepatitis because it is not metabolized to a trifluoroacetylated form and therefore does not exhibit cross-sensitivity to halothane or result in immune-mediated hepatotoxicity.

In addition to the concerns regarding direct hepatocyte injury from some of the anesthetic gases, most volatile anesthetics also decrease oxygen delivery to the liver by decreasing portal blood flow and cardiac output. Hepatic blood flow is not autoregulated as in the kidneys and brain to preserve it from variations in blood pressure. Hepatic blood flow depends on hepatic perfusion pressure. Decreases in systemic vascular resistance or cardiac output can compromise blood flow and oxygen delivery to the liver. Hepatic oxygenation depends more on hepatic arterial blood flow in patients with underlying liver disease than in healthy patients. Halothane and enflurane decrease hepatic arterial blood flow through systemic vasodilation and negative inotropic effects. The newer vaporized agents cause marked peripheral vasodilation but have less effect on cardiac contractility and thus cardiac output. Therefore, hepatic perfusion may be better preserved with isoflurane, desflurane, and sevoflurane. Nevertheless, intravascular volume and oxygen delivery should be optimized to limit intraoperative hepatic injury.

Muscle Relaxants

There are a number of significant concerns regarding the use and dosing of muscle relaxants in patients with liver disease. The duration of action of some relaxants (e.g., rocuronium and vecuronium) may be prolonged because they depend on hepatic metabolism for clearance. Another important consideration when administering a nondepolarizing agent to patients with hepatic compromise is that the increase in the volume of distribution (caused by increased fluid retention) in these patients increases the initial dose requirements for effective relaxation. Of course, higher doses also prolong paralytic effects.

The use of cisatracurium or atracurium for patients with liver disease or biliary obstruction is reasonable because these agents are metabolized via the blood-borne enzymes of the Hofmann elimination system (and in the case of atracurium, by nonspecific plasma esterases) and do not require hepatic metabolism or renal function for clearance.

Other Anesthetic Medications

Many drugs used in anesthetic practice undergo first-pass metabolism by the liver or are bound by plasma proteins synthesized by the liver. Failure of first-pass metabolism increases the potency and potential toxicity of the amide local anesthetics (e.g., lidocaine), meperidine, and diazepam. Hypoalbuminemia leads to higher free concentrations and greater potency/toxicity of barbiturates, diazepam, and warfarin. Narcotics and other sedative agents must be used with caution in patients with advanced liver disease because they can contribute to the development of hepatic encephalopathy, especially if the administered sedative depends on hepatic metabolism for clearance.

SUMMARY

1. Patients with acute liver disease should postpone elective surgery, ideally until recovery. If surgery is required, hepatotoxins should be avoided and the patient should be monitored closely in the perioperative setting for worsening hepatic dysfunction and its sequelae.
2. Patients with chronic liver disease should postpone elective surgery until the cause and severity of liver disease are known. Patients without cirrhosis may proceed to the operating room. Patients with cirrhosis should be assessed using Child's classification or the MELD score. Patients who are Child's class A may proceed to the operating room. Patients who are Child's class B should have surgery only if it is absolutely necessary. In this circumstance, avoidance of hepatotoxins and perioperative monitoring for worsening hepatic function is of paramount importance. Patients who are Child's class C should avoid surgery except for those surgical procedures designed to correct the sequelae of liver disease (e.g., shunt placement and transplantation). Although cut points have not yet been determined for the MELD score, patients whose MELD score is <10 are likely to do well postoperatively; those whose score is >20 risk significant postoperative mortality.

REFERENCES

1. Jackson FC, Christophersen EB, Peternel WW, et al. Preoperative management of patients with liver disease. *Surg Clin North Am*. 1968;48:907–930.
2. Schemel WH. Unexpected hepatic dysfunction found by multiple laboratory screening. *Anesth Analg*. 1976;55:810.
3. Harville DD, Summerskill WHJ. Surgery in acute hepatitis: causes and effects. *JAMA*. 1963;184:257–261.
4. Powell-Jackson P, Greenway B, Williams R. Adverse effects of exploratory laparotomy in patients with unsuspected liver disease. *Br J Surg*. 1982;69:449–451.
5. Hargrove MD Jr. Chronic active hepatitis: possible adverse effect of exploratory laparotomy. *Surgery*. 1970;68:771–773.
6. Higashi H, Matsumata T, Adachi E, et al. Influence of viral hepatitis status on operative morbidity and mortality in patients with primary hepatocellular carcinoma. *Br J Surg*. 1994;81:1342–1345.
7. Dixon JM, Armstrong CP, Duffy SW, et al. Factors affecting morbidity and mortality after surgery for obstructive jaundice: a review of 373 patients. *Gut*. 1983;24:845–852.
8. Greig JD, Krukowski ZH, Matheson NA. Surgical morbidity and mortality in one hundred and twenty nine patients with obstructive jaundice. *Br J Surg*. 1988;75:216–219.
9. Shirahatti RG, Alphonso N, Joshi RM, et al. Palliative surgery in malignant obstructive jaundice: prognostic indicators of early mortality. *J R Coll Surg Edinb*. 1997;42:238–243.
10. Pain JA, Cahill CJ, Bailey ME. Perioperative complications in obstructive jaundice: therapeutic considerations. *Br J Surg*. 1985;72:942–945.
11. Fogarty BJ, Parks RW, Rowlands BJ, et al. Renal dysfunction in obstructive jaundice. *Br J Surg*. 1995;82:877–884.

12. Cahill CJ. Prevention of post-operative renal failure in patients with obstructive jaundice: the role of bile salts. *Br J Surg*. 1983; 70:590–595.

13. Pain JA, Bailey ME. Experimental and clinical study of lactulose in obstructive jaundice. *Br J Surg*. 1986;73:775–778.

14. Befeler AS, Palmer DE, Hoffman M, et al. The safety of intra-abdominal surgery in patients with cirrhosis: model for end-stage liver disease score is superior to Child-Turcotte-Pugh classification in predicting outcome. *Arch Surg*. 2005;140:650–654.

15. Ferral H, Gamboa P, Postoak DW, et al. Survival after elective transjugular intrahepatic portosystemic shunt creation: prediction with model for end-stage liver disease score. *Radiology*. 2004;231:231–236.

16. Shimada M, Rikimaru T, Sugimachi K, et al. The importance of hepatic resection for hepatocellular carcinoma: originating from nonfibrotic liver. *J Am Coll Surg*. 2000;191:531–537.

17. Nagasue N, Kohno H, Tachibana M, et al. Prognostic factors after hepatic resection for hepatocellular carcinoma associated with Child-Turcotte class B and C cirrhosis. *Ann Surg*. 1999;229: 84–90.

18. Garrison RN, Cryer HM, Howard DA, et al. Clarification of risk factors for abdominal operations in patients with hepatic cirrhosis. *Ann Surg*. 1984;199:648–655.

19. Mansour A, Watson W, Shayani V, et al. Abdominal operations in patients with cirrhosis: still a major surgical challenge. *Surgery*. 1997;122:730–736.

20. Ziser A, Plevak DJ, Wiesner RH, et al. Morbidity and mortality in cirrhotic patients undergoing anesthesia and surgery. *Anesthesiology*. 1999;90:42–53.

21. Northup PG, Wanamaker RC, Lee VD, et al. Model for End-Stage Liver Disease (MELD) predicts nontransplant surgical mortality in patients with cirrhosis. *Ann Surg*. 2005;242:244–251.

22. Caldwell SH, Hoffman M, Lisman T, et al. Coagulation disorders and hemostasis in liver disease: pathophysiology and critical assessment of current management. *Hepatology*. 2006;44:1039–1046.

23. Pain JA, Cahill CJ, Gilbert JM, et al. Prevention of postoperative renal dysfunction in patients with obstructive jaundice: a multi-centre study of bile salts and lactulose. *Br J Surg*. 1991;78:467–469.

24. Rizvon MK, Chou CL. Surgery in the patient with liver disease. *Med Clin N Am*. 2003;87:211–227.

25. Patel T. Surgery in the patient with liver disease. *Mayo Clin Proc*. 1999;74:593–599.

Neurologic Disease

David L. Hepner and Angela M. Bader

Because patients with a wide variety of neurologic disorders will be evaluated, the following questions may assist the clinician in the evaluation and formulation of an anesthetic plan:

1. What is the basic pathophysiology of the particular neurologic disorder?
2. What are the patient's history, symptomatology, and neurologic deficit?
3. What current treatments are being used?
4. What testing results are available or must be ordered to evaluate the patient for the planned anesthetic?
5. What are the potential impact, risk, and benefit of particular anesthetic options based on the pathophysiology, symptoms, and treatment? Is there anything that can be done preoperatively that may improve outcome?

In all cases, accurate documentation of the responses to the above questions will greatly assist the team assigned to provide anesthesia care for patients with neurologic disease.

The following conditions will be discussed:

1. Multiple sclerosis
2. Seizure disorders
3. Acquired and inherited disorders affecting the neuromuscular junction including myasthenia gravis, Lambert-Eaton myasthenia syndrome, muscular dystrophies, and myotonic dystrophies
4. Cerebrovascular disease/strokes
5. Dementia
6. Parkinson's disease
7. Pituitary tumors
8. Brain tumors
9. Aneurysms and arteriovenous malformations

MULTIPLE SCLEROSIS

Multiple sclerosis is a significant cause of neurologic disability with a wide range of manifestations. The disease alters neurologic disability over years in two general patterns: Exacerbating-remitting, in which attacks appear and resolve over a time period, and chronic progressive (1). The etiology remains unknown, although it is generally considered an inflammatory immune disorder with a genetic predisposition mediated by T cells directed against myelin components (2). The epidemiology of the disease is of interest; onset is generally between 20 and 40 years of age. In the United States the prevalence is about 100 per 100,000, with increasing prevalence in populations farther from the equator. Factors associated with relapse include the postpartum period, infection, elevated temperature, and stress (3).

Common symptoms are motor weakness, sensory disorders, visual impairment, ataxia, bladder and bowel dysfunction, autonomic instability, and emotional instability. Cerebrospinal fluid may be abnormal, and magnetic resonance imaging (MRI) may demonstrate white matter plaques with prolongation of evoked potentials in the involved areas.

Treatment Modalities

There is no curative treatment. A number of immunosuppressive therapies have been tried, including corticosteroids, cyclosporine, azathioprine, immunoglobulin, and plasma exchange. Azathioprine has been associated with bone marrow suppression and abnormal liver function. Cyclophosphamide can result in electrolyte abnormalities because of inappropriate secretion of antidiuretic hormone. Several β-interferon class agents have been investigated, but data on long-term efficacy are sparse (4). Studies of newer agents such as glatiramer, which competes with myelin antigens, and natalizumab, a monoclonal antibody, show some benefit. Symptoms of bladder dysfunction and muscle spasticity may be treated with diazepam, dantrolene sodium, or baclofen. Dantrolene has been associated with liver function abnormalities, and baclofen may prolong the action of sedatives and hypnotics.

Table 10.1. Preanesthetic considerations for multiple sclerosis

1. Assess and document degree of compromise and pattern of deficits.
2. Consider pulmonary function tests in patients with a significant degree of respiratory compromise.
3. Consider complete blood count with platelets and liver function testing (albumin, alanine transaminase, aspartate transaminase, alkaline phosphatase, and total bilirubin) in patients taking dantrolene and azathioprine because bone marrow may be suppressed and liver function may be impaired (lesions of the venous system of the liver: Peliosis hepatis, veno-occlusive disease of the liver, perisinusoidal fibrosis, and nodular regenerative hyperplasia of the liver).
4. Consider electrolyte levels in patients taking steroids or cyclophosphamide, which can induce syndrome of inappropriate antidiuretic hormone secretion.
5. Consider blood glucose levels in patients treated with steroids, which may cause hyperglycemia.
6. Patients treated with steroids or adrenocorticotropic hormone for prolonged periods may require perioperative supplemental steroids.
7. Sensitivity to hyperthermia makes temperature management critical.
8. Despite previous controversy, general and regional anesthesia can be options depending on type of surgery and patient preference.

Preanesthetic Evaluation

Patient assessment documents history and pattern of deficits, with special attention to respiratory involvement in those more severely affected. Severely debilitated patients may be at risk for succinylcholine-induced hyperkalemia. Formerly, there was concern regarding the administration of regional anesthesia to patients with multiple sclerosis because of potential exposure of demyelinated areas of the spinal cord to the neurotoxic effects of local anesthetics, which may increase postoperative relapse and disability. The recent literature suggests that the incidence of relapse is not increased after the use of epidural anesthesia (5,6). Data on spinal anesthesia in these patients are extremely limited; however, it is our practice to consider all options for regional anesthesia in these patients. Patients are told that there is no clear association of any particular type of anesthetic with an increase in relapse rate, and the choice depends on overall medical issues and type of surgery. Patients are instructed to take their medications as scheduled up until the day of surgery. Careful attention is paid to avoid or treat factors known to be associated with relapses, such as increased temperature, infection, and postoperative pain-induced stress. Table 10.1 summarizes the preanesthetic considerations for multiple sclerosis.

SEIZURE DISORDERS

Epilepsy is a condition in which the patient experiences one of a variety of forms of recurrent seizure activity in the absence of metabolic disorders or acute brain disease. Seizures are generally classified by type based on clinical appearance and the result of laboratory and imaging studies. In the presurgical population seizures may not be caused by classic epilepsy, but by primary or metastatic intracranial lesions as well as metabolic disorders. In the elderly, 25% to 50% of new seizures are seen in patients over the age of 65 (7). Cerebrovascular disease, including strokes and transient ischemic attacks (TIAs), has been associated with seizures. Both Alzheimer and non-Alzheimer dementia are risk factors for epilepsy (8).

Treatment Modalities

Treatment is geared toward patients with increased risk for recurrent seizures; individuals with a single seizure or seizures from factors that resolve may not require long-term therapy. Choice among a variety of anticonvulsant drugs depends on seizure type and patient response to therapy.

Preanesthetic Evaluation

Assessment includes a history of seizure type, frequency, etiology, and any significant testing or imaging results. An increase in seizure frequency requires consultation with the patient's neurologist to determine if therapy is needed before the planned surgery. Other causes of increased seizure frequency, such as electrolyte disturbances, should be investigated. Documentation of drug therapies and dosages is necessary, as is knowledge of their adverse effects and potential toxicities (Table 10.2). Preoperative laboratory testing is interpreted in light of the adverse

Table 10.2. Commonly used antiepileptic therapies

Drug	Dose	Adverse Effects and Toxicities
Phenytoin	Average: 400 mg/day Therapeutic level: 10–20 μg/mL	Ataxia, drowsiness, gum hyperplasia, nystagmus, macrocytic anemia, Stevens-Johnson syndrome
Carbamazepine	Average: 600 mg/day Therapeutic level: 4–8 μg/ml	Nausea, diarrhea, rash, pruritus, dizziness, hyponatremia, leucopenia, blood dyscrasias, Stevens-Johnson syndrome
Phenobarbital	Average: 120 mg/day Therapeutic level: 10–35 μg/mL	Drowsiness, nystagmus, rash
Ethosuximide	Average: 1,000 mg/day Therapeutic level: 40–100 μg/mL	Drowsiness, nausea, rash, marrow depression
Primidone	Average: 1,000 mg/day Therapeutic level: 4–12 μg/mL	Drowsiness, nausea, rash, lupus, macrocytic anemia

effects of the particular agents the patient is taking. For example, a number of these agents are associated with electrolyte and liver function abnormalities. Accordingly, serum electrolyte levels and liver function are measured, except in the stable patient on chronic therapy. Therapeutic levels of antiepileptic drugs are usually assessed by "trough" levels just before the scheduled dose, and are documented during the initial phases of anticonvulsant therapy; usually patients who are monitored on an established dose for a period of time will have stable therapeutic levels. As long as seizures are controlled and there are no signs or symptoms of toxicity, levels are not checked before surgery. Oral therapies are continued when possible throughout the perioperative period, including the day of surgery, when they can be taken with a small amount of water (pediatric patients can take medications sprinkled on Jell-O). If the agents used are not available in parenteral forms, conversion to a parenteral agent such as phenytoin may be required during the postoperative period and levels should be monitored to ensure that they are therapeutic. Adverse effects of all of these agents should be considered; in general, these agents may have sedating properties and also induce liver enzymes, which may lead to rapid breakdown of anesthetics that depend on hepatic metabolism. Hyponatremia in particular has been associated with carbamazepine and similar agents such as oxcarbazepine. This effect is more likely to be seen within the first 3 months of treatment or in elderly patients.

There is no contraindication to the administration of regional anesthesia in patients with classic epilepsy without evidence of intracranial mass lesions. These patients are not more sensitive to the toxic effects of local anesthetics and do not require alterations in dosages for regional anesthesia. In fact, the blood concentrations achieved after epidural anesthesia may have an anticonvulsant effect in pre-eclamptic women (9). Drugs known to lower the seizure threshold are avoided or used judiciously. These drugs include ketamine, etomidate, and meperidine. Most of the inhalational agents provoke seizurelike activity to varying degrees. The agents ranked from greatest to least by their relative ability to spike activity are enflurane > sevoflurane > isoflurane > desflurane (10). Low doses of propofol also activate the electrocorticogram in epileptic patients; at higher doses, however, burst suppression is induced (11). Even fentanyl has been associated with electroencephalographic and clinical signs of epileptoid activity in some surgical patients (12). Diazepam is used as a premedicant to prevent or reduce the epileptoid phenomenon from opioid administration during the anesthetic procedure.

MYASTHENIA GRAVIS

Myasthenia gravis is an autoimmune disorder characterized by muscle weakness that worsens with activity (13). Table 10.3 lists common symptoms of this disorder.

Abnormal autoimmune regulation produces antibodies directed against the nicotinic acetylcholine receptor on the neuromuscular endplate of skeletal muscle. Antibodies destroy the receptor or block the remaining receptors; smooth and cardiac muscle are not affected. Thymic hyperplasia is common and thymic tumors are found in 10% of patients. The most common symptom is weakness, which can be exacerbated by pain, sleeplessness, infections, hypokalemia, surgery, and menses. Myasthenia is often associated with other autoimmune disorders such as rheumatoid arthritis and polymyositis. Table 10.4 shows a common classification system for this disorder originally described by Osserman.

Table 10.3. Symptoms of myasthenia gravis

Muscle weakness is typically exacerbated by exercise and resolves partially with rest.

Cranial nerves are particularly susceptible.

Ocular symptoms are extremely common, particularly diplopia and ptosis.

Bulbar involvement can lead to pharyngeal and laryngeal muscle weakness with resultant respiratory insufficiency and risk of aspiration.

**Table 10.4.   Common classification system
for myasthenia gravis**

1. Ocular myasthenia
2a. Mild generalized myasthenia with slow progression; no crises;
    drug responsive
2b. Moderate generalized myasthenia; severe skeletal and bulbar
    involvement, but no crises; drug response less than satisfactory
3. Acute fulminating myasthenia; rapid progression of severe
   symptoms with respiratory crises and poor drug response; high
   incidence of thymoma; high mortality
4. Late severe myasthenia

Treatment Modalities

Treatment includes thymectomy, anticholinesterase medications,
immunosuppressive agents, and plasmapheresis. More than 90%
of patients improve after thymectomy (14). In myasthenia gravis,
a cholinergic crisis results from an excess of muscarinic effects
of anticholinesterase therapy; a myasthenic crisis results from a
worsening of the disease. These can be distinguished with the use
of edrophonium; the symptoms will not improve if a cholinergic
crisis is present.

Preanesthetic Evaluation

Patients with myasthenia gravis are particularly sensitive to
drugs that can potentiate muscle weakness, like the neuromuscular blocking agents, propranolol, and aminoglycoside antibiotics
(15). A list of drugs and other factors that can exacerbate myasthenia gravis is provided in Table 10.5.

Preanesthetic evaluation assesses the degree of respiratory
and bulbar involvement. In patients with a significant degree
of respiratory compromise (Osserman class 3 or 4), pulmonary
function tests (PFTs) are performed. Opioids are used cautiously

**Table 10.5.   Some factors that exacerbate
myasthenia gravis**

Pain
Lack of sleep
Temperature extremes
Infections
Hypokalemia
Drugs:
  Glucocorticoids
  Antiseizure medications: Phenytoin and possibly carbamazepine
  Antibiotics including aminoglycosides, ciprofloxacin, clindamycin,
    and possibly ampicillin
  Antiarrhythmics including procainamide, propranolol, and
    possibly quinidine and verapamil
  Neuromuscular blockers

in the presence of respiratory compromise. Reduced plasma cholinesterase activity in patients taking anticholinesterase drugs potentially prolongs the effects of medications like succinylcholine and ester local anesthetic agents. Response to muscle relaxants is unpredictable; in general, muscles affected by the disease are highly sensitive to depolarizing agents, and nonaffected muscles are highly resistant (16). Volatile anesthetic agents may potentiate the effects of muscle relaxants. A recent study comparing propofol and sevoflurane anesthesia without the use of muscle relaxants in myasthenic patients found that after either technique patients could be extubated early in the operating room (17).

Table 10.6 summarizes both traditional as well as recent work attempting to identify factors that predict an increased risk for postoperative ventilation in patients with myasthenia (18). The recent studies, however, have been criticized for small numbers of patients and overlap in some categories. Perhaps the most important preoperative factor predicting the need for postoperative mechanical ventilation is the severity of bulbar involvement, usually found in patients in Osserman groups 3 and 4 (Table 10.4), the groups for which preoperative PFTs should be considered.

Patients treated with azathioprine may experience bone marrow suppression and liver function abnormalities, warranting consideration of appropriate laboratory tests for evaluation. Patients are instructed to take their usual anticholinesterase medications on the day of surgery, although the adverse effects of these medications can include bradycardia and salivation. Perioperative steroid coverage is considered in patients who are treated chronically with steroids, which includes taking their usual dose on the day of surgery. Blood glucose levels are evaluated

Table 10.6.   Factors that predict the need for postoperative ventilation in myasthenia gravis

Traditional:

1. Duration >6 years
2. History of chronic respiratory disease
3. Pyridostigmine dosage >750 mg/day
4. Preoperative vital capacity of <2.9 L

More recent:

1. Female gender
2. Forced expiratory flow (FEF) 25%–75% <3.3 L/sec and <85% predicted
3. Forced vital capacity (FVC) <2.6 L/sec and <78% of predicted
4. Maximum expiratory flow (MEF) 50% <3.9 L/sec and <80% of predicted

FEF 25%–75% = Forced midexpiratory flow between 25% and 75% of the FVC.
MEF 50% = Maximum expiratory flow at 50% of the FVC.
From Naguib M, el Dawlatly A, Ashour M, et al. Multivariate determinants of the need for postoperative ventilation in myasthenia gravis. *Can J Anaesth.* 1996;43:1006–1013.

in patients on chronic steroid therapy. Plasmapheresis, as well as intravenous immunoglobulin therapy, has been used in some patients during myasthenic crises and before surgery. Both have been shown to be equally efficacious, although improvement requires several weeks of treatment. Consultation with the patient's neurologist determines the best method of preparation for the upcoming surgical procedure.

LAMBERT-EATON SYNDROME

Lambert-Eaton syndrome is similar in pathophysiology to myasthenia, and over 60% of cases are associated with small cell lung carcinoma (19). Patients have progressive limb girdle weakness, dysautonomia, and oculobulbar palsy. In this disorder autoantibodies have been identified against voltage-gated calcium channels, which reduce calcium influx and decrease acetylcholine (Ach) release.

Treatment Modalities

Selective potassium channel blockade with a drug such as 3,4-diaminopyridine increases Ach release in these patients and may improve symptoms. Acetylcholinesterase inhibitors such as pyridostigmine have also been used. Immunologic therapies such as prednisone, azathioprine, plasmapheresis, and intravenous immune globulin are beneficial in some patients.

Preanesthetic Evaluation

These patients are sensitive to both nondepolarizing and depolarizing neuromuscular junction blockers and significantly more sensitive to nondepolarizers than patients with myasthenia gravis (20). Preanesthetic evaluation assesses the degree of respiratory compromise and otherwise is very similar to assessment of myasthenia gravis. PFTs are considered in patients with significant bulbar involvement and respiratory symptomatology. Drug therapies are continued perioperatively. The same issues noted under myasthenia gravis for laboratory testing in patients taking prednisone and azathioprine for treatment are considered as well.

DUCHENNE AND BECKER MUSCULAR DYSTROPHY

The inherited disorders affecting the neuromuscular junction include the muscular dystrophies, congenital myopathies, and central core disease (21). Duchenne and Becker dystrophies are X-linked recessively inherited diseases in which dystrophin protein is missing or in an abnormal form resulting in muscle cell necrosis. Duchenne dystrophy is the more severe form; death from pulmonary causes by age 20 is usual. Young male patients with family histories of these dystrophies who have not been tested should be considered at risk for these disorders. Both disorders are characterized by an elevation in serum creatinine phosphokinase level and a myopathic pattern on the electromyogram. There is no definitive treatment, although some evidence suggests that prednisone slows the progression of Duchenne dystrophy.

Preanesthetic Assessment

Patients with muscular dystrophies, particularly Duchenne, are evaluated for progressive cardiomyopathy, and electrocardiogram

(ECG) and echocardiogram define the extent of cardiac involvement. Because respiratory impairment is progressive, baseline PFTs are advised except in the mildest cases. In fact, otherwise normal female carriers may have a dilated cardiomyopathy (22). Evaluation of functional status and cardiac symptomatology determine the need for echocardiography in these carriers.

Use of nondepolarizers requires careful monitoring, especially in the presence of severe muscle wasting. Life-threatening responses including hyperkalemia, dysrhythmias, and rhabdomyolysis have been seen after administration of succinylcholine to these patients. Hypermetabolic syndrome similar to malignant hyperthermia is a risk when patients are exposed to succinylcholine and/or a volatile halogenated agent; therefore, triggering agents are avoided. These agents exacerbate the instability and permeability of the dystrophin-deficient muscle membranes (23).

FASCIOSCAPULOHUMERAL AND LIMB-GIRDLE DYSTROPHIES

Fascioscapulohumeral dystrophy is an autosomal dominant, slowly progressive disorder that primarily affects the muscles of the shoulder and face; cardiac arrhythmias have infrequently been reported. Limb-girdle dystrophies have a variable inheritance pattern and involve a slow degeneration of the shoulder and pelvic muscles. Facial, bulbar, and extraocular muscles are spared. Cardiac conduction disorders are found in some patients; therefore, preoperative ECGs are indicated. Cardiomyopathies are much less frequent. These dystrophies are rare and in general are treated as Duchenne and Becker muscular dystrophy in terms of anesthetic management. Most anesthesiologists avoid the use of triggering agents in these patients.

MYOTONIA AND MYOTONIC DYSTROPHIES

Myotonia is a general term that describes prolonged contraction and delay in relaxation after muscle stimulation. There are several important disorders in which myotonia is the primary symptom (24).

Myotonic dystrophy, the most common, is inherited in an autosomal dominant pattern. Symptoms may not become apparent until the 2nd or 3rd decade of life. Specific muscle wasting usually involves the hand, facial, masseter, and pretibial muscles. The range in severity is wide. Pharyngeal, laryngeal, and diaphragmatic muscles may also be affected. Cardiac conduction may be abnormal and 20% have mitral valve prolapse (MVP) or other valvular lesions.

Congenital myotonic dystrophy is a severe form of myotonic dystrophy that manifests early in infancy, often in a child of a mother with myotonic dystrophy.

Myotonia congenita, a milder familial disorder, is characterized by skeletal muscle myotonia without multisystem involvement. Because smooth and cardiac muscles are not affected, ECG and echocardiogram are not required. In all of these disorders, drugs such as quinine, procainamide, and corticosteroids may relieve myotonic symptoms.

Central core disease is a rare disorder in which muscle biopsies reveal discrete "cores" devoid of mitochondrial enzymes.

Individuals with central core disease have proximal muscle weakness and often scoliosis.

Preanesthetic Assessment

Preoperative evaluation of patients with myotonic dystrophy considers cardiac and respiratory abnormalities, pulmonary aspiration risk, associated disorders, and abnormal responses to drugs used for anesthesia.

Assessment of functional status, respiratory symptomatology, and muscular involvement determines the need for further testing. Preoperative PFTs and a chest radiograph are considered in all except the very mild cases. Cardiac dysrhythmias and conduction abnormalities are quite common and may precede other symptoms of the disease. A baseline ECG is obtained and often reveals bradycardia and intraventricular conduction delays, changes that do not correlate with the severity of skeletal muscle involvement. Death from arrhythmias is common, but the treatment of the arrhythmia may worsen cardiac conduction. Thus, antiarrhythmics are used with caution, but the need to control cardiac rhythm is anticipated because anesthesia and surgery may aggravate pre-existing conduction blockade. All patients affected with muscular dystrophy, except myotonia congenita, have some degree of cardiomyopathy and need an ECG. An echocardiogram or cardiac consultation may be indicated, especially if exercise tolerance cannot be assessed. Myocardial depression associated with anesthetic agents may be exaggerated. It is important to auscultate for a click or murmur and inquire about symptoms such as palpitations.

Gastrointestinal hypomotility, combined with weakness of pharyngeal, laryngeal, and thoracic muscles, makes these patients vulnerable to pulmonary aspiration of gastric contents. The patient is questioned about pulmonary aspiration, and prophylaxis is considered.

The risk of endocrine abnormalities is increased, which may affect the course of anesthesia. The preoperative evaluation specifically seeks diabetes mellitus, hypothyroidism, and adrenal insufficiency. Thyroid function tests, glucose level, and electrolyte levels are obtained as appropriate.

For the anesthetic plan, the patient's sensitivity to opioids and other sedatives is considered. Myotonia is an intrinsic muscle disorder that is not relieved with regional anesthesia; only local infiltration with an anesthetic relieves the myotonia. Patients are kept warm because cold triggers myotonia. Patients with myotonic dystrophy have a high incidence of pulmonary complications after general anesthesia (25). See Chapter 5 for a detailed discussion of preoperative pulmonary optimization. Depolarizing agents are avoided since fasciculation may trigger myotonia; these patients seem to respond normally to nondepolarizing muscle relaxants.

MALIGNANT HYPERTHERMIA

Malignant hyperthermia has been reported in patients with myotonia congenita, as well as with Duchenne and Becker muscular dystrophies (26). Central core disease, although rare, is associated with malignant hyperthermia (21). There is some debate regarding the susceptibility of myotonic patients to uncontrolled metabolism of muscle and severe rhabdomyolysis in a malignant hyperthermia-type pattern. Some conclude that all myopathic patients may be susceptible; others, that true predisposition has been established for very few myopathies, including central core disease (26).

CEREBROVASCULAR DISEASE AND STROKE

It is important to assess the risk of cerebral reinfarction during the upcoming preoperative period. If patients have not been fully evaluated, delay of elective procedures until evaluation has been performed is considered, since a history of stroke or TIA is a strong predictor of perioperative stroke (27). There is no definitive data on how soon after a documented stroke elective surgery can be performed. The etiology and treatment of the documented stroke or TIA are considered; the myriad causes make the development of a single guideline unlikely.

In a study of the risk of perioperative stroke in 284 patients with known carotid stenosis who underwent general anesthesia and surgery, previous history of TIA or stroke within 3 months of surgery did not significantly increase stroke rates (28). However, it has been recommended that a TIA or stroke occurring within the last 6 months be investigated and treated (27). An even more cautious approach should be utilized if the patient's neurologic status worsened after the TIA or stroke. Prophylactic carotid endarterectomy before general surgery is not indicated in patients with known carotid stenosis (28). The risk of perioperative stroke in patients without known carotid disease is approximately 0.5% (29). Evans and Wijdicks reported a perioperative stroke risk of approximately 3.6% in patients with known carotid stenosis; greater degrees of stenosis in their study did not confer significantly higher risk (28). Therefore, they suggested that the sum of the perioperative stroke risk associated with carotid endarterectomy (CEA) should be significantly lower than 3.6% to recommend prophylactic CEA before surgery in these patients. Although the risk of perioperative stroke is higher than in the general population, the risk does not appear sufficient to warrant CEA before surgery.

Over 80% of perioperative strokes occur in the postoperative period; one third of cases after embolism are associated with atrial fibrillation (AF) (30). Prevention of new cardiac arrhythmias perioperatively, therefore, seems critical to lessen the possibility of this postoperative complication. Cerebrovascular disease is often a marker for significant coexisting cardiac disease as discussed in the review of the American College of Cardiology/American Heart Association (ACC/AHA) 2007 guidelines on perioperative cardiovascular evaluation and care in Chapter 3.

Preanesthetic Assessment

Preoperative assessment of patients with a history of cerebrovascular disease, stroke, or TIA requires careful documentation of events, symptomatology, and residual deficits. The cause of stroke is defined and may be related to primary cerebrovascular disease or embolic events from atrial fibrillation, artificial valves, or right to left shunts such as a patent foramen ovale. An echocardiogram is recommended as part of the routine evaluation of a stroke or TIA. A careful history looks for symptoms of TIAs. Related testing results and treatments are documented, particularly the results of carotid ultrasounds, radiologic procedures of the head and neck (e.g., MRI, computed tomography), and cardiac echocardiography. Unfortunately, there are no specific guidelines in the literature regarding the use of diagnostic preoperative carotid ultrasound in these patients. Since patients with vascular disease often have significant comorbidities, baseline studies generally include ECG and chemistries including glucose. For example, an elevated blood urea nitrogen (BUN) and creatinine may detect renal vascular disease.

In new-onset AF, a preoperative echocardiogram will assess systolic function and diagnose an atrial thrombus, which can be a source of emboli. Anticoagulant therapy is indicated for the treatment of intracardiac thrombus, and elective procedures should be delayed for 3 months after the start of therapy. It may be important to bridge warfarin with a short-term anticoagulant such as low-molecular-weight heparin (LMWH) or unfractionated heparin in this setting (see Chapter 7). It has even been recommended to undergo minor dental, endoscopic, or orthopedic procedures without an interruption of oral anticoagulation (27).

If patients are currently treated with anticoagulants for stroke prophylaxis, the clinician consults with the physician prescribing the anticoagulant medication to establish protocols or formulate a perioperative plan (see Chapters 7 and 17).

The following issues should be considered:

- For patients at particularly high risk for stroke, discontinuing long-acting anticoagulants such as warfarin generates the need for bridging with a short-term anticoagulant such as LMWH or intravenous unfractionated heparin. Patients with artificial heart valves or those with a history of repeated TIAs are in this high-risk group.
- A physician must monitor the patient's coagulation status and be available should a problem develop between the time the anticoagulant is discontinued and the time of the planned procedure. At some institutions hospitalists or other perioperative physicians perform this function.
- A physician (this can be the surgeon, a hospitalist, or the original prescribing physician) monitors the resumption of anticoagulant therapy for adequate levels after the patient is discharged from the hospital.

If regional anesthesia is contemplated, the perioperative plan includes stopping both long-term and short-term anticoagulants in sufficient time for the regional anesthetic to be safely performed according to generally accepted guidelines. (These guidelines are included in Chapters 7 and 17). Consensus statements are also available through the Web site of the American Society of Regional Anesthesia (www.asra.com).

UNDOCUMENTED CAROTID BRUIT

During the preoperative history and physical examination, a previously unknown asymptomatic carotid bruit may be detected. Only 40% to 60% of asymptomatic patients with carotid bruits have significant carotid lesions, and the risk of stroke in patients with asymptomatic but hemodynamically significant carotid artery stenosis is approximately 1% to 2% per year (31). The incidence of stroke not preceded by a TIA is relatively low (32). There is no evidence that patients with asymptomatic carotid bruits are at increased risk for perioperative stroke. In addition, the evidence against prophylactic CEA before general surgery suggests that further preoperative evaluation of patients with asymptomatic carotid bruits is unwarranted. Still, a thorough history and physical examination evaluate and document any neurologic symptom that the patient may not report spontaneously. Some clinicians may want to investigate previously unevaluated asymptomatic bruits with carotid ultrasound, particularly if significant hemodynamic perturbations or neck manipulation are anticipated during surgery.

Patients with an asymptomatic bruit and significant carotid stenosis upon evaluation may benefit from CEA before cardiac surgery. The perioperative stroke risk during coronary artery bypass grafting (CABG) increases with the degree of carotid stenosis (27). The incidence of permanent neurologic deficit was increased in patients who had CABG alone versus those who underwent staged or combined CEA and CABG (33).

Different recommendations are provided for patients with symptomatic carotid stenosis, where evaluation with carotid ultrasound and revascularization before cardiac or major vascular surgery are encouraged due to the increased risk of stroke in this patient population (27).

DEMENTIA

Preoperative evaluation of patients with dementia requires an understanding of the type, degree of interference with independent functioning, and prevention of associated postoperative complications.

Major dementia syndromes include Parkinson disease with dementia (5%), vascular dementia (10% to 20%), and Alzheimer disease (60% to 80%) (34).

Hypertension and diabetes are risk factors for vascular dementia; uniform diagnostic criteria for this progressive disorder are lacking. Alzheimer disease, likely caused by the abnormal processing of amyloid-β protein, results in extracellular deposits, intracellular neurofibrillary tangles, and loss of neurons. Behavioral problems and cognitive impairment are common. In addition to the three major causes of dementia listed above, patients may suffer reversible dementia from medications, alcohol, metabolic disorders, depression, central nervous system neoplasms, and normal pressure hydrocephalus (35).

The pharmacologic options for dementia treatment may affect the choice of an anesthetic plan. Patients with Alzheimer disease may be taking cholinesterase inhibitors to correct a decrease in acetylcholine transferase and impaired cortical cholinergic function. Disease-modifying agents, such as memantine, affect the glutamate receptor. Selegiline, a monoamine oxidase inhibitor, and vitamin E may slow progression. Psychiatric medications often control behavioral disorders, depression, and agitation.

Preanesthetic Evaluation

The level of cognitive dysfunction in patients with dementia is extremely variable. The clinician performing the preoperative assessment makes a decision in each case regarding reliability of information and ability of the patient to give informed consent. A discussion with family members is often necessary in this regard. Accountability for medical decision making and advanced care directives are established. It is important to ensure that the patient's current medications are not contributing to the dementia, especially if the regimen has not been fully evaluated. Because patients also may be at increased risk for aspiration, respiratory symptoms are assessed and the absence of infection is verified preoperatively.

Patients with dementia are at increased risk for postoperative delirium. Delirium, which is reported in 2% to 60% of postoperative patients, depends on type of surgery and the population studied and is associated with increased mortality, postoperative complications, and longer hospital stay (36). Patients with delirium may be immobile and suffer irreversible functional decline. Precipitating factors include polypharmacy (particularly psychoactive drugs), infection, metabolic disturbances, dehydration, immobility, and the use of restraints or bladder catheters. Untreated pain and inadequate analgesia are extremely high risk factors for delirium (37). Opioids have been associated with an increased risk of delirium in some reports; the benefits of opioids to treat pain must be balanced against their potential to cause delirium. Meperidine in particular has been associated with an increased risk for delirium (38). Although regional anesthesia has not been shown to prevent or lessen delirium in these patients (39), its use in the postoperative period for analgesia is likely to minimize postoperative pain and the need for opioids, conditions known to contribute to delirium. Unless preoperative plans are made to control precipitating factors in patients with underlying dementia, dementia or delirium may worsen. Preoperative planning may include follow up by a geriatrician and possible extended postoperative rehabilitation to facilitate recovery. Options for optimal pain control, including regional blocks, should be discussed preoperatively.

PARKINSON DISEASE

Parkinson disease is a degenerative disorder of the central nervous system in which dopamine-secreting fibers regress in the basal ganglia of the brain. One of the main actions of the neurotransmitter dopamine is to inhibit the firing rate of the neurons that inhibit the extrapyramidal motor system. When the action of acetylcholine is unopposed, the classic signs and symptoms of the disorder are manifested. With diminished inhibition of the extrapyramidal motor system, spontaneous movements decrease, and rigidity and resting tremors result. Other characteristics of autonomic dysfunction are orthostatic hypotension, poor temperature control, and excessive saliva secretion. Many patients with more severe forms of the disorder have swallowing abnormalities. The respiratory muscles may also be affected by rigidity and bradykinesia, increasing the risk for postoperative pulmonary complications (40). Dementia frequently accompanies this disorder, masked by the Parkinsonian symptoms of slurred speech and facial rigidity.

Treatment Modalities

Dopamine does not cross the blood–brain barrier; however, levodopa, the precursor of dopamine, does. Levodopa, the mainstay of treatment for Parkinson disease, is often combined with carbidopa. Carbidopa inhibits the activity of the decarboxylating enzyme that converts levodopa. When the systemic breakdown of levodopa decreases, the dose can be reduced. As the disease progresses, the effect of levodopa decreases, requiring close attention to the dosing schedule. With degeneration of dopamine terminals, dopamine cannot be stored and released, decreasing its concentration in the basal ganglia and creating dependence upon the levels provided by levodopa. Unfortunately, up to 50% of patients who have taken levodopa for 5 years develop dyskinesias and motor fluctuations (41). Dyskinesias are abnormal involuntary movements that may be dystonic or myoclonic, and other drugs are often used to control symptoms. Among these drugs are anticholinergic agents, as well as dopamine agonists. Increased levels of dopamine after levodopa administration act on myocardial β-adrenergic receptors to generate arrhythmias and on α-adrenergic receptors to increase blood pressure. Renal effects of dopamine can result in orthostatic hypotension. For patients with mild symptoms, anticholinergic agents may be used. Dopamine receptor agonists such as bromocriptine and pergolide, which have longer half-lives than levodopa, are effective. The U.S. Food and Drug Administration (FDA) recalled pergolide in March 2007 because of a risk of serious damage to heart valves. Tricuspid, mitral, and aortic regurgitation are associated with the use of pergolide (42). Selegiline, a monoamine oxidase inhibitor, has been used to inhibit degradation of dopamine. Amantadine is an antiviral drug that has some efficacy in mild cases with relatively few adverse effects; it may act by altering presynaptic dopamine release and uptake. Some patients are treated with deep brain stimulation (DBS) by electrodes implanted in the brain to decrease symptoms.

Preanesthetic Assessment

Preoperative evaluation includes an assessment and documentation of disease severity, with special attention to degree of pulmonary compromise. Dysphagia is documented as it may predispose patients to pulmonary aspiration. Rigidity, especially cogwheel rigidity; a shuffling gait; and masked facies are common findings. Patients who have taken pergolide in the past (now recalled) should be evaluated for valvular abnormalities. One should inquire about shortness of breath, fatigue, and palpitations and auscultate for murmurs. If any symptoms or physical findings suggestive of valvular disease are present, an ECG and echocardiogram are indicated.

All medications for Parkinson disease are continued. Abrupt withdrawal of levodopa exacerbates symptoms; increased skeletal muscle rigidity affecting ventilation has been reported (43). Levodopa withdrawal also is associated with neuroleptic malignant syndrome, characterized by altered consciousness, autonomic instability, extrapyramidal dysfunction, and elevated temperature. Severe chest wall rigidity and dysphagia have been reported. Dosage schedules are carefully maintained throughout the perioperative period. Levodopa is not administered intravenously because systemic conversion to dopamine has cardiac and hemodynamic effects. Therefore, enteral feeding may be required perioperatively. There are few reports of adverse anesthetic events in patients with Parkinson disease. Response to muscle relaxants does not seem to be a concern. There is a single report of hyperkalemia after succinylcholine; however, succinylcholine has been used successfully in a number of other patients (44). Drugs that may exacerbate parkinsonian symptoms are avoided. These include metoclopramide, phenothiazines, and butyrophenones. Patients taking monoamine oxidase inhibitors are identified so that medications such as meperidine can be avoided (see Chapter 17). Muscle rigidity after fentanyl has been reported; rigidity responds to neuromuscular blockade and may result from presynaptic inhibition of dopamine release (46).

The manufacturers recommend disabling DBS before surgery (46). If cautery must be used, the path should be kept as far away from the electrodes as possible; bipolar cautery is recommended.

PITUITARY NEOPLASMS

Endocrine abnormalities frequently coexist with pituitary tumors. The pituitary gland consists of two parts: The anterior lobe, or adenohypophysis, and the posterior lobe, or neurohypophysis. The anterior lobe contains cells that produce and release growth hormone, prolactin, adrenocorticotropic hormone (ACTH), melanocyte-stimulating hormone, thyrotropin (thyroid-stimulating hormone [TSH]), and the gonadotrophs follicle-stimulating hormone (FSH) and luteinizing hormone (LH). The hypothalamus normally controls release of these hormones. The posterior pituitary stores and releases oxytocin and vasopressin, which are synthesized in the hypothalamus. Pituitary tumors account for about 10% of intracranial neoplasms (47). Genetics may play a role in their formation. Pituitary adenomas are the most common type of pituitary tumor, a number of them associated with inappropriate hormone secretion (48). Adenomas arise from any type of cell in the anterior pituitary and, therefore, hypersecretion of the associated hormones is possible.

Preanesthetic Assessment

Symptoms of pituitary neoplasms can include headache, visual disturbance from mass effect, and symptoms specific to hormonal hypersecretion. The preoperative assessment documents visual deficits; assesses signs of increased intracranial pressure (ICP), which include mental changes, unsteady gait, vomiting, and bladder and bowel incontinence; and evaluates the effects of excess hormone secretion.

Careful airway evaluation is necessary, as excess secretion of growth hormone causes symptoms of acromegaly: Soft tissues of the pharynx and larynx thicken, sometimes progressing to laryngeal stenosis and recurrent laryngeal palsy. Upper airway obstruction can cause sleep apnea. Growth hormone may cause thyroid goiter and subsequent tracheal compression. Difficulties with airway management and tracheal intubation have been reported (49). Left ventricular hypertrophy (LVH), hypertension, and diabetes mellitus are associated with excess growth hormone secretion as well. Therefore, the clinician considers an ECG and measurement of blood glucose levels before a surgical procedure.

Pituitary tumors that secrete ACTH lead to excess cortisol secretion and symptoms of Cushing disease. Cushing disease, which affects multiple organ systems, is characterized by impaired glucose tolerance, proximal myopathy, osteoporosis, hypertension, hypernatremia, hyponatremia, and gastrointestinal reflux, all of which may have implications for the preoperative assessment. Preoperative evaluation focuses on the metabolic as well as the cardiovascular systems. In the asymptomatic patient, the cardiovascular workup consists of the standard history, physical examination, and laboratory tests. Additional testing, including ECG and echocardiography, may be appropriate in the patient with hypertension, ischemic heart disease, and LVH. Asymmetric septal hypertrophy is reported; the cause is unknown, but the problem often resolves when cortisol levels are normalized. Coexisting obesity and the classic "buffalo hump" may make ventilation difficult. Muscle wasting may result in increased susceptibility to neuromuscular blocking agents. In most patients cortisol replacement is necessary because normal corticotrophs are heavily suppressed (48). Serum electrolyte and glucose levels are evaluated because of the associated metabolic disturbances.

Prolactin and gonadotroph-secreting tumors have little interaction with anesthetic agents. TSH-secreting pituitary tumors are extremely rare and may be associated with symptoms of hyperthyroidism, requiring preoperative management. A detailed discussion of the management of thyroid disorders is found in Chapter 6.

Non–hormone-secreting pituitary tumors may be the product of mass effect or pituitary insufficiency. In these cases, the particular problems associated with symptoms of hypoadrenalism or hypothyroidism are evaluated and managed preoperatively (see Chapter 6). In most cases baseline ECG, electrolytes, and glucose levels are obtained.

BRAIN TUMORS

Intracranial neoplasms vary in histology, presentation, and prognosis, with a yearly incidence of primary brain neoplasms of about 15 per 100,000.

Gliomas are the most common and account for about 45% of all intracranial tumors. They derive from astrocyte anaplasia and include glioblastoma multiforme, astrocytoma, ependymoma, medulloblastoma, and oligodendrocytoma. Glioblastomas are the most lethal; oligodendrocytomas have a better prognosis.

Benign meningiomas, which account for about 15% of all brain neoplasms, arise from the dura mater or arachnoid.

Pituitary adenomas account for about 7% of clinically detected brain neoplasms; the majority of pituitary adenomas are found only at autopsy.

Metastatic carcinomas account for about 6% of all brain tumors and vary widely in origin and symptoms produced.

A variety of other brain neoplasms make up the remainder, including schwannomas, craniopharyngiomas, and dermoid tumors.

Despite their disparate etiologies and presentations, brain neoplasms may share features. Mass effects from any type of tumor cause neurologic deficits. Tumor enlargement increases ICP producing papilledema, headache, and false localizing signs when impending herniation compresses the side opposite the lesion. Unsteady gait, changes in mental function, seizures, and vomiting are other symptoms. Brain edema may result from a combination of vasogenic and cytotoxic mechanisms. Brain tumors and elevated ICP create autonomic dysfunction, which manifests as bradycardia, arrhythmias, changes on the ECG, and hypertension. The potential for herniation should be considered in the presence of a mass lesion. The three basic compartments of the brain are the cerebrum, the cerebellum, and the brainstem. The cerebrum is separated into right and left halves by the falx cerebri and the tentorium separates the cerebellum. High pressure in any of the compartments can cause shifts with potential devastating effects.

Preanesthetic Assessment

The preoperative assessment of a patient with a brain tumor includes careful documentation of history, presenting symptoms, and previous therapies. Damage from radiation therapy can result in lethargy and mental status alterations and worsen cerebral edema. Patients may be given corticosteroids to attempt to ameliorate edema. Steroids can potentially cause hyperglycemia, which requires monitoring perioperatively. Anticonvulsants are generally started to prevent seizures. Chemotherapy, particularly if the tumor is a metastatic lesion, also worsens mental status. When evaluating these patients, consideration is given to stress-dose steroids. Because these patients are at risk of steroid-induced hyperglycemia and elevated blood sugars worsen outcome in patients with neurologic compromise, it is important to evaluate blood glucose preoperatively. If the patient has recently been started on anticonvulsants, therapeutic levels are likely to be established. Routine levels are not generally indicated if symptoms are controlled and there are no signs or symptoms of drug toxicity. Although general anesthesia is frequently used, some procedures, particularly those incorporating interventional MRI, are performed with intravenous sedation (monitored anesthesia care [MAC]). The patients are assured that the amount of sedation will make the procedure comfortable and that they will have little or no recall. This technique allows the surgeon to interactively perform surgery using MRI guidance and can yield data that may significantly influence intraoperative neurosurgical decision making (50).

Baseline ECGs are obtained and may show abnormalities including arrhythmias and ST-segment changes. Electrolytes and glucose tests are ordered. Anticonvulsants and steroids are continued throughout the perioperative period and the day of the surgery.

ANEURYSMS AND ARTERIOVENOUS MALFORMATIONS

The vast majority of aneurysms are not diagnosed before they have ruptured; only a small percentage is found incidentally. Before rupture, about a third of patients may have signs and symptoms from "sentinel bleeding." Asymptomatic aneurysms rupture at a rate of about 1% to 2% per year and symptomatic aneurysms at a rate of about 5% per year, often with devastating results. The incidence of aneurysms and subarachnoid hemorrhage increases in patients with a family history of aneurysms or certain systemic disorders such as polycystic kidney disease, fibromuscular dysplasia, and the vascular type of Ehlers-Danlos syndrome. A progressive increase in the incidence of aneurysmal bleeding throughout gestation is reported, probably in parallel with greater blood volume (51). Surgical management of aneurysms during pregnancy has been associated with significantly lower maternal and fetal mortality.

Arteriovenous malformations (AVMs) are associated with high blood flow and low resistance and with symptoms ranging from hemorrhage to mass effects. They are reported to bleed at a rate of about 4% per year. Whether pregnancy increases the rate of bleeding from an AVM is controversial, and the data regarding surgical management do not clearly demonstrate a beneficial effect on maternal or fetal mortality of performing this nonobstetric procedure during gestation (51).

Preanesthetic Assessment

Clinical evaluation of the patient with an aneurysm or AVM includes documentation of history, symptoms, and deficits. Associated disease states such as polycystic kidneys are also evaluated. If the patient has already suffered a subarachnoid hemorrhage, fluids may be restricted for the syndrome of inappropriate secretion of antidiuretic hormone (SIADH). Evaluation of blood pressure and heart rate preoperatively is essential in view of the hypertension and bradycardia associated with an elevated ICP. The patient may be taking steroids, nicardipine, or mannitol, warranting measurement of serum glucose and electrolyte levels.

Patients with subarachnoid hemorrhage have associated ECG abnormalities. Bradycardia, other arrhythmias, and ST- and T-wave changes are common. ECG abnormalities associated with neurologic injury were not independently predictive of postoperative cardiac morbidity and mortality (52). Although the etiology of the changes is not clear, further preoperative evaluation may be necessary to ensure that significant cardiac dysfunction is not responsible for these changes. The pathophysiology of ECG changes is controversial, but evidence exists that structural myocardial lesions are possible after subarachnoid hemorrhage. Wall motion abnormalities demonstrated by echocardiography have been reported. Assuming that ECG changes are merely manifestations of subarachnoid hemorrhage may be erroneous. If the patient has ECG changes suggestive of infarct or ischemia, cardiac evaluation is performed according to ACC/AHA guidelines (Chapter 3).

The patient's blood pressure is adequately controlled perioperatively because of the consequences of uncontrolled hypertension on aneurysm rupture.

SUMMARY

Common themes in the preoperative assessment of patients with neurologic disorders include the following:

- Knowledge of the basic pathophysiology of the disorder is essential to understand anesthetic options as well as potential interactions with particular agents.
- Current neurologic deficits must be documented preoperatively.
- Many disorders are associated with decline in respiratory function. Respiratory status is assessed and further testing is done when respiration is compromised.
- Steroid treatment is common in many disorders; preoperative electrolyte and glucose determinations are important; and perioperative steroid coverage and glucose monitoring may be necessary.
- Some neurologic disorders involve other organ systems, particularly cardiac. Other organ systems known to be associated with the particular neurologic disorder should be evaluated.

REFERENCES

1. Kurtzke JF. Patterns of neurologic involvement in multiple sclerosis. *Neurology*. 1989;39:1235–1238.
2. Weiner HL. Multiple sclerosis is an inflammatory T-cell-mediated autoimmune disease. *Arch Neurol*. 2004;61:1613–1615.
3. Mohr D, Hart SL, Julian L, et al. Association between stressful life events and exacerbation in multiple sclerosis: a meta-analysis. *BMJ*. 2004;328:731–733.
4. Filippini G, Munari L, Incorvaia B, et al. Interferons in relapsing remitting multiple sclerosis: a systematic review. *Lancet*. 2003;361:545–552.
5. Confavreaux C, Hutchinson M, Hours MM, et al. Rate of pregnancy-related relapse in multiple sclerosis. *N Engl J Med*. 1998;339:285–291.
6. Bader AM, Hunt CO, Datta S, et al. Anesthesia for the obstetric patient with multiple sclerosis. *J Clin Anesth*. 1988;1:21–24.
7. Ramsay RE, Rowan AJ, Pryor FM. Special considerations in treating the elderly patient with epilepsy. *Neurology*. 2004;62: S24–29.
8. Hesdorffer DC, Hauser WA, Annegers JF, et al. Dementia and adult-onset unprovoked seizures. *Neurology*. 1996;46:727–730.
9. Merrell DA, Koch MA. Epidural anaesthesia as an anticonvulsant in the management of hypertension and the eclamptic patient in labour. *S Afr Med J*. 1980;58:875–877.
10. Voss LJ, Ludbrook G, Grant C, et al. Cerebral cortical effects of desflurane in sheep: comparison with isoflurane, sevoflurane and enflurane. *Acta Anaesthesiol Scand*. 2006;50:313–319.
11. Smith M, Smith SJ, Scott CA, et al. Activation of the electrocorticogram by propofol during surgery for epilepsy. *Br J Anaesth*. 1996;76:499–502.
12. Cervantes M, Antonio-Ocampo A, Ruelas R, et al. Effects of diazepam on fentanyl-induced epileptoid EEG activity and increase

of multineuronal firing in limbic and mesencephalic brain structures. *Arch Med Res*. 1996;27:495–502.

13. O'Neill GN. Acquired disorders of the neuromuscular junction. *Int Anesthesiol Clin*. 2006;44:107–121.
14. Baraka A. Anaesthesia and myasthenia gravis. *Can J Anaesth*. 1992;39:476–486.
15. Barrons RW. Drug-induced neuromuscular blockade and myasthenia gravis. *Pharmacotherapy*. 1997;17:1220–1232.
16. Foldes FF, McNall PG. Myasthenia gravis: a guide for anesthesiologists. *Anesthesiology*. 1962;23:837–872.
17. Della Rocca G, Coccia C, Diana L, et al. Propofol or sevoflurane anesthesia without muscle relaxants allows the early extubation of myasthenic patients. *Can J Anesth*. 2003;50:547–552.
18. Naguib M, el Dawlatly A, Ashour M, et al. Multivariate determinants of the need for postoperative ventilation in myasthenia gravis. *Can J Anaesth*. 1996;43:1006–1013.
19. O'Neill JH, Murray NM, Newson-David J. The Lambert-Eaton myasthenic syndrome. A review of 50 cases. *Brain*. 1988;111:577–596.
20. Brown JC, Charlton JE. A study of sensitivity to curare in myasthenic disorders using a regional technique. *J Neurol Neurosurg Psychiatry*. 1975;38:27–33.
21. O'Neill GN. Inherited disorders of the neuromuscular junction. *Int Anesthesiol Clin*. 2006;44:91–106.
22. Mirabella M, Servidei S, Manfredi G, et al. Cardiomyopathy may be the only clinical manifestation in female carriers of Duchenne muscular dystrophy. *Neurology*. 1993;43:2342–2345.
23. Denborough M. Malignant hyperthermia. *Lancet*. 1998;352:1131–1136.
24. Russell SH, Hirsch NP. Anaesthesia and myotonia. *Br J Anaesth*. 1994;72:210–216.
25. Mathicu J, Allard P, Gobeil G, et al. Anesthetic and surgical complications in 219 cases of myotonic dystrophy. *Neurology*. 1997;49:1646–1650.
26. Brownell KW. Malignant hyperthermia: relationship to other diseases. *Br J Anaesth*. 1988;60:303–308.
27. Selim M. Perioperative stroke. *N Engl J Med*. 2007;356:706–713.
28. Evans BA, Wijdicks EFM. High-grade carotid stenosis detected before general surgery: is endarterectomy indicated? *Neurology*. 2001;57:1328–1330.
29. Parikh S, Cohen JR. Perioperative stroke after general surgical procedures. *NY State J Med*. 1993;93:162–165.
30. Hart R, Hindman B. Mechanisms of perioperative cerebral infarction. *Stroke*. 1982;13:766–773.
31. Wolf P, Kannel W, Sorlie P, et al. Asymptomatic carotid bruit and risk of stroke: the Framingham Study. *JAMA*. 1981;245:1442–1445.
32. Dodick DW, Meissner I, Meyer FB, et al. Evaluation and management of asymptomatic carotid artery stenosis. *Mayo Clin Proc*. 2004;79:937–944.
33. Hines GL, Scott WC, Schubach SL, et al. Prophylactic carotid endarterectomy in patients with high-grade carotid stenosis undergoing coronary bypass. Does it decrease the risk of perioperative stroke? *Ann Vasc Surg*. 1998;12:23–27.

34. Knopman DS, Boeve BF, Petersen RC. Essentials of the proper diagnoses of mild cognitive impairment, dementia, and major subtypes of dementia. *Mayo Clin Proc.* 2003;78:1290–1308.

35. Clarfield AM. The reversible dementias: do they reverse? *Ann Intern Med.* 1988;109:476–486.

36. Francis J, Martin D, Kapoor WN. A prospective study of delirium in hospitalized elderly. *JAMA.* 1990;263:1097–2011.

37. Lynch EP, Lazor MA, Gellis JE, et al. The impact of postoperative pain on the development of postoperative delirium. *Anesth Analg.* 1998;86:781–785.

38. Morrison RS, Magaziner J, Gilbert M, et al. Relationship between pain and opioid analgesics on the development of delirium following hip fracture. *J Gerontol A Biol Sci Med Sci.* 2003;58:76–81.

39. Williams-Russo P, Sharrock NE, Mattis S, et al. Cognitive effects after epidural vs. general anesthesia in older adults: a randomized trial. *JAMA.* 1995;274:44–50.

40. Paulson GD, Tafrate RH. Some 'minor' aspects of Parkinsonism, especially pulmonary function. *Neurology.* 1970;20:14–17.

41. Olanow CW, Watts RL, Koller WC. An algorithm (decision tree) for the management of Parkinson's disease (2001); treatment guidelines. *Neurology.* 2001;56:S1–88.

42. www.fda.gov/cder/drug/advisory/pergolide.htm. Accessed April 12, 2007.

43. Hetherington A, Rosenblatt RM. Ketamine and paralysis agitans. *Anesthesiology.* 1980;52:527.

44. Muzzi DA, Black S, Cucchiara RF. The lack of effect of succinylcholine on serum potassium in patients with Parkinson's disease. *Anesthesiology.* 1989;71:322.

45. Nicholson G, Pereira AC, Hall GM. Parkinson's disease and anaesthesia. *Br J Anaesth.* 2002;89:904–916.

46. http://www.medtronic.com/physician/activa/downloadablefiles/197928_b_006.pdf.

47. Freda PU, Post KD. Differential diagnosis of sellar masses. *Endocrinol Metab Clin North Am.* 1999;28:81–117.

48. Smith M, Hirsch NP. Pituitary disease and anaesthesia. *Br J Anaesth.* 2000;85:3–14.

49. Burn JM. Airway difficulties associated with anaesthesia in acromegaly. *Br J Anaesth.* 1972;44:413–414.

50. Hall WA, Liu H, Martin A, et al. Safety, efficacy and functionality of high-field strength interventional magnetic resonance imaging for neurosurgery. *Neurosurgery.* 2000;46:632–642.

51. Dias MS, Sekhar LN. Intracranial hemorrhage from aneurysms and arteriovenous malformations during pregnancy and the puerperium. *Neurosurgery.* 1990;27:855–866.

52. Zaroff JG, Rordorf GA, Newell JB, et al. Cardiac outcome in patients with subarachnoid hemorrhage and electrocardiographic abnormalities. *Neurosurgery.* 1999;44:34–39.

Musculoskeletal and Autoimmune Diseases

Parwane S. Parsa

This chapter reviews the preoperative evaluation of patients with musculoskeletal and autoimmune diseases. The autoimmune diseases discussed in this section include **rheumatoid arthritis, ankylosing spondylitis, systemic lupus erythematosus,** and **scleroderma.** Other musculoskeletal diseases included in this chapter are **osteoarthritis** and **kyphoscoliosis. Marfan syndrome** and other **inherited connective tissue diseases** are reviewed. These entities are distinguished by variable disease severity and frequent multisystem effects requiring careful preoperative investigation. This chapter discusses strategies to identify and treat patients with consequent pulmonary and cardiac involvement and also reviews newer therapies used to delay disease progression.

RHEUMATOID ARTHRITIS

Rheumatoid arthritis (RA), a common and debilitating autoimmune disease, affects up to 1% of the population, typically ranging in age from 40 to 70 years. Incidence of the disease is greater in females than in males (ratio of 2.5:1) (1). In addition to the characteristic joint inflammation, multiple organ systems are impacted by the disease, requiring careful evaluation.

General

Patients with RA may report fatigue, malaise, weight loss, and fever.

Arthropathy

The disease involves multijoint inflammation and morning stiffness of both small and large joints of the extremities. The temporomandibular joint, cervical spine, and cricoarytenoid cartilages are frequently affected. Patients may experience limited neck and jaw mobility or hoarseness. The arthropathy is progressive and disabling.

Neurologic

Sensory peripheral neuropathy associated with vasculitis and nerve entrapment occurs with RA.

Cardiac

Pericardial effusion, aortic insufficiency, and conduction abnormalities are common. The incidence of myocardial ischemia (and cardiovascular mortality) is higher in RA patients compared with non-RA patients with common risk factors (2).

Pulmonary

Decreased thoracic mobility can produce a restrictive defect; other associated pulmonary disorders include pleural effusions and interstitial fibrosis also resulting in predominantly restrictive lung disease.

Renal

Patients with RA can have renal vasculitis.

Hematologic

Anemia, leucocytosis, thrombocytosis, and splenomegaly with thrombocytopenia can be present.

Dermatologic

Rheumatoid nodules, dry eyes, vasculitis, and salivary inflammation are typical.

History

The evaluation of patients with RA assesses the onset and course of the disease, the location and severity of joint involvement, factors that exacerbate symptoms, and the best level of activity the patient can achieve. A history of neck stiffness, crepitation with neck movement, hoarseness, stridor, and any neurologic deficits is elicited. The evaluator asks about dyspnea with exertion, orthopnea, anemia, and chest pain or pressure. Extra-articular effects of RA and any recent hospital admissions are discussed. Current medications are listed along with any history of adverse drug effects.

Physical Examination

General

Observe the patient for signs of anemia (such as pallor or tachycardia) or malnutrition. Examine the extremities for degree of joint involvement so that intraoperative positioning of the patient can be anticipated.

Airway Examination

Several aspects of the airway examination are important in patients with RA. Limited neck flexion or extension from cervical spine involvement may make positioning and laryngoscopy difficult. Similarly, a limited oral aperture may hamper intubation. Atlanto-occipital subluxation caused by ligament laxity can be found in any patient with RA; the incidence is up to 46%. The direction of the subluxation is anterior in the majority of cases (3). Patients, therefore, are at risk for spinal cord compression and permanent neurologic injury with excessive movement during airway management (4) or positioning. Neurologic signs with neck movement are documented, although neurologic signs do not identify all patients at risk of this complication. Patients who report significant hoarseness may need preoperative referral to the otolaryngology clinic for fiberoptic laryngoscopy to diagnose poor mobility of the vocal cords from cricoarytenoid arthritis (5).

Cardiopulmonary

Observe the patient for cyanosis, abnormal respiratory rate or effort, and chronic cough. Auscultation of the chest may reveal evidence of a pleural effusion or pneumonia, or rales consistent with pulmonary fibrosis. Document murmurs or rubs from valvular insufficiency or pericarditis.

Diagnostic Testing

Laboratory Tests

Because anemia is a common feature of RA, a complete blood count (CBC) with platelets is ordered for patients who will have surgery with any expected blood loss. For individuals with renal or cardiac disease, blood urea nitrogen (BUN), creatinine, and electrolytes are measured.

Radiology

Because of the high incidence of atlantoaxial subluxation in patients with RA, preoperative cervical spine (C-spine) radiographs are performed in patients who are symptomatic or who will undergo anesthetic techniques involving potential airway manipulation. The x-ray examination includes the anteroposterior (AP) view of the C-spine, an AP odontoid view, and lateral flexion and extension films. Criteria for atlantoaxial subluxation are an anterior atlas—dens interval of >3 mm or a posterior atlas—dens interval of ≤14 mm (3). Patients with abnormal C-spine radiographs and/or neuralgia or myelopathy need neurology consultation and possible intervention (halo traction or surgical correction) (6).

Pulmonary Evaluation

The resting oxygen saturation is measured. Findings on history and physical examination (H&P) that suggest pneumonia, restrictive lung disease, or pleural effusion are further evaluated with a chest radiograph. For patients who have limited exercise tolerance and/or possible restrictive lung disease, an electrocardiogram (ECG) and pulmonary function tests (PFTs) are indicated. Chapter 5 contains a detailed discussion of restrictive lung disease.

Cardiac Evaluation

Basic cardiac evaluation, such as resting ECG, is warranted in RA patients. The ECG yields information about pericardial effusion, conduction abnormalities, or ischemic heart disease. Two-dimensional (2-D) echocardiography is indicated in patients with suspected pericardial effusion (e.g., muffled heart sounds, friction rub, displaced point of maximal impulse [PMI], low voltage on ECG, enlarged cardiac silhouette on chest radiograph) or valvular disease.

Ischemic heart disease is an important consideration in any patient with RA undergoing major surgery. Some patients may not be able to exercise sufficiently to develop signs or symptoms of myocardial ischemia because of joint pain and limited mobility. Evidence supports a more rapid progression of coronary artery disease (CAD) in patients with RA, although the reasons for accelerated atherosclerosis are not entirely clear (2). The preoperative

Table 11.1. Common medications, adverse effects, and preoperative management for patients with rheumatoid arthritis

Agent	Adverse Effects	Preoperative Management
Nonsteroidal anti-inflammatory drugs	Bleeding complications, gastrointestinal irritation, renal dysfunction	Stop 2 days before surgery
Methotrexate	Pancytopenia, gastrointestinal irritation, abnormal LFTs	Monitor CBC with platelets and LFTs; if tests are abnormal, discontinue medication to allow normalization before surgery
Glucocorticoids	Impaired wound healing, glucose intolerance, increased risk of infection, adrenal suppression	Continue on day of surgery; provide perioperative "stress doses" (see Chapter 17)
Leflunomide	Hepatotoxicity, hypertension, pancytopenia	Monitor CBC with platelets and LFTs; if laboratory tests are abnormal, discontinue drug to allow normalization before surgery
Anti–tumor necrosis factor agents: Etanercept Infliximab Adalimumab	Increased risk of opportunistic infection and malignancy	Preoperative management based on severity of patient's disease, duration of action of the drug, and risk of infection with the planned surgery
Interleukin-1 receptor antagonist: Anakinra	Skin irritation, increased risk of infection	Preoperative management based on severity of patient's disease and risk of infection with the planned surgery

CBC, complete blood count; LFTs, liver function tests.

evaluator can utilize stress-thallium examination or dobutamine stress echocardiography to evaluate the patient for inducible ischemia. Patients with positive stress tests may require further testing or additional medications before the surgical procedure. See Chapter 3.

Preoperative Medication and Instructions

Therapy for RA has improved with the introduction of new agents that slow progression of the disease (7). A list of common medications, adverse effects, and suggested preoperative instructions appears in Table 11.1.

Preoperative Preparation

Preoperative therapy includes treatment for any underlying pulmonary infection (pneumonia, bronchitis) as well as evaluation and treatment of pleural effusions that impair effective ventilation. Based on the results of cardiac evaluation, medical therapy (such as beta blockers) can be started in selected patients.

Anesthetic Implications

Airway Management

General anesthesia (GA) in patients with RA requires careful planning for airway management. Major concerns are the increased incidence of difficult laryngoscopy and the risk of neurologic deficit with atlantoaxial subluxation during laryngoscopy. In patients at high risk (airway examination indicating probable difficulty or positive C-spine films), preparations for awake fiberoptic intubation (FOI) are made. After successfully securing the airway, the anesthesiologist tests the patient's ability to move the extremities before induction. Using a smaller-diameter endotracheal tube facilitates placement in the presence of cricoarytenoid involvement. In the recovery room, the patient is carefully observed for acute airway obstruction caused, in rare cases, by exacerbation of cricoarytenoid arthritis (8,9).

Regional Anesthesia

Regional techniques for patients with RA have several advantages. Patients who need orthopedic surgery on the extremities can have peripheral nerve block supplemented with intravenous sedation. Regional techniques can minimize the risk of cardiovascular depression and airway management problems associated with GA. A peripheral nerve block also provides excellent postoperative analgesia. Pre-existing neuropathy or patient inability to maintain position for a peripheral nerve block may preclude this technique. Neuraxial blockade offers similar advantages for patients with RA.

ANKYLOSING SPONDYLITIS

Ankylosing spondylitis is a rheumatic disease characterized by progressive inflammation of large joints, affecting particularly the sacroiliac joints and the spine. Movement can be severely restricted by calcification of spinal ligaments. Other manifestations of ankylosing spondylitis are peripheral arthritis and uveitis. Vascular inflammation may coexist, with aortitis and aortic insufficiency (AI). Pulmonary fibrosis and poor chest wall compliance from joint fixation and kyphosis are possible. The majority of ankylosing spondylitis patients are young males.

History

Inquire about the location and severity of joint involvement. Significant cervical spine or thoracic spine disease affects airway management and patient positioning. Any history of associated ocular, cardiovascular, and pulmonary disease is also explored. To gauge the severity of cardiopulmonary impairment, patients are asked about their best level of exercise tolerance.

Physical Examination

General examination notes the presence of cyanosis, tachypnea, and asymmetric chest expansion. The range of motion of the spine is checked (flexion, extension). Airway management may be challenging because of restricted neck flexion or extension and possible thoracic kyphosis. Chest examination focuses on the presence of kyphosis and associated cardiopulmonary disease, such as a diastolic murmur associated with AI.

Diagnostic Testing

Ankylosing spondylitis patients who routinely take nonsteroidal anti-inflammatory agents (NSAIDs) for relief of pain require a preoperative BUN and creatinine level. Individuals who take leflunomide require CBC with platelets and liver function tests preoperatively.

Patients with significant kyphosis and limited exercise capacity need a chest radiograph and ECG. PFTs (spirometry and arterial blood gas [ABG] analysis) are useful to assess the severity of restrictive lung disease. AI and ventricular performance are assessed with echocardiography.

Preoperative Medication and Instructions

The first-line therapy for ankylosing spondylitis is an NSAID, which decreases pain and stiffness. These medications are discontinued 2 days prior to surgery to avoid bleeding complications. Leflunomide is employed for the treatment of arthritis in the extremities. Tumor necrosis factor (TNF)-α antagonists, such as etanercept and infliximab (see Table 11.1), have been successful treatments, improving mobility in patients and establishing partial remission in some cases (10).

Preoperative Preparation

In patients with significant spine disease, the severity of pulmonary restrictive physiology is clarified based on history, physical examination, and results of PFTs. Any active pulmonary infection needs treatment before surgery, and any coexisting bronchospasm should be well controlled (see Chapter 5).

Anesthetic Implications

Airway management in patients with potentially limited cervical spine mobility and thoracic kyphosis requires planning. Awake or asleep FOI should be discussed with patients. For procedures on the extremities, regional anesthesia can be employed. Neuraxial blockade, difficult or impossible in patients with severe spinal involvement, may be an option in patients with less severe disease. Careful positioning in the operating room (OR) is important in these patients with limited range of motion to avoid iatrogenic injury (11).

SYSTEMIC LUPUS ERYTHEMATOSUS

Systemic lupus erythematosus (SLE) is an autoimmune disease in which antinuclear antibodies (ANAs) are present in almost all cases. A significant majority of patients with SLE are younger females, with an overall population incidence of SLE of 40 cases per 100,000 persons (12). The clinical course of the disease is variable, characterized by active periods and remission.

General

Chronic fatigue and fever are features of the disease.

Arthritis

Arthritis with SLE is very common, and migratory, often involving multiple small joints in the hands and wrists. Muscle can be inflamed.

Skin

Dermatologic involvement includes photosensitive rash, "butterfly rash" on the face, subacute cutaneous lupus rash, and alopecia. Oral ulcers may also be present.

Vascular Disease

Raynaud phenomenon, characterized by episodic vasospasm in the digits, is found in patients with SLE along with atrophic changes at the fingertips. Vascular headache is also common.

Renal

Lupus nephritis with associated hypertension is a marker for poor prognosis, and declining renal function may lead to renal failure.

Pulmonary

Pulmonary disease includes pleural effusions, atelectasis, interstitial pneumonitis, and pulmonary hypertension.

Cardiac

Related cardiac disease includes pericarditis (most frequent), myocarditis, and endocarditis of the mitral or aortic valves. Patients with SLE have earlier onset of coronary atherosclerotic disease compared with the general population, even after accounting for other common CAD risk factors (13). Corticosteroid treatment of SLE may be a contributing factor. Other causes of cardiac morbidity in SLE include coronary vasculitis and possibly hypercoagulability. In rare cases, patients can have cardiomyopathy, which may improve with immunosuppressive therapy.

Neurologic

Neuropsychiatric disease manifests as cognitive dysfunction, affective disorders, neuropathy (including phrenic pathology), propensity for cerebrovascular accident (CVA), and seizures. SLE patients have carotid artery disease more frequently than age-matched members of the general population (2).

Hematologic

SLE is often associated with hematologic abnormalities including anemia, leukopenia, and thrombocytopenia. Antiphospholipid antibody syndrome in a subset of patients with SLE is associated with thromboembolic complications such as deep vein thrombosis (DVT), CVA, and pulmonary embolism (PE). Anticoagulation therapy for such patients can reduce the incidence of thrombotic events. The antiphospholipid antibody syndrome may result in a prolonged activated partial thromboplastin time (aPTT).

Infection

Immune system dysfunction or the immunosuppressive effects of medications used to treat the disease put patients at risk for serious infection.

Several drugs can induce a disease similar to SLE; however, drug-induced lupus is relatively mild and time limited (12, 25). Medications associated with this disorder are listed in Table 11.2.

History

The history includes a discussion of the patient's general condition: presence of constitutional symptoms, course of the disease, recent exacerbations, medications and side effects, and specific end-organ disease. The evaluator also inquires about chronic cough, dyspnea at rest and with exertion, and a history of recent pulmonary infections. Recent thromboembolic events or other hematologic problems are discussed. The patient is asked about the best level of exercise tolerance and symptoms consistent with ischemic heart disease. A history of neurologic events is also elicited.

Physical Examination

The preoperative physical examination documents vital signs, the general appearance of the patient, associated dermatologic signs, and airway examination. The remainder of the physical examination focuses on cardiovascular and pulmonary systems,

Table 11.2. Drugs capable of causing drug-induced lupus erythematosus

ACE inhibitors	Hydrochlorothiazide	Phenytoin
Beta blockers	Interferons	Procainamide
Carbamazepine	Isoniazid	Propylthiouracil
Chlorpromazine	Lithium	Simvastatin
Hydralazine	Lovastatin	Sulfasalazine
	Macrodantin	Anti-TNF agents

ACE, angiotensin-converting enzyme; TNF, tumor necrosis factor.

documenting displaced PMI, muffled heart sounds, murmurs, pericardial rub, carotid bruits, and evidence of pulmonary edema, pleural effusion, or lung consolidation. The clinician also examines the patient for lower extremity edema, jugular venous distension (JVD), and hepatomegaly. Neurologic examination documents sensory and motor deficits from neuropathy or CVA.

Diagnostic Testing

Laboratory Testing

Patients with SLE require certain preoperative tests to identify common abnormalities. A CBC with platelets and aPTT is obtained. If hematologic abnormalities are present, the patient is referred for further testing to his or her rheumatologist or to a hematologist. The risk of renal involvement in SLE mandates a preoperative BUN and creatinine level. Patients with heart failure or renal insufficiency should have electrolyte levels measured.

Cardiovascular Testing

An ECG is performed because patients with SLE are at significantly higher risk for ischemic heart disease, pulmonary hypertension, and other cardiac abnormalities. The ECG may show right axis deviation (RAD), right bundle branch block (RBBB), low voltage associated with pericardial effusion, Q waves, or ST-T–wave abnormalities. With the early onset of atherosclerotic disease in this patient population, the preoperative evaluator should have a low threshold for cardiology referral and exercise or pharmacologic stress testing. If pericardial effusion, pulmonary hypertension, heart failure, or a valvular abnormality is suspected, 2-D transthoracic or transesophageal echocardiography (TEE) confirms the diagnosis.

Pulmonary Testing

Patients with worsening pulmonary status who will undergo major surgery should have a chest radiograph. PFTs can determine the presence and degree of restrictive lung disease. Echocardiography may be indicated for patients with suspected or known pulmonary hypertension. See the Scleroderma section in this chapter.

Preoperative Medications and Instructions

A wide variety of medications are used to treat SLE. See Table 11.3 for common agents, adverse effects, and perioperative recommendations.

Preoperative Preparation

The patient's pulmonary status should be optimized with treatment of effusion or infection before surgery. Patients with hypertension should have controlled blood pressure (140/90 or lower) before surgery, and diagnosis and management of ischemic heart disease are needed before major procedures (see Chapter 3).

Table 11.3.   Common medications, adverse effects, and preoperative management for patients with systemic lupus erythematosus

Agent	Adverse Effects	Preoperative Management
Aspirin	Bleeding complications, gastrointestinal irritation, renal dysfunction	Stop 7 days before surgery
Nonsteroidal anti-inflammatory drugs	Bleeding complications, gastrointestinal irritation, renal dysfunction	Stop 2 days before surgery
Hydroxychloroquine, chloroquine, quinacrine	Thrombocytopenia, myopathy, neuropathy	Monitor CBC with platelets; if thrombocytopenic, discontinue drug to allow normalization before surgery
Glucocorticoids	Impaired wound healing, glucose intolerance, increased risk of infection, adrenal suppression	Continue on day of surgery; provide perioperative "stress doses" (see Chapter 17)
Cytotoxic agents: Cyclophosphamide, azathioprine, mycophenolate mofetil	Immunosuppression, pancytopenia, gastrointestinal effects	Monitor CBC with platelets; if anemic or thrombocytopenic, discontinue drug to allow normalization before surgery

CBC, complete blood count.

Patients on chronic steroids may require stress doses perioperatively (see Chapter 17).

Anesthetic Implications
Patients with severely compromised respiratory or cardiovascular function may benefit from peripheral nerve block if the procedure allows. In patients with SLE and pre-existing neurologic deficits from CVAs or neuropathy, nerve block or neuraxial blockade can be performed after documenting the neurologic examination and discussing the risks and benefits of the procedure. The management of GA is guided by the patient's coexisting end-organ effects. Keeping the patient with Raynaud phenomenon warm is important to minimize vasospasm.

SYSTEMIC SCLEROSIS (SCLERODERMA)

The prominent feature of systemic sclerosis (scleroderma), an autoimmune disease, is excessive fibrosis. Female patients outnumber males 3:1. Clinical characteristics of scleroderma subtypes (14) are contrasted in the following section.

Localized Scleroderma

In localized scleroderma the skin is thickened without other end-organ disease.

Systemic Sclerosis

Systemic sclerosis has multiple end-organ effects.

Limited Cutaneous Systemic Sclerosis

In this disease subtype, the skin of the distal aspects of the upper extremities and face is thickened. Patients may have fatigue, Raynaud phenomenon, digital ulceration, gastroesophageal reflux disorder (GERD), dysphagia, and pulmonary complications such as interstitial lung disease (ILD) and pulmonary hypertension. Pulmonary hypertension or ILD is associated with limited survival after 5 years (15) and puts patients at risk for perioperative complications (16).

Diffuse Cutaneous Systemic Sclerosis

Characteristics of the diffuse subtype of systemic sclerosis are rapid onset of generalized skin thickening (progressing distal to proximal in the extremities). End-organ involvement includes myocardial fibrosis with ventricular dysfunction, pericarditis, arrhythmias, coronary vasospasm, thickening of small coronary vessels (17), and congestive heart failure. Renal failure occurs as a consequence of severe hypertension. ILD can be present in this subtype. Patients also have Raynaud phenomenon, fatigue, GERD, and dysphagia.

Raynaud phenomenon is present in several autoimmune diseases with varying frequency (18) (Table 11.4).

History

In patients with systemic sclerosis, the history should detail the type and onset of disease. Document gastrointestinal symptoms, including GERD and dysphagia, and review the severity of Raynaud phenomenon. Discuss known pulmonary, cardiac, or renal involvement associated with systemic sclerosis. To identify

Table 11.4. The incidence of Raynaud phenomenon in autoimmune diseases

Diseases	Incidence (Percent)
Scleroderma	>95%
Sjögren syndrome	20%–30%
Systemic lupus erythematosus	20%–30%
Rheumatoid arthritis	<5%

patients with severe pulmonary involvement associated with the disease, questions regarding fatigue, exercise capacity, and dyspnea at rest or on exertion are key. Patients are queried about orthopnea, nocturnal dyspnea, chest pain, and syncopal episodes. List current medications and significant side effects.

Physical Examination

The airway examination assesses for microstomia and limitation of neck mobility from skin fibrosis and thickening. Examination of the oropharynx verifies the presence of telangiectasias. Dermal thickening, edema, scarring, loss of digits, and contractures of the extremities are noted, to plan patient positioning, vascular access, and regional anesthesia. The clinician documents diminished breath sounds, crackles (indicating pulmonary edema, ILD, or pneumonia), or wheezing. Cyanosis, tachypnea, lower extremity edema, JVD, and hepatomegaly are noted. Cardiac auscultation may reveal a murmur or splitting of the second heart sound (S_2) consistent with pulmonary hypertension with tricuspid regurgitation (TR).

Diagnostic Testing

Laboratory Testing

Preoperative tests needed for systemic sclerosis patients are electrolyte, BUN, and creatinine levels. Patients who are being treated with immunosuppressive drugs need a CBC with platelets. Individuals who are malnourished require tests for prothrombin time (PT) and albumin level.

Cardiovascular Testing

A preoperative ECG is performed for systemic sclerosis patients to search for conduction abnormalities, arrhythmia, or evidence of right ventricular (RV) or left ventricular (LV) hypertrophy. Further cardiac testing is warranted in selected patients. In general, echocardiography is useful for patients with an H&P consistent with RV or LV dysfunction; the role of echocardiography in the evaluation of pulmonary disease is discussed in the next section. Testing for myocardial ischemia may be indicated because systemic sclerosis can be associated with small vessel CAD. Individuals with a history of palpitations, syncope, or dysrhythmia on ECG need Holter monitoring.

Pulmonary Evaluation

A patient with a history of dyspnea or a limited level of physical activity and findings consistent with pulmonary disease benefits from further evaluation before surgery. Modalities such as chest radiography, PFTs, and echocardiography establish a diagnosis and assist in medical management and perioperative care. An initial chest radiograph may reveal consolidation (pneumonia), opacities consistent with ILD, or an enlarged cardiac silhouette. Subsequent PFTs can reveal restrictive disease with low lung volumes in ILD as well as poor diffusing capacity consistent with ILD or pulmonary hypertension (15). Two-dimensional echocardiography is an excellent noninvasive technique to diagnose pulmonary hypertension. The degree of pressure elevation in the pulmonary artery (PA) along with abnormalities of the RV and tricuspid valve may be assessed. An invasive option is right heart catheterization with direct pressure measurements to confirm findings on echocardiography. Figure 11.1 is a suggested algorithm for identification of severe pulmonary disease in patients with systemic sclerosis (15).

Preoperative Medication and Instructions

Medical therapy for scleroderma is supportive and aims to treat the effects of this disease.

Calcium channel blockers (e.g., nifedipine, diltiazem, nicardipine, felodipine), angiotensin-converting enzyme (ACE) inhibitors, alpha blockers, and supplements (fish oils) are used to treat **Raynaud phenomenon** (18). These agents, with the exception of supplements and ACE inhibitors (see below), can be continued on the day of surgery (DOS) (see Chapter 17).

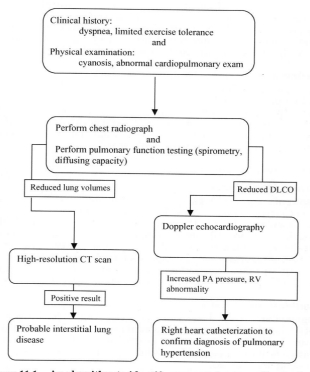

Figure 11.1.   An algorithm to identify severe pulmonary disease in patients with symptomatic scleroderma. CT, computed tomography; DLCO, diffusing capacity of the lung for carbon monoxide; PA, pulmonary artery; RV, right ventricle. (Based on information in Racz H, Mehta S. Dyspnea due to pulmonary hypertension and interstitial lung disease in scleroderma: room for improvement in diagnosis and management. *J Rheumatol.* **2006;33:1723–1725.)**

Hypertension is treated with a range of antihypertensive agents that may be continued on the day of surgery. However, ACE inhibitors and angiotensin receptor blockers (ARBs) may be omitted on the DOS to avoid intraoperative hypotension in certain situations (major procedures with significant anticipated blood loss, preoperative volume depletion, etc.). See Chapter 17.

Gastrointestinal problems are treated with histamine blockers and proton pump inhibitors, which should be continued on the DOS.

An immunosuppressive agent, such as cyclophosphamide, is used to treat early ILD. Based on the preoperative CBC with platelets, this medication is discontinued before surgery to allow blood counts to normalize. **Antifibrotic agents** such as D-penicillamine and interferons are also given to systemic sclerosis patients.

The treatment of **pulmonary hypertension** can improve the prognosis in these patients. Several agents are employed (14): prostaglandin-based agents epoprostenol, treprostinil, and iloprost; the endothelin inhibitor bosentan; and the nitric oxide potentiator sildenafil. Agents that are delivered by continuous infusion should not be interrupted during the perioperative period; similarly, oral agents are continued through the DOS.

Preoperative Preparation

Plans for airway management are explained to the patient, including possible awake FOI. Cardiopulmonary status should be stable (pulmonary and/or cardiology consults and testing completed if necessary) and patients are given optimal medical therapy. Patients with pulmonary hypertension should be managed with a specialist familiar with this disease.

Anesthetic Implications

Airway Management

If patients require GA, planning airway management is a priority. Direct laryngoscopy may be difficult or traumatic if the patient has vascular lesions in the oropharynx. Awake or asleep FOI is considered to cope with microstomia and limited neck movement. Because of the high incidence of GERD, premedication to decrease the risk of regurgitation and aspiration is considered. During GA, ventilation takes into account the presence of restrictive lung disease. The patient is kept warm to minimize vasospasm.

Regional Anesthesia

Regional anesthesia is a safe and effective option for the patient with scleroderma having a peripheral procedure. In patients with severe lung disease and/or cardiac dysfunction, spontaneous ventilation is maintained, and anesthetics that cause myocardial depression are avoided.

Intraoperative Monitoring

The use of central venous pressure (CVP), a PA catheter, or TEE is considered in patients with known pulmonary hypertension and/or ventricular dysfunction during lengthy or invasive surgery.

OSTEOARTHRITIS

Osteoarthritis (OA) is the degeneration of articular cartilage, characterized by inflammation and pain with joint motion. The elderly are particularly affected by OA, which appears frequently in the knees and hips. The spine can be involved, especially the cervical and lower lumbar regions. In contrast to RA, systemic manifestations do not accompany OA.

History

The history of joint involvement in OA is documented, along with any factors that relieve or exacerbate symptoms. Because the cervical spine may be involved, questioning the patient about neck stiffness or neurologic complaints is important. Cardiac and pulmonary history is routine as for other patients.

Physical Examination

The airway examination notes any limitation of neck flexion or extension as well as any difficulty in mouth opening. Neurologic examination includes any evidence of nerve root compression of the upper or lower extremities with sensory or motor deficits. The remainder of the examination is routine.

Diagnostic Testing

Patients with OA do not require any specific testing because of this condition. Patients who routinely take NSAIDs for relief of joint pain require a BUN and creatinine level. As the level of exercise may be limited (e.g., by knee pain) in a patient with OA, pharmacologic cardiac testing to search for ischemic heart disease may be necessary, based on the usual risk factors (see Chapter 17).

Preoperative Medication and Instructions

Patients with OA often take aspirin, NSAIDs, opioids, and non-opioid analgesic agents. Aspirin is discontinued 7 days before surgery, and NSAIDs are stopped for 2 days before to minimize the risk of bleeding complications. Other analgesic agents may be continued through the DOS. Some patients with OA take herbal medications for relief of their symptoms, and a recent review has summarized the results of clinical trials of various herbal medicines in OA (19). Patients are advised to stop herbal medicines 1 week before surgery because of the possibility of unwanted clinical effects of herbals.

Implications for Perioperative and Anesthetic Management

If a patient with OA has significant C-spine disease, neck movement to facilitate direct laryngoscopy may be impossible, or neck movement may precipitate neurologic injury. For these reasons, awake or asleep FOI is considered for cases requiring GA.

In procedures amenable to regional anesthesia, the ability of the patient to assume a position for the block is considered. In all cases, proper positioning and padding of extremities is recommended.

KYPHOSCOLIOSIS

Description

Kyphoscoliosis involves both lateral curvature and anterior flexion of the thoracic and/or lumbar spine. Most cases of kyphoscoliosis are idiopathic; however, in some patients, kyphoscoliosis is one manifestation of a syndrome or underlying disease (20) (Table 11.5). The structural abnormality of the spine limits normal ventilation, as severe spinal curvature causes an extrinsic restrictive pathology. To quantitate the degree of scoliosis, the Cobb angle is measured between lines drawn from the uppermost and lowest vertebral bodies comprising the spinal curvature. An angle >50 degrees places the patient at risk for pulmonary and cardiac compromise. Patients with severe kyphoscoliosis and pulmonary dysfunction may develop pulmonary hypertension and cardiac failure. In rare cases, the cardiac chambers may themselves be compressed by the abnormal spine and thorax (21) or there is tracheobronchial compression (22). If other interventions are not sufficient, surgical correction is necessary based on the severity of the curvature and the patient's functional status.

History

The evaluator determines the age of onset of the spinal curvature and any coexisting diseases or syndromes. The patient is questioned regarding functional status and best level of exercise tolerance, as cardiopulmonary impairment with kyphoscoliosis may be significant. Any history of fatigue, dyspnea at rest or on exertion, syncope, orthopnea, chronic cough with or without sputum production, and difficulty clearing secretions is elicited. Past or present neurologic deficits such as numbness or motor weakness are noted. If the patient with kyphoscoliosis is a child or teenager, the family is engaged in the preoperative evaluation and anesthetic planning process.

Physical Examination

Airway Examination

The cervical, thoracic, and lumbar spine are examined for curvature and mobility. Severe curvature and limited mobility may create challenges for airway management and intraoperative positioning. The upper airway is examined in the usual manner.

Table 11.5. Disease states associated with kyphoscoliosis

Neurofibromatosis
Ependymoma, astrocytoma
Cerebral palsy
Poliomyelitis
Muscular dystrophy
Friedrich ataxia
Marfan syndrome
Collagen vascular disorders

Cardiopulmonary Examination

Cyanosis, asymmetric chest expansion, coexisting sternal abnormalities (pectus excavatum), and the presence of wheezes or crackles are documented. Cardiac examination searches for murmurs consistent with valvular disease (e.g., AI in a patient with Marfan syndrome). Signs of pulmonary hypertension are sought, including JVD, peripheral edema, a TR murmur, or an accentuated pulmonic component of S_2.

Diagnostic Testing

Basic Testing

Many patients with significant kyphoscoliosis will undergo extensive surgery for correction of the spinal curvature or for other indications, and therefore require preoperative CBC and type and screen (T&S) tests. Patients with severe kyphoscoliosis with evidence of respiratory or cardiac compromise should have an ECG to reveal ventricular hypertrophy or conduction abnormalities. Such patients need a preoperative chest radiograph to reveal consolidation or cardiomegaly.

Specialized Testing

Patients with significant kyphoscoliosis and apparent pulmonary compromise require preoperative PFTs and ABG analysis. PFTs can delineate the severity of extrinsic restrictive lung disease; indicate the existence of any reversible component of bronchospasm so medical therapy can be intensified; and measure the preoperative level of carbon dioxide and oxygen to guide intraoperative and postoperative ventilation. In rare cases of tracheobronchial compression with kyphoscoliosis, preoperative computed tomography (CT) or magnetic resonance imaging (MRI) is valuable (22) (e.g., presence of stridor, wheezing that does not respond to inhalers).

Some patients with severe scoliosis and restrictive pulmonary physiology may have cardiac dysfunction as a consequence of pulmonary hypertension or coexisting cardiac disease as part of a syndrome. These patients require a preoperative ECG. Based on the H&P and ECG results, preoperative echocardiography can be performed to confirm ventricular dysfunction, quantify the degree of pulmonary hypertension, and identify valvular abnormalities.

Preoperative Medications and Instructions

No specific medical therapies are indicated for kyphoscoliosis itself. Patients may be taking medications for treatment of bronchospasm, pulmonary infection, or pain. Ordinarily these medications, with the exception of NSAIDs and aspirin, should be continued on the DOS.

Preoperative Preparation

Any reversible pulmonary conditions such as current or recent infection or bronchospasm are treated and elective surgery is postponed until resolved (see Chapter 5). Care may be best managed in conjunction with the patient's primary care physician or a pulmonologist. Medical management of pulmonary hypertension and other cardiovascular disease is optimized before surgery;

coordination with a specialist in this area is recommended. See the Scleroderma section of this chapter.

Anesthetic Implications

Induction Approach and Airway Management

Depending on the airway examination and the age of the patient, options include standard intravenous induction with direct laryngoscopy, awake FOI, or inhalation induction followed by laryngoscopy or FOI. Plans for awake (sedated) FOI are discussed with the patient to reduce the level of anxiety. In cases of airway compression from the kyphoscoliosis, equipment such as a rigid ventilating bronchoscope is available during induction. For pediatric patients, premedication before induction or arrangements for parents to accompany the child into the OR for induction can be considered (see Chapter 15).

Monitoring

Many patients with kyphoscoliosis undergo lengthy operations on the spine or for other indications. Invasive monitoring should be considered, including arterial line and CVP monitors. A PA catheter or TEE can be employed in patients with compromised cardiac function. Neurologic monitoring commonly used for spinal surgery to detect intraoperative spinal cord ischemia with traction includes monitoring somatosensory- and motor-evoked potentials, which may require special anesthesia techniques and advance planning. In selected cases, a wake-up test for motor function is performed intraoperatively. Plans for a wake-up test are discussed preoperatively with the patient so that he or she may anticipate this necessity.

Postoperative Care

Patients with severe restrictive lung disease who undergo major operations may require postoperative ICU admission with ventilatory support.

INHERITED CONNECTIVE TISSUE DISORDERS

This section reviews aspects of certain inherited connective tissue disorders pertinent to perioperative management.

Marfan syndrome is characterized by fibrillin mutations (23,24). Clinical features include tall stature, arachnodactyly, scoliosis, pectus excavatum or carinatum, ascending aortic dilation, dissection, valvular disease (AI, mitral valve prolapse [MVP], mitral regurgitation [MR] with possible pulmonary hypertension), and arrhythmias. Ocular (ectopia lentis, strabismus, glaucoma), pulmonary (blebs, spontaneous pneumothorax), and dilation of the dura with lower extremity pain can occur.

Ehlers-Danlos syndrome is a disorder of collagen synthesis and encompasses several subtypes, listed in Table 11.6. The condition includes tall stature, joint hypermobility, scoliosis, fragile and thin skin, blood vessel fragility, risk of vascular dissections, MVP, and spontaneous pneumothorax.

Osteogenesis imperfecta (OI) is a disorder of collagen production resulting in bone fragility with fractures; several subtypes of the disorder are described. Coexisting issues include

Table 11.6. Clinical features of Ehlers-Danlos syndrome subtypes (former classifications listed in brackets)

Ehlers-Danlos Subtype	Clinical Features
Hypermobility [type III]	Joint hypermobility and skin hyperextensibility
Classic [type I, II]	Joint hypermobility, skin fragility and hyperextensibility, scarring
Vascular [type IV]	Vascular and skin fragility, vascular and visceral rupture, pneumothorax, easy bruising, characteristic facial features, small joint hypermobility
Kyphoscoliosis [type VI]	Joint laxity, muscle weakness, scoliosis, ocular fragility, skin fragility, easy bruising, osteopenia
Arthrochalasia [type VIIA, VIIB]	Joint hypermobility, congenital hip dislocation, skin fragility and hyperextensibility, osteopenia, kyphoscoliosis
Dermatosparaxis [type VIIC]	Skin fragility and redundancy, easy bruising, presence of hernias
Other[a]	
Type V	Skin laxity and fragility
Type VIII	Skin fragility, scarring, bruising, periodontal disease
Type X	Joint laxity

[a]Types IX and XI are no longer included in the Ehlers-Danlos syndrome classification scheme; types V, VIII, and X are extremely rare disorders.
From Hahn BH. Systemic lupus erythematosus. In: Fauci AS, Langford CA, eds. *Harrison's Rheumatology.* New York: McGraw-Hill; 2006:69–83.

short stature, scoliosis, joint hypermobility, hearing loss, respiratory disease, muscle weakness, MVP, and platelet dysfunction.

Epidermolysis bullosa is a group of connective tissue disorders distinguished by blistering, skin fragility, and scarring because of abnormal epidermal–dermal anchoring.

History

As there is variation in clinical presentation for patients with the connective tissue diseases discussed in this section, the clinician inquires about the patient's connective tissue diagnosis, age at diagnosis, and specific complications caused by the disease. Musculoskeletal history focuses on level of chronic pain, stiffness, and recent fractures. The evaluator asks about hoarseness, chronic cough, dyspnea at rest or with exertion, orthopnea, palpitations, syncope, and activity limitations.

Physical Examination

The evaluator documents the presence of skin infection, blistering, excessive bruising, or scarring. The spine is examined for curvature and mobility. Sensory or motor neurologic deficits are noted. The upper airway is examined for features characteristic of the connective tissue disorders reviewed above. The airway examination in Marfan patients may reveal a high arched palate and retrognathia. The examination may indicate a difficult airway in a patient with OI (short neck). Blisters in the oropharynx may be evident in patients with epidermolysis bullosa.

Cyanosis, asymmetric chest expansion, sternal abnormalities, and wheezes or crackles are documented. Cardiovascular examination detects murmurs (e.g., the early diastolic murmur of AI in Marfan syndrome). Signs consistent with the presence of pulmonary hypertension and RV failure are sought, including JVD, peripheral edema, a TR murmur, and an accentuated pulmonic component of S_2.

Diagnostic Testing

In certain inherited connective tissue diseases with vascular fragility (subtypes of Ehlers-Danlos syndrome; see Table 11.6) or platelet dysfunction (OI), a preoperative CBC with platelets and T&S test is performed because of greater than normal anticipated blood loss. Patients who have potential cardiac involvement need an ECG. Arrhythmias (associated with MVP in Marfan syndrome) may be evaluated with Holter monitoring. Patients with suspected valvular abnormalities or an examination consistent with pulmonary hypertension receive 2-D echocardiography.

Patients who have severe kyphoscoliosis or pectus excavatum require preoperative diagnostic testing to determine the degree of pulmonary or cardiac compromise based on the guidelines listed in previous sections of this chapter. Preoperative C-spine radiographs are performed in patients who have joint hypermobility with neurologic signs or cervical fracture risk before undertaking anesthetic techniques involving airway manipulation. See the RA section of this chapter for specifics on C-spine evaluation.

Preoperative Medication and Instructions

Patients with Marfan syndrome may be taking beta blockers to prevent aortic dissection and these should be continued through the DOS.

Patients with OI who take calcium and vitamin D supplements to prevent osteoporosis should omit these medications on the DOS. NSAIDs are frequently given to manage pain and should be stopped 2 days before planned surgery.

Preoperative Preparation

Plans for airway management are explained to the patient. Any reversible pulmonary condition such as bronchospasm is treated. Cardiac disease is controlled with appropriate medical management preoperatively.

Anesthetic Implications

Patients with these connective tissue disorders may present for a variety of surgical procedures. Anesthetic management is based on organ systems involved and the planned surgical procedure; for a detailed discussion of anesthetic concerns with cardiac valvular disease see Chapter 4. The connective tissue disorders frequently impact airway management plans. The upper airway length may be greater than normal in Marfan patients; a longer laryngoscope blade or FOI is used to secure the airway. In patients with OI, laryngoscopy may be difficult (short neck) and can fracture the cervical spine; awake or asleep FOI may be indicated. Patients with C-spine hypermobility (Ehlers-Danlos syndrome) also benefit from FOI to avoid dislocation and oropharyngeal trauma with laryngoscopy. Avoiding direct laryngoscopy is also helpful in epidermolysis bullosa patients who require GA to minimize oropharyngeal and laryngeal injury. Some individuals with these diseases are at risk of pneumothoraces and require low airway pressures during positive pressure ventilation.

Patients with OI may develop hyperthermia under GA. Although intraoperative hypermetabolism and hyperthermia are observed in some OI patients, not all such cases are actual malignant hyperthermia (MH) episodes. Clinicians may consider administering a total intravenous anesthetic (TIVA).

Regional techniques, especially peripheral nerve blocks, can minimize the risk of cardiovascular depression, as well as airway management problems, associated with GA. Neuraxial blockade may be difficult or hazardous in some of the connective tissue disorders because of fragility of the spine, inability of the patient to position for the block, bleeding tendency, or skin breakdown. Regardless of the anesthetic technique chosen, careful positioning for all patients with connective tissue diseases helps minimize skin disruption and avoids iatrogenic fracture.

REFERENCES

1. Lee DM, Weinblatt ME. Rheumatoid arthritis. *Lancet*. 2001;358: 903–911.
2. Manzi S, Wasko MCM. Inflammation-mediated rheumatic diseases and atherosclerosis. *Ann Rheum Dis*. 2000;59:321–325.
3. Tokunaga D, Hase H, Mikami Y, et al. Atlantoaxial subluxation in different intraoperative head positions in patients with rheumatoid arthritis. *Anesthesiology*. 2006;104:675–679.
4. Takenaka I, Urakami Y, Aoyama K, et al. Severe subluxation in the sniffing position in a rheumatoid patient with anterior atlantoaxial subluxation. *Anesthesiology*. 2004;101:1235–1237.
5. Miyanohara T, Igarashi T, Suzuki H, et al. Aggravation of laryngeal rheumatoid arthritis after use of a laryngeal mask airway. *J Clin Rheumatol*. 2006;12:142–144.
6. van Asselt KM, Lems WF, Bongartz EB, et al. Outcome of cervical spine surgery in patients with rheumatoid arthritis. *Ann Rheum Dis*. 2001;60:448–452.
7. Olsen NJ, Stein CM. New drugs for rheumatoid arthritis. *N Engl J Med*. 2004;350:2167–2179.
8. Kolman J, Morris I. Cricoarytenoid arthritis: a cause of acute upper airway obstruction in rheumatoid arthritis. *Can J Anaesth*. 2002;49(7):729–732.
9. Takakura K, Hirakawa S, Kudo K, et al. Cricoarytenoid arthritis diagnosed after tracheostomy in a rheumatoid arthritis patient. *Masui*. 2005;54:690–693.
10. Clegg DO. Treatment of ankylosing spondylitis. *J Rheumatol Suppl*. 2006;78:24–31.

11. Ruf M, Rehm S, Poeckler-Schoeniger C, et al. Iatrogenic fractures in ankylosing spondylitis—a report of two cases. *Eur Spine J.* 2006;15:100–104.
12. Mills JA. Systemic lupus erythematosus. *N Engl J Med.* 1994;330: 1871–1879.
13. D'Agate DJ, Kokolis S, Soloman N, et al. Case reports: premature coronary artery disease in systemic lupus erythematosus with extensive reocclusion following coronary artery bypass surgery. *J Invasive Cardiol.* 2003;15:157–163.
14. Charles C, Clements P, Furst DE. Systemic sclerosis: hypothesis-driven treatment strategies. *Lancet.* 2006;367:1683–1691.
15. Racz H, Mehta S. Dyspnea due to pulmonary hypertension and interstitial lung disease in scleroderma: room for improvement in diagnosis and management. *J Rheumatol.* 2006;33:1723–1725.
16. Ramakrishna G, Sprung J, Ravi BS, et al. Impact of pulmonary hypertension on the outcomes of noncardiac surgery: predictors of perioperative morbidity and mortality. *J Am Coll Cardiol.* 2005; 45:1691–1699.
17. Gupta MP, Zoneraich S, Zeitlin W, et al. Scleroderma heart disease with slow flow velocity in coronary arteries. *Chest.* 1975;67: 116–119.
18. Isenberg DA, Black C. ABC of rheumatology: Raynaud's phenomenon, scleroderma, and overlap syndromes. *BMJ.* 1995;310: 795–798.
19. Long L, Soeken K, Ernst E. Herbal medicine for the treatment of osteoarthritis: a systematic review. *Rheumatology.* 2001;40:779–793.
20. Hagberg C, Welch WC, Bowman-Howard M. Anesthesia and surgery for spine and spinal cord procedures. In: Albin MS, ed. *Textbook of Neuroanesthesia.* New York: McGraw-Hill; 1997: 1052–1075.
21. Alexianu D, Skolnick ET, Pinto AC, et al. Severe hypotension in the prone position in a child with neurofibromatosis, scoliosis and pectus excavatum presenting for posterior spinal fusion. *Anesth Analg.* 2004;98:334–335.
22. Donnelly LF, Bisset GS III. Airway compression in children with abnormal thoracic configuration. *Radiology.* 1998;206:323–326.
23. Ho NCY, Tran JR, Bektas A. Marfan's syndrome. *Lancet.* 2005; 366:1978–1981.
24. Wordsworth P, Halliday D. The real connective tissue diseases. *Clin Med.* 2001;1:21–24.
25. Hahn BH. Systemic lupus erythematosus. In: Fauci AS, Langford CA, eds. *Harrison's Rheumatology.* New York: McGraw-Hill; 2006:69–83.
26. Beighton P, de Paepe A, Steinmann B, et al. Ehlers-Danlos syndromes: revised nosology, Villefranche 1997. *Am J Med Genet.* 1998;77:31–37.

Psychiatric Disease, Chronic Pain, and Substance Abuse

Jane C. Ballantyne

The anesthetist regularly encounters patients with psychiatric disease, chronic pain, and substance use disorders. It is no coincidence, in fact, that these three states are presented together in this chapter since two of them, and sometimes all three, coexist in many patients, and each state is a risk or comorbid factor for the others. Although the three states are presented separately here, when preparing patients with one of the conditions for surgery and anesthesia, we probe for the existence of the others.

Many of the anesthetic considerations for psychiatric disease, chronic pain, and substance abuse are drug related. Psychoactive drugs used for the treatment of psychiatric disorders have become safer and better tolerated. They are widely used even in the absence of a formal psychiatric diagnosis. Anesthetists find that concerns about drug therapy for psychiatric disease arise less frequently than those about chronic use of opioids, either illicit or legitimate.

PSYCHIATRIC DISEASE

Depression and anxiety are common. Major depression has a point prevalence of 2% to 4% in adults and a lifetime prevalence of 10% in men and 20% in women (1,2). It is one of the leading causes of disability worldwide. Criteria for major depression are listed in Table 12.1. Minor depression has been difficult to classify, define, and quantify. Mood and cognitive symptoms predominate more than the neurovegetative symptoms (e.g., loss of appetite, sleep disorders) associated with major depression (3). Antidepressants, especially the new generation of selective serotonin reuptake inhibitors (SSRIs), anticonvulsants, and anxiolytics (benzodiazepines) are the treatment for depression and anxiety, which frequently coexist with chronic pain and substance use disorders (4). Other psychiatric disorders, such as obsessive compulsive disorder, phobias, and panic disorders, are similarly treated. Bipolar disease is treated with mood stabilizers, including anticonvulsants and lithium, or antidepressants during depressive episodes. The psychoses, such as classic schizophrenia, are treated with antipsychotics. New-generation antipsychotics are markedly safer with fewer neurologic (extrapyramidal) adverse effects than traditional antipsychotics.

Preoperative Preparation

The preoperative interview establishes trust and rapport, even if another physician is to manage anesthesia. An empathetic and caring anesthesiologist can have tremendous influence on a patient's emotional state. Nonfearful patients have lower pre- and

**Table 12.1. Diagnostic characteristics
of major depression**[a]

Depressed mood
Diminished pleasure or interest in activities
Significant weight loss or gain
Insomnia or hypersomnia
Psychomotor agitation or retardation
Fatigue or loss of energy
Feelings of worthlessness
Diminished ability to think or concentrate
Recurrent thoughts of death
Symptoms in the absence of delusions or hallucinations

[a]At least five of the symptoms must be present for at least a 2-week period.
Reprinted with permission from American Psychiatric Association. *Diagnostic and Statistical Manual of Mental Disorders.* 4th ed. Washington, DC: American Psychiatric Association Press; 1994.

intraoperative medication requirements and a smoother anesthetic course (5).

Despite the best efforts of the caregiver, a patient who is depressed, delusional, or combative may be unable to provide an accurate history or cooperate with procedures. In such cases, information is obtained from collateral sources, such as the patient's primary care physician, a family member, or staff from a group home. Medical care of psychiatric patients often is fragmented, and many family members may have distanced themselves or are estranged from the patient. Ideally, patients should be involved in discussions of their physical health or should at least verify information obtained from outside sources. Even combative and highly agitated patients may be able to cooperate with focused questions.

A patient's obvious psychiatric symptoms may be affected by certain medications or diseases (Table 12.2). Symptoms of major depression can result from clinically significant hypothyroidism. Patients with brain tumors may have personality changes, delusions, and social impairment like those associated with schizophrenia.

Schizophrenia is characterized by psychotic episodes manifested by hallucinations, delusions, and inappropriate affect. If a schizophrenic patient needs surgery during an acute psychotic episode, speaking with the patient's caregivers before meeting with the patient is advisable. This meeting gives the clinician the opportunity to understand the patient's delusional system and determine the best way to conduct the interview and physical examination, without becoming entrapped in the patient's psychosis. Schizophrenic patients may be unable to read social cues, often appear unkempt, and have difficulty getting organized (6). The incidence of cigarette smoking is high in these patients with a consequent increase in smoking-related illnesses (7).

Drug Considerations

Drug treatment of psychiatric disease is complex and often confounding to nonpsychiatrists. From the point of view of anesthetic

Table 12.2. Medical problems that can cause psychiatric symptoms

Hypothyroidism and hyperthyroidism
Cushing syndrome
AIDS
Seizure disorders
Brain tumors
Encephalitis
Nutritional deficiency
Toxic substance poisoning
Drug dependency

management, an understanding of the mechanisms of action and potential interactions of psychotropic medications is more important than an understanding of why these medications have been prescribed by the treating mental health professional. Table 12.3 summarizes the problems, interactions, and anesthetic considerations for drugs used to treat psychiatric disorders.

Selective Serotonin Reuptake Inhibitors (see Table 12.3 for examples)

- Treatment with this relatively safe class of drugs is not confined to patients with major depression.
- The drugs selectively block the uptake of serotonin from the synaptic cleft; activity on other neurotransmitter systems is negligible (8,9).
- SSRIs should be continued perioperatively. Abrupt discontinuation has been associated with a syndrome characterized by dizziness, irritability, headache, nausea, visual disturbance, and electric shock sensations. Fluoxetine (Prozac) is the least likely to produce the syndrome because of its relatively long half-life and a long-acting active metabolite.
- SSRIs are potent inhibitors of cytochrome P-450 enzymes, especially the 2D6 isoenzyme (8), but the clinical significance of this inhibition during anesthesia is unknown.

Tricyclic Antidepressants (see Table 12.3 for examples)

- Tricyclic antidepressants (TCAs) exert antidepressant effects by blocking the reuptake of norepinephrine and serotonin from the synaptic cleft.
- They block α_1-adrenergic, muscarinic, and histamine receptors and slow cardiac conduction (major side effects), and can have potential interactions with anesthetic agents (8,9). An electrocardiogram (ECG) is usually obtained periodically during chronic antidepressant therapy (high dose) and should be reviewed or repeated preoperatively.
- In patients taking high antidepressant doses, pressors may exaggerate responses. Lower doses used in chronic pain treatment are less toxic and less problematic. The tricyclics are not first-line antidepressants and are rarely used at high dose.

Table 12.3. Common interactions and anesthetic considerations for drugs that treat psychiatric disorders

Drug	Problems and Interactions	Recommendations
Selective serotonin reuptake inhibitors (SSRIs) Fluoxetine (Prozac) Paroxetine (Paxil) Sertraline (Zoloft) Citalopram (Celexa) Escitalopram (Lexapro)	Favorable side effect profile. Limited sedation Weak anticholinergic effects	Do not withdraw abruptly. No added serotonergic drugs (e.g., tramadol, meperidine) to avoid serotonergic syndrome
Tricyclic antidepressants (TCAs) Imipramine (Tofranil) Amitriptyline (Elavil) Doxepin (Sinequan) Desipramine (Norpramin) Nortriptyline (Pamelor)	SSRIs preferred because of better side effect profile. Inhibit metabolism of catecholamines. May produce postural hypotension, dysrhythmias. Anticholinergic effects worsen bowel slowing Potentiates the CNS effects of epinephrine	Possible exaggerated pressor responses
Monoamine oxidase inhibitors (MAOIs) Phenelzine (Nardil) Isocarboxazid (Marplan) Tranylcypromine (Parnate)	Rarely used because of unsafe interactions and dietary restrictions. React with meperidine—coma, twitching, CNS excitement. Severe hypertensive response especially to indirectly acting pressors (ephedrine)	

Atypical antidepressants Bupropion (Wellbutrin) (NDRI) Venlafaxine (Effexor) (SNRI) Duloxetine (Cymbalta) (SNRI) Mirtazapine (Remeron) (NASA) Trazodone (Desyrel) (SARI)	Drug interactions listed in PDR or other resource Can lower seizure threshold
Anticonvulsants	Most induce liver enzymes (except valproate). Possible increased requirements for hypnotics. Abrupt discontinuation can cause withdrawal seizures	Preoperative evaluation should include LFTs and blood count
Phenytoin		Possible increased requirement for muscle relaxants
Sodium valproate (Epilim) Carbamazepine (Tegretol) Oxcarbazepine (Trileptal)	May slow metabolism of other drugs Hematologic and hepatic toxicities possible Hyponatremia possible	Measure sodium level
Topiramate (Topamax) Lamotrigine (Lamictal)	Steven-Johnson syndrome, possibly fatal, can arise with rapid dose escalation	
Gabapentin (Neurontin) Pregabalin (Lyrica)	Usually well tolerated Usually well tolerated	
Anxiolytics Alprazolam (Xanax) Clonazepam (Klonopin) Diazepam (Valium) Lorazepam (Ativan) Oxazepam (Serax) Buspirone (BuSpar) (nonbenzodiazepine)	Compound sedating effects of anesthetics and opioids	Continue perioperatively. Additional doses may be needed

(Continued)

Table 12.3. *Continued*

Drug	Problems and Interactions	Recommendations
Atypical neuroleptics	Less dopamine antagonism than typical neuroleptics. Also block serotonin and α_2-adrenergic receptors. Less propensity to produce adverse neurologic effects. Can be associated with insulin resistance	Continue therapy perioperatively. Exaggerated hypotension possible
Risperidone (Risperdal) Clozapine (Clozaril)	Because of 0.4%–2% risk of potentially fatal agranulocytosis, only used in treatment-refractory psychosis	Delayed recovery possible
Olanzapine (Zyprexa) Quetiapine (Seroquel)		
Typical neuroleptics (antipsychotics)	Atypical (second-generation) neuroleptics preferred because of better side effect profile. Typical neuroleptics have extrapyramidal, hormonal, and anticholinergic side effects	
Phenothiazine Chlorpromazine (Thorazine) Haloperidol (Haldol)		
Mood stabilizers Lithium	Impairs renal concentrating ability. Impairs thyroid hormone production. Discontinuation associated with suicide. Potentiates nondepolarizing relaxants	If possible, discontinue 48–72 hours before anesthesia, but re-establish after surgery. Check electrolytes, urea, creatinine, and thyroid function
Anticonvulsants (see above)		

CNS, central nervous system; LFTs, liver function tests; NASA, norepinephrine antagonist/serotonin antagonist; NDRI, norepinephrine-dopamine reuptake inhibitor; PDR, *Physicians Desk Reference*; SARI, serotonin antagonist/reuptake inhibitor; SNRI, serotonin-norepinephrine reuptake inhibitor.
NOTE: Psychiatric drugs as a group act by a variety of mechanisms, and although common problems and cautions are listed here, a large number of other adverse effects and interactions can arise. The reader should refer to more comprehensive resources when he or she is not familiar with a medication and its potential adverse effects and interactions.

Monoamine Oxidase Inhibitors (see Table 12.3 for examples)

- Monoamine oxidase inhibitors (MAOIs) interact with vasoactive amines such as tyramine (imposing dietary restrictions) to produce hypertensive crisis. They remain useful for refractory depression, and they have re-emerged as options for treating major depression.
- MAOIs interact with meperidine to produce "serotonin syndrome": Hypertension, coma, and possibly death. Use with pressors, especially indirect sympathomimetics (e.g., ephedrine), can cause hypertensive crisis.
- If the MAOI has been the only effective treatment, the current recommendation is that it should be continued preoperatively to avoid the complications associated with discontinuation (e.g., risk of suicide). Otherwise, withdraw (at least 3 weeks before surgery) and substitute another antidepressant.

Atypical Antidepressants (see Table 12.3 for examples)

- Atypical antidepressants belong to an eclectic group of medications whose receptor-binding and side effect profiles should be reviewed when they are encountered.
- Bupropion hydrochloride (Zyban) is also approved as an aid to smoking cessation. Bupropion is associated with a dose-dependent increase in the incidence of seizures in patients with a history of head trauma, seizure, central nervous system tumor, or concomitant use of medications that lower the seizure threshold (10).
- Duloxetine (Cymbalta) is efficacious for chronic pain (specifically neuropathic pain and fibromyalgia) (11,12).

Anticonvulsants (see Table 12.3 for examples)

- Anticonvulsant drugs are effective mood stabilizers whose efficacy has been demonstrated in controlled, double-blind trials.
- The four most commonly used drugs for this indication are sodium valproate, carbamazepine, lamotrigine, and gabapentin.
- Anticonvulsants, especially gabapentin and pregabalin, which are well tolerated, are also used frequently for the treatment of chronic neuropathic pain.
- Gabapentin and pregabalin are cleared largely unmetabolized by the kidney. The other drugs are metabolized by the liver and can induce hepatic enzymes with possible effects on the metabolism of anesthetics and an increased requirement for hypnotics.
- Preoperative evaluation should include liver function tests and blood count (except for gabapentin and pregabalin).
- Abrupt discontinuation can result in withdrawal seizures (10).

Anxiolytics (see Table 12.3 for examples)

- Most of the anxiolytics are benzodiazepines, which compound the sedating effects of anesthetics and opioids.
- It is usual to continue or even supplement anxiolytic therapy during the perioperative period.

- Buspirone, a nonbarbiturate, nonaddictive, 5HT1A antagonist, is used with SSRIs to treat obsessive-compulsive disorders. It has also been used successfully in the treatment of posttraumatic stress disorder.

Atypical Neuroleptics (see Table 12.3 for examples)

- These drugs antagonize dopamine less than typical neuroleptics and therefore produce fewer extrapyramidal adverse effects (parkinsonism, akathisia, and tardive dyskinesia).
- They also block serotonin and α_2-adrenergic receptors, which can exaggerate hypotension during surgery and anesthesia, notably spinal anesthesia (13–15).
- Treatment should be continued perioperatively.

Typical Neuroleptics (see Table 12.3 for examples)

- Rarely used, the typical neuroleptics have extrapyramidal, hormonal, and anticholinergic adverse effects.

Mood Stabilizers (see Table 12.3 for examples)

- Both anticonvulsants and lithium are used as mood stabilizers.
- Lithium impairs renal concentrating ability, producing nephrogenic diabetes insipidus, possibly increasing fluid requirements (10). It may impair thyroid hormone production and produce hypothyroidism and goiters. Check thyroid function, electrolytes, urea, and creatinine. Discontinuation has been associated with suicide (16).
- Lithium may potentiate nondepolarizing relaxants.
- If possible, lithium should be discontinued for 48 to 72 hours before surgery, then restarted after surgery.

The majority of psychiatric disorders are mild and well controlled with or without medication. Even patients with serious psychiatric disorders are rational, cooperative, and calm before surgery. For the few with serious disorders who may be unable to cooperate, not only is it necessary to obtain consent from the next of kin or the person with power of attorney, but also it may be necessary to use measures such as a ketamine dart (intramuscular ketamine) to calm the patient sufficiently to induce and maintain general anesthesia. The other difficulty with treating uncooperative patients is managing postoperative pain: Pain levels can only be guessed since the patients are unable to provide reliable information about their pain. If a caregiver is present, this person should be reassured that pain will not be neglected, and it may be helpful to involve this person in the pain treatment plan.

CHRONIC PAIN

Chronic pain is ubiquitous in the general population, and even more likely to be found in the surgical population. Over the last two decades it has become commonplace to treat chronic pain aggressively, with physical and behavioral interventions or medical interventions including opioids, injections, and operations. Medication issues predominate as anesthetic considerations. Chronic opioid use produces real difficulties for the perioperative management of acute pain and the success of continued management of the chronic pain.

Preoperative Preparation

All members of the team (anesthetists, surgeons, and nurses) looking after surgical patients with chronic pain benefit from a well-documented pain history taken at the time of the preoperative visit. It is helpful to know how the pain evolved, which treatments have worked and which have not, and what the patient's expectations are for pain treatment during the perioperative period and after the recovery phase. The history must include a full list of medications and current doses, as well as medication allergies and intolerances. Chronic pain patients often have psychiatric comorbidities, notably depression, anxiety, somatoform disorder, or posttraumatic stress disorder (17). Many chronic pain patients are being treated with psychotropic medications for psychiatric disorders as well as for pain. It is important to establish whether or not these conditions accompany chronic pain so that they can be managed properly during the perioperative period.

It is always helpful to discuss the pain management plan with the patient and, if relevant, the patient's relatives. Patients with chronic pain tend to be especially fearful of pain, and it is reassuring to them to learn that their caregivers understand this and will make every effort to optimize pain management. The perioperative period is not the time to ration pain medications. Patients, especially those taking opioids, may need exceptionally large opioid doses. They can also benefit from opioid-sparing measures such as regional anesthesia, catheter treatments, and nonsteroidal anti-inflammatory drugs (NSAIDs) to reduce opioid requirements. These options should be offered and discussed if appropriate.

Drug Considerations

Chronic treatment with opioids produces many problems for the management of acute surgical pain. Chronic pain patients may also take neuropathic pain medications in the antidepressant, anticonvulsant, and membrane-stabilizing classes, as well as possibly acetaminophen or NSAIDs. There are anesthetic considerations for all these drug types.

Opioids

- The standard μ-receptor agonists include morphine, oxycodone, hydromorphone (Dilaudid), meperidine (Demerol), and codeine.
- The constipating effect of codeine restricts its dosage. It is only used for chronic pain when combined with acetaminophen in Tylenol 3, and then only for moderate pain because of the ceiling dose for acetaminophen. Dosage for the other standard opioids can be titrated upward as required, and there is no strict ceiling dose.
- Although there is much debate about the safety and efficacy of prolonged high-dose opioid therapy (18), patients who take high doses still need surgical procedures.
- It becomes difficult to adequately manage acute pain in opioid-treated patients who have become markedly opioid tolerant or

who may also display opioid-induced hyperalgesia, especially when the new pain requires doses that produce withdrawal because opioid requirements are difficult to match (19–22). These factors must be understood so that a reasonable strategy for perioperative pain management can be outlined and agreed upon.

- The simplest approach is to supplement chronic therapy with additional opioids (even if exceptionally high additional doses are needed). Supplementation can be with patient-controlled analgesia (PCA) when there is an inpatient stay or with additional oral opioids for outpatient surgery. If the patient is unable to take oral medications, then the usual oral dose can be converted to a parenteral dose as a continuous infusion on the PCA. If bolus dose requirements become excessive, the basal infusion dose can be increased.

- Opioid-sparing analgesia interventions can minimize opioid requirements. Regional anesthesia, especially when prolonged with continuous catheter infusions (e.g., in epidurals and in the brachial plexus and femoral nerve sheath), is one example. NSAIDs are also opioid sparing, if tolerated. These analgesic interventions must be discussed and agreed upon before surgery so that contraindications can be determined.

Methadone

- Methadone has long been the choice for maintenance treatment of opioid addiction because it has a long half-life and maintains a steady state with once-daily dosing.

- More recently, methadone has been adopted as an option for the treatment of chronic and cancer pain. For reasons that are not fully understood, methadone works well in opioid rotations. A rotation or "switch" is undertaken when tolerance to one opioid is insurmountable; rotating to a different opioid restores analgesic efficacy because of incomplete cross-tolerance between opioids. Thus, methadone is often used for the treatment of opioid refractory pain.

- There are some problems, however, with methadone. The metabolism of methadone, though prolonged, is variable and idiosyncratic. The degree to which the drug accumulates varies from patient to patient. Deaths from respiratory depression have occurred because of this unpredictability.

- Serious interactions, notably with antibiotics and antifungals, have been found, as well as rare but dangerous prolongation of the QTc interval on the electrocardiogram (23). Preoperative ECG can help identify prolonged QTc.

- When patients taking methadone come for surgery, its use perioperatively depends on whether the drug is a maintenance treatment for addiction or for pain. In either case, it may prove difficult to control pain unless methadone is continued. If possible, the oral methadone dose should be continued with a standard opioid added to treat acute pain (e.g., PCA morphine). For patients who are unable to take oral medications perioperatively, either methadone or an alternative opioid can be given by continuous intravenous infusion (e.g., through the PCA pump).

- It will sometimes be difficult to overcome severe pain with alternative opioids, especially when methadone has been used to treat opioid-refractory pain. In this case, methadone PCA is the best option, and large doses may be needed.
- Most patients who are taking methadone have developed tolerance to it and can safely be sent home with the preoperative dose or a slightly higher dose and an additional opioid to treat acute pain. For patients started on methadone de novo during hospitalization (e.g., for opioid refractory pain), the drug can accumulate more than expected, if time in the hospital has been insufficient to reach a steady state.
- When methadone-treated patients are evaluated for surgery, methadone usage, reason for treatment, dose, and dosing history are documented. These patients may need reassurance about the management of their pain. Methadone maintenance patients may be concerned that opioid treatment of pain might result in addiction relapse, in which case they are reassured that hospital treatment of acute pain rarely reinstates addiction (24).

Buprenorphine

- Buprenorphine, a partial μ-agonist and an alternative for maintenance treatment of addiction, has recently been approved in the United States for clinic- and office-based treatment of addiction (in large part to avoid the regulatory onus and stigma of methadone) (25,26).
- Buprenorphine is marketed in the United States as Suboxone (with naloxone) or Subutex (without naloxone). Naloxone is added as an antiabuse measure. If the drug is abused by snorting or injecting (i.e., taken parenterally instead of orally), the effect is reserved by the naloxone. Oral naloxone is rapidly cleared by the liver, so there is no such reversal when the drug is taken as prescribed. Naloxone has no significance perioperatively since it is rapidly cleared.
- Buprenorphine, like methadone, has an established record of utility for the treatment of pain, largely from the European experience, since the drug has only been popularized more recently in the United States and currently can be used there only off-label for pain.
- Buprenorphine has certain limitations in terms of pain treatment. While it is useful for the treatment of mild to moderate pain, its partial agonism results in a ceiling effect that may limit its utility in severe pain. Its μ-opioid receptor occupancy is prolonged and difficult to displace; therefore, it compromises the ability of added potent agonists such as morphine and fentanyl to provide greater analgesia. This factor does not seem to be a problem when standard opioids are used for breakthrough pain during chronic buprenorphine treatment for pain or addiction (27). It can be a problem when severe acute pain (e.g., surgery or trauma) intervenes (28).
- Because it may not be possible to overcome the partial agonist effect of buprenorphine, it is recommended that chronic buprenorphine treatment be discontinued or substituted for a week before surgery.

- For emergency surgery, when there has not been an opportunity to discontinue the treatment, it may prove difficult to control severe pain during the perioperative period. Opioid-sparing interventions may need to be maximized.

Neuropathic Pain Medications

- The two main classes of drugs used as neuropathic pain medications are the antidepressants and the anticonvulsants.
- Gabapentin is currently the most popular choice because of its relative safety compared to the tricyclic antidepressants (the original neuropathic pain medications, and still widely used for this indication). Newer antidepressants such as duloxetine (Cymbalta) are being adopted as neuropathic pain medications.
- In general, it is advisable to continue neuropathic pain medications during the perioperative period, at least when patients can take oral medications. Cautions and restrictions associated with these medications are described in the Drug Considerations section in the discussion of psychiatric disease and summarized in Table 12.3.

Nonsteroidal Anti-Inflammatory Drugs and Acetaminophen

- The NSAIDs and acetaminophen, over-the-counter analgesics, have a long history of use for mild to moderate pain. They are also combined with opioids in oral formulations. Many patients with chronic pain take these medications, either under or without medical supervision. Prolonged treatment with NSAIDs is not recommended.
- The newer cyclo-oxygenase (COX)-2 inhibitors were developed in the hope of reducing the adverse effects of NSAIDs, particularly the damaging gastrointestinal (GI) effects. The steady emergence of evidence shows that deleterious cardiovascular and thrombotic effects preclude the use of these drugs in many patients (29,30). Most drugs in this class are now withdrawn, and the only selective COX-2 inhibitor on the market in the United States at the time of this writing is celecoxib (Celebrex).
- The adverse effects of NSAIDs in surgical patients include bleeding risk (especially gastrointestinal and closed cavity), renal dysfunction, and delayed bone fusion. Acetaminophen is relatively safe and not associated with bleeding, renal dysfunction, or delayed bone fusion. The COX-2 inhibitors are less likely to cause bleeding (platelet effects), particularly GI bleeding (unprotected GI mucosa), but carry the same risk as standard NSAIDs of renal dysfunction. Their effect on bone healing is largely unknown.
- Patients should be advised to stop taking standard NSAIDs before surgery, chiefly because of their platelet effects and their propensity to increase surgical bleeding. Aspirin, whose platelet effects are not reversible, should be discontinued for 7 days before elective surgery. Other NSAIDs have rapidly reversible platelet effects, and 24 hours' cessation is probably sufficient, although 2 to 3 days' cessation is usual. Acetaminophen and COX-2 inhibitors can be continued because they do not have platelet effects.

Other Anesthetic Implications

It may be extremely challenging to manage pain during and after surgery in patients being treated for chronic pain. Largely, this is because of opioid tolerance confined to patients receiving long-term opioids. Neuropathic pain medications also have anesthetic implications, as described above, but because they provide additional analgesia, they can be continued during the perioperative period and may even be helpful in managing pain and anxiety. Opioid tolerance may be overcome only by utilizing alternative analgesic strategies or with unusually large opioid doses.

Surgery sometimes presents a chance of reversing the painful condition (e.g., replacement joint surgery). Immediate reversal of pain would be rare, and acute pain should be treated as aggressively as necessary. The operative period is not the right time to wean patients off high-dose opioid therapy. It may, however, be helpful to have a conversation with the patient's primary physicians to discuss long-term pain treatment plans, the transition from acute to chronic management, and the intention to reduce the dose of opioids once acute pain has resolved.

SUBSTANCE ABUSE

Substance abuse[1] is becoming a societal problem of unprecedented proportions, especially in liberal states such as the United States, where regulations have failed to control illicit drug use. Statistics suggest a steady increase in illicit drug use over the past decade. For example, findings from drug abuse–related visits to emergency departments show an increase from 700,000 events in 1992 to 900,000 events in 2000 (32). Perhaps of greatest relevance to anesthesiologists is the fact that some of this increase in substance abuse stems from an increase in prescription drug abuse, much of this being abuse of prescription analgesics (opioids). For example, the numbers of new abusers of prescription opioids increased from <500 in 1967 to >2,500 in the year 2000 (33,34). A large portion of this increase can be accounted for by criminal diversion from pharmacies (35) or from patients, with only a small proportion from opioid abuse or dependence in opioid-treated pain patients de novo. As opioids have been prescribed in greater and greater quantities because of their popularity for treatment of chronic pain, opioid addicts have chosen prescription opioids such as OxyContin over heroin. In the year 2002, prescription opioids were second only to marijuana in illicit drug dependence and abuse by individuals aged 12 or over (marijuana 4.23, pain relievers 1.51, cocaine 1.49, and heroin 0.21 million) (36). Anesthesiologists will encounter substance use, abuse, and dependence in their patients in growing numbers, often involving opioids, which interfere profoundly with pain and stress management both intra- and postoperatively.

[1] The term *substance abuse* will be retained here since it is widely understood to mean aberrant use of illicit substances and/or controlled substances. Strictly, though, *substance abuse* has narrow criteria by the *Diagnostic and Statistical Manual of Mental Disorders,* 4th ed. (DSM-IV) classification (31), and by this classification is a lesser form of *substance dependence*, the main difference being that *abuse* is erratic and not associated with tolerance and dependence. *Substance use disorder* is the blanket term used in the DSM-IV for *substance abuse* and *substance dependence*.

Preoperative Preparation

Substance abuse should not be considered in isolation since many substance abusers will have a psychiatric history, and others will be receiving treatment for chronic pain. Anesthetic issues depend on the medical condition of these patients as well as possible drug interactions, tolerance to anesthetics and opioid analgesics, and the likelihood of a withdrawal syndrome. Whether the drug abuse is remote or current and whether there is polysubstance abuse must be determined.

Many of the disease sequelae of substance abuse follow from lifestyle issues such as nutrition, hygiene, sexual behavior, and use of dirty needles. For example, injected drugs and high-risk sexual behaviors present a high risk of blood-borne diseases such as HIV/AIDS and hepatitis C (37). Osteomyelitis and bacterial endocarditis are other possible consequences of hematogenous spread of bacteria from dirty needles. Drug-abusing pregnant women present particular challenges: Drug use can mimic abnormal pregnancy (e.g., cocaine use can mimic preeclampsia). Many substance abusers are also smokers with smoking-related diseases. A thorough review of the systems and extensive laboratory evaluation is always warranted in current or past drug abusers to identify or exclude related medical conditions.

The history must also include as accurate an assessment as possible of current and past drug use. Substance abusers are usually honest about the fact that they have used illicit substances, since they recognize that the anesthesiologist wants to avoid potentially dangerous interactions. Abusers will, however, often tell half-truths, especially with regard to dosage. Half-truths are particularly told by alcoholics who frequently underestimate their real usage even in their own minds.

Drug Considerations

Table 12.4 summarizes some of the concerns in treating patients with a history of substance abuse and illicit drug use.

Alcohol

- Alcohol abuse appears to be widespread throughout most cultures worldwide and affects at least 10 million to 15 million Americans (38).
- It may be difficult to diagnose alcohol abuse during a preoperative evaluation. Although alcoholic patients usually admit to drinking daily, they may not admit that they have a problem, and evidence of it sometimes comes instead from medical problems linked to alcoholism.
- Medical complications of excessive alcohol intake involve every organ system.
- Central nervous system effects include cerebral atrophy and cerebellar degeneration with associated amnestic blackouts and tremor.
- The cardiovascular system may show signs of a dilated cardiomyopathy, dysrhythmias, peripheral vascular insufficiency, and hypertension.
- Gastritis, esophagitis, esophageal varices, gastric ulcers, pancreatitis, hepatitis, and hepatic cirrhosis are common among chronic alcohol abusers.

Table 12.4. Common interactions and anesthetic considerations for abused substances

Drug	Interactions	Recommendations
Alcohol	*Acute intoxication*	
	Effects of opioids and hypnotics enhanced. Caution with dosage. Will delay gastric emptying	Measure serum alcohol level. Aspiration precautions needed
	Chronic use	
	Full workup needed to identify alcohol-related disease. Hepatic enzyme induction results in tolerance to effects of opioids and hypnotics. May need increased anesthetic doses	Watch for delirium tremens (withdrawal from heavy drinking), which is a medical emergency. Benzodiazepines mainstay of symptomatic treatment
Marijuana	Easy to detect because of slow elimination (up to 1 week). Tachycardia associated with chronic or moderate use. Hypotension and bradycardia associated with toxicity. Chronic smoking produces lung disease	Advise discontinuation of use before surgery, preferably for at least 1 week
Cocaine	Interferes with presynaptic uptake of sympathomimetic neurotransmitters producing excitatory state. Rapid metabolism, but inactive metabolites can be detected late. Toxicity (overdose) can result in cardiac death	General anesthesia is generally safe in nontoxic cocaine users. During active use, general anesthesia preferred to regional because of unpredictable responses to pressors (when needed) and because agitation may be difficult to control in awake intoxicated patients
		(Continued)

Table 12.4. *Continued*

Drug	Interactions	Recommendations
Heroin	Opioid tolerance	For current users, be prepared for opioid refractoriness due to opioid tolerance. Watch for opioid withdrawal syndrome
Hallucinogens and "club drugs"	During use, high risk of autonomic dysregulation and coronary or cerebral vascular spasm. Overdose can kill through respiratory depression, seizures, and coma. May be exaggerated obtundation with opioids. Cardiomyopathy may develop in repeat users	During intoxication, exaggerated responses to pressors possible. Interference with cholinesterase activity may alter responses to muscle relaxants
Lysergic acid diethylamide (LSD)		
3,4-methylenedioxy-methamphetamine (MDMA); "ecstasy"	Water hunger can lead to cerebral/pulmonary edema	Can be associated with overheating, in which case inhalation agents and succinylcholine should be avoided
γ-Hydroxybutyrate (GHB); "liquid ecstasy"	Difficult to detect because rapidly eliminated	
Solvents	Toxicity produces possible cardiac dysrhythmias, pulmonary/hepatic toxicity, cerebral/pulmonary edema. Chronic use can cause central nervous system degeneration or diffuse brain atrophy	During acute intoxication, general endotracheal anesthesia is often the best option because of respiratory compromise, nausea, and vomiting

- Nutritional and metabolic effects include Wernicke-Korsakoff syndrome, hypoalbuminemia, hypomagnesemia, pellagra, and beriberi (38).
- The majority of alcoholics are heavy smokers.
- Currently, no laboratory test exists that is specific for alcohol abuse or dependence, but elevated liver enzymes and mean corpuscular volume of red blood cell ≥94 fL can be associated with chronic alcohol ingestion.
- Preoperatively, alcoholic patients need an ECG and chest radiograph. Prothrombin time, hematocrit, albumin, glucose, bilirubin, serum alanine aminotransferase, aspartate aminotransferase, and alkaline phosphatase levels should be determined. Acutely intoxicated patients need a serum alcohol level determination.
- For current heavy drinkers, one should anticipate and treat withdrawal or delirium tremens. Delirium tremens is a medical emergency that occurs in 5% of patients who experience alcohol withdrawal symptoms. It is manifested as altered consciousness, confusion, hallucinations (usually visual and tactile), hypertension, hyperthermia, and grand mal seizures. It is potentially fatal. Benzodiazepines are the primary intervention for treating delirium tremens. Once symptoms are under control, benzodiazepine dosage should be gradually tapered. The use of beta blockers is controversial because these drugs can mask symptoms of inadequate benzodiazepine coverage.
- Acutely intoxicated patients have delayed gastric emptying and should be treated with histamine-2 receptor blockers, sodium citrate, and metoclopramide. They also have a decreased requirement for anesthesia and, because of alcohol-induced vasodilation, are prone to hypotension.
- Patients being treated with disulfiram may require less anesthetic medication because of disulfiram sedation. Disulfiram users are acutely sensitive (experiencing flushing, nausea, and tachycardia) to small amounts of alcohol (skin preparations, medications).

Marijuana

- Marijuana, also known as pot, hash, grass, or weed, is one of the most popular recreational drugs. It is obtained from the plant *Cannabis sativa,* which contains various cannabinoids, including the active ingredient delta-9-tetrahydrocannabinol and the tobacco carcinogen benzopyrene.
- Acute toxicity and major interactions with anesthesia are rare, but chronic use of this drug can affect numerous body systems including the autonomic nervous system (increased sympathetic tone with tachycardia and increased cardiac output), the cardiovascular system (increase in dysrhythmias and ST-segment and T-wave abnormalities), and the pulmonary system (smoking-related lung disease). Chronic marijuana use can also reduce uteroplacental perfusion and restrict fetal intrauterine growth.
- Marijuana can increase the sedative effects of other sedative drugs and hypnotics (37).

- Acute intoxication can be associated with myocardial depression and bradycardia or tachycardia, possibly exacerbating similar effects from anesthetic agents.
- Marijuana has a very long half-life and prolonged effects on cognitive function. It is detectable in urine for up to 1 week after use. Marijuana users should be advised to discontinue use for at least 1 week before surgery to avoid interactions with anesthetics.

Cocaine

- Cocaine is extracted from the leaves of *Erythroxylum coca,* a South American plant. The commercially available hydrochloride form can be converted back to its alkalinized form by adding baking soda or ammonia and water, and heating. The alkalinized form is known as "crack" or "rock" and is smoked, injected, snorted, or swallowed.
- Cocaine has a short half-life (0.5 to 1.5 hours) and is metabolized by plasma and liver cholinesterases. A small amount is excreted unchanged in the urine and is detectable in urine for up to 6 hours. Metabolites can be detected in the urine for 3 to 5 days.
- Cocaine inhibits the uptake of sympathomimetic neurotransmitters including norepinephrine, serotonin, and dopamine. It produces a powerful euphoria by stimulation of the sympathoadrenal axis and prolongation of dopaminergic activity in the limbic system and adrenal cortex.
- At high doses, cocaine can depress ventricular function and slow electrical conduction of the heart.
- Pathologic changes such as contraction-band necrosis and ventricular hypertrophy can contribute to the potentially lethal effects of cocaine associated with continued use (39).
- Other adverse effects include infection or perforation of the nasal septum, anxiety, restlessness, irritability, confusion, seizures, tachycardia, vasoconstriction, hypertension, angina, and myocardial infarction (37).
- It seems that general anesthesia is safe in nontoxic users (i.e., those with detectable metabolites but no immediate use, or with a remote usage history) (40), although it has also been argued that some of the cardiac effects of chronic cocaine abuse can persist even years after discontinuing use (37).
- Any number of abnormal potentially serious cardiac events can occur during anesthesia in patients who are acutely intoxicated with cocaine. β- and α-adrenergic blockers are often needed to reverse cocaine's sympathomimetic effects on the heart and vasculature, and sympathomimetic and dysrhythmogenic agents such as ketamine should be avoided.
- It is reasonable to recommend a cocaine-free interval of 1 week before surgery.

Heroin

- Heroin (diamorphine) is rapidly converted to morphine in plasma. Clinically, then, this drug behaves like other standard μ-opioid receptor agonists described in the Chronic Pain section. The reader should refer to this section for a full description of the anesthetic considerations for patients who use opioids, which will be similar to those for chronic heroin (diamorphine) abuse.

- One major difference in the anesthetic management of heroin abusers compared with other chronic opioid users is that heroin is not permitted for medical use in the United States (unlike in many other countries). Therefore, it is not possible to treat pain or withdrawal using diamorphine. A different opioid must be substituted to treat pain and withdrawal (should this arise), and very high doses may be needed for patients who have developed opioid tolerance through heroin abuse.
- The principle of using opioid-sparing analgesic strategies whenever possible applies equally to opioid-tolerant heroin abusers and chronic pain patients using opioids.
- Some heroin abusers and recovered abusers are treated with methadone or buprenorphine, and the anesthetic considerations for patients who take these drugs are also described under Chronic Pain.
- General medical considerations for heroin abusers are the same as those for other drugs of abuse.

Other Anesthetic Implications

A few other substances of abuse will be encountered by the anesthesiologist rarely. The hallucinogens, sometimes called "club" or "rave" drugs, are party drugs used mainly by young people. The effects of acute ingestion last about 12 hours. Preanesthetic considerations arise mainly in the case of emergency surgery. An exact account of drug use should be elicited so that appropriate measures can be taken to counter the adverse effects of these drugs, effects being different for each drug (see Table 12.4) (41). When there is a suggestion of solvent abuse, preoperative evaluation includes a comprehensive workup and a full panel of laboratory tests (see Table 12.4) (41).

It cannot be overemphasized that substance abusers may have complex medical and psychiatric comorbidities requiring careful workup before surgery. Substance abuse also has an association with psychiatric disease and chronic pain. The association between chronic pain and substance abuse is especially strong for opioid-treated chronic pain patients. It is not always clear whether psychiatric comorbidity and substance abuse precede or follow chronic pain, but regardless of the exact progression, the end result is that patients can be difficult to manage during and after surgery because their chronic drug use alters responses to anesthetic drugs, especially to opioids. All these factors must be considered during the preoperative workup, and in particular, the drug history must be carefully documented.

REFERENCES

1. Murray DJL, Lopez AD. Alternating visions of the future: projecting mortality and disability, 1990-2020. In: Murray DJL, Lopex AD, eds. *The Global Burden of Disease*. Cambridge, MA: Harvard University Press; 1996.
2. Depression Guideline Panel. Depression in primary care. Clinical Practice Guideline, no 5. Vol. 1: Detection and Diagnosis. Agency for Health Care Policy and Research publication #93-0550. Rockville, MD: U.S. Department of Health and Human Services.
3. Rapaport MJ, Judd LL, Schettler PJ, et al. A descriptive analysis of minor depression. *Am J Psychiatry*. 2002;159:637–643.

4. Fishbain D, Cutler R, Rosomoff H, et al. Chronic pain-associated depression: antecedent or consequence of chronic pain? A review. *Clin J Pain*. 1997;113:116–137.

5. Klafta JM, Roizen MF. Current understanding of patients' attitudes toward and preparation for anesthesia: a review. *Anesth Analg*. 1996;83:1314–1321.

6. Pinals DA, Breier A. Schizophrenia. In: Tasman A, Kay J, Lieberman JA, eds. *Psychiatry*. Philadelphia: WB Saunders; 1997: 927–965.

7. Dalack GW, Healy DJ, Meador-Woodruff JH. Nicotine dependence in schizophrenia: clinical phenomena and laboratory findings. *Am J Psychiatry*. 1998;155:1490–1501.

8. Gruenberg AM, Goldstein RD. Depressive disorders. In: Tasman A, Kay J, Lieberman JA, eds. *Psychiatry*. Philadelphia: WB Saunders; 1997: 990–1019.

9. Kellar MB, Boland RJ. Antidepressants. In: Tasman A, Kay J, Lieberman JA, eds. *Psychiatry*. Philadelphia: WB Saunders; 1997: 1606–1639.

10. *Physicians Desk Reference*. 61st ed. Thomson PDR; Montvale, New Jersey; 2007. Available at: www.PDR.net.

11. Arnold LM, Rosen A, Pritchett YL, et al. A randomized, double-blind, placebo-controlled trial of duloxetine in the treatment of women with fibromyalgia with or without major depressive disorder. *Pain*. 2005;119:5–15.

12. Wernicke JF, Pritchett YL, D'Souza DN, et al. A randomized controlled trial of duloxetine in diabetic peripheral neuropathic pain. *Neurology*. 2006;67:1411–1420.

13. Tarres AA. Severe hypotension following spinal anesthesia in a patient treatment with risperidone. *Can J Anesth*. 2005;52:334–335.

14. Buckley NA, Sanders P. Cardiovascular adverse effects of antipsychotic drugs. *Drug Saf*. 2000;23:215–228.

15. Williams JH, Hepner DL. Risperidone and exaggerated hypotension during a spinal anesthetic. *Anesth Analg*. 2004;98:240–241.

16. Post RM, Denicoff KD, Frye MA. A history of the use of anticonvulsants as mood stabilizers in the last two decades of the 20th century. *Neuropsychobiology*. 1998;38:152–166.

17. Fishbain D, Goldberg M, Meagher B, et al. Male and female chronic pain patients categorized by DSM-III psychiatric diagnostic criteria. *Pain*. 1986;26:181–197.

18. Ballantyne J, Mao J. Opioid therapy for chronic pain. *N Engl J Med*. 2003;349:1943–1953.

19. Mao J. Opioid-induced abnormal pain sensitivity: implications in clinical opioid therapy. *Pain*. 2002;100:213–217.

20. Mitra S, Sinatra R. Perioperative management of acute pain in the opioid-dependent patient. *Anesthesiology*. 2004;101:212–227.

21. Angst MS, Clark JD. Opioid-induced hyperalgesia: a qualitative systematic review. *Anesthesiology*. 2006;104:570–587.

22. Wilder-Smith O, Arendt-Nielsen L. Postoperative hyperalgesia: its clinical importance and relevance. *Anesthesiology*. 2006;104: 601–607.

23. Fishman SM, Wilsey B, Mahajan G, et al. Methadone reincarnated: novel clinical applications with related concerns. *Pain Med*. 2002;3:339–348.

24. Porter J, Jick H. Addiction rare in patients treated with narcotics (letter). *N Engl J Med*. 1980;302:123.
25. Fiellin DA, O'Connor PG. Office-based treatment of opioid-dependent patients. *N Engl J Med*. 2002;347:817–823.
26. Krantz M, Mehler P. Treating opioid dependence. Growing implications for primary care. *Arch Intern Med*. 2004;164:277–288.
27. Mercadante S, Villari P, Ferrera P, et al. Safety and effectiveness of intravenous morphine for episodic breakthrough pain in patients receiving transdermal buprenorphine. *J Pain Symptom Manage*. 2006;32:175–179.
28. Alford DP, Compton P, Samet JH. Acute pain management for patients receiving maintenance methadone or buprenorphine therapy. *Ann Intern Med*. 2006;144:127–134.
29. Weir M, Sperling R, Reicin A. Selective COX-2 inhibition and cardiovascular effects: a review of the rofecoxib development program. *Am Heart J*. 2003;146:591–604.
30. FitzGerald GA. Coxibs and cardiovascular disease. *N Engl J Med*. 2004;351:1709–1711.
31. American Psychiatric Association. *Diagnostic and Statistical Manual of Mental Disorders*. 4th ed. Washington, DC: American Psychiatric Association; 1994.
32. Year-end 2000 emergency department data from the Drug Abuse Warning Network. DAWN series D-18. DHHS publication no. (SMA) 01-3532. Rockville, MD: Substance Abuse and Mental Health Services Administration; 2001. Available at http://www.samhsa.gov/oas/dawn/200yrend.pdf.
33. Office of Applied Studies. National Survey on Drug Use and Health. Substance Abuse and Mental Services Administration (SAMHSA); Rockville, Maryland, 2004. Available at: http://oas.samhsa.gov/NHSDA/2k3NSDUH/2keresults.htm.
34. National Institute of Drug Abuse (NIDA). Prescription pain and other medications, 2006. Available at: http://nida.nih.gov/Infofacts/PainMed.html. Accessed October 12, 2006.
35. Joranson DE, Gilson AM. Wanted: a public health approach to prescription opioid abuse and diversion. *Pharmacoepidemiol Drug Saf*. 2006;15:632–634.
36. Department of Health and Human Services, Substance Abuse and Mental Health Services Administration. National Household Survey on Drug Abuse Main Findings. Series H-11. Washington, DC: U.S. Department of Health and Human Services; 1998.
37. Hernandez M, Birnbach DJ, Van Zundert AAJ. Anesthetic management of the illicit-substance-using patient. *Curr Opin Anaesthesiol*. 2005;18:315–324.
38. O'Connor P, Schottenfeld R. Patients with alcohol problems. *N Engl J Med*. 1998;338:592–601.
39. Schindler CW. Cocaine and cardiovascular toxicity. *Addict Biol*. 1996;1:31–47.
40. Hill GE, Ogunnaike BO, Johnson ER. General anaesthesia for the cocaine abusing patient. Is it safe? *Br J Anaesth*. 2006;97:654–657.
41. Passik SD, Kirsh KL, Whitcomb L, et al. A new tool to assess and document pain outcomes in chronic pain patients receiving opioid therapy. *Clin Ther*. 2004;26:552–561.

Miscellaneous Issues

James B. Mayfield and Benjamin E. McCurdy

This chapter addresses the preoperative assessment of patients with various medical conditions and issues. The topics covered are assessment of patients with latex allergy; patients who are breastfeeding; patients who refuse blood transfusion; and geriatric patients, including those presenting for cataract surgery. In addition, patients with active do-not-resuscitate orders, extreme obesity, sleep apnea syndrome, cancer, and human immunodeficiency virus are discussed.

PATIENTS WITH LATEX ALLERGY

First described in the American literature in 1933, latex-induced allergic reactions saw a marked increase in the late 1980s with the adoption of universal precautions by the Centers for Disease Control and Prevention (CDC). The desired properties of natural rubber latex (deformability, elasticity, tactile sensitivity, high tensile strength, and excellent barrier qualities), a mixture of polyisoprene, lipids, phospholipids, and proteins, are accentuated by the addition of various chemicals, accelerators, and vulcanizing compounds during the manufacturing process. The protein content triggers most generalized allergic reactions.

There are three distinct reactions in latex-sensitive patients: Irritant contact dermatitis, type IV delayed hypersensitivity, and type I immediate hypersensitivity (1,2). Irritant contact dermatitis, which is the most frequently observed reaction, is not immune mediated. It is caused by the drying action of cornstarch and other chemicals in gloves. Type IV delayed hypersensitivity is an immune-mediated allergic response to chemical additives (accelerators). Skin reactions appear 6 to 72 hours after initial contact and may develop into oozing skin blisters. Type IV may progress to a type I reaction. In type I immediate hypersensitivity the immune-mediated (IgE) response begins within minutes of exposure. Symptoms range from mild (skin redness and hives) to life threatening (bronchospasm and cardiovascular collapse).

There are several populations at risk for latex allergy. Among them are patients with a history of multiple surgical procedures (congenital genitourinary tract anomalies and spina bifida); those exposed at work (health care and rubber industry workers, hairdressers); those with a history of atopy, hay fever, rhinitis, asthma, or eczema; those with food allergy to tropical fruits (kiwi, banana, avocado), chestnuts, or stone fruits; and those with severe hand dermatitis who wear latex gloves. Figure 13.1 gives a list of questions for evaluation of possible latex allergy.

Several methods are used to obtain an accurate diagnosis. If careful medical history and physical examination determine that the patient is at risk, patch testing, the definitive test for

1. Sex: . . . . ☐ Male . . . . ☐ Female

2. Race: . . . . ☐ Caucasian . . ☐ Black
   ☐ Hispanic . . . . ☐ Other

3. Have you ever been told by a doctor
   that you are allergic to latex? . . . . ☐ yes . . . . ☐ no

4. How many surgeries have you had in the past? . . . . _____

5. Do you suffer from:
   Seasonal hay fever? . . . . ☐ yes . . . . ☐ no
   Asthma? . . . . ☐ yes . . . . ☐ no
   Eczema? . . . . ☐ yes . . . . ☐ no
   Autoimmune disease? . . . . ☐ yes . . . . ☐ no

6. Do you have on-the-job exposure to latex? . . . . ☐ yes . . . . ☐ no

7. Were you born with problems involving your spinal cord? . . . . ☐ yes . . . . ☐ no

8. Do you catheterize yourself to urinate? . . . . ☐ yes . . . . ☐ no

9. Do you have any food allergies? . . . . ☐ yes . . . . ☐ no

10. Are you allergic to bananas? . . . . ☐ yes . . . . ☐ no
    Kiwi fruit? . . . . ☐ yes . . . . ☐ no
    Avocados? . . . . ☐ yes . . . . ☐ no
    Guacamole? . . . . ☐ yes . . . . ☐ no
    Chestnuts? . . . . ☐ yes . . . . ☐ no

11. Are you allergic to latex or products containing rubber? . . . . . ☐ yes . . . . ☐ no
    If yes, are the symptoms a rash? . . . . ☐ yes . . . . ☐ no
    Hives? . . . . ☐ yes . . . . ☐ no
    Itching? . . . . ☐ yes . . . . ☐ no
    Wheezing? . . . . ☐ yes . . . . ☐ no
    Difficulty breathing? . . . . ☐ yes . . . . ☐ no
    Watery eyes? . . . . ☐ yes . . . . ☐ no
    Anaphylaxis? . . . . ☐ yes . . . . ☐ no

12. Do you have allergic symptoms while:
    Blowing up balloons? . . . . ☐ yes . . . . ☐ no
    During dental examinations? . . . . ☐ yes . . . . ☐ no
    On contact with diaphragms/condoms? . . . . ☐ yes . . . . ☐ no
    During vaginal or rectal exams? . . . . ☐ yes . . . . ☐ no
    While wearing rubber gloves? . . . . ☐ yes . . . . ☐ no

(Prepared by the ASA Task Force on Latex Sensitivity, 1999.)

Figure 13.1. Screening questionnaire for latex sensitivity. From ASA Committee on Occupational Health of Operating Room Personnel. Task Force on Latex Sensitivity. Natural Rubber Latex Allergy: Considerations for Anesthesiologists. Park Ridge. IL: American Society of Anesthesiologists; 2005.

diagnosis of type IV delayed hypersensitivity, can be performed. A standardized patch test screen or a fragment of the offending latex is used. The radioallergosorbent test (RAST) or the enzyme allergosorbent test (EAST) can be used to run one of the four serum tests approved by the Federal Drug Administration (FDA) for latex-specific IgE responses: Ala-STAT, Immunolite, Pharmacia coated allergen particle test (CAP), or HY-TEC. A skin-prick test using antigens extracted from various glove products is considered the gold standard for diagnosis of type I hypersensitivity.

For an elective surgery, consultation with an allergist for a definitive diagnosis (using the aforementioned tests) should be considered. All patients with a high likelihood or definite latex allergy should be given a latex-free perioperative course. Careful coordination among anesthesia, surgical, and nursing teams is necessary to identify such patients and avoid patient contact with the many latex products present in an operating room (OR). A warning sign should be placed on the patient's chart, bed, and both inside and outside the OR.

MOTHERS WHO ARE BREASTFEEDING

Little reliable information is available on the effects on the babies and infants of women who are administered drugs while breastfeeding. The effects on infants of drugs ingested from breast milk depend on the drug itself, the variability of the composition of human milk, and infant factors. Wilson (3) developed a three-compartment model of the way drugs move from blood to breast milk: The central compartment receives the drug, the second compartment is composed of interstitial and intracellular water, and the third compartment contains breast milk. A drug moves from each compartment in both directions at variable rates. The elimination rate is constant from the central compartment. An infant-modulated rate is constant for removal of drug from breast milk. The rate constants vary for different drugs, depending on other factors. The unbound form of a drug crosses freely into the mammary cells, so medications with less protein binding enter milk in greater amounts (4). Drug factors that determine the ease with which a drug crosses into the mammary cells include fat solubility, degree of ionization, and molecular weight. Highly fat-soluble drugs readily cross the lipid boundary of the mammary cell membrane. Because milk contains a lipid phase that is lacking in plasma, highly lipid-soluble drugs can partition into milk fat and achieve higher concentrations in milk than in plasma. Nonionized drugs are excreted in the milk more readily than are ionized ones. Given the pH difference between plasma (pH 7.4) and milk (pH 6.8 to 7.3, average 7.0), weakly acidic drugs ionize more, and weak bases less, in plasma than in milk. Under normal pH conditions, the concentration of weak acids is lower in milk than in plasma, although the free concentration of basic drugs in milk may exceed concentration in plasma. Drugs with molecular weights <500 daltons are more likely to transfer into human milk. Most clinically useful drugs range in weight between 200 and 500 daltons (4).

The breast also affects the movement of drugs from blood to breast milk. Blood flow into the mammary glands is affected by their metabolic activity and release of lactogenic hormones in response to suckling. The pores between mammary cells, which are completely open at delivery and gradually tighten in the following days, are responsible for the bulk of fluid changes across the epithelium.

A drug excreted with breast milk must be absorbed by the infant's gastrointestinal (GI) tract. Absorption varies with transit time across the GI tract, and transit time varies with age, drug ionization, and lipid solubility. The younger the infant and the younger the gestational age are, the more likely that a drug will be poorly tolerated because the detoxification pathways in the infant liver are immature. At birth, renal function is not fully developed, but the kidney matures rapidly so that glomerular filtration approaches adult levels in 2 months. With decreased elimination rates drugs present in only small quantities in breast milk may accumulate significantly in plasma.

Lastly, drug accumulation in milk is affected by the pH and composition of milk, which vary over time. In the first few days after delivery colostrum has a pH of 7.45 and contains no fat. Several days later and up until the third month milk has a pH of 7.0 and contains fat. After the third month, pH, lactose concentration, and fat increase so that the concentration of lipophilic drugs can increase (5). The American Academy of Pediatrics Committee on Drugs has categorized medications for breastfeeding mothers according to their safety (Table 13.1) (6).

Preoperative Assessment

Breastfeeding mothers are identified so that general or regional anesthetic regimens can be selected with little or no risk to the suckling infant. In elective cases, mothers are advised to pump milk preoperatively. This milk is used in the first 24 hours after surgery to substitute for suckling. Breast milk is pumped and discarded in the immediate postoperative period. Normal breastfeeding resumes 24 hours after surgery, when anesthetics have dropped to safe levels. In emergent cases, when prepumping of milk is not an option, anesthetic agents are selected with care and mothers are advised to discard their breast milk in the 24 hours after surgery. Nonsteroidal anti-inflammatory drugs (NSAIDs), morphine, codeine, hydrocodone, and fentanyl are considered safe in low to moderate maternal doses for postoperative pain (4).

PATIENTS WHO REFUSE BLOOD TRANSFUSION

In 1945, the leadership of the Jehovah's Witnesses outlawed the transfusion of blood or blood products, basing their decision on a strict, literal interpretation of certain passages in the Bible (Genesis 9:3–4, Leviticus 17:14, Acts 15: 28–29) (7) that they believed threatened the loss of eternal life if the commandments on blood were not followed. Many Jehovah's Witnesses are convinced that they forfeit a chance for eternal life and risk excommunication from their church and religious community if they receive blood. Although it is generally assumed that all patients who refuse blood transfusions are Jehovah's Witnesses who do so on the

Table 13.1. Medication effects on nursing infants

Drugs for which the effect on nursing infants is unknown but may be of concern[a]

Drug	Reported or Possible Effect
Antianxiety	
Alprazolam	None
Diazepam	None
Lorazepam	None
Midazolam	—
Perphenazine	None
Prazepam[b]	None
Quazepam	None
Temazepam	—
Antidepressants	
Amitriptyline	None
Amoxapine	None
Bupropion	None
Clomipramine	None
Desipramine	None
Dothiepin	None
Doxepin	None
Fluoxetine	Colic, irritability, feeding and sleep disorders, slow weight gain
Fluvoxamine	—
Imipramine	None
Nortriptyline	None
Paroxetine	None
Sertraline[b]	None
Trazodone	None
Antipsychotic	
Chlorpromazine	Galactorrhea in mother; drowsiness and lethargy in infant; decline in developmental scores
Chlorprothixene	None
Clozapine[b]	None
Haloperidol	Decline in developmental scores
Mesoridazine	None
Trifluoperazine	None
Others	
Amiodarone	Possible hypothyroidism
Chloramphenicol	Possible idiosyncratic bone marrow suppression
Clofazimine	Potential for transfer of high percentage of maternal dose; possible increase in skin pigmentation
Lamotrigine	Potential therapeutic serum concentrations in infant

(Continued)

Table 13.1. *(Continued)*

Drug	Reported or Possible Effect
Metoclopramide[b]	None described; dopaminergic blocking agent
Metronidazole	In vitro mutagen; may discontinue breastfeeding for 12–24 hours to allow excretion of dose when single-dose therapy given to mother
Tinidazole	See metronidazole

Drugs that have been associated with significant effects on some nursing infants and should be given to nursing mothers with caution[c]

Drug	Reported Effect
Acebutolol	Hypotension; bradycardia; tachypnea
5-Aminosalicylic acid	Diarrhea (one case)
Atenolol	Cyanosis; bradycardia
Bromocriptine	Suppresses lactation; may be hazardous to the mother
Aspirin (salicylates)	Metabolic acidosis (one case)
Clemastine	Drowsiness, irritability, refusal to feed, high-pitched cry, neck stiffness (one case)
Ergotamine	Vomiting, diarrhea, convulsions (doses used in migraine medications)
Lithium	One-third to one-half therapeutic blood concentration in infants
Phenindione	Anticoagulant: Increased prothrombin and partial thromboplastin time in one infant; not used in United States
Phenobarbital	Sedation; infantile spasms after weaning from milk containing phenobarbital, methemoglobinemia (one case)
Primidone	Sedation, feeding problems
Sulfasalazine (salicylazosulfapyridine)	Bloody diarrhea (one case)

Maternal medication usually compatible with breastfeeding[d]

Drug	Reported Sign or Symptom in Infant or Effect on Lactation
Acetaminophen	None
Acetazolamide	None
Acitretin	—
Acyclovir[e]	None
Alcohol (ethanol)	With large amounts, drowsiness, diaphoresis, deep sleep, weakness, decrease in linear growth, abnormal weight gain; maternal ingestion of 1 g/kg daily decreases milk ejection reflex

(Continued)

Table 13.1. *(Continued)*

Drug	Reported Sign or Symptom in Infant or Effect on Lactation
Allopurinol	—
Amoxicillin	None
Antimony	—
Atropine	None
Azapropazone (apazone)	—
Aztreonam	None
B_1 (thiamin)	None
B_6 (pyridoxine)	None
B_{12}	None
Baclofen	None
Barbiturate	See Table 13.5
Bendroflumethiazide	Suppresses lactation
Bishydroxycoumarin (dicumarol)	None
Bromide	Rash, weakness, absence of cry with maternal intake of 5.4 g/day
Butorphanol	None
Caffeine	Irritability, poor sleeping pattern, excreted slowly; no effect with moderate intake of caffeinated beverages (two to three cups per day)
Captopril	None
Carbamazepine	None
Carbetocin	None
Carbimazole	Goiter
Cascara	None
Cefadroxil	None
Cefazolin	None
Cefotaxime	None
Cefoxitin	None

Drug	Reported or Possible Effect
Cefprozil	—
Ceftazidime	None
Ceftriaxone	None
Chloral hydrate	Sleepiness
Chloroform	None
Chloroquine	None
Chlorothiazide	None
Chlorthalidone	Excreted slowly
Cimetidine[e]	None
Ciprofloxacin	None
Cisapride	None
Cisplatin	Not found in milk
Clindamycin	None
Clogestone	None
Codeine	None

(Continued)

Table 13.1. *(Continued)*

Drug	Reported or Possible Effect
Colchicine	—
Contraceptive pill with estrogen/progesterone	Rare breast enlargement; decrease in milk production and protein content (not confirmed in several studies)
Cycloserine	None
D (vitamin)	None; follow up infant's serum calcium level if mother receives pharmacologic doses
Danthron	Increased bowel activity
Dapsone	None; sulfonamide detected in infant's urine
Dexbrompheniramine maleate with *d*-isoephedrine	Crying, poor sleeping patterns, irritability
Diatrizoate	None
Digoxin	None
Diltiazem	None
Dipyrone	None
Disopyramide	None
Domperidone	None
Dyphylline[e]	None
Enalapril	—
Erythromycin[e]	None
Estradiol	Withdrawal, vaginal bleeding
Ethambutol	None
Ethanol (cf. alcohol)	—
Ethosuximide	None, drug appears in infant serum
Fentanyl	—
Fexofenadine	None
Flecainide	—
Fleroxacin	One 400-mg dose given to nursing mothers; infants not given breast milk for 48 hours
Fluconazole	None
Flufenamic acid	None
Fluorescein	—
Folic acid	None
Gadopentetic (gadolinium)	None
Gentamicin	None
Gold salts	None
Halothane	None
Hydralazine	None
Hydrochlorothiazide	—
Hydroxychloroquine[e]	None
Ibuprofen	None
Indomethacin	Seizure (one case)
Iodides	May affect thyroid activity; see iodine
Iodine	Goiter

(Continued)

Table 13.1. *(Continued)*

Drug	Reported or Possible Effect
Iodine (povidone-iodine, e.g., in a vaginal douche)	Elevated iodine levels in breast milk, odor of iodine on infant's skin
Iohexol	None
Iopanoic acid	None
Isoniazid	None; acetyl (hepatotoxic) metabolite secreted but no hepatotoxicity reported in infants
Interferon-α	—
Ivermectin	None
K_1 (vitamin)	None
Kanamycin	None
Ketoconazole	None
Ketorolac	—
Labetalol	None
Levonorgestrel	—
Levothyroxine	None
Lidocaine	None
Loperamide	—
Loratadine	None
Magnesium sulfate	None
Medroxyprogesterone	None
Mefenamic acid	None
Meperidine	None
Methadone	None
Methimazole (active metabolite of carbimazole)	None
Methohexital	None
Methyldopa	None
Methyprylon	Drowsiness
Metoprolol[e]	None
Metrizamide	None
Metrizoate	None
Mexiletine	None
Minoxidil	None
Morphine	None; infant may have measurable blood concentration
Moxalactam	None
Nadolol[e]	None
Nalidixic acid	Hemolysis in infant with glucose-6-phosphate dehydrogenase (G6PD) deficiency
Naproxen	—
Nefopam	None
Nifedipine	—
Nitrofurantoin	Hemolysis in infant with G6PD deficiency
Norethynodrel	None
Norsteroids	None

(Continued)

Table 13.1. *(Continued)*

Drug	Reported or Possible Effect
Noscapine	None
Ofloxacin	None
Oxprenolol	None
Phenylbutazone	None
Phenytoin	Methemoglobinemia (one case)
Piroxicam	None
Prednisolone	None
Prednisone	None
Procainamide	None
Progesterone	None
Propoxyphene	None
Propranolol	None
Propylthiouracil	None
Pseudoephedrine[e]	None
Pyridostigmine	None
Pyrimethamine	None
Quinidine	None
Quinine	None
Riboflavin	None
Rifampin	None
Scopolamine	—
Secobarbital	None
Senna	None
Sotalol	—
Spironolactone	None
Streptomycin	None
Sulbactam	None
Sulfapyridine	Caution in infant with jaundice or G6PD deficiency and ill, stressed, or premature infant; appears in infant's milk
Sulfisoxazole	Caution in infant with jaundice or G6PD deficiency and ill, stressed, or premature infant; appears in infant's milk
Sumatriptan	None
Suprofen	None
Terbutaline	None
Terfenadine	None
Tetracycline	None; negligible absorption by infant
Theophylline	Irritability
Thiopental	None
Thiouracil	None mentioned; drug not used in United States
Ticarcillin	None
Timolol	None
Tolbutamide	Possible jaundice
Tolmetin	None
Trimethoprim/ sulfamethoxazole	None

(Continued)

Table 13.1. *(Continued)*

Drug	Reported or Possible Effect
Triprolidine	None
Valproic acid	None
Verapamil	None
Warfarin	None
Zolpidem	None

[a]Psychotropic drugs, the compounds listed under antianxiety, antidepressant, and antipsychotic categories, are of special concern when given to nursing mothers for long periods. Although there are very few case reports of adverse effects in breastfeeding infants, these drugs do appear in human milk and, thus, could conceivably alter short-term and long-term central nervous system function (56). See discussion in text of psychotropic drugs.

[b]Drug is concentrated in human milk relative to simultaneous maternal plasma concentrations.

[c]Blood concentration in the infant may be of clinical importance.

[d]Drugs listed have been reported in the literature as having the effects listed or no effect. The word *none* means that no observable change was seen in the nursing infant while the mother was ingesting the compound. Dashes indicate no mention of clinical effect on the infant. It is emphasized that many of the literature citations concern single case reports or small series of infants.

[e]Drug is concentrated in human milk.

Adapted from American Academy of Pediatrics. Committee on Drugs. Transfer of drugs and other chemicals into human milk. *Pediatrics.* 2001;108:776–789.

basis of their faith, adopted policies should also accommodate those who refuse on nonreligious grounds.

Every institution and clinical department should have a policy, compliant with the applicable state law, to guide clinicians in dealing with such patients. Some key court rulings include *Schloendorff v. Society of New York Hospital,* which established a competent adult's right to refuse care; *Cruzan v. Missouri,* which established the right of any individual to refuse medical therapy; a Georgetown case that upheld a court order to transfuse a Jehovah's Witness patient for the sake of her 7-month-old infant; and *Powell v. Columbia Presbyterian Medical Center,* which ordered a transfusion in a competent woman with minor children to avoid their posing an undue burden on the state (8).

When treating Jehovah's Witnesses for elective procedures, the following guidelines are useful. Allow ample time to discuss all issues with the patient and clinicians involved. It is imperative to interview patients in private so that they are not influenced, however inadvertently, by the presence of relatives or church elders. Verify that the patient would rather die than receive blood. Occasionally, a patient's faith may not be sufficient for them to risk death and they will accept blood. Discuss with the patient which blood alternatives, if any, are acceptable (9). For blood components and procedures usually accepted or refused by Jehovah's Witnesses, see Table 13.2. Identify anesthesiology faculty ethically comfortable with caring for Jehovah's Witnesses. Determine if the patient has minor children and, if so, document that a willing caregiver has been identified and obtain a signature on a release-of-liability form. Seek a legal opinion and a court order if

Table 13.2.   Blood components and procedures usually accepted and usually refused by Jehovah's Witnesses

Usually refused	Whole blood
	Erythrocytes
	Platelets
	Fresh frozen plasma
	Granulocytes
	Predeposited autologous blood
Usually accepted	Normovolemic hemodilution[a]
	Intraoperative red blood cell salvage[a]
	Erythropoietin[b]
	Hemodialysis[c]
	Cardiopulmonary bypass[c]
	Veno-veno bypass[c]
Individual decision	Albumin
("conscience item")	Cryoprecipitate
	Immune globulins
	Factor concentrates
	Organ and tissue transplants

[a]Usually accepted if patient remains continuously in contact with blood.
[b]Synthetic hormone frequently suspended in albumin.
[c]Provided that a nonblood prime is used.
Reproduced, with permission, from Doyle JD. Blood transfusions and the Jehovah's Witness patient. *Am J Ther.* 2002;9:417–424.

the patient is a pregnant Jehovah's Witness with a viable child or a minor child of a Jehovah's Witness. Most courts favor the state's interest in preserving the life of the child and will authorize blood transfusion. However, such a transfusion can have serious consequences for the child of a Jehovah's Witness, including parental rejection. Transfusion is given only if necessary to preserve life.

When emergency circumstances do not allow for discussion with patients or relatives before surgery, institute transfusions on the ethical principle of beneficence and worry about the legal position later. If in doubt about a particular case and if surgery can be delayed for a few hours, obtain a legal opinion. Court orders can be granted in a few hours if necessary on a 24-hour basis. Damages have been awarded to at least one Jehovah's Witness who was transfused even though he carried a card proclaiming his refusal of blood and blood products in keeping with his faith (10).

GERIATRIC PATIENTS

The geriatric population, generally is somewhat arbitrarily classified as those over the age of 65 years, is the fastest-growing segment in the United States and other developed countries. Yet, because some people age better than others (i.e., have a slower rate of biologic decline), the primary focus of the preoperative assessment is on "physiologic," not chronologic, age, as determined by an assessment of age-associated pathophysiology. Aging affects various systems in the body. Tables 13.3 through 13.7 outline

Table 13.3.　Cardiovascular system changes associated with aging

Overall decline in ventricular function due to decreased myocytes and increased collagen	Reduced ventricular compliance ($\downarrow$ elasticity and fibrotic change) resulting in $\downarrow$ left ventricular (LV) end-diastolic volume and $\uparrow$ LV end-diastolic pressure resulting in pulmonary congestion and diastolic dysfunction	$\downarrow$ responsiveness to sympathetic stimulation making cardiac output maintenance dependent upon preload and stroke volume rather than increased heart rate (HR)	Decrease in maximum HR (Maximum HR = 220 − age)
Concentric LV hypertrophy secondary to reduced elasticity and stiffening of the outflow tract with increased peripheral vascular resistance	Conduction abnormalities due to fibrotic infiltration of internodal tracts and His bundle	Greater frequency of coronary artery disease	Increased incidence of aortic stenosis. Estimated 2%–9% of patients over the age of 65[a]

[a]Christ M, Sharkova Y, Gelder G, et al. Preoperative and perioperative care for patients with suspected or established aortic stenosis facing noncardiac surgery. *Chest.* 2005;128:2944–2953.

Table 13.4. Respiratory system changes associated with aging

↓ elastic recoil of lungs. ↑ alveolar compliance with collapse of small airways, uneven ventilation, and air trapping	↓ oxygenation; PaO_2 (mm Hg) = 102 – (age/3). Normal range 60–100 mm Hg. Decrease likely due to increase in closing capacity relative to functional residual capacity (FRC)	Decline in strength of respiratory muscles resulting in a decrease of as much as 50% in forced expiratory volume in 1 second (FEV_1) and maximum inspiratory force	↓ diffusing capacity	↓ vital capacity by 20 mL/y
↓ compliance of chest wall secondary to kyphosis and vertebral collapse	↓ ventilatory responses to hypoxia and hypercarbia	↓ ciliary function and cough	↑ closing capacity and residual volume	Unchanged or slightly ↑ functional residual capacity

Table 13.5. Nervous system changes associated with aging

↓ brain size (cerebral/cortical neuron loss: 30% by age 80, particularly gray matter)	↓ density of pain-sensing Meissner corpuscles in the skin	↑ plasma catecholamines at rest and in response to stress. However, they do not trigger "hyperadrenergic" responses secondary to ↓ end-organ responsiveness
↓ cerebral blood flow as tissue mass ↓ (autoregulation maintained)	↓ numbers of peripheral, motor, sensory, and autonomic nerve fibers (auditory, visual, tactile, vibratory, hypothalamic temperature regulation). ↓ conduction velocity along nerve pathways	↑ incidence of dementia. Prevalence doubles approximately every 5 yr starting at 65–70 yr. Nearly 25% in those over age 85. Dementia at baseline is the most significant risk factor for delirium postoperatively[a]

[a]Rosenthal RA, Kavic SM. Assessment and management of the geriatric patient. *Crit Care Med.* 2004;32:S92–S105.

Table 13.6.   Renal system changes associated with aging

Renal blood flow is reduced by roughly 50% from age 25 to 85; profound effect on renal vasculature	Skeletal muscle mass decline leads to steady or only slightly decreased serum creatinine levels in spite of a progressive decline in creatinine clearance
Approximate 45% reduction in glomerular filtration rate (GFR) by 80 yr of age. GFR decrease by 6%–8% per decade of life beginning at age 30. GFR (mL/min) = (140 − age)(wt in kg)/(serum creatinine) (72)	↓ sodium conservation and hydrogen ion excretion reduce renal tubular function by upsetting the acid–base and fluid balance

the changes occurring in the cardiovascular, respiratory, nervous, renal, and hepatobiliary systems.

Preoperative Assessment

The focus is on evaluating perioperative risk by relying on the patient's physiologic as opposed to chronologic age. Comorbid conditions are identified. The functional reserves of specific organ systems are assessed. Surgical risk is inversely correlated with the patients' ability to perform routine activities of daily living such as feeding, dressing, and bathing themselves. Patients functioning at <4 metabolic equivalents (METs) are at an increased perioperative cardiac risk (11–13). One MET equals basal oxygen consumption (3.5 mL/kg/minute) of a 70-kg, 40-year-old male at rest. Targeted and cost-effective preoperative testing is based on a thorough patient history and physical examination after assessment of the patient's physical status, disease manifestations, and planned surgical procedure. Cost-effective tests in this population often include hematocrit, electrocardiogram (ECG), chest radiograph, albumin, glucose (or hemoglobin A1c), and creatinine levels. Unwarranted preoperative testing of the elderly based on age alone has not proven clinically productive or cost effective. Such tests often reveal borderline abnormalities and false positives that must be followed up with further tests of little clinical significance to avoid medicolegal problems. The Centers for Medicare and Medicaid Services (CMS) mandate that a supporting diagnosis be provided to justify preoperative tests. "Age-based" testing alone is not sufficient for proper reimbursement. For further information visit www.cms.gov.

While physiologic age, as opposed to chronologic age, is the primary focus in the elderly, the very elderly (>85 years old) may be at increased risk. In a study of 564,267 outpatient surgical procedures, Fleisher et al. identified that age >85 years, previous inpatient hospital admission within 6 months, surgery at a physician's office or outpatient hospital, and invasiveness of surgery identified patients at increased risk of inpatient hospital admission or death within 7 days of surgery (14).

Table 13.7.   Hepatobiliary system and drug metabolism changes associated with aging

↓ number of hepatocytes resulting in reductions in size and weight of liver	↓ hepatic synthesis of plasma cholinesterase; little clinical significance	↓ hepatic blood flow beginning at age 60 and falling 1% per year thereafter	↑ incidence of gallstones and gallstone-related complications
↓ drug clearance, meaning that elderly patients usually need lower dosages of drugs	↓ minimum alveolar concentration (MAC) of all volatile anesthetics	Reduction in hepatic drug clearance secondary to ↓ liver blood flow and size resulting in accumulation of drugs. Start any drug at a low dose and increase slowly, monitoring for beneficial and adverse effects	

The preoperative assessment of this population should consider the many social issues in the perioperative period. Many geriatric patients will have advanced directives or do-not-resuscitate (DNR) orders. Appropriate discussions regarding these should take place in the preoperative setting (see section on DNR orders in this chapter). Consultation with social services may prove beneficial in this fragile and often needy population. Many geriatric patients will need prolonged postoperative care through a home health agency or rehabilitation or extended-care facility following surgery. Consideration of these issues in the preoperative clinic will allow for better perioperative care and avoid delays on the day of surgery or prolonged hospitalizations.

CATARACT SURGERY

Cataract surgery, which is a low-risk procedure even in a geriatric population suffering from comorbid conditions, is usually performed under regional or topical anesthesia. The mortality risk of cataract surgery is much lower than that for other surgeries, even for patients with previous myocardial infarction (15). Though unlikely, serious perioperative complications are possible. They are minimized by identifying patients who are unable to lie flat (e.g., shortness of breath from congestive heart failure or severe lung disease) or still (e.g., demented or with very frequent coughing) and postponing surgery for them until those conditions have been reversed or lessened. Patients who do not speak the language of the caregivers in the room should have a hospital-employed translator present during cases when communication is necessary. All but the sickest patients tolerate regional or topical anesthesia. The risk/benefit ratio is considered carefully before opting for general anesthesia (GA).

A large, randomized trial showed that routine medical testing before cataract surgery does not measurably increase safety. Perioperative morbidity and mortality are not reduced by routine use of commonly ordered preoperative medical tests. The study population was relatively healthy and had to have been seen by an internist prior to enrolling in the study. Most patients did not have GA and their primary care physician could order appropriate tests preoperatively (16). Stable patients undergoing cataract surgery likely do not need routine preoperative tests. This does not mean that medical testing is unhelpful or not indicated for all patients. Testing is appropriate when the history or physical examination indicates the need.

There is no need to stop antiplatelet agents or warfarin prior to cataract surgery (no blood vessels involved) if general or topical anesthesia is used. Patients with end-stage renal disease should receive dialysis the day before surgery to optimize fluid and electrolyte status. Poorly controlled hypertension should be optimized prior to surgery. Implantable cardiac defibrillators (ICDs) need to be deactivated to avoid unplanned defibrillation during surgery and external modes of cardioversion/defibrillation should be available. Patients with pacemakers should have the device interrogated with a programmer for evaluating lead performance and obtaining current program information. Preoperative interrogation is now part of the American College of Cardiology (ACC) guidelines (13). Certain functions, such as rate-adaptive pacing, need to be programmed off because of possible interference from mechanical ventilators or monitors.

PATIENTS WITH DO-NOT-RESUSCITATE ORDERS

Do-not-resuscitate orders are meant to give patients or their legal representatives the choice to forego certain resuscitative procedures and their benefits because of the burdens they may impose (17). The applicability of DNR orders to anesthetized patients has been challenged, because anesthesia itself evokes changes in physiology and involves many of the elements of cardiopulmonary resuscitation (CPR) (e.g., intubation and use of vasoactive medications), and because resuscitation from cardiac arrest during anesthesia has a significantly higher success rate than in other clinical scenarios (18). Anesthesiologists may think that they cannot provide excellent anesthetic care if their normal armamentarium is limited by a DNR order.

The original 1993 ethical guidelines for DNR orders developed by the American Society of Anesthesiologists (ASA) were procedure directed, spelling out which resuscitative functions were permitted, but they fail to adequately consider the patient's desired end-of-life goals and outcomes. In 2001, the guidelines were revised to reflect a more flexible, goal-directed approach with an emphasis on outcome rather than procedures. This goal-directed approach places a greater ethical burden upon the anesthesiologist, who must know beforehand a patient's values and objectives, but also allows a procedural flexibility in response to physiologic changes under anesthesia. Patient autonomy and self-determination are leading principles in modern medical ethics and respecting the patient's right to choose is vitally important. A "required reconsideration" of DNR orders is mandatory for surgical patients.

The patient's right to choose and act intentionally is respected by obtaining informed consent. A discussion with the patient or patient's representative and surgeon to establish an understanding of the patient's wishes is necessary. The institutional policy regarding perioperative DNR orders is followed. The discussion of the required reconsideration of the DNR order is documented. Three options for perioperative DNR orders are provided below (18).

1. Full resuscitation: "I, _____, desire that full resuscitative measures be employed during my anesthesia and in the postanesthesia care unit regardless of the clinical situation."
2. Limited resuscitation (procedure directed): "During anesthesia and in the postanesthesia unit, I _____, refuse the following procedures" (<u>procedures are listed</u>).
3. Limited resuscitation (goal directed): "I, _____, desire attempts to resuscitate me during my anesthesia and in the postanesthesia care unit only if, in the clinical judgment of the attending anesthesiologist and surgeons, such resuscitative efforts will support the following goals and values of mine" (<u>goals are listed</u>).

EXTREMELY OBESE PATIENTS

Extreme obesity is defined as weight 100 pounds above ideal body weight (IBW) or as a body mass index (BMI = weight/height^2 or kg/m^2) of $\geq$40. The BMI cutoff for obesity is $\geq$30 (19). Various Web sites are available to assist in the calculation of BMI. Two that are helpful are http://www.cdc.gov/nccdphp/dnpa/bmi/index.htm and http://www.nhlbisupport.com/bmi/. In the United States, >50% of adults are currently 20% above their IBW. To minimize perioperative risk, physiologic and pathophysiologic changes associated with obesity are identified in the preoperative assessment. Common changes to the pulmonary and cardiovascular system are found in Tables 13.8 and 13.9.

Gastrointestinal and Hepatic Systems

Obese patients may have more gastric juice volume and a lower gastric pH. These changes put them at risk for regurgitation and aspiration, a risk magnified by intra-abdominal pressure and a greater incidence of hiatus hernia. A recent study (20), however, in otherwise healthy, nondiabetic, fasting patients showed that obese surgical patients had a lower incidence of combined high-volume and low-pH stomach contents than did lean patients. Further studies are needed to shed light on the issue of resting gastric contents in obese patients. Obese patients may have elevation of transaminase levels due to a fatty liver. This is a diagnosis of exclusion and can only be confirmed with a liver biopsy. Other etiologies need to be considered. Hepatic function is usually normal. Drug metabolism may be altered in obese patients. More free fluoride ions are found after exposure to methoxyflurane, enflurane, and, in some studies, halothane (no definitive data on sevoflurane). Obesity is a risk factor for halothane-induced hepatotoxicity.

Renal and Endocrine

Elimination of medications is faster because of increased renal blood flow and glomerular filtration rate (GFR). Because some highly lipophilic drugs, including barbiturates and benzodiazepines, may have large volumes of distribution, the serum concentration from a dose and the rate of elimination is slower. With less lipophilic medications, little change is observed in the volume of distribution in obese patients. For example, fentanyl and propofol seem to behave similarly in obese and nonobese patients. An unpredictable behavior of drugs may occur in obese patients. The extremely obese have impaired glucose tolerance and a high prevalence of type 2 diabetes. Peripheral adipose tissues are resistant to insulin.

Weight Reduction Drugs

Certain anti-obesity drugs affect the heart and pulmonary vasculature. In the late 1960s and early 1970s, a small epidemic of pulmonary hypertension with some deaths resulted from the use of aminorex for weight reduction. Fenfluramine and dexfenfluramine are associated with pulmonary hypertension, and even a brief course of combined fenfluramine and phentermine

Table 13.8. Pulmonary system changes associated with obesity

↓ functional residual capacity (FRC), possibly resulting in lung volumes below closing capacity leading to small airway closure, ventilation-perfusion mismatch, and hypoxemia	↓ expiratory reserve volume (primary cause of reduced FRC)	↑ oxygen consumption and carbon dioxide production secondary to increased metabolic activity of excess adipose
↓ vital and/or total lung capacity	↑ work of breathing	↑ risk of hypoxia during anesthesia or after surgery when the patient is in the supine or Trendelenburg position

Table 13.9. Cardiovascular system changes associated with obesity

Expanded blood volume	↑ cardiac output	↑ preload leading to dilation and eccentric left ventricular hypertrophy with reduced compliance and eventual diastolic dysfunction and biventricular failure	↑ risk of coronary artery disease; whether secondary to age alone or disease process is unclear	↑ incidence of hypertension. Systemic vascular resistance is normal but many patients display a 3–4 mm Hg increase in systolic and a 2 mm Hg increase in diastolic blood pressure per 10-kg weight gain. Pathophysiology is poorly understood
↑ stroke volume	↑ left ventricular stroke work	Pulmonary hypertension and increased pulmonary artery occlusion pressure	Higher perioperative risk of deep venous thrombosis and pulmonary embolism[a]	Decreased maximum attainable heart rate (HR). Maximum HR = 220 – age

[a]Demaria EJ, Carmody BJ. Perioperative management of special populations: obesity. *Surg Clin North Am.* 2005;85:1283–1289.

(fen-phen) has been associated with fatal pulmonary hypertension (21). In 1997, reports emerged that valvular heart disease (mostly left-sided and regurgitant lesions) was associated with use of fen-phen (22). Fenfluramine and dexfenfluramine have subsequently been removed from the market, but phentermine remains available. The U. S. Department of Health and Human Services recommends a cardiovascular examination and complete history for persons exposed to either drug for any period. If valvular disease is suspected, patients need an ECG and a two-dimensional (2-D) echocardiogram (echo), and if significant valvular lesions are present, cardiology consultation is appropriate.

Preoperative Assessment

In taking the medical history or conducting the physical examination of an obese patient, the physician should pay particular attention to several areas. What is the patient's tolerance of exercise and ability to lie flat, especially while sleeping? The inability to walk four blocks on level ground or climb two flights of stairs due to cardiopulmonary symptoms suggests poor exercise tolerance. Using metabolic equivalents is useful for quantifying a patient's functional capacity. A level of ≥ 4 METs is desirable. Exertional dyspnea or angina may or may not be discovered because of limited mobility and sedentary lifestyle. Symptoms of sleep apnea are often present and should be appropriately evaluated (see the Sleep Apnea Syndrome section in this chapter). Has the patient used diet tablets, particularly fenfluramine, dexfenfluramine, and even phentermine?

To measure blood pressure, the cuff should have a width approximately two-thirds that of the arm and a length sufficient to encircle the arm. Oxygen saturation while the patient breathes room air is measured. If signs of cardiac failure (increased jugular venous pressure, added heart sounds, pulmonary crackles, hepatomegaly, and peripheral edema) are present, an ECG and 2-D echo are needed.

Extremely obese patients may have challenging airways. Check for limited flexion and extension of the cervical spine, restricted mouth opening from submental fat, an enlarged tongue, and redundant oral tissue. The thyromental distance also should be assessed. Neck circumference may be the single most reliable predictor of problematic intubation. A patient with a neck circumference of 40 cm has a 5% probability of difficult intubation, and one with a neck circumference of 60 cm, a 35% probability (23). A BMI >30 has been shown to be a predictor of difficult mask ventilation and intubation (24). If a difficult airway is suspected, discussions regarding awake fiberoptic intubation (FOI) should take place with the patient. If the patient is scheduled for surgery in an ambulatory surgery center, the surgeon should be notified of the potential difficult airway and consideration given to moving the surgery to a facility where inpatient and intensive care is available.

Pulmonary function tests (PFTs) have very limited usefulness in non–lung resection surgeries. PFTs are only indicated if the etiology of dyspnea (a common complaint of these patients due to obesity or deconditioning) is unclear or to optimize therapy in patients with known lung disease. PFTs do not predict postoperative pulmonary complications.

Possible difficulty obtaining peripheral intravenous access requiring central access should be discussed. Standard OR table weight capacities are 300 to 400 pounds. Arrangements are made to accommodate the extremely obese patient with appropriate equipment. Weight reduction should be emphasized. There is increasing evidence that weight loss may improve cardiac morphology. Most hemodynamic parameters, left ventricular (LV) systolic function, and LV diastolic filling are better after weight loss (25).

Obesity Hypoventilation Syndrome

Among extremely obese patients, 5% to 8% have obesity hypoventilation syndrome (OHS), originally dubbed pickwickian syndrome by Osler. The classic description of pickwickian syndrome includes obesity, excessive daytime sleepiness, snoring, and cor pulmonale. In OHS daytime hypoxemia ($PaO_2 \leq 65$ mm Hg) is chronic and hypoventilation ($PaCO_2 \geq 45$ mm Hg) is found without the diagnosis of chronic obstructive pulmonary disease (COPD) (26). Pickwickian patients often suffer from obstructive sleep apnea, but the two are distinct syndromes. Other characteristics of OHS are hypercapnia, severe hypoxemia, periodic breathing, biventricular enlargement (especially of the right ventricle), pulmonary hypertension, dependent edema, polycythemia, and pulmonary edema. Pulmonary compliance is reduced dramatically, which increases the work of breathing more than in simply obese individuals. Impaired central ventilatory drive, decreased respiratory system compliance, and inefficiency and fatigue of respiratory muscles are believed to play a part in the syndrome. These patients are sensitive to the respiratory depressant effects of GA. In a preoperative assessment of a patient with OHS, cardiopulmonary systems are thoroughly evaluated. Weight reduction is emphasized before elective surgery because anesthetic risk is high. A relatively minor weight loss can drastically improve physiologic status. Continuous positive airway pressure (CPAP) should be instituted via consultation with a pulmonologist. ECGs detect rhythm disturbances (sinus bradycardia, sinus arrest, sinus arrhythmia, wandering pacemaker, premature ventricular and supraventricular contractions), ventricular hypertrophy, right axis deviation, and right bundle branch block. Chest radiographs exclude cardiomegaly and atelectasis or other pulmonary processes. Symptoms of cardiac disease warrant 2-D echo for evaluation of hypertrophy, contractility, pulmonary artery pressures, and tricuspid valve integrity. Evidence of pulmonary hypertension should be evaluated and optimized by a cardiopulmonary specialist prior to elective surgery.

PATIENTS WITH SLEEP APNEA SYNDROME

Often underdiagnosed, sleep apnea syndrome (SAS) is defined as ≥ 5 apneic events (airflow stops for ≥ 10 seconds despite continued respiratory effort) or ≥ 15/hour hypopneic events (airflow lessens >50% for ≥ 10 seconds) during a 7-hour sleep study. There are three types of SAS, obstructive, central, and mixed. In obstructive SAS airflow is impeded in spite of normal respiratory muscle function because of upper airway obstruction. In central SAS, there is no respiratory muscle activity during periods of apnea. Both patterns are found in the same patient in mixed SAS. Apneic episodes are more frequent during rapid eye movement (REM) than deep non-REM sleep. They are associated with arterial desaturation, which is worse in the obstructive pattern. Besides disrupting sleep, they may lead to daytime somnolence, naps, and reduced performance of daily activities. Apneic episodes are associated with snoring (loud enough to be heard through a closed door) and may produce pulmonary hypertension and cardiac arrhythmias.

A patient with SAS is identified by reviewing the medical record and by interviewing the patient and/or family. The interview is the most efficient and cost-effective means of screening patients. The Berlin questionnaire, developed in 1996, includes a series of questions about risk factors for sleep apnea, including snoring behavior, waketime sleepiness or fatigue, and obesity or hypertension. Netzer et al. evaluated the usefulness of the Berlin questionnaire to identify patients with SAS and concluded that it provides a means of identifying patients who are likely to have SAS (27). See Figure 13.2 for the entire Berlin questionnaire. The physical examination includes a thorough airway examination, similar to that for an extremely obese patient. A BMI >35, neck circumference of 17 inches (men) or 16 inches (women), craniofacial abnormalities affecting the airway, anatomic nasal obstruction, and tonsils nearly touching or touching in the midline all suggest the possibility of OSA. Before proceeding with surgery, in nonurgent situations, a sleep specialist is consulted, who can perform the definitive diagnostic test, polysomnography. The severity of the disease may be determined by a sleep study. If a sleep study is not available, patients should be treated as though they have moderate SAS unless one or more of the signs or symptoms is markedly severe (e.g., extremely increased BMI or neck circumference). If patients use CPAP at home, they should bring their system with them to the hospital. Because SAS patients seem to be markedly more sensitive to the effects of sedatives, opioids, and GA (28), anesthesiologists need to review the guidelines developed by the ASA for the perioperative management of such patients (29). The ASA guidelines emphasize that patient selection for surgery depends on the severity of OSA, coexisting disease, type of anesthesia, nature of surgery, and anticipated postoperative opioid requirement. Preoperative preparation is to optimize a patient's physical status by use of CPAP or bilevel positive airway pressure (BiPAP), weight loss, and use of mandibular advancement devices. Uvulopalatopharyngoplasty and tracheotomy may be considered for severe cases. Suitability of patients with moderate to severe SAS for ambulatory surgery remains controversial and scientific literature is limited. It is agreed that patients believed to be at increased risk from SAS can safely undergo outpatient procedures when local or regional anesthesia is administered. When patients with SAS undergo GA as outpatients, the facility should have equipment necessary to manage a difficult airway, respiratory equipment (CPAP, ventilators), radiology, and laboratory facilities (blood gas and electrolyte measurement). Transfer arrangements with an inpatient facility should be in place

The Berlin Questionnaire

Question	Response
Has your weight changed?	Increased Decreased No change
Do you snore?	Yes No Do not know
Snoring loudness	Loud as breathing Loud as talking Louder than talking Very loud
Snoring frequency	Almost every day 3 to 4 times per week 1 to 2 times per week 1 to 2 times per month Never or almost never
Does your snoring bother other people?	Yes No
How often have your breathing pauses been noticed?	Almost every day 3 to 4 times per week 1 to 2 times per week 1 to 2 times per month Never or almost never
Are you tired after sleeping?	Almost every day 3 to 4 times per week 1 to 2 times per week 1 to 2 times per month Never or almost never
Are you tired during waketime?	Almost every day 3 to 4 times per week 1 to 2 times per week 1 to 2 times per month Never or almost never
Have you ever fallen asleep while driving?	Yes No
Do you have high blood pressure?	Yes No Do not know

Adapted with permission from Netzer NC, Stoohs RA, Netzer CM, et al. Using the Berlin Questionnaire to identify patients at risk for the sleep apnea syndrome. Ann Intern Med 1999;131:488.

Figure 13.2. Berlin questionnaire.

for ambulatory centers. The guidelines recommend monitoring of SAS patients for a median of 3 hours longer than their non-SAS counterparts prior to discharge. Patients who are at significantly increased risk of perioperative complications are generally not good candidates for surgery in a freestanding ambulatory center. In the OR these patients often are difficult to mask ventilate and intubate. Plans should be made for possible FOI. Caution is advised when planning for deep sedation or monitored anesthesia care (MAC).

CANCER PATIENTS

The physician's first impulse on conducting a preoperative assessment of a cancer patient is to concentrate on the effects of anticancer drugs and radiotherapy on anesthesia and surgery. Undoubtedly, these are important aspects of preoperative assessment. However, equally important are the physiologic disturbances that can occur with some cancers as well as other complications that can arise because of location of the tumors.

Radiation therapy to the thyroid may result in primary or central hypothyroidism, thyroiditis, Graves disease, euthyroid Graves ophthalmopathy, benign adenomas, multinodular goiter, and radiation-induced thyroid carcinoma. Primary hypothyroidism is the most common radiation-induced thyroid dysfunction. Approximately half of these occur within the first 5 years after therapy. Patients are assessed for lethargy, intolerance to cold, weight gain, and generalized decrease in metabolic activity. Radiotherapy for head and neck cancer may result in laryngeal edema, dental decay, salivary gland degeneration, and dysphagia. Chondroradionecrosis of the larynx and fibrosis with stricture of the pharyngoesophageal segment is a recognized complication of radiation therapy usually occurring within the first year. Fibrosis and contractures of the face, mouth, and neck may alter airway anatomy and make conventional management with mask ventilation and intubation difficult.

Radiation pneumonitis is a well-described complication of irradiation to the breast and mediastinum. Characterized by interstitial pulmonary inflammation, it develops in 5% to 15% of patients within 1 to 6 months of radiation. Early diagnosis is made with chest radiography and the treatment of choice is corticosteroids. Consultation with a radiation oncologist and pulmonologist is advised. Pericarditis with and without effusion, accelerated coronary atherosclerosis, valvular dysfunction, myocardial fibrosis, and conduction abnormalities are associated with radiation to the chest, breast, or mediastinum. Cardiovascular disease is the second most common cause of mortality in survivors of Hodgkin disease. One study found that 88% of patients had echocardiographic abnormalities 5 to 20 years posttreatment, most of them asymptomatic (7). Treatment at a younger age increases risk. These risk factors were not considered in the ACC/American Heart Association (AHA) Guidelines for Cardiac Evaluation for Noncardiac Surgery, but they may be clinical predictors of coronary artery disease (CAD) (13), ECG, echocardiography, and stress testing may be indicated.

Chemotherapy with doxorubicin and daunorubicin increases the risk for cardiomyopathy. Indeed, the total dose of doxorubicin is the most significant risk factor for cardiomyopathy. A total dose of <550 mg/m^2 minimizes the chance of cardiac toxicity. Symptoms of cardiac distress including shortness of breath, chest pain, nonproductive cough, weight gain, and ankle swelling (30) should be evaluated with ECG, chest radiography, and 2-D echo. These drugs produce nonspecific ST-T changes, sinus tachycardia, premature ventricular and atrial contractions, and low-voltage QRS complexes on ECG.

Bleomycin may produce pulmonary toxicity, adding to the risk of pulmonary fibrosis, especially at doses >500 units. Symptoms include a dry, hacking cough, and dyspnea on exertion. For the patient who has been given bleomycin, serial PFTs are indicated.

Cyclophosphamide, procarbazine, melphalan, methotrexate, mitomycin C, and carmustine have been cited as pulmonary toxins. Hepatic toxicity results from nitrosourea compounds carmustine, lomustine, and streptozocin. The patient has mildly elevated serum transaminases, alkaline phosphatase, and bilirubin levels, which generally return to normal once the agent is discontinued. Methotrexate elevates aspartate aminotransferase and lactate dehydrogenase levels. Upon discontinuation, hepatic inflammation may resolve but hepatic cirrhosis will not. Azathioprine and 6-mercaptopurine may cause intrahepatic cholestasis and parenchymal cell necrosis. Cytosine arabinoside can elevate liver enzymes. L-asparaginase causes fatty changes, decreases levels of serum proteins and coagulation factors, and elevates liver enzymes. Cisplatin, methotrexate, and streptozocin may cause major renal toxicity depending on the dose and administration schedule. Cyclophosphamide and ifosfamide may lead to hemorrhagic cystitis, which normally resolves within 2 to 6 weeks after the agent is discontinued. The condition can sometimes be avoided with aggressive hydration. Neurologic toxicity, usually reversible, is an effect of vincristine. Its manifestations are distal paresthesias and loss of deep tendon reflexes. At high cumulative doses it produces cranial nerve palsy, autonomic neuropathy, and syndrome of inappropriate antidiuretic hormone (SIADH) secretion. Cisplatin and carboplatin cause symmetric sensory neuropathy at high cumulative doses. 5-fluorouracil (5-FU) may cause cerebellar ataxia, L-asparaginase may cause lethargy, confusion, and disorientation. Doxorubicin, daunorubicin, dactinomycin, mitomycin C, carmustine, dacarbazine, nitrogen mustard, vincristine, vinblastine, and vinorelbine may cause severe tissue inflammation and necrosis that persist over months from local infiltration of the drug; necrosis may necessitate excision and skin grafting.

Bone marrow suppression is a dose-limiting side effect of nearly all chemotherapeutic agents. It can result in infection (sepsis) from drug-induced leucopenia or bleeding because of thrombocytopenia. Chemotherapy-induced neutropenia typically occurs 3 to 7 days following chemotherapy and continues for several days before returning to normal. The type and dose of chemotherapy affects how low the neutrophil count drops and how long it will take to recover. Filgrastim and pegfilgrastim can prevent neutropenia. Though challenged by some clinicians, platelet counts $<100,000$ mm^3 are a contraindication to regional anesthesia. Anemia is most common and preoperative blood transfusion may be necessary.

Breast Cancer

Breast cancer is the second most common cause of cancer death in women. The 5-year survival rate has increased from 72% in the 1940s to 95% today as a result of earlier detection and improved treatment. This type of cancer most frequently metastasizes to bone, lung, liver, and brain (31). Regional (thoracic epidural, paravertebral block), general, or local with intravenous sedation are anesthetic options. However, preliminary data have suggested that survival is improved in patients avoiding GA. Patients are often anxious, which can be allayed through preoperative education.

Colorectal Cancer

Colorectal cancer is the third most common cancer in men and women and the second leading cause of cancer death. Patients with colorectal cancer are often asymptomatic but may experience nausea, vomiting, dehydration, weight loss, anemia, or bowel obstruction. In the early stages of the disease, primary resection is the principal treatment. Adjuvant chemotherapy is employed in the more advanced stages. The disease may metastasize to the liver, abdomen, lungs, bone, and brain. A complete blood count (CBC) is indicated in these patients even without advanced disease as occult gastrointestinal bleeding is often present. Hepatic and coagulation profiles are considered if the disease is advanced. Patients need to be informed of the possible benefits of epidural analgesia.

Head and Neck Cancer

The incidence of this cancer is highest in patients >60 years of age and twice as high in men as in women. Patients may experience dysarthria, dysphagia, or dyspnea and often have a history of heavy alcohol and tobacco use. Head and neck cancer can metastasize to liver, lung, and bone. The head and neck are examined for evidence of airway compression or obstruction. Pharyngeal, laryngeal, thyroid, or base-of-tongue tumors may obstruct the upper airway. Wheezing and stridor are typically ominous signs. Computed tomography (CT) scans may be necessary to evaluate the extent of disease. The airway is managed via FOI or awake tracheostomy in some cases. When a difficult airway is anticipated, the management plan is to be discussed with the patient preoperatively. Morbidities include an intermediate (generally <5%) risk for perioperative myocardial infarction (13), cerebral vascular accident (4.8% with resection of head and neck tumors) (32), pneumothorax, and venous air embolism (33).

Lung Cancer

Lung cancer is the number one cause of cancer-related mortality in the United States. Cigarette smoking remains the most significant risk factor. The patient with lung cancer may have cough, dyspnea, hemoptysis, and postobstructive pneumonia. Complications include airway obstruction, pneumonia, pleural and pericardial effusions, and ectopic hormone production. Lung cancer metastasizes to brain, pleura, bone, liver, adrenal glands, the contralateral lung, and mediastinum.

Lymphomas, thymomas, teratomas, and retrosternal goiters are common anterior mediastinal masses. Mediastinal masses need complete evaluation for possible airway compromise. Mediastinal tumors may be associated with pulmonary artery, superior vena cava (SVC), and cardiac compression. SVC syndrome develops when tumor prevents venous drainage in the upper thorax. Dilation of collateral veins in the neck and thorax; edema and cyanosis of the face, neck, and upper chest; edema of the conjunctiva; evidence of increased intracranial pressure (ICP); and dyspnea are present. Preoperative evaluation of a mediastinal mass includes chest radiography, flow-volume loops, CT, and clinical evaluation for airway obstruction (dyspnea with or without exertion, shortness of breath or cough while lying flat). However, the degree of pulmonary symptoms while awake may not correlate with respiratory compromise experienced under anesthesia. Flow-volume loops may help to identify obstruction and whether it is intra- or extrathoracic (Fig. 13.3). The degree of tracheal

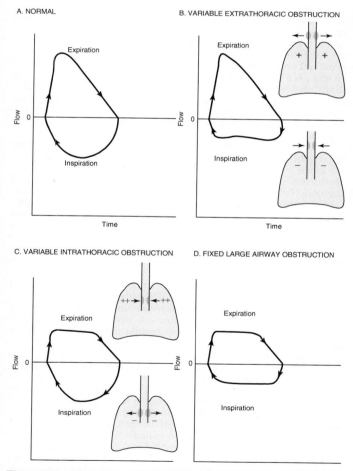

Figure 13.3. Flow-volume loops of intrathoracic and extrathoracic obstruction. (From Morgan GE, Mikhail MS, Murray MJ. *Clin Anesthesiol.* 2002;3:542.)

compression on CT is useful when evaluating the airway. FOI is discussed with the patient preoperatively and a thoracic surgeon and rigid bronchoscope should be readily available prior to induction of GA.

PFTs are useful in patients scheduled for lung resection. Patients with a forced expiratory volume in 1 second (FEV_1) $>70\%$ will be able to tolerate pneumonectomy. Generally, a predicted postresection FEV_1 of 800 mL or 33% is necessary. See Chapter 5 for a more detailed discussion of PFTs.

Paraneoplastic syndromes such as hypercalcemia, syndrome of inappropriate antidiuretic hormone (SIADH), Eaton-Lambert syndrome, or Cushing syndrome are possible. Eaton-Lambert, also known as myasthenic syndrome, was originally described in patients with small cell carcinoma of the lung. It is an autoimmune disease in which IgG antibodies to presynaptic calcium channels are produced, resulting in skeletal muscle weakness. Proximal muscle weakness (legs more than arms) improving with exercise is a distinguishing feature. Males are affected more often than females. Patients are sensitive to the effects of nondepolarizing and depolarizing neuromuscular blocking drugs. Antagonism with anticholinesterase may be inadequate. The need to decrease doses of muscle relaxants should be considered in patients with known or suspected lung cancer.

Hypercalcemia from osteolytic activity of bony metastases may be present. Parathyroid-related protein is the most common cause of humoral-mediated hypercalcemia in lung cancer patients. Hypercalcemia may cause somnolence, vomiting, dehydration, and polyuria. Total serum calcium (Ca^+) levels >10 mEq/L are considered elevated. Increased serum Ca^+ concentrations can cause prolonged PR and shortened QT intervals and wide QRS complexes on ECG. Hydration with normal saline allows sodium (Na^+) to inhibit renal tubular absorption of Ca^+. Furosemide, 40 to 80 mg every 2 to 4 hours, promotes diuresis and delivery of Ca^+ to the renal tubules. Thiazide diuretics may enhance renal tubular reabsorption of Ca^+ and are contraindicated.

SIAD is characterized by hyponatremia (Na^+ <136 mEq/L) and normal extracellular fluid volume. Patients with Na^+ concentrations >125 mEq/L are usually asymptomatic. Complications of hyponatremia include anorexia, nausea, weakness, lethargy, confusion, seizure, and coma. Hyponatremia needs to be corrected before elective procedures. Asymptomatic and stable patients are treated with water restriction. Iso- or hypertonic saline is indicated for symptomatic hyponatremia. Demeclocycline antagonizes antidiuretic hormone (ADH) activity and can be used as adjunct treatment. Rapid correction of hyponatremia can cause central pontine myelinolysis. Cushing syndrome results from ectopic corticotropin production stimulating the adrenal cortex to produce excessive amounts of cortisol, and is most often associated with small cell lung cancer. Sudden onset of weight gain, usually central and associated with facial fat (moon facies); hypertension; edema; hypokalemia; glucose intolerance; and abnormal menses are present. Depression and insomnia are common. Preoperative evaluation of the patient's airway, blood pressure, electrolytes, and glucose is important.

Prostate Cancer

Preoperative assessment of patients with prostate cancer notes symptoms of urinary obstruction, anemia, pancytopenia, or metastatic disease to the bones. It is important to be familiar with the patient's chemotherapy, hormonal, and radiation treatment history.

PATIENTS WITH HUMAN IMMUNODEFICIENCY VIRUS

Human immunodeficiency virus type 1 (HIV-1) is the etiologic agent for acquired immunodeficiency syndrome (AIDS). First described in 1981, this disease has now reached epidemic proportions worldwide and poses a risk to health care providers. A retrovirus of the Lentivirus group of viruses, it attaches to CD4 receptors on host cells by means of its envelope of proteins. The host produces antibodies to the virus (providing a basis for tests), but they are unprotective. As it replicates, the virus damages or destroys T lymphocytes, leaving the host immunocompromised and vulnerable to infectious diseases and cancer. The virus can remain dormant for long periods, but continues to replicate, and can suddenly multiply rapidly, leading to cell death. The clinical spectrum of AIDS ranges from asymptomatic but infective to life-threatening infection. The CDC expanded its classifications of AIDS in 1993 and recognized the prognostic importance of CD4 counts. There are three stages of disease progression. The initial stage displays mononucleosis-like symptoms that gradually resolve, leaving the patient feeling well but infective. The second stage, chronic lymphadenopathy, lasts 3 to 5 years before reaching the third stage, cell-mediated immune deficiency. The third stage is characterized by a wide variety of opportunistic infections; the appearance of tumors such as Kaposi sarcoma and non-Hodgkin lymphoma; and death, usually as a result of opportunistic infections, wasting, or cancer.

The risk factors for AIDS include sexual contact with an infected individual or blood-borne contamination. High-risk contacts include men who have sex with men (MSM), sexual workers, and those having contact with sexual workers. In the United States there is one HIV infection per 1.5 to 2 million blood donor exposures. The risk in the early 1980s was 1 per 100; in 1997, 1 per 400,000. Infected mothers can transmit HIV to their infants. Health care workers exposed to HIV-infected blood have a 0.3% seroconversion rate, but a much lower rate with mucous membrane exposure. HIV is transmitted via intravenous illicit drug use. Tattoos and body piercing carry a theoretical risk of transmission if instruments contaminated with blood are not sterilized or disinfected appropriately between clients. No documented cases of transmission have been reported to date. The CDC recommends that single-use instruments intended to penetrate the skin be used only once.

The enzyme-linked immunosorbent assay (ELISA) is the primary screening test. It detects the antibody to an extract of a tissue culture growth of HIV. It is >99% sensitive but generates a number of false-positive results. The Western blot technique is used to confirm ELISA results. HIV infection causes a wide spectrum of complications affecting all organ systems. Complications may be the direct infection of a specific organ system by HIV or secondary to the immunodeficiency associated with HIV infection. Aseptic meningitis and AIDS-related dementia occur with central nervous system (CNS) involvement. Myelopathies, peripheral neuropathies, and opportunistic CNS infections and neoplasms occur. Increased ICP may occur with CNS involvement. Headaches, visual disturbances, nausea and vomiting, and decreased consciousness suggest increased ICP and can be detected by CT scanning.

Pericardial disease with effusion and tamponade; nonspecific or infectious myocarditis; dilated cardiomyopathy with global left ventricular dysfunction; valvular disease due to marantic or infective endocarditis; pulmonary hypertension; and neoplastic invasion are possible. Antiretroviral-induced lipodystrophy leads to coronary artery disease and dyslipidemia. Drug-related cardiotoxicity and autonomic dysfunction are prevalent. The presence of chest pain, orthopnea, dyspnea at rest or on exertion, and decreased exercise tolerance or physical findings of a murmur, pericardial rub, jugular venous distention, pulmonary crackles, or lower extremity edema raise suspicion of cardiac disease and prompt cardiology consultation. Diagnostic tools include chest radiography, ECG, and 2-D echo.

Opportunistic pulmonary infection with *Pneumocystis carinii*, *Mycobacterium avium* complex, *Mycobacterium tuberculosis*, cytomegalovirus, and cryptococcosis are common. Typically of limited duration in immunologically intact patients, such infections can become insidious and protracted in immunologically compromised AIDS patients. Lymphoma, Kaposi sarcoma, and lymphoid interstitial pneumonitis occur. Preoperative chest radiography is ordered for evaluation in patients with dyspnea, cough, and fever. Supraglottic Kaposi sarcoma may cause problematic ventilation and intubation. Non-Hodgkin lymphoma can cause mediastinal masses that may compromise large airways (see section on cancer for management of mediastinal masses). Useful diagnostic tools include chest radiography, ECG, and 2-D echo.

Hematologic disorders range from simple anemia to coagulation problems, either from the disease itself or due to various treatments, such as zidovudine (AZT). The major dose-limiting toxicity of AZT is suppression of erythropoiesis and myelopoiesis. Anemia and granulocytopenia occur as drug dosage increases with progression of disease. Chronic diarrhea, dysphagia, and esophagitis are caused by the virus itself or by opportunistic infections. They can lead to malnutrition, dehydration, and electrolyte imbalance.

Renal function should be carefully assessed in AIDS patients. HIV patients are susceptible to acute tubular necrosis, glomerular nephritis, renovascular disease, and HIV-associated nephropathy (HIVAN). HIVAN consists of: Proteinuria, azotemia, normal to large kidneys on ultrasonography, normal pressure, and focal segmental glomerulosclerosis on renal biopsy. Patients present with a nephrotic syndrome consisting of proteinuria (>3.5 g/dL), azotemia, hyperlipidemia, and hypoalbuminemia. Electrolyte abnormalities, such as hyponatremia and hyperkalemia, occur with HIVAN and may reflect an increase in total body water (from the nephrotic syndrome, SIAD, or hyporeninemic hypoaldosteronism).

HIV medications are generally well tolerated, even in the presence of renal insufficiency. The potential toxicity of the nucleoside reverse transcriptase inhibitors (i.e., zidovudine, didanosine, zalcitabine, stavudine, lamivudine, abacavir, emtricitabine) is lactic acidosis. Didanosine may cause electrolyte abnormalities, such as hypokalemia, hyponatremia, hypermagnesemia, and hyperuricemia. Stavudine may cause hyperuricemia. Except for nevirapine, which may cause lactic acidosis, the nonnucleoside reverse transcriptase inhibitors (i.e., nevirapine, delavirdine, efavirenz) have no reported significant renal toxicity.

There is limited information about the risk of anesthesia and surgery in HIV/AIDS patients. As far as can be determined, surgical interventions do not increase the postoperative risk for complications or death and should not be withheld. The laboratory workup should include CBC, clotting functions, glucose, and liver and renal function tests. Verification of the immunologic status with the $CD4^+$ lymphocyte cell count and viral load during the previous 3 months is important. Regardless of the surgical procedure, there is a 13.3% mortality rate 6 months postoperatively when the $CD4^+$ count is <50 mm^{-3} and a 0.8% mortality rate when the $CD4^+$ count is >200 mm^{-3} (34). Chest radiography and ECG are needed in all patients. Patients with a history or signs of cardiac or pulmonary dysfunction should undergo a more thorough evaluation. Antiretroviral therapy should be continued perioperatively. Anesthesiologists should be aware of the toxic side effects and possible interaction of antiretrovirals with anesthetics. See Tables 13.10, 13.11, and 13.12 for antiretroviral drugs and side effects. Protease inhibitors, such as ritonavir, impair the metabolism of many medications, such as midazolam, fentanyl, and amiodarone, by inhibiting CYP-450, requiring dose adjustments. Nevirapine, an inducer of CYP-450, requires increased doses of anesthetics. Etomidate, atracurium, remifentanil, and desflurane are independent of CYP-450 metabolism and optimal choices for anesthetics.

Logistics, cost, and ethical considerations make it impractical to test all patients preoperatively for HIV. The CDC recommends that health care workers institute "universal precautions" as though every patient has a communicable disease (35). If health care workers are stuck by a contaminated needle or have extensive areas of broken skin come into contact with a patient's body fluids, they should immediately clean exposed surfaces (by washing the skin with soap and water, or irrigating the mucous membranes with sterile normal saline or water), apply first aid to the local wound as needed, and immediately contact the employee health department so that HIV testing can be conducted and prophylactic treatment discussed. A sample of the patient's blood is to be tested if not known to be HIV positive. This incident is to be treated as a medical emergency. The CDC recommendations for HIV postexposure prophylaxis (PEP) include a basic 4-week regimen of two drugs (ZDV and lamivudine [3TC]; 3TC and stavudine [d4T]; or didanosine [ddI] and d4T) for most HIV exposures. An expanded regimen includes the addition of a third drug for HIV

Table 13.10. Antiretroviral drugs (nucleoside analog reverse transcriptase inhibitors (NRTIsl) and side effects

Generic Name	Trade Name	FDA Pregnancy Category	Dose	Adverse Side Effects
Zidovudine (AZT)	Retrovir	C	100 mg 6×/day	Anemia, neutropenia, pancytopenia, headache, neuropathy, myopathy
Didanosine (ddi)	Videx	B	200 mg bid	Peripheral neuropathy, pancreatitis, gastrointestinal disturbances
Stavudine (d₄T)	Zerit	C	40 mg bid	Peripheral neuropathy, pancreatitis
Zalcitabine (ddC)	Hivid	C	0.75 mg tid	Peripheral neuropathy, pancreatitis
Abacavir	Ziagen	C	300 mg tid	Gastrointestinal disturbances, skin rash, myalgia
Lamivudine (3Tc)	Epivir	C	300 mg bid	Peripheral neuropathy, skin rash, gastrointestinal disturbances
Zidovudine plus lamivudine	Combivir	C	300 mg bid	Peripheral neuropathy, pancreatitis
Adefovir	Hepsera	C	120 mg/day	Gastrointestinal disturbances, increased liver enzymes, renal toxicity

Food and Drug Administration (FDA) Pregnancy Category: B, animal reproduction studies failed to demonstrate a risk to the fetus; C, safety in human pregnancy has not been determined.

Table 13.11. Antiretroviral drugs (nonnucleoside reverse transcriptase inhibitors) and side effects

Generic Name	Trade Name	FDA Pregnancy Category	Dose	Adverse Side Effects
Nevirapine	Viramune	C	200 mg qd	Gastrointestinal disturbances, increased liver enzymes, skin rash, P-450 enzyme induction
Efavirenz[a]	Sustiva	C	600 mg qd	Skin rash, gastrointestinal disturbances, increased liver enzymes
Delavirdine	Rescriptor	C	400 mg tid	Skin rash, gastrointestinal disturbances, increased liver enzymes

Food and Drug Administration (FDA) Pregnancy Category: C, safety in human pregnancy has not been determined.
[a]Efavirenz should be avoided during the first trimester of pregnancy.

Table 13.12. Antiretroviral drugs (protease inhibitors) and side effects

Generic Name	Trade Name	FDA Pregnancy Category	Dose	Adverse Side Effects
Saquinavir	Invirase Fortovase	C	600 mg tid	Gastrointestinal disturbances, hyperglycemia, lipodystrophy, inhibits cytochrome P-450-isoenzyme (CYP$_3$A)
Indinavir	Crixivan	B	800 mg tid	Gastrointestinal disturbances, hyperglycemia, skin rash, nephrolithiasis, renal failure, unusual distribution of fat, inhibits cytochrome P-450
Ritonavir	Norvir	B	600 mg bid	Gastrointestinal disturbances, hyperglycemia, increased liver enzymes, lipodystrophy, inhibits cytochrome P-450
Nelfinavir	Viracept	C	750 mg tid	Gastrointestinal disturbances, hyperglycemia, lipodystrophy, inhibits cytochrome P-450
Amprenavir	Agenerase	C	1,200 mg bid	Skin rash, inhibits cytochrome P-450

Food and Drug Administration (FDA) Pregnancy Category: B, animal reproduction studies failed to demonstrate a risk to the fetus; C, safety in human pregnancy has not been determined.

exposures that pose an increased risk for transmission. When the source person's virus is known or suspected to be resistant to one or more of the drugs considered for the PEP regimen, the selection of drugs to which the source person's virus is unlikely to be resistant is recommended. Special circumstances (e.g., delayed exposure report, unknown source person, pregnancy in the exposed person, resistance of the source virus to antiretroviral agents, or toxicity of the PEP regimen) require consultation with local experts and/or the National Clinicians' Post-Exposure Prophylaxis Hotline (PEPline: 1-888-448-4911). For more information on this topic visit www.cdc.gov.

REFERENCES

1. ASA Committee on Occupational Health of Operating Room Personnel. Task Force on Latex Sensitivity. Natural Rubber Latex Allergy: Considerations for Anesthesiologists. Park Ridge, IL: American Society of Anesthesiologists; 2005.
2. Hepner DL, Castells MC. Latex allergy: an update. *Anesth Analg.* 2003; 96:1219–1229.
3. Wilson JT. Determinants and consequences of drug excretion in breast milk. *Drug Metab Rev.* 1983;14:619–652.
4. Hale T. Maternal medications during breastfeeding (management of breastfeeding). *Clin Obstet Gynecol.* 2004;47:696–711.
5. Rathwell JP, Visconti CM, Ashburn MA. Management of nonobstetric pain during pregnancy and lactation. *Anesth Analg.* 1997;85:1075–1087.
6. American Academy of Pediatrics. Committee on Drugs. Transfer of drugs and other chemicals into human milk. *Pediatrics.* 2001;108:776–789.
7. Harris AL, Engel TP. Anesthetic challenges and the Jehovah's Witness patient. June 5, 2001. Gasnet Anesthesiology. Available at: http://www.gasnet.org. Accessed December 8, 2006.
8. *Powell vs. Columbia Presbyterian Medical Center,* 49 Misc 2d 215, 216, 267 NYS 2d 450, 452 (Sup Ct NY County, 1965).
9. Associated Jehovah's Witnesses for Reform on Blood. New Light on Blood [homepage]. 2006. Available at: http://www.ajwrb.org. Accessed December 8, 2006.
10. In re EG, a minor. Supreme Court of Illinois No. 66089, November 13, 1989.
11. Christ M, Sharkova Y, Gelder G, et al. Preoperative and perioperative care for patients with suspected or established aortic stenosis facing noncardiac surgery. *Chest.* 2005;128: 2944–2953.
12. Rosenthal RA, Kavic SM. Assessment and management of the geriatric patient. *Crit Care Med.* 2004;32:S92–S105.
13. Fleisher LA, Beckman JA, Brown KA, et al. ACC/AHA guidelines for perioperative cardiovascular evaluation and care for noncardiac surgery. *J Am Coll Cardiac.* 2007;50:e159–241. Available at: http://www.acc.org. Accessed September 28, 2007.
14. Fleisher LA, Pasternak R, Anderson GF. Inpatient hospital admission and death after outpatient surgery in elderly patients: importance of patient and system characteristics and location of care. *Arch Surg.* 2004;139:67–72.

15. Backer CL, Tinker JH, Robertson DM. Myocardial reinfarction following local anesthesia for ophthalmic surgery. *Anesth Analg*. 1980;59:257–262.

16. Schein OD, Katz J, Bass EB, et al. The value of routine preoperative medical testing before cataract surgery. *N Engl J Med*. 2000;342:168–175.

17. Waisel DB. Perioperative do-not-resuscitate orders. *Curr Opin Anaesthesiol*. 2000;13:191–194.

18. Truog RD, Waisel DB. Do-not-resuscitate orders: from the ward to the operating room; from procedures to goals. *Int Anesthesiol Clin*. 2001;30:53–65.

19. Demaria EJ, Carmody BJ. Perioperative management of special populations: obesity. *Surg Clin North Am*. 2005;85:1283–1289.

20. Harter RL, Kelly WB, Kramer MG, et al. A comparison of the volume and pH of gastric contents of obese and lean surgical patients. *Anesth Analg*. 1998;86:147–152.

21. Mark EJ, Patalas ED, Chang HT, et al. Fatal pulmonary hypertension associated with the short-term use of fenfluramine and phentermine. *N Engl J Med*. 1997;337:602–606.

22. Connolly HM, Crary JL, McGoon MD, et al. Valvular heart disease associated with fenfluramine-phentermine. *N Engl J Med*. 1997;337:581–588.

23. Brodsky JB, Lemmens HJ, Brock-Utne JG, et al. Morbid obesity and tracheal intubation. *Anesth Analg*. 2002;94:732–736.

24. Kheterpal S, Han R, Tremper K, et al. Incidence and predictors of difficult and impossible mask ventilation. *Anesthesiology*. 2006;105:885–891.

25. Alpert MA, Fraley MA, Brichem JA, et al. Management of obesity cardiomyopathy. *Expert Rev Cardiovasc Ther*. 2005;3: 225–230.

26. Cartagena R. Preoperative evaluation of patients with obesity and obstructive sleep apnea. *Anesthesiol Clin North Am*. 2005;23: 463–478.

27. Netzer NC, Stoohs RA, Netzer CM, et al. Using the Berlin questionnaire to identify patients at risk for the sleep apnea syndrome. *Ann Intern Med*. 1999;131:485–491.

28. Jain S, Dhand R. Perioperative treatment of patients with obstructive sleep apnea. *Curr Opin Pulm Med*. 2004;10:482–488.

29. American Society of Anesthesiology. Practice guidelines for the perioperative management of patients with obstructive sleep apnea. *Anesthesiology*. 2006;104:1081–1093. Available at: http://www2.asahq.org/publications/p-111-practice-guidelines-for-the-perioperative-management-of-patients-with-obstructive-sleep-apnea.aspx. Accessed December 11, 2006.

30. Desai DM, Kuo PC. Perioperative management of special populations: immunocompromised host (cancer, HIV, transplantation). *Surg Clin North Am*. 2005;85:1267–1282.

31. Schmiesing CA, Fischer SP. The preoperative assessment of the cancer patient. *Curr Opin Anaesthesiol*. 2001;14:721–729.

32. Selim M. Perioperative stroke. *N Engl J Med*. 2007;356:706–713.

33. Lefor AT. Perioperative management of the patient with cancer. *Chest*. 1999;115(Suppl 5):165S–171S.

34. Evron S, Glezerman M, Harow E, et al. Human immunode-ficiency virus: anesthetic and obstetric considerations. *Anesth Analg*. 2004;98:503–511.
35. 2001 Updated U.S. Public Health Service Guidelines for the Management of Occupational Exposures to HBV, HCV, and HIV and Recommendations for Postexposure Prophylaxis. 2001 *MMWR Morb Mortal Wkly Rep*. 50(RR11);1–42.

The Pregnant Patient for Nonobstetric Surgery

Robert Gaiser

Caring for the parturient is one of the most rewarding and challenging aspects of anesthesia as one must consider two patients, the mother and the fetus. Both patients require evaluation in the preoperative period. The mother is the primary patient; the fetus is secondary. In general, optimal evaluation and care of the mother ensures good care of the fetus. Given that many conditions requiring surgery surface during the childbearing years, it is not surprising that the anesthesia care provider is called upon to adequately prepare the parturient for surgery. Pregnancy alters maternal physiology. These changes must be considered when evaluating the pregnant patient and planning the anesthetic.

INCIDENCE OF SURGICAL CONDITIONS

Abdominal pain during pregnancy is not uncommon. Many nonobstetric conditions may result in pain. It is estimated that 1 in 500 pregnancies is complicated by a nonobstetric surgical condition, most commonly appendicitis, cholecystitis, pancreatitis, and bowel obstruction (1). Based on abdominal conditions alone, the predicted incidence would be 0.2%. Nonabdominal conditions that require surgical intervention during pregnancy yield an estimated incidence of 1.5% to 2.0% (2). Unlike other operations in which the patient is primarily concerned with her own safety, the parturient is very concerned about her baby's welfare. This concern must be discussed in the preoperative interview.

EVALUATION OF THE MOTHER

The mother undergoes various changes to meet the increased metabolic demands of pregnancy. Every organ system is affected.

Cardiovascular

Pregnancy increases cardiac output to meet the demands of oxygen consumption of the developing fetus. Cardiac output increases by 40% during pregnancy, increasing most during the first trimester (3). When cardiac output increases, uterine blood flow increases from approximately 50 mL/minute to 500 to 700 mL/minute at term. Cardiac output increases because stroke volume and heart rate increase. Despite the increase in cardiac output, systolic, diastolic, and mean arterial pressures decrease during midpregnancy, returning toward baseline as the pregnancy approaches term. So blood pressure should not increase during pregnancy (4). An increase in blood pressure is abnormal and requires further investigation to rule out preeclampsia (Fig. 14.1).

Maternal blood volume increases during pregnancy by 35% over nonpregnant levels, or an additional 1,500 mL, beginning

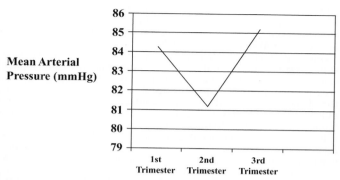

Figure 14.1. Maternal mean arterial pressure decreases during the first trimester and nadirs during the second trimester at which point it returns to normal. (Based on data from Iwasaki R, Ohkuchi A, Furuta I, et al. Relationship between blood pressure level in early pregnancy and subsequent changes in blood pressure during pregnancy. *Acta Obstet Gynecol Scand.* 2002;81:918–925.)

during the first trimester and continuing until mid–third trimester (5). The increase provides a reserve to protect the mother during the blood loss that accompanies childbirth. As the blood volume increases, total peripheral vascular resistance decreases. The central venous pressure and pulmonary artery pressures are similar to those during nonpregnant states (6).

Important preoperative considerations include an awareness that changes in the cardiac physical examination and laboratory studies are normal and have no clinical implications. One may hear a grade II systolic ejection murmur, a murmur that reflects benign flow from increases in intravascular volume and cardiac output. On physical examination, the point of maximal cardiac impulse is displaced cephalad and leftward by the uterus. Because diaphragmatic elevation displaces the heart leftward, it may appear enlarged on chest radiographs. The electrocardiogram shows left axis deviation, again from displacement by an expanding uterus (7).

In the supine position, up to 15% of pregnant patients develop nausea, hypotension, and vomiting (supine hypotensive syndrome) after 24 weeks' gestation. The gravid uterus compresses the inferior cava, restricting venous return to the right atrium and reducing cardiac output. A decrease in blood pressure decreases cerebral perfusion (nausea and lightheadedness) and uterine blood flow. Uterine blood flow decreases if the uterus compresses the aorta, as the uterine artery is a branch of the hypogastric artery. During physical examination, position the patient so that the uterus is displaced off the vena cava and aorta, by placing a wedge underneath her right hip.

Respiratory

The maternal airway changes during gestation. Vascular engorgement of the airway swells the larynx and pharynx. When parturients had their airways examined at 12 weeks' gestation and then again at 36 weeks' gestation, the percentage of patients with a Mallampati class 4 airway had doubled (8). As gestation advances, the airway examination reveals less visible structures and a higher Mallampati score (Fig. 14.2).

A gravid uterus elevates the diaphragm 4 cm, decreasing expiratory reserve volume and residual volume (both are components of functional residual capacity). Diaphragmatic elevation may increase lung markings, mimicking mild congestive heart failure on the chest radiograph (9). Minute ventilation increases by 30% during the first trimester and peaks at 70% during the third trimester (10). This increase results primarily from increased tidal volume and increased respiratory rate. Arterial blood gas analysis reveals hypocarbia but minimal respiratory alkalosis because the kidneys compensate by excreting more bicarbonate. A decline in bicarbonate concentration is evident on the preoperative chemistry panel. On physical examination, parturients appear dyspneic from an increased respiratory rate. In fact, 60% to 70% of parturients have mild intermittent dyspnea.

Gastrointestinal

The enlarged gravid uterus displaces the stomach cephalad. Displacement changes the angle of the gastroesophageal junction, decreasing competence of the gastroesophageal sphincter. The uterus also displaces the pylorus upward and posteriorly, delaying gastric emptying. Elevated concentrations of progesterone decrease gastrointestinal motility and food absorption. Given these changes, many anesthesia care providers treat all pregnant women as if they had a full stomach and give appropriate prophylaxis preoperatively (nonparticulate antacids, metoclopramide, cimetidine/ranitidine). Not all providers agree with this position.

In 1946, Mendelson reported 66 cases of aspiration of stomach contents during obstetric anesthesia (11). Of these patients, five aspirated solid material and were excluded from further analysis; 21 were subsequently diagnosed as having aspirated (the

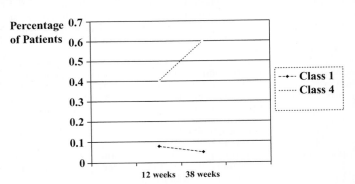

Figure 14.2.   The percentage with Mallampati score 1 decreases as the pregnancy progresses. The exact opposite occurs with Mallampati score 4 increases. (Based on data from Pilkington S, Carli F, Dakin MJ, et al. Increase in Mallampati score during pregnancy. *Br J Anaesth.* 1995;74:638–642.)

delayed diagnosis also excluded the group from further analysis), and 40 aspirated liquid material. The 40 parturients who aspirated liquid material had a stormy course for 36 to 48 hours, but all survived. The term *Mendelson syndrome* is used to describe pneumonitis accompanying aspiration. Researchers then focused on quantifying the volume and pH of a solution that causes fatality in an animal model. This research led to the development of strategies to reduce gastric volume and increase gastric pH.

Recent studies question the theory that gastric emptying is delayed and gastrin concentration is increased. When gastric emptying times were measured in 11 women during the first trimester, third trimester, and postpartum, there was no difference between first trimester and postpartum (12). Gastrointestinal transit time was significantly longer in the third trimester. Thus, despite hormonal changes, it seems that gastric emptying is affected only in the third trimester and during labor, not earlier in pregnancy. In another study, the gastric contents of 100 term parturients were aspirated via a nasogastric tube before cesarean section and compared with the contents from 100 nonpregnant women scheduled for gynecologic surgery. The gastric volume in the pregnant group at term was greater than that in the nonpregnant group. However, serum gastrin levels did not differ between the groups (13). Unlike previously thought, serum gastrin levels are not more elevated in the parturient.

The Closed Claims Database contains most malpractice claims that have been settled involving anesthesiologists. When obstetric claims were compared to nonobstetric claims, aspiration was more common in the former (14). In fact, 5% of the obstetric claims were for aspiration as compared to 1% of nonobstetric claims. There are several shortcomings to this database. Only complications resulting in a malpractice claim are included and because complications that do not result in a lawsuit are not included, actual incidence is not represented. Some conclusions to be drawn from these data are that the incidence of aspiration in the parturient is increased and that obstetric patients are more likely to sue or general surgical patients are less likely to sue. The important point is that this type of research does not confirm a higher incidence of aspiration in pregnant patients.

A 4-year audit of gynecologic and obstetric patients who developed aspiration pneumonitis was performed (15). Aspiration pneumonitis was diagnosed if an episode of gastric contents entering the trachea was witnessed or an intraoperative episode made pulmonary aspiration likely. Eleven cases were identified, four in parturients and seven in women undergoing gynecologic procedures, yielding an incidence of developing aspiration pneumonitis of 0.11% in the obstetric population and 0.04% in the gynecologic population.

Another study examined obstetric procedures performed in the peripartum period, excluding cesarean section. The study identified 1,870 patients who had general anesthesia but were not intubated (16). In this series, there was only a single case of mild aspiration. This incidence, 0.053%, is comparable to that in the general surgical population. These results challenge the idea that pregnant women who undergo general anesthesia (excluding cesarean section) require an endotracheal tube. All pregnant patients undergoing nonobstetric surgery do not require rapid sequence induction and intubation.

Gastric emptying is not delayed until the third trimester. At term, gastric volume is greater but not early in the pregnancy. Serum levels of gastrin are not elevated. During their first and second trimester, parturients should be treated like nonpregnant women. If the parturient has symptomatic reflux, aspiration prophylaxis is required. If the patient is asymptomatic, aspiration prophylaxis is not required. During the third trimester, it is prudent to administer aspiration prophylaxis, although the literature does not support this recommendation.

Hematologic Changes

Plasma volume increases 45%, but the red cell mass increases only 20%, leading to the dilutional anemia of pregnancy. The maternal hemoglobin concentration is lower than in the nonpregnant state, but it should not be <11 g/dL. A maternal hemoglobin concentration <11 g/dL is abnormal. The most common cause of anemia during pregnancy is iron deficiency (17).

Platelet counts are usually elevated but decreases are possible without other hematologic pathology. Gestational thrombocytopenia results when platelets are destroyed. This normal response becomes exaggerated in patients with gestational thrombocytopenia (18). Given this risk, a platelet count should be obtained in all parturients. Pregnancy produces a hypercoagulable state as evident from the increase in deep vein thrombosis and pulmonary embolism. All coagulation factors except factors XI and XIII increase in concentration (19). Parturients undergoing nonobstetric surgery probably will receive anticoagulation prophylaxis postoperatively for deep vein thrombosis. This prophylaxis must be incorporated in the preoperative anesthesia plan.

Endocrine

In the majority of parturients, serum glucose concentration remains within the normal range. The placenta secretes human placental lactogen, a hormone that renders the parturient relatively resistant to insulin. The thyroid gland enlarges 50% to 70% during pregnancy, which may be detected upon physical examination (20). Concentrations of total thyroxine increase, but concentrations of free thyroxine and triiodothyronine do not change because thyroid-binding globulin increases.

Renal

Renal plasma flow and glomerular filtration rate (GFR) increase during the first trimester, achieving a level 50% over normal by the fourth month. The increases in renal plasma flow and GFR result in an increased creatinine clearance and decreased blood urea nitrogen (BUN) and creatinine (Cr) (21). BUN decreases 40% to 8 to 9 mg/dL; Cr decreases to 0.4 to 0.5 mg/dL. A BUN of 15 mg/dL, a serum Cr of 1.0 mg/dL, or a Cr clearance of 100 mL/minute suggest abnormal renal function in pregnant women who are near term and the need for further evaluation. Proteinuria, up to 300 mg/day, is common.

A summary of the preoperative considerations is presented in Table 14.1.

Table 14.1.   Preoperative implications of the physiologic changes of pregnancy

Organ System	Physiologic Change	Preoperative Implication
Cardiovascular	Increased cardiac output	Possible grade II systolic ejection murmur
	Enlarging uterus	1. Displaced point of maximal cardiac impulse
		2. Supine hypotensive syndrome
Respiratory	Swelling of the airway	Increased probability of Mallampati class III or IV airway
	Enlarging uterus	1. Displaced diaphragm cephalad
		2. Increased lung markings on radiography
	Increased minute ventilation	1. Increased respiratory rate
		2. Possible dyspnea
		3. Decreased $PaCO_2$
Gastrointestinal	Enlarging uterus	Full stomach precautions during third trimester
Hematologic	Increased plasma volume and red cell mass	Anemia (Hemoglobin = 11 g/dL)
	Increased coagulation factors (except XI and XIII)	Deep venous thrombosis prophylaxis postoperatively
Renal	Increased renal plasma flow and glomerular filtration rate	Decreased blood urea nitrogen (8–9 g/dL) and creatinine (0.4–0.5 g/dL)

PREOPERATIVE EVALUATION OF THE FETUS

There are many ways to evaluate the fetus. With an ultrasound the fetus can be examined and the amount of amniotic fluid can be determined. The most common means for evaluating the fetus is by fetal heart rate (FHR) monitoring, whose purpose is to ensure that the fetus is well oxygenated. In the fetus, the brain modulates the heart and hypoxemia is reflected in the FHR. The FHR is monitored in two ways, external or internal. The external monitor uses a Doppler device that is placed on the maternal abdomen. When properly placed over the fetal heart, a computerized program interprets and counts Doppler signals. The internal monitor has an electrode that is applied to the fetal scalp to record the heart rate. Internal monitoring requires rupture of the amniotic membranes and is only used during labor.

In 1997, the National Institute of Child Health and Human Development proposed definitions for the interpretation of the FHR (22). This group classified various decelerations in FHR during uterine contraction: Early—nadir with peak of the contraction; late—onset and nadir after onset and peak of contraction; variable—an abrupt decrease in FHR. The other important criterion was baseline variability or the amplitude of peak-to-trough in beats per minute (Fig. 14.3). Three decades earlier, Lee and Hon had demonstrated that variable decelerations of FHR were associated with umbilical cord compression. In their study of babies delivered via cesarean section, the umbilical cord was delivered first and then compressed. FHR dropped markedly with compression. The association of depressed neonates with late decelerations in the FHR led to the proposed mechanism of uteroplacental insufficiency. Pressure on the neonate's head, which induced a decrease in heart rate, led to the association of head compression and early deceleration (23).

The purpose of FHR monitoring is to ensure the well-being of the fetus. A normal tracing (i.e., a baseline of 110 to 160 bpm, regular rate, presence of accelerations, presence of variability, and

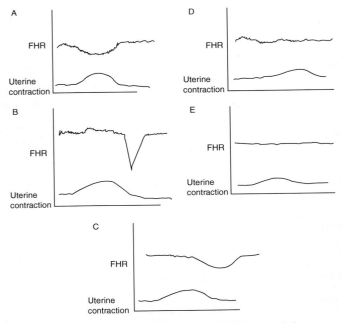

Figure 14.3.   A: Early decelerations are a mirror image of the contraction. B: Variable decelerations have an abrupt onset and offset and can occur in any relation to the contraction. C: Late decelerations are delayed with respect to the uterine contraction. D: Fetal variability is an indicator of fetal well-being. E: Absence of variability is a possible indicator of poor fetal status.

absence of periodic decelerations) is associated with a healthy, well-oxygenated fetus (24). A question arises when the tracing is not perfect because FHR patterns that accurately predict asphyxia have not been specified. A nonreassuring tracing as an indication of fetal hypoxia has a false-positive rate >99% (25).

The use of continuous FHR monitoring was compared to intermittent auscultation during labor in 504 patients. Auscultation was applied every 15 minutes during or immediately following a uterine contraction. No significant difference was found between the two groups in neonatal deaths, Apgar scores, maternal and neonatal morbidity, and cord blood gases. The only difference was the higher cesarean section rate in the continuously monitored group (26). Certain fetal patterns were associated with fetal acidosis, decreased uterine perfusion, and fetal hypoxemia (27). The presence of late decelerations correlated with fetal acidosis (28). Finally, another FHR parameter associated with acidosis is decreased baseline variability. In 186 term gestations subjected to continuous FHR monitoring, decreased variability in the 1 hour before delivery was significantly correlated with low pH (29). Despite these strong associations with fetal acidosis, the role of FHR monitoring in reducing morbidity and mortality remains to be proven.

Given the lack of proven efficacy in decreasing birth injury and in reducing neonatal morbidity, the use of fetal monitoring during maternal surgery is a hotly debated topic. After 18 to 20 weeks' gestation, the FHR can be monitored. The argument for intraoperative fetal monitoring is that it can improve fetal outcome. When changes in the FHR signal compromise of the uteroplacental circulation, the anesthesia provider can take steps to improve uteroplacental perfusion and fetal oxygenation. The maneuvers may include increasing left uterine displacement, increasing inspired concentration of oxygen, adjusting maternal ventilation, augmenting maternal circulating blood volume, or managing hypotension with drugs. Despite these possible interventions, no study has examined FHR monitoring during surgery. Still, if FHR monitoring has no effect on neonatal outcome during labor (except for increasing the cesarean section rate), it probably has little impact on fetal outcome during maternal surgery. The use of FHR monitoring during surgery is not universally applied. When hospitals in the United States were surveyed regarding monitoring, 184 hospitals responded and 60% routinely used fetal monitors; 40% did not (30). In another study that reviewed case reports of nonobstetric surgery during pregnancy, the authors concluded that intraoperative monitoring by obstetric personnel was unnecessary, recommending instead that the FHR and uterine activity be checked before and after surgery (31). Checking the FHR preoperatively documents a live fetus. It also ensures that the fetus is doing well. The American College of Obstetricians and Gynecologists endorses the consideration of FHR monitoring for preoperative evaluation (32): "It is important for physicians to obtain obstetric consultation before performing nonobstetric surgery because obstetricians are uniquely qualified to discuss aspects of maternal physiology and anatomy that may affect intraoperative maternal and fetal well-being. The decision to use fetal monitoring should be individualized and if used, may be based on gestational age, type of surgery, and facilities available. Ultimately, each case warrants a team approach for optimal safety of the woman and her baby." According to the guideline, the obstetrician must be consulted preoperatively. This important step is often forgotten. The obstetrician will evaluate the fetus for the anesthesia provider by measuring FHR and by ultrasound.

COUNSELING THE PARTURIENT PREOPERATIVELY

Teratogenicity of Anesthetic Agents

The greatest concern for the parturient is the effect of anesthetic agents on the fetus and on the risk of congenital anomalies. All anesthetic agents have been implicated as a teratogen in animals. For a teratogenic effect, the mother must be exposed to a given level of drug for a specific time period at a specific point in the gestation. It is clear that the animal model does not replicate the clinical situation because these studies document exposures at amounts greater than would be used clinically. To assess the teratogenicity of general anesthesia, population studies are needed.

Snider and Webster were the first to study the effect of anesthesia and surgery during pregnancy (33). They evaluated the medical records of 9,073 women who delivered infants between July 1959 and August 1964. Of these women, 147 parturients (1.6%) had surgery during pregnancy. Incidence of congenital anomalies in the surgical group did not increase, but the authors noted that the majority of parturients received anesthesia during the second or third trimester (after the period of organogenesis in the first trimester). For those parturients who had surgery during the first trimester, multiple techniques and agents were used, making conclusions difficult. Brodsky et al. had a different approach, mailing a questionnaire to dentists and dental assistants to identify pregnant women who underwent surgery during pregnancy or who had occupational exposure to nitrous oxide or volatile agents (34). Of the 287 women who had surgery during pregnancy, 187 had surgery during the first trimester. A larger number, 3,624 parturients, had occupational exposure only. There was no major difference in the incidence of congenital anomalies in infants born to women who had surgery during pregnancy or those born to a control group who did not have surgery. Congenital anomalies in infants born to women with occupational exposure did not increase. Duncan et al. reviewed the health insurance data from the province of Manitoba from 1971 to 1978 (35). They matched 2,565 women who had surgery during pregnancy to those of similar height and weight who did not. There was no difference in the rate of congenital anomalies between the two groups. When Mazze and Kallen examined cases from three Swedish health care registries for the years 1973 to 1981, they identified 5,405 women who underwent surgery during pregnancy. Among these women, 65% received general anesthesia. Of these parturients, 2,248 had surgery during the first trimester (36). In this study, which represents the largest examination of surgery during the period of organogenesis (the period of the greatest risk of teratogenicity), no increased incidence of congenital anomalies was found.

Another method to determine the effect of anesthetic agents on congenital anomalies is to consider anomalies to find a link to anesthesia (37). Of the 20,830 pregnant women who had offspring with a congenital anomaly, 31 patients had surgery and anesthesia. This fraction did not differ when compared to the 35,727 women who had babies without defects, of whom 73 had surgery during pregnancy. There was no higher incidence of surgery and anesthesia for any group with congenital anomaly.

Despite these data, the status of nitrous oxide as a reproductive toxin continues to be debated. Nitrous oxide, a teratogen in animals, inhibits methionine synthetase, an enzyme necessary for folate metabolism (38). In their database, Kallen and Mazze noted six infants with neural tube defects (39). This number, is much higher than the expected incidence of 1 per 1,000 births. The authors postulated nitrous oxide as a possible cause, although the numbers and exposure do not support this proposition. Another study examined infants born with central nervous system defects in Atlanta between 1968 and 1980 who were matched to controls by race, birth hospital, and period of birth (40). Of the 694 mothers of infants with central nervous system defects, 12 reported first-trimester anesthesia exposure. Of the 2,984 mothers in the control group, 34 reported such exposure, yielding an odds ratio of 1.7, confidence interval (CI) 0.8 to 33 (not statistically significant). The odds ratio increased to 39.6 (CI, 7.5 to 208.2), however, when infants with hydrocephalus and eye defects were examined. There were eight infants with this defect, three of whom had first-trimester exposure to anesthetic agents. The suggested link is based on extremely small numbers.

In a study in rats exposed to normal amounts of anesthesia for a normal period, widespread apoptotic neurodegeneration was noted in the developing brain (41). The rats were exposed to midazolam, nitrous oxide, and isoflurane in doses sufficient to maintain a surgical plane of anesthesia for 6 hours. The greatest risk was during the synaptogenesis period, also known as the brain growth spurt period. In a fetus, this period starts in the third trimester. If the study in rats can be applied to women, anesthesia during the third trimester may affect the fetal brain.

There is scant literature supporting a risk of anesthesia on congenital anomalies. No population study has ever been able to find a link. Only two studies suggest a possible cause, both with extremely low numbers of affected children. It seems unlikely that a link exists. When discussing the risk of anesthesia with pregnant women scheduled for surgery, the anesthesia provider should remind the patient that there is a 3% baseline incidence of fetal anomalies among all pregnant women.

Preterm Labor

Preterm labor remains a problem after abdominal or pelvic surgery. The increase in preterm labor is more a consequence of the surgical procedure than the anesthetic because no increase follows orthopedic or neck surgery. In the preoperative period, it may be helpful to monitor uterine contraction frequency with a tocodynamometer. If the patient is in labor before the surgical procedure, the obstetrician may consider the administration of tocolytics.

The first to report an increased risk of preterm labor or miscarriage with surgery during pregnancy was Duncan et al., who reviewed health insurance data from the province of Manitoba from 1971 to 1978 (35). These authors matched 2,565 women who had surgery during pregnancy with those of similar height and weight who did not. The risk of spontaneous abortion increased in those undergoing surgery for gynecologic procedures in the first or second trimester. Mazze and Kallen examined cases from three Swedish health care registries for the years 1973 to 1981 (36). Of the 5,405 women who underwent surgery during pregnancy, the incidence of low-birth-weight infants increased, primarily from premature delivery. Given this large database, the authors were able to examine a specific procedure, appendectomy, the most common surgical procedure performed on parturients. In the group of 778 parturients who underwent appendectomy, the risk of delivery increased, especially the week after surgery (42). The authors proved that the procedure, rather than the anesthetic, increased the risk of premature labor. Further studies have verified their results. In a study of 77 consecutive parturients who had abdominal surgery, preterm labor was most common in patients with appendicitis or after adnexal surgery. The risk was greatest for third-trimester surgeries (43). Parturients counseled preoperatively should be made aware that they have the greatest risk of developing preterm labor after abdominal surgery. This risk is highest for patients in the third trimester but is elevated for both the first and second trimester.

CONCLUSIONS

Parturients will continue to require surgery during pregnancy. A firm knowledge of the physiologic changes of pregnancy is necessary for effective evaluation of the parturient. An obstetrician must be consulted preoperatively to evaluate the fetus. The obstetrician may do an ultrasound and will examine the fetal heart rate. To appropriately counsel the mother, the anesthesia provider should have an understanding of teratogenicity and preterm labor because these two conditions represent the major concern of the parturient.

REFERENCES

1. Angelini DJ. Obstetric triage revisited: update on non-obstetric surgical conditions in pregnancy. *J Midwifery Women Health*. 2003;48:111–118.
2. Kuczkowski KM. Nonobstetric surgery during pregnancy: what are the risks of anesthesia? *Obstet Gynecol Surv*. 2003;59: 52–56.
3. Capeless EL, Clapp JF. Cardiovascular changes in early phase of pregnancy. *Am J Obstet Gynecol*. 1989;161:1449–1453.
4. Iwasaki R, Ohkuchi A, Furuta I, et al. Relationship between blood pressure level in early pregnancy and subsequent changes in blood pressure during pregnancy. *Acta Obstet Gynecol Scand*. 2002;81:918–925.
5. Lund CJ, Donovan JC. Blood volume during pregnancy. Significance of plasma and red cell volumes. *Am J Obstet Gynecol*. 1967;98:394–403.
6. Cotton DB, Benedetti TJ. Use of the Swan-Ganz catheter in obstetrics and gynecology. *Obstet Gynecol*. 1980;56:641–645.

7. Sullivan JM, Ramanathan KB. Management of medical problems in pregnancy—severe cardiac disease. *N Engl J Med*. 1985;313:304–309.

8. Pilkington S, Carli F, Dakin MJ, et al. Increase in Mallampati score during pregnancy. *Br J Anaesth*. 1995;74:638–642.

9. Pilsczek FH, George L. Unilateral paralysis of the diaphragm during pregnancy: case report and literature review. *Heart Lung*. 2005;34:282–287.

10. Martin C, Varner MW. Physiologic changes in pregnancy: surgical implication. *Clin Obstet Gynecol*. 1994;37:241–255.

11. Mendelson CL. The aspiration of stomach contents into the lungs during obstetric anesthesia. *Am J Obstet Gynecol*. 1946;52:191–204.

12. Chiloiro M, Darconza G, Piccioli E, et al. Gastric emptying and orocecal transit time in pregnancy. *J Gastroenterol*. 2001;36:538–543.

13. Hong JY, Park JW, Oh JI. Comparison of preoperative gastric contents and serum gastrin concentrations in pregnant and nonpregnant women. *J Clin Anesth*. 2005;17:451–455.

14. Chadwick HS. Obstetric anesthesia closed claims update II. *ASA Newsletter*. 1999;63:6.

15. Soreide E, Bjornestad E, Steen PA. An audit of perioperative aspiration pneumonitis in gynaecological and obstetric patients. *Acta Anaesthesiol Scand*. 1996;40:14–19.

16. Ezri T, Szmuk P, Stein A, et al. Peripartum general anesthesia without tracheal intubation: incidence of aspiration pneumonia. *Anaesthesia*. 2000;55:421–426.

17. Schwartz WJ III, Thurnau GR. Iron deficiency anemia in pregnancy. *Clin Obstet Gynecol*. 1995;38:443–454.

18. Sainio S, Kekomaki R, Riikonen S, et al. Maternal thrombocytopenia at term: a population-based study. *Acta Obstet Gynecol Scand*. 2000;79:744–749.

19. Hellgren M. Hemostasis during normal pregnancy and puerperium. *Sem Thromb Hemost*. 2003;29:125–130.

20. Sack J. Thyroid function in pregnancy—maternal-fetal relationship in health and disease. *Pediatr Endocr Rev*. 2003;1(Suppl 2):170–176.

21. Dafnis E, Sabatini S. The effect of pregnancy on renal function: physiology and pathophysiology. *Am J Med Sci*. 1992;303:184–205.

22. Electronic fetal heart rate monitoring: research guidelines for interpretation. National Institute of Child Health and Human Development Research Planning Workshop. *Am J Obstet Gynecol*. 1997;177:1385–1390.

23. Goodlin RC. History of fetal monitoring. *Am J Obstet Gynecol*. 1979;133:323–352.

24. Ellison PH, Foster M, Sheridan-Pereira M, et al. Electronic fetal heart monitoring: auscultation and neonatal outcome. *Am J Obstet Gynecol*. 1991;164:1281–1289.

25. American College of Obstetricians and Gynecologists. ACOG Practice Bulletin Number 62. Intrapartum Fetal Heart Rate Monitoring. *Obstet Gynecol*. 2005;105:1161–1167.

26. Kelso IM, Parsons RJ, Lawrence GF, et al. An assessment of continuous fetal heart rate monitoring: a randomized trial. *Am J Obstet Gynecol*. 1978;131:526–532.

27. Hadar A, Sheiner E, Hallak M, et al. Abnormal fetal heart rate tracing patterns during the first stage of labor: effect on perinatal outcome. *Am J Obstet Gynecol.* 2001;185:863–868.

28. Sheiner E, Hadar A, Hallak M, et al. Clinical significance of fetal heart rate tracings during the second stage of labor. *Obstet Gynecol.* 2001;97:747–752.

29. Williams KP, Galerneau F. Fetal heart rate parameters predictive of neonatal outcome in the presence of a prolonged deceleration. *Obstet Gynecol.* 2002;100:951–954.

30. Kendrick JM, Woodard CB, Cross SB. Surveyed use of fetal and uterine monitoring during maternal surgery. *AORN J.* 1995;62:386–392.

31. Horrigan TJ, Villarred R, Weinstein L. Are obstetrical personnel required for intraoperative fetal monitoring during nonobstetric surgery? *J Perinatol.* 1999;19:124–126.

32. American College of Obstetricians and Gynecologists. ACOG Committee Opinion 284. Nonobstetric surgery in pregnancy. *Obstet Gynecol.* 2003;102:431.

33. Shnider SM, Webster GM. Maternal and fetal hazards of surgery during pregnancy. *Am J Obstet Gynecol.* 1965;92:891–900.

34. Brodsky JB, Cohen EN, Brown BW, et al. Surgery during pregnancy and fetal outcome. *Am J Obstet Gynecol.* 1980;138:1165–1167.

35. Duncan PG, Pope WDB, Cohen MM, et al. Fetal risk of anesthesia and surgery during pregnancy. *Anesthesiology.* 1986;64:790–794.

36. Mazze RI, Kallen B. Reproductive outcome after anesthesia and operation during pregnancy: a registry study of 5405 cases. *Am J Obstet Gynecol.* 1989;161:1178–1185.

37. Czeizel AE, Pataki T, Rockenbauer M. Reproductive outcome after exposure to surgery under anesthesia during pregnancy. *Arch Gynecol Obstet.* 1998;261:193–199.

38. Koblin DD, Waskel L, Watson JE, et al. Nitrous oxide inactivates methionine synthetase in human liver. *Anesth Analg.* 1982;61:75–78.

39. Kallen B, Mazze RI. Neural tube defects and first trimester operations. *Teratology.* 1990;41:717.

40. Sylvester GC, Khoury MJ, Lu X, et al. First-trimester anesthesia exposure and the risk of central nervous system defects: a population based case-control study. *Am J Public Health.* 1994;84:1757–1760.

41. Jevtovic-Todorovic V, Hartman RE, Izumi Y, et al. Early exposure to common anesthetic agents causes widespread neurodegeneration in the developing rat brain and persistent learning deficits. *J Neurosci.* 2003;23:876–882.

42. Mazze RI, Kallen B. Appendectomy during pregnancy: a Swedish registry study of 778 cases. *Obstet Gynecol.* 1991;77:835–840.

43. Visser BC, Glasgow RE, Mulvihill KK, et al. Safety and timing of nonobstetric abdominal surgery in pregnancy. *Dig Surg.* 2001;18:409–417.

15

The Pediatric Patient

Lynne R. Ferrari

The objective of the preoperative evaluation of the pediatric surgical patient is to gather medical information and alleviate the fear and anxiety of the child and family. Parents are often more concerned with the risks and administration of anesthesia for their children than for themselves. The preoperative visit is an opportunity for the anesthesiologist to evaluate the child's psychological status and family interactions.

PSYCHOLOGICAL PREPARATION

Diseases carry with them different psychosocial aspects for children than for adults. For many healthy children who undergo elective surgery, the emotional disruption may surpass the medical issues (1). Children respond to the prospect of surgery in a varied and age-dependent manner, and the anesthesiologist must consider this during the preoperative interview.

The understanding of and response to illness is affected by a child's maturity. The medical practitioner should anticipate the child's needs and concerns and be able to interpret the child's nonverbal expressions and actions when the child's communication skills are not highly developed. The toddler's greatest fear is the loss of control of actions and choices. Helping a child make choices in the health care setting is important. A choice as simple as "What flavor air would you like in the mask?" puts the toddler in control. The preschooler fears injury, loss of control, the unknown, and abandonment. The preschooler interprets words literally and is unable to differentiate between what is heard and what is implied. The words adults use with children are as important as the messages they try to convey. Telling a preschooler that he or she is going to be "put to sleep" for an operation may be scary and confusing for a child whose pet was recently "put to sleep." Because preschoolers are unable to distinguish between reality and fantasy and exist in a world of magical thinking, they cannot recognize the difference between safe sleep during anesthesia and the kind of "sleep" from which their animal did not awaken. The school-aged child fears loss of control, injury, inability to meet the expectations of adults, and death. Between the ages of 6 and 12, children begin to think more logically; yet they may nod with understanding and listen intently, when in fact they do not fully grasp the explanation. These children may fail to ask questions or admit a lack of knowledge because they feel that they should know the information. Adolescents fear loss of control, an altered body image, and segregation from peers. They are usually convinced that the anesthesiologist will not be able to put them to sleep and that, if the anesthesiologist does succeed, they will never wake up (2) (Table 15.1).

Table 15.1. Developmental considerations during preoperative preparation

Characteristics	Strategy for Preparation
1- to 4-year-olds	
• Magical thinking • Ability to understand, but perhaps not able to verbalize thoughts • Egocentric • Preoccupied with guilt and blame • Trust in primary caregiver	• Due to limited sense of time, offer preparation no more than 2 days in advance. • Use of real objects helps build mastery of the situation. • Repetition of key ideas and words is essential. • Reinforcement of good behavior is necessary. • Keep parent with child at all times if possible.
4- to 10-year-olds	
• Beginning to think logically and understand that there is an inside to the body • Communicate verbally with ease • Mastery of skills • Seek control of decisions • Enthusiastic learner	• Preparation can be offered 1–2 weeks in advance. • Offer time for questions. • Use simplistic, but somewhat medical, terms. • Use concrete teaching materials and equipment, such as diagrams and pictures. • Offer reassurance that although one part of the body is sick, the whole body is not sick.
10-year-olds and older	
• Thought is technical • Need for independence • Search for privacy • May oppose or disagree with parents • Peer pressure • Angry at illness • May fight authority, but seek reassurance and approval	• Prepare the patient as soon as the diagnosis is made. • Involve teen in the process of decision making. • Respect privacy issues. • Respect body image and fear of being seen nude. • Offer explanations in clear, technical terms. • Support need for control and independence. • Encourage confidentiality (even the exclusion of parents from certain information). • Allow control within limits.

**Table 15.2.   Minor anesthesia-related risks
in pediatric patients**

Event	Risk per 1,000
Laryngospasm	
0–9 yr of age	17
Concomitant respiratory infection	96
Previous anesthetic complications	55
Bronchospasm	
0–9 yr of age	4
Concomitant respiratory infection	41
ASA physical status score 3 or 4	24
Aspiration pneumonia	1.7
Postoperative vomiting	60

ASA, American Society of Anesthesiologists.

RISKS OF ANESTHESIA

Parents may ask about the risks of anesthesia for their child. As with all patients, this matter must be considered on an individual basis, with the child's age, type of surgery, and other confounding factors taken into account (3) (Table 15.2). Parents are most concerned with the risk of death, which occurs at a rate of 1 in 185,000 healthy children. Most deaths in children due entirely to anesthesia occur in the first week of life (3).

HISTORY AND REVIEW OF SYSTEMS

The medical history for pediatric patients begins with a description of the **prenatal period** since events during pregnancy and delivery may influence the current state of health (Table 15.3).

- If the child was admitted to the neonatal intensive care unit after birth, specific conditions should be ruled out (4) (Tables 15.4 and 15.5).
- Previous surgical experiences or medical admissions to the hospital should be noted. A complete review of systems should be completed, with particular attention to the items listed in Table 15.6 (5).

The child's **prior anesthetic experience** should be explored during the preoperative visit.

- What was the child's reaction to previous anesthetics?
- Which techniques were successful or which should be avoided?
- Was anesthesia induced with a mask?
- Was the parent present during induction?
- Was the induction difficult?
- Were any sequelae noted after the hospital experience, such as nightmares, bad dreams, regression to earlier behavior, or new fears of odors?
- Will the child probably require premedication?

Table 15.3. Neonatal problems commonly associated with maternal history

Neonatal Problem	Maternal History
Hemolytic anemia	Rh-ABO incompatibility
Hyperbilirubinemia	
Kernicterus	
Small for gestational age	Toxemia, drug addiction
Drug withdrawal	Drug addiction
Sepsis	Maternal infection
Thrombocytopenia	
Viral infection	
Anemia	Hemorrhage
Hypotension	
Shock	
Hypoglycemia	Maternal diabetes mellitus
Birth trauma	
Large for gestational age	
Tracheoesophageal fistula	Polyhydramnios
Anencephaly	
Multiple anomalies	
Renal hypoplasia	Oligohydramnios
Pulmonary hypoplasia	
Birth trauma	Cephalopelvic disproportion
Hyperbilirubinemia	
Fractures	
Hypoglycemia	Alcoholism
Congenital malformations	
Fetal alcohol syndrome	
Small for gestational age	

Adapted with permission from Cote C, Ryan J, Todres ID, et al., eds. *A Practice of Anesthesia for Infants and Children*. Philadelphia: WB Saunders; 1993.

Family history regarding anesthesia-related events should be explored.

- Is there a history of hepatitis or liver problems after anesthesia in a family member?
- Is there a history of malignant hyperthermia in a family member?
- Is there a history of prolonged paralysis or mechanical ventilation after general anesthesia in family members indicating a possibility of pseudocholinesterase deficiency? Simple blood tests can measure plasma cholinesterase levels and dibucaine number to determine if that child is at risk (see Chapter 16).
- Is there a history of unexpected death, sudden infant death syndrome, genetic defects, or familial conditions such as muscular dystrophy, cystic fibrosis, sickle cell disease, bleeding tendencies, or human immunodeficiency virus infection?

Table 15.4. Problems in the premature infant

Problem	Anesthetic Concern
Intraventricular hemorrhage	Presence of ventriculoperitoneal shunt
Retinopathy of prematurity	Strict attention to inspired oxygen concentration
Patent ductus arteriosus	Need for prior surgical intervention
Bronchopulmonary dysplasia	Respiratory compromise
Necrotizing enterocolitis	Ostomy/malabsorption
Anemia	Perioperative oxygen-carrying capacity
Hypoglycemia	Choice of intravenous fluid
Hyperbilirubinemia	Possibility of prior transfusion
Sepsis	Hemodynamic instability, respiratory compromise, multiorgan failure
Hypothermia	Adjustment of operating room environment
Apnea and bradycardia	Postanesthetic monitoring
Social problems	Parental concerns

Table 15.5. Potential medical problems associated with admission to the neonatal intensive care unit

Condition	Potential Problem
Esophageal atresia	Tracheoesophageal fistula
	Esophageal dysmotility
Diaphragmatic hernia	Pulmonary hypertension
	Hypoplastic lungs
	Congenital heart disease
Myelodysplasia	Hydrocephalus
	Urogenital disease
	Latex allergy
Omphalocele/gastroschisis	Associated midline defects
	Congenital cardiac abnormalities
	Small abdominal cavity
	Poor body temperature maintenance
Tracheoesophageal fistula	Cardiac defects
	Musculoskeletal abnormalities

Adapted from Badgwell JM, ed. *Clinical Pediatric Anesthesia*. Philadelphia: Lippincott–Raven Publishers; 1997.

Table 15.6.   Systems approach to questioning

System	Focus of Questions	Possible Anesthetic Concerns
Respiratory	Cough, asthma, recent cold	Irritable airway, bronchospasm, atelectasis, pneumonia
Cardiovascular	Murmur, cyanosis, history of squatting, hypertension, rheumatic fever, exercise intolerance	Avoidance of air bubbles in IV, right-to-left shunt, tetralogy of Fallot, coarctation, renal disease, congestive heart failure, cyanosis, infective endocarditis prophylaxis
Neurologic	Seizures, head trauma, swallowing problems	Medication interactions, metabolic derangement, increased intracranial pressure, aspiration, neuromuscular relaxant sensitivity, hyperpyrexia
Gastrointestinal/hepatic	Vomiting, diarrhea, malabsorption, black stool, gastroesophageal reflux, jaundice	Electrolyte imbalance, dehydration, full stomach considerations (rapid-sequence induction), anemia, hypovolemia, hypoglycemia
Genitourinary	Frequency, time of last urination, frequency of urinary tract infections	Infection, hypercalcemia, hydration status, adequacy of renal function
Endocrine-metabolic	Abnormal development, hypoglycemia, steroid therapy	Endocrinopathy, hypothyroidism, diabetes mellitus, hypoglycemia, adrenal insufficiency
Hematologic	Anemia, bruising, excess bleeding	Transfusion requirement, coagulopathy, thrombocytopenia, hydration status, possible exchange transfusion
Allergy	Medications	Drug interactions
Dental	Loose teeth, carious teeth	Aspiration of loose teeth, infective endocarditis prophylaxis

Adapted with from Cote C, Ryan J, Todres ID, et al., eds. *A Practice of Anesthesia for Infants and Children*. Philadelphia: WB Saunders; 1993.

MEDICATIONS AND ALLERGIES

Currently prescribed and previously ingested medications can have significant effects on the outcome of general anesthesia. Queries should be made regarding the use and frequency of the following:

- Nonprescription cold remedies, which contain aspirin or aspirinlike compounds that interfere with platelet function and coagulation.
- Nonsteroidal antiinflammatory drugs, which should be discontinued 5 days before surgery.
- In children who have been treated for a malignancy, specific chemotherapeutic regimens should be determined. The anthracycline drugs (doxorubicin hydrochloride [Adriamycin] and daunomycin) cause myocardial dysfunction, which may require further preoperative investigation with an echocardiogram. Use of mitomycin and bleomycin sulfate may result in pulmonary dysfunction, which may require further evaluation with pulse oximetry and pulmonary function tests and avoidance of high inspired oxygen concentrations.
- Adjunct therapies such as the use of herbal remedies should be documented. The use of herbal substances such as St. John's wort and weight loss agents such as fenfluramine hydrochloride, phentermine hydrochloride, and dexfenfluramine hydrochloride may alter physiology, which may complicate the course of a general anesthetic. Children should be questioned regarding allergies to antibiotics.
- Latex allergy can be detected by asking about sensitivity to bananas, the rubber dam used by dentists and oral surgeons, or latex balloons (6,7).
- Exposure to tobacco smoke should be investigated during the preoperative interview and should be documented (8,9). Children with long-term exposure to tobacco smoke may experience an increased incidence of airway complications under general anesthesia.

PHYSICAL EXAMINATION

The physical examination should focus on the airway, respiratory and cardiovascular systems, neurologic evaluation, and the specific organ system that is involved in the surgical procedure.

One of the key features of the physical examination in children is simple observation, because approaching the child may cause inconsolable crying.

- The color of the skin and the presence of pallor, cyanosis, rash, jaundice, unusual markings, birthmarks, and scars from previous operations should be noted.
- Abnormal facies might be an indication of a syndrome or constellation of congenital abnormalities (Table 15.7). One congenital anomaly often is associated with others.
- The rate, depth, and quality of respirations should be evaluated.
- Nasal or upper respiratory obstruction is indicated by noisy or labored breathing.
- The color, viscosity, and quantity of nasal discharge should be documented.

Table 15.7.   Craniofacial deformities and associated conditions

Name	Deformity	Associated Conditions	Anesthetic Implications
Apert syndrome	Craniosynostosis, hypoplastic midface	Polysyndactyly, possible mental compromise	Difficult intravenous access
Crouzon disease	Craniosynostosis, hypoplastic maxilla, hypertelorism, exophthalmos	Conductive hearing loss, possible mental compromise	Possible upper airway obstruction
Goldenhar syndrome	Unilateral mandibular hypoplasia, cleft palate, micrognathia	Vertebral anomalies	Possible difficult intubation
Hemifacial microsomia	Unilateral ear anomalies, unilateral mandibular hypoplasia	None	Possible difficult intubation
Möbius syndrome	Micrognathia, limited mandibular mobility	Possible cranial nerve VI and VII palsy, ptosis, limited tongue movement	Difficult intubation
Pfeiffer syndrome	Brachycephaly, hypoplastic maxilla	Broad thumbs and toes, syndactyly, possible mental compromise	Difficult intubation
Pierre Robin syndrome	Mandibular hypoplasia, micrognathia, glossoptosis, cleft palate	None	Difficult intubation
Treacher Collins syndrome	Mandibular hypoplasia, zygomatic arch hypoplasia, ear malformations	Compromised hearing	Difficult intubation

Adapted from Badgwell JM, ed. *Clinical Pediatric Anesthesia.* Philadelphia: Lippincott–Raven Publishers; 1997.

- If the child is coughing, the origin of the cough (upper vs. lower airway) and the quality (dry or wet) can be evaluated even before auscultation of the lungs.
- Is wheezing or stridor audible, or are retractions visible?
- The airway should be evaluated for ease of intubation. If the child will not open his or her mouth, a manual estimation of the thyrohyoid distance should be made. Children with micrognathia, as in Pierre Robin syndrome or Goldenhar syndrome, may be especially difficult to intubate.
- The presence of loose teeth should be documented.

The child with a heart murmur or a history of a murmur warrants special consideration.

- Is the murmur innocent or pathologic?
- Is hemodynamic compromise apparent?
- Innocent or nonpathologic heart murmurs can be identified by four characteristics: The murmur is early systolic to midsystolic; it is softer than grade III or VI; the pitch is low to medium; and the sound has a musical, not harsh, quality (10).
- Is the child at risk for paradoxic air embolus?
- Is prophylaxis for infective endocarditis required (11)?

The child with significant or active cardiac disease might require an evaluation by a cardiologist before general anesthesia. Cardiac catheterization data and recommendations should be included in the preoperative evaluation (12).

Neurologic status should be assessed by the following:

- Associated congenital syndromes, neurologic deficits, metabolic disorders, or seizure disorders should be noted.
- Nausea, vomiting, difficulty concentrating, headaches, gait disorders, hypotonia, altered mental status, and inability to protect the airway may be the result of increases in intracranial pressure.
- Neurologic impairment may manifest as an increase in head circumference, hypotonia, spasticity, or flaccidity.
- The physical examination should include an evaluation of the level of consciousness, ability to swallow, intactness of the gag reflex, and an adequate cervical spine range of motion, hypotonia, spasticity, or flaccidity.

DIAGNOSTIC TESTING

Few, if any, diagnostic laboratory tests are routinely necessary in the pediatric population. Diagnostic studies should be individualized to the patient's medical condition and the surgical procedure being performed. Determination of hemoglobin level before elective surgery is unnecessary for most healthy children (13). Mild abnormalities in white blood cell and platelet counts have no significant impact on the perioperative outcome in healthy children. The routine measurement of coagulation parameters is controversial, and a history of "excess bruising" is subjective. A history of abnormal coagulation, prolonged epistaxis, and bleeding from circumcision or a tooth extraction and the presence of hematomas and large bruises are better predictors of abnormal coagulation. If an otherwise healthy child has a negative history for bruising, no further testing is required, because commonly used screening tests such as bleeding time, activated partial thromboplastin time, prothrombin time, and platelet count do not reliably predict surgical bleeding (14).

- Hemoglobin determination is indicated for premature infants and infants <6 months, and when significant surgical blood loss is anticipated.
- Coagulation screening may be indicated in children who have a history of abnormal bleeding or are scheduled for surgery in which abnormal coagulation might be induced (cardiopulmonary bypass) or procedures in which adequate hemostasis is essential (tonsillectomy, neurosurgical procedures).
- A urinalysis is not needed before surgery for most children.
- Serum chemistry measurements are indicated only to confirm a *suspected* abnormality. Serum medication levels are measured when specifically indicated (e.g., for seizure medications).
- Chest radiographs and electrocardiograms (ECGs) are indicated only when abnormalities are suspected.
- Pregnancy testing has caused a great deal of controversy. A *confidential* interview with a postmenarchal female should disclose current sexual activity, the use of birth control, or the possibility of pregnancy. Often parents refuse pregnancy testing for their child because it assumes that the child either is sexually active or is not truthful about her sexual activities. The legality of such testing is not clear and practice is dictated by hospital policy.

In summary, because most laboratory examinations are painful and distressing to children, an attempt should be made to minimize psychological and physical pain. A child who has been traumatized preoperatively may show problematic behavior during the anesthetic induction.

SPECIAL CIRCUMSTANCES

Upper Respiratory Infection

The child with a recent, full-blown, or early upper respiratory infection (URI) poses a clinical dilemma for the anesthesiologist. Because most children can have up to six URIs per year, no absolute rules exist for this common problem. The child who has an active cold or is recovering from a recent one is at risk preoperatively for atelectasis, oxygen desaturation, bronchospasm, croup, and laryngospasm (15). Most children with URIs may be anesthetized for short procedures; however, the decision to perform a lengthy or invasive procedure must be made with caution. Decisions to cancel or postpone surgery should be made in conjunction with the surgeon based on the procedure, its urgency, and the child's overall medical condition. Because bronchial hyperreactivity may exist for up to 7 weeks after the resolution of URI symptoms, delaying surgery for this length of time is often impractical. Most practitioners would agree that surgery may be scheduled after the acute symptoms have resolved and no sooner than 2 weeks after the initial evaluation.

When a child with symptoms of an URI is examined, the presence of secretions and their color should be noted. Clear secretions usually indicate a viral illness, whereas green or yellow secretions suggest a bacterial infection. Cough is a sign of lower respiratory involvement and should be evaluated for origin (upper airway or bronchial) and quality (wet or dry). Most children have clear breath sounds during quiet respirations. Crackles are best detected during coughing and crying.

Premature Birth

Former premature infants may require a variety of surgical procedures, some seemingly minor. The anesthetic management can be challenging, however. Chronic lung disease and the possibility of postoperative apnea are conditions that require planning for appropriate postprocedural monitoring. Coexisting conditions, such as gastroesophageal reflux, patent ductus arteriosus, and hydrocephalus, should be documented.

The degree of respiratory compromise in former premature infants may range from no residual lung disease to serious bronchopulmonary dysplasia. The signs of bronchopulmonary dysplasia are variable and range from mild radiographic changes in an asymptomatic patient to pulmonary fibrosis, emphysema, reactive airway disease, chronic hypoxemia and hypercarbia, tracheomalacia or bronchomalacia, and increased pulmonary vascular resistance with cor pulmonale. If pulmonary hypertension and cor pulmonale are suspected, an ECG is useful to confirm the diagnosis and guide medical therapy. Diuretics, bronchodilators, and corticosteroids—medications that many of these patients require—should be continued up to and including the day of surgery. Measurement of serum electrolyte levels to evaluate hypokalemia and compensatory metabolic alkalosis may be valuable, especially if therapy has been altered recently. A hematocrit and chest radiograph are useful in evaluating these infants. Administration of pharmacologic "stress doses" of steroids should be considered in infants treated with steroids.

Postoperative apnea has been reported in preterm and full-term infants after anesthesia (16,17). No agreement exists on which infants are at risk. Reports are not consistent in identifying the gestational age of at-risk patients, the methods used to detect apnea or periodic breathing, the surgical procedure, other confounding medical conditions, or even the definition of apnea. One review has summarized available information (17). The definition of apnea used in this analysis was cessation of breathing or no detection of air flow for 15 seconds or more or for 15 seconds or less with bradycardia (heart rate <80 beats per minute). The cause of apnea is central in 70% of cases, obstructive in 10%, and mixed in 20%. The risk of apnea is significant for infants of 35 weeks' gestation until they reach 48 weeks postconceptual age. In infants under 35 weeks' gestational age, this risk is significant until they reach 50 weeks postconceptual age. Infants with anemia, apnea in the recovery room, apnea at home (as measured with home apnea-monitoring equipment), and a history of apnea and bradycardia are at increased risk for apnea. Any child considered to be at risk for postoperative apnea should be admitted for overnight observation and monitoring. A recent hematocrit or hemoglobin determination is required for a former preterm infant because anemia is associated with an increased incidence of postanesthesia apnea that is unaffected by postconceptual age.

Apnea of prematurity and postanesthetic apnea have no relationship to sudden infant death syndrome.

Asthma

The management of children with asthma is similar to management of adult patients with asthma. Asthma treatment should be optimized and all medications, both oral and inhaled, should be continued up to and including the day of surgery. Oral medications may be taken with clear fluids up to 2 hours before the induction of anesthesia. Patients with particularly severe asthma may benefit from short-term corticosteroid therapy for several days before surgery. Therapy should be optimized with the input of a pulmonologist.

Surgery should generally be postponed for children with an acute exacerbation of asthma or an acute URI superimposed on chronic asthma. Asthmatic children are at increased risk for bronchospasm during general endotracheal anesthesia. The incidence of bronchospasm in asthmatic patients during anesthesia is between 8.4 and 71.0 per 1,000, compared with 0.2 to 8.0 per 1,000 in the general population. Acute exacerbations increase the incidence of bronchospasm.

Cystic Fibrosis

Children with cystic fibrosis have a multisystem disease, and each of these systems should be considered during the preoperative period. Pulmonary function should be optimized through the use of antibiotic and bronchodilator therapy and vigorous chest physical therapy to clear secretions and enhance airflow. Many children have some degree of malnutrition and may need parenteral or supplemental enteral nutrition before undergoing general anesthesia and surgery. Many cystic fibrosis patients should be admitted to the hospital for medical management before their surgical procedures. All medications should be continued up to and including the day of surgery.

Cardiac Disease

Children with cardiac disease can be divided into two categories: Those who have structural congenital heart disease (corrected and uncorrected) and those who have a heart murmur (previously diagnosed or new). The child who is evaluated regularly by a cardiologist should be evaluated in the preoperative period to detect and document any interval change. When the child has had a surgical repair of congenital heart disease, a description of the repair and current anatomy should be made available to the anesthesia team. If a defect still exists, management recommendations should be requested from the cardiologist. All current cardiac catheterization data should be reviewed.

Heart murmurs in children should be identified as innocent or pathologic. An ECG may be necessary. If a murmur is pathologic, the degree of physiologic and hemodynamic compromise should be determined. The need for antibiotic prophylaxis should be assessed during the preoperative visit; current guidelines are outlined in Chapter 17.

Central Nervous System Disorders

Myelomeningocele

Most children who are born with a myelomeningocele have other abnormalities, and a thorough investigation is necessary. Many of these children return to the operating room (OR) frequently, so the current perioperative management may influence patients' future behavior and concerns. Myelomeningocele patients may have associated urogenital and musculoskeletal system dysfunction leading to frequent urinary tract infections, ureteral reflux, scoliosis, and respiratory compromise. Patients and families should be questioned regarding abnormalities in these organ systems. These children are often sensitive to latex with reactions ranging from mild to anaphylaxis. For this reason, an attempt is made to minimize their exposure to latex. The notation "Latex Alert" or "Latex Allergy" should be written on the chart of every myelomeningocele patient going to the OR.

Seizure Disorders

A description of the type, frequency, and characteristics of seizure activity should be obtained during the preoperative evaluation. Current medications and, if applicable, serum levels of anticonvulsant medications should be noted. Medications that were ineffective in controlling seizure activity should be included. Patients should take all seizure medications up to and including the day of surgery. Oral medications may be taken with clear fluids up to 2 hours before the time of surgery.

Cervical Spine Instability

Several groups of pediatric patients are at risk for cervical spine instability. Children with Hurler syndrome and Morquio syndrome as well as other mucopolysaccharidoses may have abnormalities of the odontoid process, which may result in cervical spine instability. Atlantoaxial instability and superior migration of the odontoid process can occur in patients with rheumatoid arthritis. Approximately 15% of children with Down syndrome are likewise affected. Although no uniform guidelines exist regarding preoperative testing in these children, the suggestion has been made that children who are symptomatic (e.g., have gait disturbances, incontinence problems) should undergo flexion-extension radiography of the cervical spine and should have a neurologic consultation (18). If cervical abnormalities are noted, intubation in a neutral head position or somatosensory-evoked potential monitoring of the upper extremities may be required (19).

Hematologic Disorders

Sickle cell disease is one of the most common hematologic diseases in children in the United States. Sickle cell disease is a genetically transmitted autosomal recessive disease that is found in the heterozygous form with a frequency of 8% in African Americans and in the homozygous form in 0.16% of patients who are susceptible. Heterozygous sickle cell trait does not influence anesthetic management or perioperative outcome, but homozygous sickle cell disease, sickle cell–hemoglobin C disease, and hemoglobin

S–thalassemia disease carry implications for anesthetic management. Acute chest syndrome, stroke, myocardial infarction, and sickle cell crises are of concern to the anesthesiologist. To minimize these risks, patients are vigorously hydrated preoperatively. To optimize intravascular flow the OR temperature is kept elevated. In severe cases, partial exchange transfusion to decrease the level of hemoglobin S to <40% or transfusion to a hemoglobin of 10 g/dL is performed. Consultation with a hematologist for management of these patients is recommended. Coordination of care among the anesthesiologist, surgeon, pediatrician, and hematologist is essential and must begin in the preoperative period.

Diabetes Mellitus

The incidence of diabetes mellitus in the pediatric population is approximately 1.9 in 1,000 school-aged children, with age of onset peaking at 5 to 7 years and again at puberty. Consultation with the pediatrician and pediatric endocrinologist is advisable. Information regarding the typical range of serum glucose control and medication regimen should be included in the preoperative evaluation. Any suggestions for perioperative glucose management (insulin infusion, split-dose insulin injection) should be documented. Patients with diabetes mellitus are scheduled for surgery early in the morning, and a fasting serum glucose measurement is obtained in the immediate preoperative period before insulin or glucose administration.

Oncologic Disease

Children with malignant disease—either active, in remission, or cured—may have received radiation or chemotherapy that will directly affect the anesthetic outcome. Information regarding the course of the disease, prior surgery, and a list of chemotherapeutic agents and doses should be included in the preoperative evaluation. Children suspected of having an anterior mediastinal mass require flow-volume loop examination in the supine and upright positions before anesthetic induction. Clinical findings should dictate the need for other laboratory examinations, such as an ECG, hemoglobin measurement, and platelet count.

Minimally Invasive Surgery

Minimally invasive endoscopic surgery is becoming more and more prevalent in the pediatric population (20). Due to the specific requirements of this type of intervention, unique physiologic changes must be considered during the preoperative evaluation process. Among the contraindications for minimally invasive surgery are the following pre-existing conditions:

- Respiratory difficulty, which may increase airway pressure and decrease airway compliance intraoperatively
- Pulmonary hypertension, which may worsen as a result of CO_2 that is absorbed from the peritoneum
- Cardiomyopathy, because abdominal insufflation of CO_2 decreases cardiac output

PREOPERATIVE MEDICATIONS AND BEYOND

Fasting Guidelines

Fasting guidelines for children before general anesthesia have been modified so that restricting children to fasting after midnight is no longer common practice (21). Liberalization of oral intake results in a less anxious child, calmer parents, better maintenance of hemodynamic parameters, and less risk of intraoperative hypoglycemia.

Gastric volume and gastric emptying times are age related, and many surgical facilities have age-specific guidelines. In general, many institutions allow the ingestion of clear fluids until 2 to 3 hours before the time of surgery. These include water, electrolyte solutions (Pedialyte), glucose water, apple juice, white grape juice, frozen pops without fruit pulp, and gelatin. Clear fluids are defined as any fluid through which a newspaper can be read. Frozen pops that contain fruit solids; ciders; nectar juices that contain pulp and particulate material; and clear broth, which may contain animal proteins, are not considered clear liquids. No evidence exists that volume has an impact on gastric emptying time or residual volume; therefore, the quantity of clear fluids is not limited.

Formula and breast milk are not clear fluids. Breast milk is considered to be an intermediate between clear fluids and formula. Some institutions consider formula less restricted than a solid, whereas other institutions consider it to have solidlike properties. Clear policies should be established regarding formula, breast milk, and solids (Table 15.8) (22).

Induction Choices

During the preoperative interview the options that are available for the induction of general anesthesia can be introduced. It must be made clear that the choice is ultimately the responsibility of the attending anesthesiologist, who will consider the input of the child and family members.

For children <8 years, anesthesia is best induced with a volatile anesthetic agent administered by mask. With this method, the onset of unconsciousness is rapid, and a child's needle phobia is circumvented. When the child is calm and cooperative, increasing concentrations of anesthetic are administered by mask until unconsciousness is achieved. For the anxious or uncooperative child, a "single-breath" inhalation induction technique delivers a high concentration of anesthetic. The single-breath inhalation induction is less pleasant for the child because of the pungent odor of

Table 15.8. Fasting guidelines from the American Society of Anesthesiologists

Time Prior to Surgery (Hours)	Food or Fluid
2	Clear fluids
4	Breast milk
6	Formula or solids
8	Fat-containing solids

the anesthetic, but it is much faster. Children >8 years occasionally are anesthetized by mask induction, and cooperative children may choose a single-breath induction technique. The choices are based on the most appropriate method for each child and situation.

Anesthesia is usually induced in older children in the same manner as in adult patients, via an intravenous route. Topical anesthetic cream is applied to intact skin providing analgesia so an intravenous line can to be inserted without pain. The procedure should be explained to children in advance so that they are prepared.

For mentally challenged children, who are uncooperative and difficult to reason with, anesthesia may be induced with an intramuscular injection of ketamine hydrochloride, midazolam hydrochloride, or a combination of the two. This method is fast and effective for bringing the children into the OR, and discussion of this option is reassuring to parents who are concerned about an uncooperative or combative child.

Parent-Present Induction

When patients and families are prepared for anesthesia, a common concern of many parents and caretakers is, "How will my child be taken into the OR?" The presence of the parents is often the most effective premedication for a young child, especially a toddler, because the separation from parents is eliminated (23). A parent may accompany the child into the OR, and this should be an accepted practice (24). In the United Kingdom, parents are present during induction of anesthesia in 75% of cases, compared to 25% in the United States (25).

Parents are most effective if they are well prepared. They are not helpful during induction of anesthesia when the child is <8 months of age. The clinician must remember that most parents have not been in an OR, and the sounds of surgical instruments being prepared and of anesthesia monitors are new and can be frightening to both parents and children (26).

Parents may remain with the child until he or she is unaware of their presence. They should be warned that their child might not look as he or she does during natural sleep. Parents should be given a *brief* description of eye and body movements during stage 2 of anesthesia. During the excitement stage the eyes may roll back, random body movements may occur, and vocalization is common. These occurrences are normal and expected. When a parent-present induction is unsuccessful, the cause often is inadequate preparation of parents. Parents may express their desire *not* to accompany their child into the OR, and this sentiment should be respected. Alternatives to parent-present induction should be explored.

When presenting options for anesthetic induction, the clinician must not promise that a specific technique or medication will be used unless he or she is actually going to administer the anesthetic. Alternatively, an acceptable course is to explain that the final decision will be made by the anesthesiologist on the day of surgery and that all factors and requests will be taken into consideration.

Special Anesthetic Considerations

One phrase that the OR team shudders to hear is, "By the way, the patient is. . . ." The sentence may be completed with phrases such as "a Jehovah's Witness" or "do not resuscitate (DNR)." These circumstances have complicated ethical and legal ramifications for the anesthesiologist and require careful preoperative planning among the surgeon, anesthesiologist, pediatrician, family, parents or guardian, hospital administrators, and attorneys. Frequently, medical decisions are influenced by nonmedical considerations. Therefore, planning takes place before arrival in the OR, and all parties must be in agreement to prevent cancellation of surgery.

Jehovah's Witnesses

Although adult patients who are Jehovah's Witnesses may choose to refuse lifesaving blood transfusions, pediatric patients are minor children and do not have that right. The anesthesiologist, the surgeon, and hospital officials are responsible for developing a plan with the parents in the event that blood is required. The anesthesiologist and surgeon should explore the unique beliefs of the family, because some Jehovah's Witnesses will allow the use of blood conservation in an attempt to minimize intraoperative blood loss and transfusion. Perioperative volume expanders (albumin, hydroxyethyl starch), hemodilution, and blood salvage are acceptable to some individuals, depending on their interpretation of biblical passages (27,28). In an emergency, most medical personnel agree that it is unacceptable for a parent to make a decision that could result in a minor child's death. In such a case, appropriate medical therapy, including transfusion of blood and blood products, is administered against the wishes of the family. In most circumstances, the courts have intervened to allow blood transfusions over the religious objections of the parents. So that no child of Jehovah's Witness parents should die for lack of transfused blood, the physician must seek a court order to administer the blood. A petition to the appropriate court is made for judicial declaration that the minor is a "neglected child" and that a guardian be appointed, usually the hospital or hospital administrator. Evidence in support of the need for blood transfusion is made to the judge, either in person or by telephone by the pediatrician, surgeon, anesthesiologist, or all three. If the petition is granted, the new guardian consents to transfusion of blood or blood products, and a formal petition to the court is made.

"Do-Not-Resuscitate" Orders for Children

DNR orders are implemented to prevent long-term dependence on life-support systems when no reversal or resolution of a disease process is anticipated and to avoid prolongation of an inevitable death. The issue of procedure arises when a child with a DNR order comes to the OR because general anesthesia is a continuous state of cardiopulmonary resuscitation. Determining where anesthesia ends and resuscitation begins is difficult. Orders directing DNR status outside the OR are not applicable during surgery and anesthesia unless the family has specifically indicated that they should continue.

Each institution should have a policy regarding suspension of DNR orders during surgery, and that policy should be understood and agreed on by all involved parties. This matter should be discussed with the family before surgery, and written documentation of the plan either to maintain or to suspend DNR orders should be made. A distinction exists between goal-directed resuscitation and procedure-directed resuscitation (29). Most determinations of DNR outline the specific interventions that may or may not be carried out. Because these procedures often are part of the normal administration of general anesthesia, the definition becomes meaningless. Perhaps more useful is an understanding of outcome expectations. The anesthesiologist can decide what intervention will result in the desired postoperative outcome and determine which therapy is acceptable and in keeping with parental wishes. If a child requires emergency surgery and the parent or legal guardian is unavailable, the recommendation is that the DNR status be suspended.

REFERENCES

1. McGraw T. Preparing children for the operating room: psychological issues. *Can J Anaesth*. 1994;41:1094–1103.
2. Moynihan R, Kurker C. Bridging the gap to the operating room and beyond. In: Ferrari LR, ed. *Preoperative Evaluation and Pain Management of Pediatric Patients*. Baltimore: Johns Hopkins University Press; 1998.
3. Morray JG, Ramamoorthy C, Haberkern CM, et al. Anesthesia-related cardiac arrest in children. *Anesthesiology*. 2000;93:6–14.
4. Holzman RS. Morbidity and mortality in pediatric anesthesia. *Pediatr Clin North Am*. 1994;41:239–256.
5. Means LJ. Preoperative evaluation. In: Badgwell JM, ed. *Clinical Pediatric Anesthesia*. Philadelphia: Lippincott–Raven Publishers; 1997:1–13.
6. Cote CJ, Todres ID, Ryan JF. Preoperative evaluation of pediatric patients. In: Cote CJ, Ryan JF, Todres ID, et al., eds. *A Practice of Anesthesia for Infants and Children*. 2nd ed. Philadelphia: WB Saunders; 1993.
7. Means LJ, Fescorla FJ. Latex anaphylaxis: report of occurrence in two pediatric surgical patients and review of the literature. *J Pediatr Surg*. 1995;30:748–751.
8. Skolnick ET, Vomvolakis MA, Buck KA, et al. Exposure to environmental tobacco smoke and the risk of adverse respiratory events in children receiving general anesthesia. *Anesthesiology*. 1998;88:1144–1153.
9. Koop CE. Adverse anesthesia events in children exposed to environmental tobacco smoke. *Anesthesiology*. 1998;88:1141–1142.
10. Harris JP. Evaluation of heart murmurs. *Pediatr Rev*. 1994;15:490–493.
11. Wilson W, Taubert KA, Gewitz M, et al. Prevention of infective endocarditis. Guidelines from the American Heart Association. *Circulation* published online April 19, 2007. http://circ.ahajournals.org.
12. Means LJ, Ferrari LR, Fisher QA, et al. American Academy of Pediatrics. Evaluation and preparation of pediatric patients undergoing anesthesia. *Pediatrics*. 1996;98:502–508.

13. Baron MJ, Gunter J, White P. Is the pediatric preoperative hematocrit determination necessary? *South Med J*. 1992;85:1187–1189.
14. Burk CD, Miller L, Handler SD, et al. Preoperative history and coagulation screening in children undergoing tonsillectomy. *Pediatrics*. 1992;89:691–695.
15. Rolf N, Cote CJ. Frequency and severity of desaturation events during general anesthesia in children with and without upper respiratory infections. *J Clin Anesth*. 1992;4:200–203.
16. Noseworthy J, Duran C, Khine HH. Postoperative apnea in a full term infant. *Anesthesiology*. 1988;97:879–880.
17. Cote CJ, Zaslavsky A, Downes JJ, et al. Postoperative apnea in former premature infants after inguinal herniorrhaphy. A combined analysis. *Anesthesiology*. 1995;82:809–822.
18. Williams JP, Somerville GM, Miner ME, et al. Atlanto-axial subluxation and trisomy 21: another perioperative complication. *Anesthesiology*. 1987;67:253–254.
19. Cunningham MJ, Ferrari LR, Kerse L, et al. Intraoperative somatosensory evoked potential monitoring in achondroplastic dwarfs. *Paediatr Anaesth*. 1994;4:129–132.
20. Holzman RS. Special anesthetic considerations. In: Smith AD, Badlani GH, Bagley DH, et al., eds. *Smith's Textbook of Endourology*. St. Louis: Quality Medical Publishing, Inc.; 1996:1293–1306.
21. Cote CJ. NPO after midnight for children—a reappraisal. *Anesthesiology*. 1990;72:589–592.
22. Practice guidelines for preoperative fasting and the use of pharmacologic agents to reduce the risk of pulmonary aspiration: application to healthy patients undergoing elective procedures. A Report by the American Society of Anesthesiologists Task Force on Preoperative Fasting. *Anesthesiology*. 1999;90:896–905.
23. Kain ZN, Caldwell-Andrews AA, Mayes LC, et al. Family-centered preparation for surgery improves perioperative outcomes in children: a randomized controlled trial. *Anesthesiology*. 2007;106:65–74.
24. Kam, PC, Voss TJ, Gold PD, et al. Behavior of children associated with parental participation during induction of general anesthesias. *J Paediatr Child Health*. 1998;34:29–31.
25. Kain ZN, Fernandes LA, Touloukin RJ. Parental presence during induction of anesthesia: the surgeon's perspective. *Eur J Pediatr Surg*. 1996;6:323–327.
26. Kain ZN, Mayes LC, Wang SM, et al. Parental presence during induction of anesthesia versus sedative premedication: which intervention is more effective? *Anesthesiology*. 1998;89:1147–1156.
27. Benson KT. The Jehovah's Witness patient: considerations for the anesthesiologist. *Anesth Analg*. 1989;69:647–656.
28. *Jehovah's Witnesses and the Question of Blood*. Brooklyn, NY: Watch Tower Bible and Tract Society; 1977:1–64.
29. Truog R, Rockoff MA. Ethical issues in pediatric anesthesia. *Semin Anesth*. 1991;10:187–194.

Anesthetic-Specific Issues

P. Allan Klock, Jr.

This chapter discusses the preoperative evaluation and management of patients with **pseudocholinesterase deficiency, malignant hyperthermia, postoperative nausea or vomiting,** and a potentially **difficult airway.** The common thread of these issues is that they only pose a problem to individuals who have these conditions when anesthesia is administered to them. The chapter concludes with a case study of a preoperative encounter.

PSEUDOCHOLINESTERASE DEFICIENCY

Succinyldicholine is the only depolarizing muscle relaxant commonly used during general anesthesia. It is metabolized by plasma cholinesterase (pseudocholinesterase) or, more specifically, by butyryl cholinesterase and by the liver. Acetylcholinesterase, cell-bound or true cholinesterase, plays no role in the metabolism of succinyldicholine. Prolonged apnea and paralysis may occur after the administration of succinylcholine chloride (succinyldicholine) (1) if the patient has quantitative or qualitative abnormalities in pseudocholinesterase (2,3). Recovery from mivacurium chloride and ester-linked local anesthetics, which are also metabolized by pseudocholinesterase, may be a problem in patients with pseudocholinesterase abnormalities. Pseudocholinesterase activity may be reduced permanently by expression of abnormal genotypes or temporarily by disease states or drug effects and in parturients, neonates, and infants (Table 16.1).

Genetic analysis has demonstrated the existence of three allelic variants in addition to the wild type. The phenotypes that relate to these four alleles have been named differently by investigators and can be distinguished using plasma cholinesterase inhibitors such as chloride, fluoride, and dibucaine in vitro. Names include *atypical, dibucaine sensitive, fluoride sensitive,* and *silent gene* (4,5). These four alleles give rise to ten genotypes. Pharmacogenetic studies suggest that allelic predominance differs with ethnicity (5–8). Table 16.2 summarizes information on the common North American variants of pseudocholinesterase.

Davies et al. demonstrated that normal and variant pseudocholinesterase differed in at least two important ways (9). The normal enzyme W-W has a much greater affinity for choline substrate, and cholinesterase activity in normal plasma is inhibited to a greater extent by cholinesterase inhibitors than in those with an abnormal enzyme. These researchers published a method for detecting individuals with atypical plasma cholinesterase using the local anesthetic dibucaine. Dibucaine inhibits the metabolism of a choline substrate by plasma cholinesterase in vitro. The percentage inhibition of plasma cholinesterase by dibucaine is termed the *dibucaine number*. Normal individuals

Table 16.1. Causes of decreased plasma cholinesterase activity

Disease states	Hepatic failure
	Uremia
	Malnutrition
	Myxedema
	Collagen vascular diseases
	Acute myocardial infarction
	Acute infection
	Carcinoma
	Tuberculosis
Drug therapies	Echothiophate iodide
	Neostigmine
	Chlorpromazine
	Oral contraceptives
	Cyclophosphamide
	Pancuronium bromide
	Phenylzine
	Trimethaphan camsylate
Expected alterations in enzyme activity	Third trimester of pregnancy
	Newborns and infants

Data from Whittaker M. Plasma cholinesterase variants and the anaesthetist. *Anaesthesia.* 1980;35:175; and Morgan GE, Mikhil MS. *Clinical Anesthesiology.* 2nd ed. Norwalk, CT: Appleton & Lange; 1996:190.

Table 16.2. Genetic classification, frequency of occurrence, and response to succinylcholine chloride

Genotype	Phenotype	Frequency	Dibucaine Number	Expected Apnea Time (min)
W-W	Typical homozygote	96 in 100	80	10
W-A	Heterozygote	1 in 40	60	20–30
A-A	Atypical homozygote	1 in 2,000	20	480 (8 hours)

A, atypical gene; W, wild-type gene.
Data from Barash PG, Cullen BF, Stoelting RK. *Clinical Anesthesia.* 2nd ed. Philadelphia: JB Lippincott Co.; 1992:605; Morgan GE, Mikhail MS. *Clinical Anesthesiology.* 2nd ed. Norwalk, CT: Appleton & Lange; 1996:152, 154; Whittaker M. Plasma cholinesterase variants and the anaesthetist. *Anaesthesia.* 1980;35:178; and Thompson JS, Thompson MW. *Genetics in Medicine.* 4th ed. Philadelphia: WB Saunders; 1980:104.

are homozygous for the wild type, and dibucaine causes inhibition of substrate metabolism by 80%, resulting in a dibucaine number of 80.

In those who are homozygous for the atypical genes, inhibition is only 20%, resulting in a dibucaine number of 20. In individuals heterozygotic for the atypical genes, inhibition is approximately 60%, resulting in a dibucaine number of 60.

The assessment of an individual thought to have a genetic variant of this enzyme should begin with the determination of a dibucaine number. This result yields important information regarding the *quality* of the individual's plasma cholinesterase. Inhibition of the enzyme in vitro by fluoride and chloride further delineate phenotypes.

In addition to the qualitative assessment obtained using dibucaine, a quantitative assessment of the enzyme can be obtained by determining the absolute plasma cholinesterase activity. It is important to measure *plasma* cholinesterase activity (which may also be called butyrylcholinesterase or pseudocholinesterase) rather than cholinesterase activity, which is also known as red blood cell (RBC) or erythrocyte cholinesterase activity. The combination of dibucaine number and pseudocholinesterase activity help differentiate genetic from nongenetic causes for prolonged apnea after administration of succinylcholine or mivacurium chloride. Some patients suffering from prolonged paralysis after receiving mivacurium or succinylcholine have a transient decrease in pseudocholinesterase activity caused by drug interactions or other unidentified causes. Therefore, it is important to not draw a specimen for pseudocholinesterase activity until after the event is over. Given that there is no urgency to these test results, one may want to wait several days in case a drug interaction or other toxin caused the event.

MALIGNANT HYPERTHERMIA

Malignant hyperthermia (MH) is a fulminant hypermetabolic state characterized by tachycardia, hypertension, hypercarbia, arterial hypoxemia, mixed venous oxygen desaturation, metabolic acidosis, hyperkalemia, muscle rigidity, hyperthermia, renal failure, disseminated intravascular coagulation, and death if the condition is untreated. Individuals are genetically predisposed to the development of MH and are asymptomatic until they are exposed to either succinylcholine or potent volatile anesthetics such as desflurane, sevoflurane, or isoflurane. The incidence of MH is three times higher in the pediatric population than in adults; MH occurs in 1 of every 12,000 pediatric anesthesia cases (10). A number of neuromuscular diseases have been associated with the development of MH (Table 16.3). Sixty percent of susceptible individuals manifest MH when exposed to triggering drugs on first exposure, especially when succinylcholine is combined with potent volatile anesthetics (11). Those in whom no response is triggered initially may develop MH with subsequent anesthetic administration.

MH results from the activation of skeletal muscle due to an increase in intracellular sarcoplasmic calcium concentration caused by the aforementioned triggers. Calcium-selective microelectrode studies have demonstrated that individuals who are

Table 16.3.   Conditions possibly associated with susceptibility to malignant hyperthermia

Duchenne muscular dystrophy
Becker muscular dystrophy
King-Denborough syndrome
Central core disease
Carnitine palmityl transferase deficiency
Periodic paralysis
Myotonia congenita
Osteogenesis imperfecta
Schwartz-Jampel syndrome
Fukuyama-type congenital muscular dystrophy
Mitochondrial myopathy

Possibly associated:
  Strabismus
  Scoliosis
  Burkitt lymphoma
  Neuroleptic malignant syndrome
  Myelomeningocele
  Congenital hip dislocation

Based on data from Kaplan R. Malignant hyperthermia. In: *Refresher Courses in Anesthesiology.* Vol. 22. Philadelphia: JB Lippincott Co.; 1994:177; and Stoelting RK, Dierdorf SF. *Anesthesia and Co-existing Disease.* 3rd ed. New York: Churchill Livingstone; 1993:613.

susceptible to MH have increased resting levels of sarcoplasmic calcium and develop excessive levels when exposed to specific triggers (12).

Excitation–contraction coupling with subsequent muscle contraction requires the rapid release of calcium from the sarcoplasmic reticulum. With exposure to ryanodine, a toxin, a marked alteration occurs in excitation–contraction coupling in striated muscle, which leads to skeletal muscle contraction (13). Extensive genetic studies have been performed on family members susceptible to MH. Although mutations in the gene encoding for the ryanodine receptor have been identified in certain families, no single mutation segregates with all susceptible patients (14,15). The inheritance pattern in humans appears to be autosomal dominant.

In vitro studies show that the slow sodium current in cultured human muscle cells is altered in cells from patients with MH; this finding implies that sodium channels, in addition to the ryanodine receptor, are defective (16). These data suggest that susceptibility to MH is multifactorial.

Testing for MH is usually performed on individuals who are thought to have experienced an episode of MH, have a family history of MH, had an anesthetic-related event that could have been MH, or have a disorder that puts them at higher risk for developing MH (Table 16.3).

Although many tests for MH have evolved, the caffeine-halothane contracture test (CHCT) remains the gold standard in North America. It is performed at six institutions in the United States and one in Canada (17). A positive result occurs when muscle biopsy tissue, usually taken from the quadriceps femoris, develops at least 200 mg tension when challenged with 0.2 mmol caffeine or 3% halothane. Under good conditions the test has a sensitivity of 97% and a specificity of 78% (18). The disadvantages of the test are that it requires the patient to travel to the testing center to undergo a muscle biopsy; it costs $6,000, which may not be covered by third-party insurers; and it requires anesthesia. This is particularly problematic with pediatric patients as the biopsy itself will almost certainly require general anesthesia.

Genetic testing for mutations in the ryanodine receptor (RYR1) can be a supplement to, or a substitute for, the CHCT. Because known RYR1 mutations are found in only 25% to 30% of MH-susceptible individuals, the test has relatively low sensitivity. However, the test has an extremely high positive predictive value. One advantage of genetic testing is that it can be performed on a blood sample shipped to one of two laboratories in the United States. The cost varies from $740 to $1,690 depending on the number of exons that need to be sequenced (19). If the proband is found to have a RYR1 mutation linked to MH, then the proband is MH susceptible and no further testing is needed. Relatives can be tested for the same mutation as the proband for approximately $200. If the proband has high clinical risk for MH (likely prior episode or relative with MH) and has a negative genetic test, then the patient may still be MH susceptible and the CHCT should be considered. In 2005 Litman wrote an excellent review on MH susceptibility testing outlining the role of the CHCT and genetic testing (20).

Because no current test has 100% sensitivity, some patients at risk may choose to not undergo testing. In addition, many anesthesiologists may choose to deliver a nontriggering anesthetic to any patient with a personal or family history suggestive of MH regardless of the patient's test results. Ideally, the MH-susceptible patient should be scheduled for the first case of the day to minimize trace anesthetic levels in the operating and recovery rooms. The anesthesia machine should be properly prepared and triggering agents avoided. It is important to communicate well ahead of the date of surgery with the surgeon and the anesthesia providers if an MH-susceptible patient is scheduled. This can allow for proper scheduling, anesthesia machine preparation, and planning of the anesthetic and immediate recovery phase (Table 16.4).

It is the standard of care to have 36 vials of dantrolene sodium available in all facilities where triggering agents (i.e., potent

Table 16.4.　Anesthesia machine preparation for patients susceptible to malignant hyperthermia

Change the rubber bellows.
Change the carbon dioxide absorbent.
Use a new breathing circuit and bag.
Consider changing the fresh gas line.
Flush the new system with oxygen at 10 L/min for 15 to 20 min.
Consider removing potent volatile anesthetic vaporizers from the machine.

inhalation agents or succinylcholine) are available. In addition, it is recommended to have dantrolene available for patients at risk for MH even if the plan is to deliver a nontriggering anesthetic (Table 16.5). The Malignant Hyperthermia Association of the United States (MHAUS) recommends that ambulatory surgery patients be monitored in phase 1 recovery (including vital signs at least every 15 minutes) for at least 1 hour. The patient should then be monitored in phase 2 recovery for at least 1.5 hours before being discharged (21).

The management of patients who have had masseter muscle rigidity on induction of anesthesia remains controversial because this may be a risk factor for MH during subsequent anesthetics. Most commonly, this rigidity occurs in children in whom anesthesia has been induced with a combination of halothane and succinylcholine. However, masseter muscle rigidity has been reported with succinylcholine alone. The most difficult aspect of this clinical presentation is the lack of a uniform definition for rigidity. Therefore, evaluation of the patient who reports a history of "tight jaw" with anesthesia is difficult. Obtaining prior anesthesia records for details is key in determining what might have occurred. Only those patients whose mouths could not be opened after the rest of the body was relaxed should be described as having masseter muscle rigidity. Fifty percent of children and 25% of adults who fall into this group are MH susceptible (22,23). Although opinions differ as to how best to anesthetize these patients, the most conservative approach is to use a nontriggering technique (24).

The management of MH crises centers on prompt recognition of the syndrome and administration of dantrolene sodium intravenously. Active cooling and supportive care play roles if the patient becomes hyperthermic, oliguric, or coagulopathic or shows other metabolic abnormalities. Each vial of dantrolene

Table 16.5. Agents that <u>DO NOT</u> trigger malignant hyperthermia

All local anesthetics
Anticholinergics
Anticholinesterases
Barbiturates
Benzodiazepines
Calcium
Digoxin
Droperidol
Epinephrine
Etomidate
Ketamine
Nitrous oxide
Nondepolarizing muscle relaxants
Opioids
Potassium
Procainamide hydrochloride
Propofol
Sympathomimetics

sodium (a lyophilized mixture) contains 20 mg of dantrolene and 3 g of mannitol. The effective dose in 90% of patients is a bolus intravenous injection of 2.5 mg/kg, but up to 10 mg/kg of dantrolene sodium may be required to fully treat an MH episode. The drug acts by inhibiting the release of calcium from the sarcoplasmic reticulum and is the specific therapy for MH. It is not recommended to prophylactically administer dantrolene to MH-susceptible patients who are planning to have anesthesia.

The MHAUS maintains a 24-hour telephone hotline (at 1-209-634-4917) for questions regarding the management of MH. Their Web site, www.mhaus.org, is an excellent resource for patients and clinicians.

POSTOPERATIVE NAUSEA AND VOMITING

Postoperative nausea and vomiting (PONV) remains a significant problem for patients receiving general anesthesia and their care providers. It occurs in approximately 30% of patients receiving general anesthesia and up to 70% of high-risk patients (25). Postoperative nausea and vomiting is a major dissatisfier and increases postoperative length of stay. It is also a leading anesthesia-related cause of hospital admission following planned ambulatory surgery (26). In addition, the act of vomiting or retching can increase intracranial, intraocular, intra-abdominal, intrathoracic, and central venous pressure. Many consider postoperative vomiting to be a risk factor for bleeding or hematoma formation following head and neck surgery.

Risk factors for PONV can be related to the patient, the procedure, and the anesthetic (Table 16.6). Significant attention has

Table 16.6. Key risk factors for postoperative nausea and vomiting (PONV)

Patient-related	Female gender (postpubescent)
	Nonsmoking status
	History of PONV
	History of motion sickness
	Age: Child to young adult
Surgery-related: Well-established factor	Increased duration of surgical procedure
Surgery-related: Possible risk factors	Surgical site: Breast; laparoscopic; ear, nose, and throat; strabismus surgery; and others
Anesthesia-related	Volatile anesthetics
	Nitrous oxide
	Balanced anesthetic (rather than total intravenous anesthetic)
	Large neostigmine dose (>2.5 mg)
	Intraoperative or postoperative opioids (risk increases with larger doses)

Data from Gan TJ. Risk factors for postoperative nausea and vomiting. *Anesth Analg.* 2006;102:1884–1898.

been paid to the subject of PONV risk stratification. Patient risk factors include female gender, prior history of PONV or motion sickness, being a nonsmoker, and anticipated use of postoperative opioids for pain control. The risk of PONV increases with the number of risk factors. There is a 10% risk of PONV with no risk factors, 21% with one risk factor, 39% with two risk factors, 61% with three risk factors, and 79% with four risk factors (27). PONV risk is also affected by surgical factors and anesthetic technique and medications (28). There are no specific physical findings or laboratory studies that aid in PONV risk stratification.

Patients who receive regional anesthesia or sedation are at much lower risk of PONV than patients who receive general anesthesia. This should be kept in mind when counseling patients about the risks and benefits of alternative anesthetic techniques. It is worthwhile to identify patients at high risk so that an appropriate anesthetic plan can be developed and prophylactic antiemetics can be rationally allocated.

Healthcare providers working in a preoperative clinic should be aware of the transdermal scopolamine patch. The patch effectively reduces the risk of PONV but it has a very delayed onset of action and a relatively high rate of adverse effects (29). If a patient is at increased risk of PONV, one may wish to prescribe this patch (1.5 mg, applied to hairless area behind the ear), which can be worn for 3 days. After the patch is applied, there is a 4-hour delay before plasma levels of scopolamine are detected and peak levels occur 24 hours after application. It is recommended that the patch be applied the evening before surgery, with at least 4 hours between patch application and the end of surgery. Patients should be warned that they may experience a dry mouth and blurred vision due to dilation of the pupils. Patients should be instructed to remove the patch if they experience difficulty urinating. Scopolamine should not be prescribed to patients with narrow angle glaucoma and should be used with caution in patients with wide angle glaucoma.

DIFFICULT AIRWAY

Adverse respiratory events remain the major cause of injury and the leading cause of malpractice claims in anesthetic practice. In Caplan's 1990 closed claims analysis, inadequate ventilation was the largest class of adverse events (30). The introduction and widespread acceptance of the difficult airway algorithm of the American Society of Anesthesiologists (ASA), championed by Benumoff (31), have reduced the proportion of airway misadventures associated with induction of anesthesia compared with the intraoperative and postoperative periods (32). Despite the lack of definitive research, preoperative evaluation, intraoperative preparation, and adherence to accepted guidelines can reasonably be assumed to lead to improved outcomes.

The goals of this section are to provide a systematic approach to airway evaluation based on history, physical examination, and commonly used airway classification systems. In addition, planning for the management of a patient with a suspected difficult airway is discussed.

Recognition of a potentially difficult airway begins with an understanding of normal airway anatomy. A full description of the

Table 16.7. Modified Mallampati classification[a]

Class	Oropharyngeal Components Visualized
1	Soft palate, uvula, tonsillar pillars
2	Base of the tongue obscures the tonsillar pillars, but the posterior pharyngeal wall is visible below the soft palate
3	Soft palate
4	Essentially nothing visualized, not even soft palate

[a]The original Mallampati system had only three classes. The Samsoon and Young (37) modification includes the fourth class.

anatomic structures of the human airway is beyond the scope of this chapter but has been reviewed superbly by Roberts (33) and Moore (34). A number of specific features play a role in the identification of patients at risk for failed intubation, which are reviewed below.

The human airway can be divided into upper and lower segments. Anatomic abnormalities in each of these segments present different problems for the anesthesiologist. The anatomic components of the upper airway form the basis of the popular Samsoon-Young modification of the Mallampati pharyngeal classification, which is referred to as the "Mallampati class" (Table 16.7), and of the Cormack-Lehane laryngeal grading system (Table 16.8) (35–38).

As noted in Table 16.9, significant differences exist between pediatric and adult airways. Figure 16.1 reviews these and other differences. Appropriate airway management of the newborn and infant requires recognition of these important differences.

There are two major classes of airway problems the anesthesia provider may encounter: Difficulty with mask ventilation and difficulty with direct laryngoscopy or tracheal intubation. Difficulty with mask ventilation ranges from easy ventilation to impossible ventilation, even with two individuals (one "working the mask" and the other "working the bag") and appropriate use of naso- and oropharyngeal airways. A functional definition of difficult mask ventilation (DMV) was proposed by Langeron et al. in 2000. They defined DMV as the inability of an unassisted anesthesiologist to maintain an oxygen saturation >92% or to prevent or reverse signs of inadequate ventilation during general anesthesia. They

Table 16.8. Cormack-Lehane grading system of the glottic view during direct laryngoscopy

Grade	Glottic Structures Visualized
I	Entire glottic opening
II	Posterior glottic structures
III	Epiglottis
IV	Soft palate only

Reprinted with permission from Cormack RS, Lehane J. Difficult tracheal intubation in obstetrics. *Anaesthesia.* 1984;39:1105–1111.

Table 16.9. Key anatomic components of the adult and pediatric airway

Component	Description
Larynx	Cartilaginous and muscular structure housing the vocal apparatus
Vocal cords	Most narrow portion of the *normal* adult airway
Cricoid ring	Only complete cartilaginous ring in the airway; just below the thyroid cartilage; most narrow portion of the pediatric airway
Cricoid membrane	Membrane connecting the cricoid with the thyroid cartilage
Trachea	12 cm in length in the adult; 4.5 cm in the newborn
Carina	Tracheal bifurcation point; opposite the fourth thoracic vertebra

Data from Desoto H. Difficult airway recognition and management in childhood. In: *Refresher Courses in Anesthesiology.* Vol. 25. Philadelphia: JB Lippincott Co.; 1997:31–33; and Gaiser R. Airway evaluation and management. In: *Clinical Anesthesia Procedures of the Massachusetts General Hospital.* 4th ed. Boston: Little, Brown and Company; 1993:171.

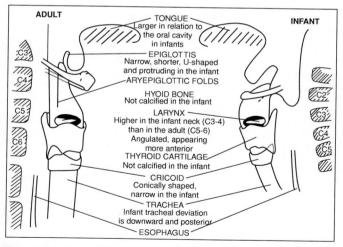

Figure 16.1. Comparison of adult and infant airway anatomic differences. (Reprinted with permission from Ho M. The pediatric airway. In: Bell C, Hughes C, Oh T, eds. *The Pediatric Anesthesia Handbook.* St. Louis: Mosby–Year Book; 1991:130.)

reported an incidence of difficulty with mask ventilation of 5% (39). The ability to predict difficulty with mask ventilation before the induction of anesthesia is important, so the anesthesia practitioner can have airway tools available should problems be encountered. Multivariate analysis reveals five independent risk factors for difficult mask ventilation: Age >55 years, body mass index >26, presence of a beard, lack of teeth, and a history of snoring. The presence of two risk factors is highly suggestive of DMV (sensitivity 72%, specificity 73%). Additional univariate risk factors include Mallampati class 2 or greater, macroglossia, and smaller thyromental distance.

Of the many anatomic features, three have been identified as helpful in predicting possible difficulty with laryngoscopy and tracheal intubation. These include tongue size relative to the pharynx, thyromental distance (the distance between the thyroid cartilage and the tip of the mandible), and atlanto-occipital extension (38). The Mallampati airway classification system is based on the extent to which the oropharyngeal structures are obscured by the patient's tongue. To assign a Mallampati class, the patient is examined in the upright and sitting position, mouth fully open with the tongue maximally protruding. The oropharyngeal structures identified with the patient in this position are the basis for the pharyngeal classes (Table 16.7). The patient should not vocalize during the test, because vocalization raises the soft palate and alters the relationship of the soft palate to the tongue.

In 1984, Cormack and Lehane (38) described four grades of the glottic view with direct laryngoscopy (Table 16.8). The incidence of difficult tracheal intubation varies with the Cormack-Lehane laryngeal grade. Both Mallampati and Samsoon have published a correlation between Mallampati pharyngeal class and ease of laryngoscopy and tracheal intubation. In summary, patients found to have Mallampati pharyngeal class 1 airway examinations have Cormack-Lehane grade I laryngoscopic views 99% to 100% of the time. Those with Mallampati pharyngeal class 4 airways have Cormack-Lehane laryngoscopic grades of III and IV up to 100% of the time (36,37,40). Unfortunately, most patients present with Mallampati class 2 or 3 airways, and these patients have been found to have Cormack-Lehane laryngeal grades ranging from I through IV. Thus, the ability to rely solely on the Mallampati airway classification system as a predictor of difficult laryngoscopy and tracheal intubation is faulty, at least for the majority of patients whose airways are Mallampati class 2 or 3.

The likely explanation for the wide range in Cormack-Lehane laryngeal grade versus Mallampati pharyngeal class, at least for Mallampati class 2 and 3 airways, lies not only in interobserver variability (41), but also in specific anatomic features of the airway that are not included in the modified Mallampati airway classification, including atlanto-occipital extension, thyromental distance, and a number of other features (Table 16.10). Frerk (42) studied whether a combination of the modified Mallampati class and measurement of the thyromental distance could be used to predict difficult laryngoscopy and tracheal intubation. Specifically, he demonstrated the individual and combined sensitivities and specificities of these two easily performed bedside tests. He

Table 16.10. Physical findings suggestive of possible difficulty with tracheal intubation

Trismus
Poor cervical spine mobility
Airway and maxillofacial trauma
Congenital facial and upper airway deformities
Facial and airway tumors and abscesses
Face and neck fibrosis (burns, radiation exposure)
Postsurgical facial and neck deformity
Large tonsils
Micrognathia
Macroglossia
Poor dentition or prominent incisors
Short neck
Large breasts
Morbid obesity

found that categorization into modified Mallampati class 3 or 4 had a sensitivity and specificity of 81% for predicting a difficult tracheal intubation. The finding of a thyromental distance of <7 cm alone showed 91% sensitivity and 81.5% specificity. Use of the two tests together had 81.2% sensitivity and 97.8% specificity. In summary, he found that patients whose airways were categorized as modified Mallampati class 3 or 4 and who had a thyromental distance of <7 cm could be expected to have difficult laryngoscopy and tracheal intubation. Of note, thyromental distance was measured with the patient's head in maximum extension. A major limitation of this study was the limited number of patients evaluated.

A number of disease states and craniofacial and cervical spine abnormalities are associated with difficult intubation. These can be identified by history (Table 16.11), physical examination (Table 16.10), and radiographic techniques (chest radiography, neck

Table 16.11. History suggestive of possible difficulty with tracheal intubation

Congenital abnormalities	Down syndrome, Treacher Collins syndrome, Pierre Robin syndrome, Goldenhar syndrome, Klippel-Feil syndrome
Endocrine disorders	Obesity, acromegaly, dwarfism, Cushing disease
Infection	Epiglottitis, Ludwig's angina
Immune and collagen vascular disease	Scleroderma, rheumatoid arthritis, cervical spine degeneration, cervical disc disease
Burns, trauma, foreign body	
Neoplasms	Cancer, lingual hemangioma, mucopolysaccharidoses

and chest computed tomography, cervical spine imaging, tracheal tomogram).

In addition, obtaining previous operative records is critical. Patients often do not know the details of their difficult airway event, if they know of the event at all. Prior anesthesia records may be especially helpful for patients who meet criteria for possible difficulty with tracheal intubation or mask ventilation.

In summary, tongue size relative to the pharynx, atlanto-occipital extension, thyromental distance, craniofacial and cervical spinal deformities, and various disease states influence both prediction of possible difficult intubation and actual difficulty in intubating the trachea. No single factor, except perhaps a history of difficult intubation, has proven absolutely reliable in predicting difficulty with direct laryngoscopy. That being said, proper preoperative evaluation is the key to minimizing the risk of an unanticipated difficult airway situation. Once the patient is inside the operating room, optimizing head position and having access to a number of airway devices as outlined in the ASA difficult airway management algorithm further enhance successful intubation of the trachea.

Many patients may appear to be at risk for difficult direct laryngoscopy but do not have risk factors for DMV or contraindications to mask ventilation. It is reasonable to induce general anesthesia in these patients and then secure the airway after the patient is anesthetized. The anesthetized patient may be intubated using a fiberoptic bronchoscope, an intubating laryngeal mask (LMA), or one of many other devices. The airway may also be managed with a supraglottic device such as an LMA or the case may be done with anesthesia delivered via a face mask only. In these "difficult intubation/easy mask ventilation" cases the patients usually do not need special instructions prior to surgery. However, **it is extremely important that the possibility of difficult laryngoscopy or intubation be well documented in the preoperative assessment** and the need for special airway equipment communicated to the necessary parties.

Other patients who appear to be at risk for difficult direct laryngoscopy or intubation and have increased risk for DMV as outlined above or contraindications to mask ventilation, such as active gastroesophageal reflux disease (GERD), morbid obesity, or pregnancy, are often best managed with an awake fiberoptic intubation (FOI). Many patients may have mild dyspepsia after a large or spicy meal, for which they take H_2 blockers or proton pump inhibitors. If they have no symptoms while being treated, many anesthesia providers would consider it safe to mask ventilate the patient. Patients who report reflux symptoms not associated with a meal or who awaken at night with a choking sensation or the sensation of fluid in the back of their mouth have active GERD and should have their airway secured via awake FOI if the anesthesia provider is not highly confident that the first attempt at direct laryngoscopy and intubation will be successful.

In addition to communicating with the anesthesia providers the need for special equipment, it is very helpful for the preoperative consultant to psychologically prepare the patient for the awake intubation. The patient should be informed of the rationale for the awake intubation. It should be explained that after the induction of general anesthesia there is limited time to secure the airway. The patient should be informed that the safest course is to allow him or her to continue to breathe and protect his or her airway from aspiration. The patient should be assured that proper sedation will be provided and that local anesthetics or "numbing medicines" will be used to prevent any gagging or unpleasant sensations. The author often explains to patients that the normal method of an asleep intubation uses a stainless steel spatula with a light bulb to push the tongue out of the way, while an FOI uses a flexible scope to gently steer the breathing tube behind the tongue and into the windpipe. When presented with this description and assurances that more sedation and numbing medicine can be provided if requested, most patients are comfortable proceeding with the airway management plan.

This chapter demonstrates that there is no simple way to identify a patient at risk for difficult airway management. Careful history taking and physical examination and review of radiographic data and previous anesthetic records are critical to the preoperative evaluation. Finally, communication between the individual who performs the preoperative evaluation and the individual who is to deliver the anesthetic is paramount if patients are to be cared for in an optimal way.

Any patient whose airway was difficult to manage, because of either poor mask ventilation or difficulty with tracheal intubation, should be encouraged to obtain a MedicAlert bracelet. MedicAlert can be reached at 2323 Colorado Avenue, Turlock, CA 95382, and at 1-800-432-5378 or www.medicalert.org.

Case Study

A 25-year-old woman with a lump in her neck is to undergo a partial thyroidectomy. She has no significant medical or surgical history and is on no medications. When asked whether anyone in the family has had problems with anesthesia, she presents a card containing the word *succinylcholine*. She says that her father had a bad "allergy" to this medication and previously had to stay in the intensive care unit after a surgical procedure. Unfortunately, she has no records.

Could he have had MH? Was he in need of ventilation due to pseudocholinesterase deficiency? Perhaps he had received too much succinylcholine and required ventilation for a phase II block? When pressed, she states that her father had received a single dose of this drug, and on completion of the operation he "could hear everything but could not move." He was ventilated in the intensive care unit for several hours with no other problems. She has never heard of MH but states that her father's anesthesiologist had said that no one in the family should receive succinylcholine.

With a likely family history of pseudocholinesterase deficiency, this patient and her children should be tested to determine whether they are at risk for prolonged apnea with use of succinylcholine and mivacurium chloride. Her dibucaine level should be determined. All close relatives should be evaluated. All affected persons need to be advised to obtain a MedicAlert bracelet and registration. She should be reassured that neither succinylcholine nor mivacurium chloride is necessary for anesthesia or surgery.

This case highlights the importance of obtaining medical records before elective surgery, because patients often are unaware of the specific details regarding medical care.

REFERENCES

1. Donati F, Bevan DR. Long-term succinylcholine infusion during isoflurane anesthesia. *Anesthesiology*. 1983;58:6–10.
2. Kalow W, Genest K. A method for the detection of atypical forms of human serum cholinesterase. Determination of dibucaine numbers. *Can J Biochem Physiol*. 1957;35:339–346.
3. Viby-Mogensen J. Succinylcholine neuromuscular blockade in subjects homozygous for atypical plasma cholinesterase. *Anesthesiology*. 1981;55:429–434.
4. Lehmann H, Lidell J. Pseudocholinesterase: genetic variants and their recognition. *Br J Anaesth*. 1969;41:235–243.
5. Krause A, Lane AB, Jenkins T. Pseudocholinesterase variation in southern Africa populations. *S Afr Med J*. 1987;71:298–301.
6. Hanel HK, Viby-Mogensen J, de Muckadell OB. Serum cholinesterase variants in the Danish population. *Acta Anaesthesiol Scand*. 1978;22:505–507.
7. Gutsche BB, Scott EM, Wright RC. Hereditary deficiency in pseudocholinesterase in Eskimos. *Nature*. 1965;215:322–323.
8. Rosenberg H, Fletcher J, Seitman D. *Pharmacogenetics in Clinical Anesthesia*. 2nd ed. Philadelphia: JB Lippincott Co.; 1992:604.
9. Davies RO, Marton AV, Kalow W. The action of normal and atypical cholinesterase upon a series of esters of choline. *Can J Biochem Physiol*. 1960;38:545–551.
10. Stoelting RK, Dierdorf SF. *Anesthesia and Co-existing Disease*. 3rd ed. New York: Churchill Livingstone; 1993:612.
11. Ording H. Incidence of MH in Denmark. *Anesth Analg*. 1985;64:700–704.
12. Lopez JR, Alamo L, Caputo C, et al. Intracellular ionized calcium concentration in muscles from humans with malignant hyperthermia. *Muscle Nerve*. 1985;8:355–358.
13. Hymel L, Inui M, Fleischer S, et al. Purified ryanodine receptor of skeletal muscle sarcoplasmic reticulum forms calcium activated oligomeric calcium channels in planar bilayers. *Proc Natl Acad Sci U S A*. 1988;85:441–445.
14. Lai FA, Erickson HP, Rousseau E, et al. Purification and reconstitution of the calcium release channel from skeletal muscle. *Nature*. 1988;331:315–319.
15. Jenden DJ, Fairhurst AS. The pharmacology of ryanodine. *Pharmacol Rev*. 1969;21:1–25.
16. Wieland SJ, Fletcher JE, Rosenberg H, et al. Malignant hyperthermia: slow sodium current in cultured human muscle cells. *Am J Physiol*. 1989;257:759–765.
17. MH Biopsy testing centers resource page. Malignant Hyperthermia Association of the United States Web Site. Available at http://www.mhaus.org. Accessed April 27, 2007.

18. Allen GC, Larach MG, Kunselman AR. The sensitivity and specificity of the caffeine-halothane contracture test: a report from the North American Malignant Hyperthermia Registry. *Anesthesiology*. 1998;88:579–588.

19. Prevention Genetics Clinical DNA test price list. Available at: http://www.preventiongenetics.com. Accessed April 14, 2007.

20. Litman RS, Rosenberg H. Malignant hyperthermia: update on susceptibility testing. *JAMA*. 2005;293:2918–2924.

21. Medical Professionals FAQ page. Malignant Hyperthermia Association of the United States Web Site. Available at: http://www.mhaus.org/index.cfm/fuseaction/Content.Display/PagePK/MedicalFAQs.cfm. Accessed June 2, 2007.

22. Rosenberg H, Fletcher J. Masseter muscle rigidity and malignant hyperthermia susceptibility. *Anesth Analg*. 1998;65:161–164.

23. Allen GC, Rosenberg H. Malignant hyperthermia susceptibility in adult patients with masseter muscle rigidity. *Can J Anaesth*. 1990;37:31–35.

24. Kaplan R. Malignant hyperthermia. In: *Refresher Courses in Anesthesiology*. Vol. 22. Philadelphia: JB Lippincott Co.; 1994:169–180.

25. Gan TJ. Postoperative nausea and vomiting—can it be eliminated? *JAMA*. 2002;287:1233–1236.

26. Shnaider I, Chung F. Outcomes in day surgery. *Curr Opin Anaesthesiol*. 2006;19:622–629.

27. Apfel CC, Laara E, Koivuranta M, et al. A simplified risk score for predicting postoperative nausea and vomiting: conclusions from cross-validations between two centers. *Anesthesiology*. 1999;91:693–700.

28. Gan TJ. Risk factors for postoperative nausea and vomiting. *Anesth Analg*. 2006;102:1884–1898.

29. Kranke P, Morin AM, Roewer N, et al. The efficacy and safety of transdermal scopolamine for the prevention of postoperative nausea and vomiting: a quantitative systematic review. *Anesth Analg*. 2002;95:133–143.

30. Caplan RA, Posner KL, Ward RJ, et al. Adverse respiratory events in anesthesia: a closed claims analysis. *Anesthesiology*. 1990;723:828–833.

31. Benumof JL. Management of the difficult airway. *Anesthesiology*. 1991;75:1087–1110.

32. Peterson GN, Domino KB, Caplan RA, et al. Management of the difficult airway: a closed claims analysis. *Anesthesiology*. 2005;103:33–39.

33. Roberts JT. *Clinical Management of the Airway*. Philadelphia: WB Saunders; 1994:3–17.

34. Moore KL. *Clinically Oriented Anatomy*. 2nd ed. Baltimore: Williams & Wilkins; 1984:1033–1062.

35. Mallampati SR. Clinical sign to predict difficult tracheal intubation (hypothesis). *Can Anaesth Soc J*. 1983;30:316–317.

36. Mallampati SR, Gatt SP, Gugino LD, et al. A clinical sign to predict difficult tracheal intubation: a prospective study. *Can Anaesth Soc J*. 1985;32:429–434.

37. Samsoon GLT, Young JRB. Difficult tracheal intubation: a retrospective study. *Anaesthesia*. 1987;42:487–490.

38. Cormack RS, Lehane J. Difficult tracheal intubation in obstetrics. *Anaesthesia*. 1984;39:1105–1111.

39. Langeron O, Masso E, Huraux C, et al. Prediction of difficult mask ventilation. *Anesthesiology*. 2000;92:1229–1236.
40. Cohen SM, Zaurito CE, Segil LJ. Oral exam to predict difficult intubations: a large prospective study. *Anesthesiology*. 1989;71:A937.
41. Charters P, Horton WA. Soft tissues and difficult intubation. *Anaesthesia*. 1991;45:996–997.
42. Frerk CM. Predicting difficult intubation. *Anaesthesia*. 1991;46:1005–1008.

Perioperative Management Issues

Stephen D. Small and BobbieJean Sweitzer

The complexity of patients and their medical regimens is growing along with the number of options and information that the anesthesiologist must manage preoperatively. Knowledge about new perioperative risks is emerging, and recommendations from experts and professional societies are changing. This chapter provides a resource for preoperative management of chronic medication schedules as well as guidelines for adding medications, such as beta blockers. Risks and benefits of continuation of antiplatelet agents in the perioperative period, especially in patients with coronary stents, are presented. Recently released changes to guidelines for prophylaxis against infective endocarditis are discussed in detail. Other topics include a review and update of fasting recommendations, and nutritional evaluation and management. A discussion of patient- and procedure-specific risks such as awareness under anesthesia, and blindness or nerve injury during surgery is included.

FASTING

Pulmonary aspiration of gastric contents is a relatively rare event. The incidence is approximately 1 in 3,000 cases of general anesthesia (1 in 895 for emergency surgery), according to two large retrospective studies over 20 years ago (1,2), and as many as 1 in 500 cesarean sections (0.15% to 0.22%) (3) in an older study. In a more recent study that examined general anesthesia without an endotracheal tube for peripartum procedures such as placental extraction, suturing of vaginal and cervical tears, and examination of the uterus for postpartum bleeding and internal massage (cesarean section was excluded), only 1 in nearly 2,000 patients suffered a mild case of aspiration (4). Although morbidity and mortality from aspiration are even less frequent, there is an intense focus in daily anesthesia practice to minimize these types of events.

Patients with conditions predisposing them to an increased risk of aspiration (Table 17.1), such as a history of incompetence of the lower esophageal sphincter with reflux, hiatal hernia, diabetes mellitus, gastric motility disorders, intra-abdominal masses (including the gravid uterus), and bowel obstruction, are specifically excluded from the following discussion on liberalized nil per os (NPO) or nothing-by-mouth guidelines for elective surgery. A thorough preoperative screening history reveals such conditions and should be obtained for every patient who will have anesthesia. Obesity was once thought to increase a patient's risk for aspiration because of increased volume and low pH of gastric contents. Harter et al. (5), however, demonstrated that obese patients, if otherwise healthy (and fasting for 10 to 12 hours),

Table 17.1. Risk factors for pulmonary aspiration

History of incompetence of the lower esophageal sphincter with reflux
Symptomatic hiatal hernia
Diabetes mellitus
Gastric motility disorders
Intra-abdominal masses (including the gravid uterus)
Bowel obstruction

actually had a lower incidence of combined high-volume, low-pH stomach contents than did lean patients.

The most current guidelines (Table 17.2) for preoperative fasting for the adult patient recommend that "fasting from solids (and) nonhuman milk should exceed a period of 6 hours before procedures requiring general anesthesia, regional anesthesia, or sedation/analgesia" (6). A small prospective study supported the offering of clear liquids (including coffee or tea, excluding any containing fat, oil, or alcohol) in the amount desired up to 2 hours before the procedure (7) and reviewed a number of studies reporting similar conclusions. In fact, liberalization of preoperative fasting rules to include clear liquids up to 2 hours before surgery may have benefits such as increased patient satisfaction, prevention of caffeine withdrawal, enhanced gastric emptying, and reduction of patient "cheating."

The American Society of Anesthesiologists (ASA) Task Force on Preoperative Fasting (6) does not recommend the routine use of gastrointestinal stimulants (in patients who have no apparent increased risk) to decrease the risk of pulmonary aspiration because of insufficient published evidence to support their effectiveness. Likewise, because of insufficient evidence demonstrating effectiveness in preventing the consequences of aspiration in low-risk patients, histamine-2 receptor antagonists and proton pump inhibitors are not recommended for routine use in patients with no apparent increased risk for aspiration. Patients who are at

Table 17.2. Guidelines for food and fluid intake before elective surgery

Time Before Surgery	Food or Fluid Intake
Up to 8 hours	Food and fluids as desired
Up to 6 hours[a]	Light meal (e.g., toast and clear liquids[b]); infant formula; nonhuman milk
Up to 4 hours[a]	Breast milk
Up to 2 hours[a]	Clear liquids[b] only; no solids or foods containing fat in any form
During the 2 hours	No solids, no liquids

[a]This guideline applies only to patients who *are not* at risk for delayed gastric emptying. Patients with the following conditions *are* at risk for delayed gastric emptying: Morbid obesity, diabetes mellitus, pregnancy, a history of gastroesophageal reflux, a surgery limiting stomach capacity, a potential difficult airway, and opiate analgesic therapy.
[b]Clear liquids are water, carbonated beverages, sports drinks, coffee, or tea (without milk). The following *are not* clear liquids: Juice with pulp, milk, coffee or tea with milk, infant formula, and any beverage with alcohol.

risk (Table 17.1) should be given nonparticulate antacids such as sodium citrate to increase mixing with gastric contents and avoid the potential risk particulate antacids (such as aluminum and magnesium hydroxide) may have of worsening pulmonary injury during aspiration (6).

Guidelines for the pediatric patient allow healthy, normal children clear liquids up to 2 hours before surgery. Infants taking human breast milk may feed until 4 hours before surgery. NPO status is 6 hours preoperatively for children consuming formula or nonhuman milk (6).

It is likely that many technical factors during induction of general anesthesia or deep sedation influence the occurrence and nature of pulmonary aspiration. These include achieving an appropriate depth of anesthesia for the type of airway manipulation, avoiding overdistention of the stomach with gas during positive pressure mask or laryngeal mask airway (LMA) ventilation, and making expert decisions for patients with difficult airways or risk factors for aspiration.

PREVENTION OF DEEP VENOUS THROMBOSIS

Although relatively rare in the general population, deep venous thrombosis (DVT) and pulmonary embolism (PE) are significant causes of morbidity and mortality in those hospitalized for serious illness or major surgery. Yearly, pulmonary emboli are responsible for the mortality of 50,000 to 100,000 hospitalized patients with an otherwise favorable prognosis and account for 5% to 10% of all deaths in U.S. hospitals (8). Determining figures for the total incidence and fatality rates for venous thromboembolism is difficult because typical signs and symptoms (leg pain and swelling, shortness of breath, chest pain) are absent in >50% of affected patients, including a majority of those who die of PE (8). Estimates are that the prevalence of clinically significant venous thromboembolism is 200,000 to 600,000 cases per year in the United States, with a possible decrease in PE over time but an unchanging incidence of DVT in men and an increasing incidence of DVT in women (9). Please refer to Chapter 7 for further information, including important discussion of consequences of anticoagulation for regional anesthesia procedures.

PREVENTION OF BACTERIAL INFECTIVE ENDOCARDITIS

Anesthesiologists must be acquainted with conditions and operations requiring antibiotic prophylaxis to prevent bacterial infective endocarditis (IE). Newly updated recommendations of the American Heart Association (AHA) (10) replace those in use since 1997 (11,12). The nine AHA position papers since 1955 encompass new scientific knowledge and the realities of health policy, dealing with problems such as microbial resistance from prolonged antibiotic prophylaxis and the medicolegal implications of incorrectly viewing the guidelines as a standard of care. The main reasons for revision of the 1997 guidelines were too high a reliance on expert opinion, a need to incorporate findings from a systematic review of the evidence in the literature, and the balance of potential benefits with potential and known risks. Experts have long acknowledged that the evidence to support the effectiveness of IE prophylaxis is not compelling due to the conclusion that bacteremia and most cases of IE result from daily activities and oral hygiene issues and not procedures.

Several major changes in the new guidelines will alter current practice. First, prophylaxis is recommended only for patients with cardiac conditions with the highest risk of major adverse outcomes from IE (Table 17.3), not necessarily the highest risk of acquiring IE. For patients with valvular or congenital heart diseases not listed, prophylaxis is not recommended. Mitral valve prolapse (MVP) has replaced rheumatic heart disease as the most common underlying condition predisposing to IE in industrialized countries, yet IE in the setting of MVP is not generally associated with severe adverse outcomes. The absolute risk rate for IE with MVP is thought to be 1 per 1.1 million procedures. Coupled with a $<100\%$ effectiveness of prophylactic regimens and the emergence of multidrug-resistant viridans group streptococci and enterococci, prophylaxis is no longer recommended for patients with MVP.

Antibiotic prophylactic regimens are given in Table 17.4. No studies have shown however, that therapy will prevent enterococcal IE. A single 2 g dose of ampicillin or amoxicillin given 30 to 60 minutes before the procedure is the regimen of choice. Vancomycin is an alternative in patients unable to tolerate ampicillin. Consultation with an infectious diseases expert is recommended

---

Table 17.3. Cardiac conditions associated with the highest risk of adverse outcome from endocarditis for which prophylaxis with at-risk procedures is recommended[c]

Prosthetic cardiac valve

Previous infective endocarditis

Congenital heart disease (CHD)[a]

    Unrepaired cyanotic CHD, including palliative shunts and conduits

    Completely repaired congenital heart defect with prosthetic material or device, whether placed by surgery or by catheter intervention, during the first 6 months after the procedure[b]

    Repaired CHD with residual defects at the site or adjacent to the site of a prosthetic patch or prosthetic device (which inhibited endothelialization)

Cardiac transplantation recipients who develop cardiac valvulopathy

---

[a]Antibiotic prophylaxis is no longer recommended for forms of CHD not listed in this table. See text for "at-risk procedures."

[b]Prophylaxis is recommended because prosthetic material is endothelialized within 6 months after the procedure.

[c]See text for "at-risk" procedures.

Wilson W, Taubert K, Gewitz M, et al. Prevention of infective endocarditis. Guidelines from the American Heart Association. A guideline from the American Heart Association Rheumatic Fever, Endocarditis, and Kawasaki Disease Committee, Council on Cardiovascular Disease in the Young, and the Council on Clinical Cardiology, Council on Cardiovascular Surgery and Anesthesia, and the Quality of Care and Outcomes Research Interdisciplinary Working Group. *Circulation.* Published online April 19, 2007. DOI: 10.1161/CIRCULATIONAHA.106.183095. Available at: http://circ.ahajournals.org. Accessed May 19, 2007.

Table 17.4. Recommended antibiotic regimens for prophylaxis of infective endocarditis[a]

Situation	Agent	Regimen: Single Dose 30–60 Min before Procedure	
		Adults	Children
Oral	Amoxicillin	2 g	50 mg/kg
Unable to take oral medication	Ampicillin	2 g IM or IV	50 mg/kg IM or IV
	or		
	Cefazolin or ceftriaxone	1 g IM or IV	50 mg/kg IM or IV
Allergic to penicillins or ampicillin—oral	Cephalexin[b,c]	2 g	50 mg/kg
	or		
	Clindamycin	600 mg	20 mg/kg
	or		
	Azithromycin or clarithromycin	500 mg	15 mg/kg
Allergic to penicillins or ampicillin and unable to take oral medications	Cefazolin or ceftriaxone[c]	1 g IM or IV	50 mg/kg IM or IV
	or		
	Clindamycin	600 mg IM or IV	20 mg/kg IM or IV

[a]These recommendations apply to patients with the medical conditions listed in Table 17.3 and for very limited procedures as outlined in the text.
[b]Or other first- or second-generation oral cephalosporin in equivalent adult or pediatric dosage.
[c]Do not use cephalosporins if history of anaphylaxis, angioedema, or urticaria with penicillins or ampicillin; use vancomycin instead.
Wilson W, Taubert K, Gewitz M, et al. Prevention of infective endocarditis. Guidelines from the American Heart Association. A Guidline from the American Heart Association Rheumatic Fever, Endocarditis, and Kawasaki Disease Committee, Council on Cardiovascular Disease in the Young, and the Council on Clinical Cardiology, Council on Cardiovascular Surgery and Anesthesia, and the Quality of Care and Outcomes Research Interdisciplinary Working Group. *Circulation*. Published online April 19, 2007. DOI: 10.1161/CIRCULATIONAHA.106.183095. Available at: http://circ.ahajournals.org. Accessed May 19, 2007.

for documented or suspected resistant enterococcal infection. Antibiotic administration should be timed to ensure adequate concentrations in the serum during and after the procedure. The concentrations can be readily achieved by giving the antibiotic intravenously at the time of induction of anesthesia. Antibiotic administration should not be continued for more than 6 to 8 hours after a procedure to minimize the risks of microbial resistance. If, for whatever reason, the preprocedure dose of antibiotics is not administered, it may be given up to 2 hours after the procedure. Anyone with fever and symptoms and signs compatible with IE should have blood cultures drawn before antibiotic administration to prevent delays in diagnosis and appropriate therapy.

For patients with the conditions listed in Table 17.3, prophylaxis should be given only before incision or biopsy of respiratory tract mucosa; procedures on infected skin or musculoskeletal structures; or dental procedures that involve manipulation of gingival tissues or the periapical region of teeth or perforation of the oral mucosa.

For procedures on the respiratory tract, prophylaxis is recommended *only* for patients with conditions in Table 17.3 who have incision or biopsy of the respiratory mucosa (e.g., tonsillectomy, adenoidectomy). Bronchoscopy is not included unless it requires incision of respiratory mucosa. For invasive procedures, treating established infections of the respiratory tract and coverage against viridans streptococci as well as suspected or documented *Staphylococcus aureus* are recommended. Patients unable to tolerate a β-lactam or who have methicillin-resistant *S. aureus* infection need vancomycin.

Patients having procedures on infected skin or musculoskeletal tissues (and with the conditions listed in Table 17.3) should receive prophylaxis as outlined in Table 17.4. Although these infections are often polymicrobial, IE is likely to be caused by either staphylococci or β-hemolytic streptococci. Vancomycin may be used for patients with allergies to β-lactams and for resistant organisms.

Many procedures involving the gastrointestinal (GI) and genitourinary (GU) tracts may cause transient bacteremia, most commonly with enterococcus. However, reports of IE-associated GI or GU procedures are anecdotal. Enterococci are increasingly resistant to penicillins, vancomycin, and aminoglycosides—antibiotics previously recommended for prophylaxis against IE. The new guidelines recommend prophylaxis *only* for patients with conditions in Table 17.3 *and* urinary tract procedural manipulation (e.g., cystoscopy) *in the presence of* enterococcal urinary infection or colonization. If the GU procedure is elective, it is recommended to eradicate enterococcus before the procedure. A regimen effective against enterococci is recommended *if* a patient has a condition in Table 17.3 *and* an established GI or GU infection, *and* will receive antibiotics to prevent wound infection or sepsis from the procedure (i.e., *not for IE prevention*). First-line prophylaxis is ampicillin or amoxicillin, with vancomycin as a second choice in patients unable to tolerate a β-lactam.

No prophylaxis is recommended for upper and lower GI diagnostic endoscopic procedures. Procedures *not recommended for prophylaxis* in the 1997 guidelines remain in that category (11), with the addition of ear and body piercing, tattooing, vaginal delivery, and hysterectomy (not recommended). Antibiotic prophylaxis is not recommended based solely on an increased lifetime risk of acquisition of IE—the recommendations focus only on preventing severe adverse IE outcomes in high-risk patients (Table 17.3).

In sum, the population-based and individual risks of antibiotic use exceed the benefits in most situations in which prophylaxis for IE is currently used. No convincing data exist that conclusively show that prophylactic antibiotics prevent IE associated with bacteremia from an invasive procedure (10). As a result, fewer patients will receive prophylactic antibiotics as the guidelines come into common usage. Patients accustomed to receiving and physicians used to prescribing antibiotics may be uncomfortable with these changes and no longer feel safe. To aid in transition to the new guidelines, the AHA includes evidence that prophylaxis may prevent a very small number of cases of IE, if any, in the now excluded categories, and the risks of antibiotics (adverse events, allergic reactions, growth of resistant organisms) outweigh putative benefits.

Several special cases deserve mention. If patients are already taking an oral antibiotic that is the same as the IE-recommended therapy, a drug from another class is given rather than an increased dose of the same antibiotic. Patients taking antibiotics orally have relatively low blood levels that can induce resistance. If patients are receiving parenteral therapy for ongoing IE and will undergo procedures, doses of established antibiotics should be given 30 to 60 minutes before the procedure. Low-level resistance that may have developed will be managed by the high levels of antibiotics achieved through parenteral dosing.

Patients receiving anticoagulants immediately preoperatively should not receive intramuscular antibiotics for prophylaxis against IE.

For cardiac valve surgery, no single regimen is effective against all of the possible organisms causing IE. Thus, therapy targeting the most common—*S. aureus*—is recommended, as is considering patterns of local infection and resistance. Prophylaxis commences just before the procedure, is repeated during prolonged procedures, and is limited to 48 hours postoperatively.

Antibiotic prophylaxis is not recommended for patients with coronary stents, bypass grafts, pacemakers, or implanted cardiac defibrillators. In the absence of reliable data on heart transplantation patients, prophylaxis is limited to patients with postoperative cardiac valvulopathy (Table 17.3). All patients with planned cardiac valve surgery, replacement, or correction of congenital heart disease should have a preoperative dental consultation so that any required dental treatment may be performed before surgery.

PREOPERATIVE MEDICATION MANAGEMENT

The patient's comorbidities and the nature of the procedure must be considered when managing medications preoperatively. Some medications have beneficial effects during surgery, others are detrimental, and in some cases stopping therapy suddenly has a negative effect. Table 17.5 outlines the medications to continue

Table 17.5. Medication instructions

Instruct patients to take these with a small sip of water EVEN IF OTHERWISE NPO.

1. **Antihypertensive medications**
   Continue on the day of surgery (DOS)

   o **Exceptions:**
   For patients undergoing certain procedures or who have medical conditions where hypotension is particularly dangerous, it may be prudent to discontinue angiotensin-converting enzyme inhibitors (ACEIs) or angiotensin receptor blockers (ARBs) before surgery.
   The following are possible indications (especially if more than one apply to any given patient) to hold ACEIs and ARBs 12–24 hours before surgery:
      - Patients on multiple antihypertensive medications
      - Patients with well-controlled blood pressure
      - General anesthesia planned
      - Lengthy surgery planned
      - Procedures involving significant blood loss or fluid shifts

2. **Cardiac medications (e.g., digoxin)**
   Continue on the DOS.

3. **Antidepressant, antianxiety, and psychiatric medications**
   Continue on the DOS.

4. **Thyroid medications**
   Continue on the DOS.

5. **Birth control pills**
   Continue on the DOS.

6. **Eye drops**
   Continue on the DOS.

7. **Heartburn or reflux medications (e.g., Prilosec, Zantac)**
   Continue on the DOS.

8. **Narcotic pain medications**
   Continue on the DOS.

9. **Antiseizure medications**
   Continue on the DOS.

10. **Asthma medications**
    Continue on the DOS.

11. **Steroids (oral or inhaled)**
    Continue on the DOS.

12. **Statins (e.g., Zocor, simvastatin)**
    Continue on the DOS.

13. **Aspirin**
    Continue aspirin unless the risk of bleeding outweighs the risk of thrombosis. If reversal of platelet inhibition is necessary, then aspirin must be stopped 7 days before surgery. There is no need to stop aspirin in patients having cataract surgery with topical or general anesthesia. Do NOT discontinue aspirin in patients who have drug-eluting coronary stents (DESs) until they have completed 12 months of antiplatelet therapy unless the patient, surgeon, and cardiologist have discussed the risks of discontinuation. The same applies to patients with bare-metal stents (BMSs) until they have completed 1 month of antiplatelet therapy.

(Continued)

Table 17.5. Medication instructions (*Continued*)

14. **Antiplatelet agents; thienopyridines (e.g. clopidogrel, Plavix, ticlopidine)**
    Continue antiplatelets unless the risk of bleeding outweighs the risk of thrombosis. If reversal of platelet inhibition is necessary, then antiplatelets must be stopped 7 days before surgery. There is no need to stop antiplatelets in patients having cataract surgery with topical or general anesthesia. Do NOT discontinue antiplatelets in patients who have DESs until they have completed 12 months of antiplatelet therapy unless the patient, surgeon, and cardiologist have discussed the risks of discontinuation. The same applies to patients with BMSs until they have completed 1 month of antiplatelet therapy.

15. **Insulin**
    For all patients, discontinue all short-acting (e.g., regular) insulins on DOS (unless administered via continuous pump). Type 2 diabetics should take none or up to a half-dose of long-acting or combination (70/30 preparations) insulins on DOS. Type 1 diabetics should take a small amount (usually one third) of their usual morning long-acting insulin (e.g., lente or NPH) on the DOS. Patients with an insulin pump should continue their basal rate ONLY.

16. **Vitamins, minerals, iron**
    Discontinue on the DOS.

17. **Topical medications (e.g., creams and ointments)**
    Discontinue on the DOS.

18. **Oral hypoglycemic agents**
    Discontinue on the DOS.

19. **Diuretics**
    Discontinue on the DOS (exception is triamterene or hydrochlorothiazide [HCTZ], when taken for hypertension, should be continued on the DOS).

20. **Viagra or similar drugs**
    Discontinue 24 hours before surgery.

21. **Cyclooxygenase-2 inhibitors**
    Continue on the DOS unless surgeon is concerned about bone healing.

22. **Nonsteroidal anti-inflammatory drugs**
    Discontinue 48 hours prior to the DOS.

23. **Warfarin (Coumadin)**
    Discontinue 4–5 days before surgery except for patients having cataract surgery without a bulbar block.

24. **Herbals and nonvitamin supplements**
    Discontinue 7 days before surgery.

25. **Monoamine oxidase inhibitors**
    Continue these medications and adjust anesthesia accordingly.

or discontinue preoperatively. Several drug classes and emerging controversies deserve special mention.

Medications for hypertension should generally be continued preoperatively. Stopping beta blockers or centrally acting α_2 agonists (e.g., clonidine) may be associated with rebound hypertension. For patients who cannot tolerate hypotension, angiotensin-converting enzyme inhibitors (ACEIs) or angiotensin receptor blockers (ARBs) may be discontinued 12 to 24 hours before the day of surgery (13). Hypotension may be refractory to fluid administration and require ephedrine and/or phenylephrine in patients taking these drugs. Vasopressin has been used successfully to treat hypotension in these instances. These drugs may be discontinued 12 to 24 hours preoperatively when procedures involve significant blood loss or fluid shifts, patients are taking multiple antihypertensive medications, patients have a history of well-controlled blood pressure, the intraoperative positioning of the patient may impair blood pressure, or the procedure is complex spine surgery.

ARBs and ACEIs may have protective effects in patients with coronary artery disease (CAD) and protective renal effects in taken long term. The negative consequences if ARBs and ACEIs are abruptly stopped are not clear, especially in patients with heart failure (HF). The potential for refractory hypotension must be balanced against the positive therapeutic impact of continuing these agents perioperatively on a case-by-case basis. A suggested approach is to continue ACEIs and ARBs and alter the anesthetic plan, especially induction dosages and drugs, and have vasopressin available to prevent or mitigate significant hypotension.

Diuretics are generally discontinued preoperatively, with the exception of hydrochlorothiazide if taken for hypertension, especially if it is the only antihypertensive drug. Potent loop diuretics, which may cause volume depletion and hypokalemia, should generally be discontinued on the day of surgery. It may be best to continue diuretics in patients with significant volume overload, severe HF, or ascites, especially if the scheduled procedure is minor and not likely to result in fluid shifts or blood loss. These drugs can always be administered intravenously during the procedure.

Patients with heart disease or with cardiovascular risk factors may be taking a variety of medications such as beta blockers, statins, antiplatelet agents, digoxin, and antiarrhythmics. These medications should be continued up until surgery because of their beneficial effects and potential for negative effects if discontinued. Perioperative administration of beta blockers may reduce adverse cardiac events in patients who need intermediate- to high-risk surgery and have clinical predictors for cardiac events (14,15). The American College of Cardiology (ACC)/AHA recommends (class I indications) that beta blockers should be continued in patients undergoing surgery who are receiving beta blockers to treat angina, symptomatic arrhythmias, or hypertension (16).

The ACC/AHA recommends perioperative beta blockers (a class I indication) for patients with a positive stress test who need major vascular surgery. In patients with a history of CAD but without ongoing ischemia or undergoing procedures other than major vascular surgery the ACC/AHA endorses using perioperative beta blockers as a class IIa recommendation (conditions for which there is conflicting evidence and/or a divergence of opinion about the usefulness/efficacy of a procedure or treatment but the weight of evidence/opinion is in favor of usefulness/efficacy) (16).

Minimizing risk for high-risk patients scheduled for elective surgery may entail postponing surgery to optimize beta blockers and statin therapy (14). Table 17.6 provides a protocol for inclusion and exclusion criteria for starting preoperative beta blockers, and suggests dosing regimens. The optimal regimen, type of beta blockers, doses, timing, and degree of heart rate (HR) control have not been conclusively determined. Studies suggest that beta blockers may not be effective if target HR (<70 bpm) is not achieved or if patients are at low risk (17). Longer-acting agents may be superior because of a lower incidence of subtherapeutic blood levels. One study showed that patients receiving atenolol versus metoprolol had a lower incidence of perioperative myocardial infarction (MI) and death (18).

Beta blockers are not contraindicated for patients with stable, mild to moderate chronic obstructive pulmonary disease, asthma, or diabetes (19). Beta blockers should not be started in patients with an acute or recent (within 1 month) exacerbation of heart failure (although they are beneficial for patients with chronic heart failure), in patients with high-degree heart block or significant bradycardia, or in patients with reactive airway disease who are dependent on daily β agonists or have an acute exacerbation of bronchospasm.

Starting beta blockers preoperatively provides an opportunity to titrate these agents to the desired HR and identify adverse effects and intolerance. Preoperative anesthesia clinics are ideal settings to deal with these challenges, identify high-risk patients who may benefit from starting or escalating beta blocker therapy, and then implement and monitor administration (20).

Beyond simply lowering cholesterol, statins have multiple modulating effects on ischemic heart disease, including anti-inflammatory and coronary plaque stabilizing properties. Statins (3-hydroxyl-3-methylglutaryl coenzyme A reductase inhibitors) reduce oxidative stress by scavenging oxygen free radicals, augment nitric oxide production, inhibiting smooth muscle proliferation, improve endothelial function, and inhibit platelet aggregation. Multiple studies have shown a benefit of statins in reducing stroke, renal dysfunction, myocardial infarction, death, and even hospital length of stay (21–23). The benefits of statins started shortly before surgery have not been extensively studied. One small trial in patients having vascular surgery showed a significant reduction in cardiac complications in those given atorvastatin regardless of serum cholesterol levels (24).

Statins are generally well tolerated with only minor side effects such as myalgias. Hepatotoxicity and rhabdomyolysis can occur but are exceedingly rare and generally develop soon after initiation of therapy. No study of perioperative statin therapy has reported significant risks with the use of these drugs (25). Abruptly stopping statins may be associated with an increase in risk, including death (26).

Statins should be continued in the perioperative period and serious consideration given to starting them in patients with known or with increased risk of atherosclerotic disease.

Table 17.6.   Preoperative beta (β)-blocker protocol

Inclusion criteria:
1. Patients undergoing surgical procedures of moderate to high risk
   a. All vascular surgical procedures: aortic, carotid, peripheral
   b. Major orthopedic, e.g., total joints, open spine surgery
   c. Open abdominal, pelvic, gastrointestinal, urologic, gynecologic
   d. Open thoracic surgeries or those requiring one-lung ventilation
   e. Major head and neck

And
2a. Patients with known coronary artery disease

Or
2b. Patients with at least two of the following risk factors for coronary artery disease:
   a. Age >70 years
   b. Diabetes mellitus
   c. Poorly controlled hypertension (systolic > 160 mmHg; diastolic > 100 mmHg)
   d. Peripheral vascular or carotid arteriosclerosis
   e. Renal insufficiency (creatinine $\geq$2.0 mg/dL)
   f. Cerebrovascular disease (stroke, transient ischemic attack)
   g. Poor functional capacity (<5 METs; i.e., unable to walk up a flight of stairs or walk 2 blocks without stopping)

Exclusion criteria:
Acute or recent (<1 month) exacerbation of heart failure
Severe left ventricular dysfunction (<30% ejection fraction) unless already taking a β-blocker
Significant bradycardia
Second or third degree heart block
Reactive airway disease and dependence on daily beta-agonists, or bronchospasm exacerbation
Allergy to β-blockers
Systolic blood pressure <100 mmHg or heart rate <50 beats/minute (bpm)

Preoperative instructions for β-blocker therapy:
1. Start atenolol or metoprolol 25–50 mg/day titrating to HR <65 bpm
2. If the patient is already taking a β-blocker, titrate to HR of 65–80 bpm and continue therapy until day of surgery.
3. Toprol XL 50 mg by mouth on the day of surgery if the patient has missed her usual β-blocker dose.
4. The anesthesiologist may also titrate intravenous β-blocker therapy in small increments (e.g., metoprolol 2.5 mg, propranolol 1 mg) on the day of surgery if the patient has missed her usual β-blocker dose, being careful to avoid hypotension.

MET = metabolic equivalent, a measure of a patient's functional status.

Chronic administration of aspirin is commonly used to lower risk of events in patients with known vascular disease or risk factors such as diabetes, renal insufficiency, or simply advanced age. The U.S. Preventative Services Taskforce recommends aspirin for patients with CAD, other atherosclerotic disease, and those at increased risk for the development of CAD (27). Traditionally aspirin has been withdrawn in the perioperative period because of concern over increased bleeding. However, this practice has come under scrutiny. A meta-analysis involving almost 50,000 patients undergoing a variety of noncardiac surgeries (30% on perioperative aspirin) found that aspirin increased bleeding complications by a factor of 1.5 (28). Aspirin did not increase the severity of bleeding complications except in patients undergoing intracranial surgery and possibly transurethral resection of the prostate. Additionally, acute coronary syndromes occurred 8.5 ± 3.6 days and acute cerebral events 14.3 ± 11.3 days after aspirin cessation. When surgeons are blinded to aspirin administration, they cannot identify patients on or off aspirin based on bleeding (29). Several studies support an increased risk of vascular events when chronic aspirin is stopped perioperatively (30–32).

There may be a rebound hypercoagulable state when chronic aspirin is withdrawn with promotion of prothrombogenic changes (33). This coupled with the hypercoagulable state of many surgeries is likely to pose significant risk. For many minor, superficial procedures such as cataract extraction, endoscopies, and peripheral procedures, the risk of withdrawing aspirin in high-risk patients is clearly greater than the risk of bleeding. Many patients are unknowingly taking aspirin. Many cold preparations and over-the-counter drugs (e.g., Alka-Seltzer and Pepto-Bismol) may contain aspirin (Table 17.7). Studies support the safety of neuraxial and peripheral anesthesia in patients taking chronic aspirin and the American Society of Regional Anesthesia (ASRA) endorses this opinion (34–36).

Aspirin may be continued or withheld for the shortest amount of time. Since new platelets formed after aspirin dosing is stopped will not be affected and surgical bleeding should be minimally affected with a count of normally functioning platelets >50,000, stopping aspirin for 3 to 4 days should be sufficient. If aspirin is stopped, doses should be resumed as soon as possible. The American College of Chest Physicians has recommended *preoperative* aspirin therapy for patients scheduled to have peripheral revascularization, especially carotid endarterectomy and infrainguinal bypass (37).

There is limited information on the safety or risks of continuing other antiplatelet therapies, such as the thienopyridines, clopidogrel and ticlopidine, or glycoprotein (GP) IIb/IIIa inhibitors. Case reports of bleeding and traditions of aspirin cessation have influenced practice so that most patients are advised to stop these medications 7 to 10 days before procedures. One study concluded that therapy with either aspirin *or* clopidogrel alone was generally safe (38). The actual risk of spinal hematoma with ticlopidine, clopidogrel, and the GP IIb/IIIa antagonists is unknown. Based on labeling, ASRA guidelines, and surgical reviews, the suggested time interval between discontinuation of thienopyridine therapy

Table 17.7. Medications containing aspirin

Adprin-B	Goody's Powders
Aggrenox	Lortab
Alka-Seltzer	Magnaprin
Anacin	Meprobamate
Ascriptin	Methocarbamol
Aspergum	Micrainin
Azdone	Norgesic
B-A-C	Oxycodone
BC Powder	P-A-C
Bufferin	Pepto-Bismol
Butalbital Compound	Percodan
Carisoprodol	Propoxyphene
Cope	Rhinocaps
Darvon	Robaxisal
Disalcid	Roxiprin
Easprin	Salsalate
Ecotrin	Sine-Off
Empirin	Soma
Endodan	Supac
Equagesic	Sureprin
Excedrin	Synalgos
Fiorinal	Talwin Compound
Fiortal	Trigesic
Fortabs	Vanquish
Gelpirin	ZORprin
Genacote	

This is not a complete listing of all aspirin-containing products. Many of these drugs are available in different varieties with combinations of other compounds.

and neuraxial blockade is 14 days for ticlopidine and 7 days for clopidogrel (36).

A scientific advisory from major national cardiovascular professional associations, the ACC, and the AHA provides recommendations for managing patients with coronary stents (Table 17.8) (39). For patients with drug-eluting stents (DESs), 1 uninterrupted year of dual antiplatelet therapy with aspirin plus a thienopyridine (e.g., ticlopidine or clopidogrel [Plavix]) is needed. Elective procedures that risk significant blood loss and necessitate interrupting dual antiplatelet therapy should be delayed during this 1-year period. If surgery must be performed, aspirin should be continued throughout the perioperative period if at all possible, and the thienopyridine restarted as soon as possible after surgery. For patients with bare metal stents (BMSs), as opposed to DESs, antiplatelet therapy is continued for a minimum of at least 1 month after stent placement.

Premature discontinuation of dual antiplatelet therapy can cause catastrophic stent thrombosis, MI, and/or death. No large prospective studies of patients with coronary stents and noncardiac surgery have been performed, but increased bleeding during cardiac surgery (including off-pump grafting) has been reported. Schouten and Poldermans recommended that until

Table 17.8.   Recommendations for perioperative management of antiplatelet agents in patients with coronary stents

- Health care providers who perform invasive procedures must be aware of the potentially catastrophic risks of premature discontinuation of thienopyridine (e.g., clopidogrel or ticlopidine) therapy. Such professionals should contact the patient's cardiologist to discuss optimal strategies if issues regarding antiplatelet therapy are unclear.

- Elective procedures involving risk of bleeding should be deferred until an appropriate course of thienopyridine therapy (12 months after drug-eluting stents [DESs] and 1 month after bare-metal stents [BMSs]) has been completed.

- Patients with DESs who must undergo procedures that mandate discontinuing thienopyridine therapy should continue aspirin if at all possible and have the thienopyridine restarted as soon as possible.

Adapted from reference 39.

more evidence is available, antiplatelet therapy should be continued during surgery unless absolutely contraindicated (40). This was based on their finding a significant increase in major adverse cardiac events in patients with percutaneous coronary interventions (PCIs) and stents (both DES and BMS) who discontinued (31%) versus continued (0%) antiplatelet agents. This study was small and retrospective, but they found no difference in transfusions or number of blood units transfused.

Low-molecular-weight heparin (LMWH) should be held at least 12–24 hours (therapeutic doses 24 hr.; prophylactic doses 12 hr.) before surgery or planned neuraxial block (36). Monitoring of the anti-Xa level is not recommended. The anti-Xa level is not predictive of the risk of bleeding and is, therefore, not helpful in the management of patients receiving LMWH. During subcutaneous (mini-dose) heparin prophylaxis, there is no contraindication to the use of neuraxial techniques (36). Combining neuraxial techniques with intraoperative anticoagulation with heparin during vascular surgery seems acceptable if patients have no other coagulopathies and heparin administration is delayed for 1 hour after needle placement (36).

Warfarin may be associated with increased bleeding except for minor procedures such as cataract surgery without bulbar blocks. There is no consensus on the optimal perioperative management of patients on warfarin. The usual recommendation is to withhold four doses of warfarin before operation (if the international normalized ratio [INR] is 2.0 to 3.0) to allow the INR to decrease to <1.5, a level considered safe for surgical procedures (36). If the INR is >3.0, it is necessary to withhold warfarin longer than four doses. If the INR is measured the day before surgery and remains >1.8, a small dose of vitamin K (1.0 to 5.0 mg orally or subcutaneously) can reverse anticoagulation (41).

Substitution with shorter-acting anticoagulants such as unfractionated or LMWH, referred to as bridging, is controversial and should be individualized (41). Kearon recommends preoperative bridging with intravenous heparin only for patients who have had an acute arterial or venous thromboembolism within 1 month before operation, if the procedure cannot be postponed (41).

Caution should be used when performing neuraxial techniques in patients recently discontinued from chronic warfarin therapy. The anticoagulant therapy must be stopped (ideally 4 to 5 days before the planned procedure) and the prothrombin time (PT)/INR measured prior to initiation of neuraxial block. Early after discontinuation of warfarin therapy, the PT/INR reflect predominantly factor VII levels, and in spite of acceptable factor VII levels, factor II and X levels may not be adequate for normal hemostasis. Adequate levels of II, VII, IX, and X may not be present until the PT/INR is within normal limits. For patients receiving an initial dose of warfarin prior to surgery, the PT/INR should be checked prior to neuraxial block if the first dose was given >24 hours earlier or a second dose of oral anticoagulant has been administered (36).

Preoperative evaluation should determine whether fibrinolytic or thrombolytic drugs have been administered preoperatively or have the likelihood of being used intra- or postoperatively. Patients receiving fibrinolytic and thrombolytic drugs should be cautioned against receiving spinal or epidural anesthetics except in highly unusual circumstances (36). Platelet GP IIb/IIIa inhibitors exert a profound effect on platelet aggregation. Following administration, the time to normal platelet aggregation is 24 to 48 hours for abciximab and 4 to 8 hours for eptifibatide and tirofiban. Neuraxial techniques should be avoided until platelet function has recovered (36).

Nonsteroidal anti-inflammatory drugs (NSAIDs) have *reversible* antiplatelet effects, so once the drug has been eliminated coagulation returns to normal. Table 17.9 lists examples of generic and trade names of various NSAIDs. Discontinuation of NSAIDs may benefit patients at risk for renal insufficiency.

Table 17.9. Examples of generic and trade names of various nonsteroidal anti-inflammatory drugs

Aclin (sulindac)	Lodine (etodolac)
Act-3C (ibuprofen and codeine)	Mobic (meloxicam)
Advil (ibuprofen)	Motrin (ibuprofen)
Aleve (naproxen)	Naprogesic (naproxen)
Arthrexin (indomethacin)	Naprosyn SR (naproxen)
Butazolidin (phenylbutazone)	Orudis (ketoprofen)
Clinoril (sulindac)	Oruvail SR (ketoprofen)
Daypro (oxaprozin)	Ponstel (mefenamic acid)
Dolobid (diflunisal)	Sine-aid (ibuprofen)
Feldene (piroxicam)	Surgam (tiaprofenic acid)
Fenac (diclofenac)	Synflex (naproxen)
Indocid (indomethacin)	Tilcotil (tenoxicam)
Indocin (indomethacin)	Toradol (ketorolac)
Inza (naproxen)	Voltaren (diclofenac)

NSAIDs appear to represent no added significant risk for the development of spinal hematoma in patients having epidural or spinal anesthesia (36). NSAIDs are generally discontinued before the day of surgery and should be stopped 24 to 72 hours before surgery. Stopping NSAIDs for longer periods does not increase safety and will be burdensome to many patients with significant arthritis or chronic painful conditions. Cyclooxygenase-2 inhibitors have minimal effect on platelet function and can be continued in the perioperative period.

Glycemic control perioperatively has been receiving increased scrutiny because of the adverse effects of hyperglycemia on wound healing and other outcomes. The three goals of diabetic glucose control preoperatively are to prevent hypoglycemia during fasting, to prevent extreme hyperglycemia, and to prevent ketosis. Type 1 diabetics have an absolute insulin deficiency and require insulin even if they are not hyperglycemic. Insulin facilitates transport of glucose into cells, inhibits protein breakdown, prevents ketoacidosis, and has effects beyond energy metabolism, including actions on steroidogenesis, vascular function, fibrinolysis, and growth. Type 2 diabetics are usually insulin resistant, may be overweight, and are more prone to extremes of hyperglycemia than ketoacidosis.

Both type 1 and 2 diabetics should discontinue short-acting insulins. An exception to this rule is in diabetics managed with continuous subcutaneous insulin infusions via pumps. Patients with an insulin pump should continue their lowest basal rate only. Lowest basal rates are usually nighttime fasting rates during sleep. Type 2 diabetics should take none or up to a half dose of intermediate to long-acting (e.g., lente or NPH) or combination (70/30 preparations) insulins on the day of operation. Patients taking half of their usual dose of intermediate- or long-acting or combination insulins on the day of surgery have improved preoperative glycemic levels compared to those taking no insulin (42). Type 1 diabetics should take a small amount (usually one third to one half) of their usual morning intermediate- to long-acting insulin (e.g., lente or NPH) on the day of surgery to avoid diabetic ketoacidosis.

Metformin does not need to be discontinued before the day of surgery. There is a very rare risk of lactic acidosis in patients who develop renal and hepatic failure while taking metformin. Therefore, metformin should not be restarted in patients postoperatively until any such risk has passed. There are no data to support the recommendation to stop metformin 24 to 48 hours before surgery. Stopping metformin before the day of surgery increases the chance of poor perioperative glycemic control. Sulfonylurea agents with very long half-lives (e.g., chlorpropamide) can cause hypoglycemia in the fasting patient. Several newer oral agents (acarbose, pioglitazone) used as single-agent therapy do not carry a risk of hypoglycemia in the fasting patient. However, to avoid confusion, oral hypoglycemic agents should generally be held the day of surgery to avoid hypoglycemia. Perioperative blood sugars are best managed with insulin.

Patients taking steroids regularly should take their usual dose on the day of surgery. Stress-associated adrenal insufficiency may occur in patients taking steroids chronically unless additional steroid therapy is instituted perioperatively. Approximately 5 to 7.5 mg of prednisone is equivalent to a normal daily adrenal output of cortisol (30 mg). The hypothalamic-pituitary-adrenal (HPA) axis is not suppressed in patients who take <5 mg/day of prednisone or its equivalent. In patients who take >5 to 20 mg/day of prednisone or its equivalent for >3 weeks, the HPA axis may or may not be suppressed. More than 20 mg/day of prednisone or its equivalent for >3 weeks will suppress the HPA axis. The risk of adrenal insufficiency remains for up to 1 year after the cessation of high-dose steroid therapy. Surgery, trauma, or infection may be stressful and an intact HPA will respond by increasing adrenal output of glucocorticoids. The circulating cortisol concentration is normal within 24 to 48 hours in most patients (43). Surgeries induce a variety of stress from minimal to severe. The amount of supplementation should depend on the estimated amount of stress, the duration and severity of surgery, and the chronic daily dose of steroid (Table 17.10). The risk of infection, psychosis, decreased wound healing, and hyperglycemia outweigh the benefits of extremely high doses of perioperative steroids, which are rarely necessary (43).

Postmenopausal hormone replacement therapies containing estrogen increase the risk of perioperative thromboembolic complications and should be discontinued before operation (44). Estrogens must be stopped approximately 1 month before surgery to return coagulation to baseline. Most modern oral contraceptives contain low doses of estrogen that minimally increase thromboembolic risk. The risk of unanticipated pregnancy may outweigh the benefits of discontinuing oral contraceptives. Therefore, it is our practice to continue oral contraceptives in the perioperative period.

Herbals and supplements may interact with anesthetic agents, alter the effects of prescription medications, and increase bleeding. Many patients do not consider supplements medications and do not include them in a list of their medications unless asked. Gingko, echinacea, garlic, ginseng, kava, St. John's wort, and valerian may be associated with increased bleeding or a resistance or increased sensitivity to anesthetic and sedative agents. There is no wholly accepted test to assess adequacy of hemostasis in the patient reporting preoperative herbal medications. The use of herbal medications alone does not preclude performing neuraxial blocks (36). Data on the combination of herbal therapy with other forms of anticoagulation are lacking. However, the concurrent use of other medications affecting clotting mechanisms, such as oral anticoagulants or heparin, may increase the risk of bleeding complications in these patients.

It is generally recommended to discontinue herbals and supplements 7 to 14 days before surgery. The exception is valerian, a central nervous system depressant that may cause a benzodiazepine-like withdrawal when discontinued. If the time until surgery permits, valerian should be tapered before a planned anesthetic. Mandatory discontinuation of these medications, or cancellation of surgery in patients in whom these medications have been continued, is not supported by available data.

Most medications for neurologic, psychiatric, and psychological problems are continued on schedule in the preoperative

Table 17.10. Recommendations for perioperative glucocorticoid coverage

Surgical Stress	Target Hydro-cortisone Equivalent	Preoperative Steroid Dose	Intraoperative Steroid Dose	Postoperative Steroid Dose[b]	Postoperative Steroid Dose Day 1[b]	Postoperative Steroid Dose Day 2[b]
Minor (e.g. inguinal herniorrhaphy)	25 mg/day for 1 day	Usual daily dose of steroid	None[a]	None[a]	Usual daily dose[a]	
Moderate (e.g. colon resection, total joint replacement, lower extremity revascularization)	50–75 mg/day for 1–2 days	Usual daily dose of steroid	50 mg hydrocortisone	20 mg hydrocortisone every 8 hours	20 mg hydrocortisone every 8 hours	
Major (e.g. pancreatoduodenectomy, esophagectomy)	100–150 mg/day for 2–3 days	Usual daily dose of steroid	50 mg hydrocortisone	50 mg hydrocortisone every 8 hours	50 mg hydrocortisone every 8 hours	50 mg hydrocortisone every 8 hours

[a] If the postoperative course is uncomplicated, patients can resume their usual steroid dose on postoperative day 1.
[b] If postoperative complications occur, continued glucocorticoid administration will be necessary commiserate with the level of stress.
Salem M, Tainsh RE, Bromberg J, et al. Perioperative glucocorticoid coverage. A reassessment 42 years after emergence of a problem. *Ann Surg.* 1994;219:416–425.

Table 17.11. Monoamine oxidase inhibitors (brand names in parentheses)

Isocarboxazid (Marplan)
Moclobemide (Aurorix, Manerix, Moclodura)
Phenelzine (Nardil)
Tranylcypromine (Parnate, Jatrosom)
Selegiline (Selegiline, Eldepryl, Emsam)
Nialamide
Iproniazid (Marsilid, Iprozid, Ipronid, Rivivol, Propilniazida)
Iproclozide
Teloxantrone

period. Antiepileptics, anti-Parkinson medications, antidepressants including monoamine oxidase inhibitors (MAOIs), antipsychotics, benzodiazepines, and drugs to treat myasthenia gravis are best maintained to avoid exacerbations of symptoms. Anxiolytics should be continued up until the time of the procedure. Communication is crucial to alert the day-of-surgery caregivers because alterations in anesthesia may be necessary when caring for patients on these medications, especially for patients taking MAOIs (Table 17.11). Patients taking MAOIs should not be given meperidine or indirect-acting vasopressors such as ephedrine. Historically, MAOIs were discontinued before surgery but these drugs must be stopped for at least 3 weeks because of their long duration of inhibition. Case reports of suicides and/or severe depression have appeared in the literature when patients discontinued MAOIs. The safest approach is to continue these drugs and adjust the anesthetic plan.

Highly active antiretroviral therapies (HAART) for HIV infection require regular dosing to prevent drug resistance. It is important to maintain these as scheduled. Antibiotics are taken to complete a prescribed course of therapy. Patients continue narcotic pain medications to prevent withdrawal symptoms and discomfort during preoperative processing before intravenous catheter placement. Drugs used to treat addiction such as methadone, clonidine, and nicotine replacement therapies should be continued on the day of surgery. Inhalers and long-term medications for asthma or chronic obstructive disease are continued on the day of surgery (45). Thyroid replacement drugs and thyroid suppressant medications should continue on schedule (46).

Patients who are particularly anxious should be offered a prescription for a short course of benzodiazepines such as lorazepam to be taken in the days preceding surgery as well as on the day of surgery.

NUTRITIONAL EVALUATION AND MANAGEMENT

Patients who need surgery may be malnourished, either because of a chronic disease process (e.g., cancer or difficulty swallowing after a stroke) or because of a medical condition, such as intermittent bowel obstruction. Malnutrition is associated with postoperative complications, which range from prolonged hospital stay for patients undergoing total hip replacement (47) to more major morbidity, such as wound breakdown, abscesses, infections, anastomotic breakdowns, respiratory failure, and death (48).

Therefore, the patient's nutritional status is evaluated preoperatively with the goal of improving the nutrition of a severely malnourished patient before surgery, if possible. Reasonable agreement exists about significant factors of the patient's nutritional status: Weight loss >10% in the 6 months before surgery; change in dietary intake relative to normal; gastrointestinal symptoms that persist for >2 weeks; decreased functional capacity (from lethargic to bedridden); and other physical factors such as loss of subcutaneous fat, muscle wasting, ankle edema, sacral edema, and ascites. Detsky et al. (49) have incorporated these factors into the Subjective Global Assessment scale (Table 17.12).

Table 17.12.   Features of Subjective Global Assessment

History

1. Weight change
   Overall loss in past 6 months: Amount = _____ kg: _____%
   Change in past 2 weeks: _____ increase
                             _____ no change
                             _____ decrease

2. Dietary intake change (relative to normal)
   _____ no change
   ___ change ___ duration = ___ weeks
               ___ type: ___ suboptimal solid diet ___ full liquid diet
                         ___ hypocaloric liquids   ___ starvation

3. Gastrointestinal symptoms (that persisted for >2 weeks)
   _____none _____nausea _____vomiting _____diarrhea _____anorexia

4. Functional capacity
   _____no dysfunction (e.g., full capacity)
   _____ dysfunction _____duration = _____ weeks
                     _____ type: _____ working suboptimally
                               _____ ambulatory
                               _____ bedridden

Physical (for each trait specify: 0 = normal, 1 + = mild, 2+ = moderate, 3+ =severe)
   _____ loss of subcutaneous fat (triceps, chest)
   _____ muscle wasting (quadriceps, deltoids)
   _____ ankle edema
   _____ sacral edema
   _____ ascites

Subjective Global Assessment rating (select one)
   _____ A = well nourished
   _____ B = moderately (or suspected of being) malnourished
   _____ C = severely malnourished

Class A indicates those with <5% weight loss or >5% total weight loss but recent gain and improvement in appetite; class B, those with 5%–10% weight loss without recent stabilization or gain, poor dietary intake, and mild (1+) loss of subcutaneous tissue; and class C, ongoing weight loss >10% with severe subcutaneous tissue loss and muscle wasting often with edema.
Derived from Detsky AS, Smalley PS, Chang J. Is this patient malnourished? *JAMA.* 1994; 271:54–58.

The physical factors are rated as normal (0), mild (1+), moderate (2+), or severe (3+). The best places to look for loss of subcutaneous fat are the triceps region of the arms, the midaxillary line at the costal margin, the interosseous and palmar areas of the hand, and the deltoid region of the shoulder. Muscle wasting is best examined in the quadriceps femoris and deltoid region. Detsky classifies the nutritional status of patients as well nourished (class A), moderately malnourished (class B, weight loss of 5% to 10% without stabilization or weight gain, poor dietary intake, and mild loss of subcutaneous tissue), or severely malnourished (class C, ongoing weight loss of >10%, severe subcutaneous tissue loss, muscle wasting, and edema).

Among laboratory tests, a serum albumin level of <3.5 g/dL in the general surgical population or <3.9 g/dL in patients who need total hip replacement is an accurate predictor of malnutrition (47,48). The combination of history and physical examination and serum albumin level provides slightly improved accuracy in predicting malnutrition than either indicator alone.

When possible, nutritional status should be improved preoperatively in severely malnourished patients. Enteral nutrition is the preferred means, but if the gut cannot be used because of enterocutaneous fistulas or severe pancreatitis, total parenteral nutrition (TPN), although not without its own risks, is acceptable. Severely malnourished patients who received TPN had fewer noninfectious complications than controls (5% vs. 43%), with no concomitant increase in infectious complications (48).

MITIGATION OF RISKS WHILE UNDER ANESTHESIA

Several situations present specific real and potential risks that may be ameliorated by appropriate preoperative planning. Patients may have experienced an episode of awareness under anesthesia or think that they had such an experience. They may not have discussed the awareness or they may have raised the issue and been treated dismissively. Although it is not standard practice to query patients specifically for episodes of awareness under anesthesia, it is advisable to set the right climate and create the right structure during the preoperative interview to obtain the most value from discussion with the patient. When searching for information about any problems with prior anesthetics, provide enough time for patients to respond, show concern for their views, and probe for additional information when necessary. There may have been a break in anesthetic technique, or the patient may have a predisposition to awareness that requires adjustment of dosing of amnestic, narcotic, or anesthetic drugs. It is important to allay patients' fears and communicate the situation to caregivers providing anesthesia on the day of the procedure. The ASA publishes an educational brochure for use by patients titled "What is Patient Awareness Under General Anesthesia?" It can be accessed at http://www.asahq.org/patientEducation/Awarenessbrochure.pdf.

Transient numbness, weakness, or muscle soreness may have resulted from positioning during a past anesthetic or from a reaction to succinylcholine. The underlying cause might be spinal stenosis, nerve root compression, or arthritis. Attention to cervical spine disease and motion should be a part of every preoperative anesthetic interview whether or not intubation or unusual positioning is planned, since unexpected circumstances may necessitate manipulation of the neck. Obtaining old records is often useful. These outcomes may not have been mentioned to other caregivers or noted in records but can be elicited during a careful, unhurried preoperative interview. It is important to discuss with patients future risks from positioning and assure them that every precaution will be taken to avoid injury. It is important to document conversations with the patient and efforts to coordinate care. Certain positions requiring prone, lateral, or change of position while under anesthesia deserve special consideration.

Patients with a history of radical mastectomy, axillary lymph node dissection, or similar procedures predisposing to lymphedema or poor drainage should probably not have intravenous line placements in those extremities. Patients with arteriovenous (AV) shunts and/or fistulas for dialysis access are similarly treated. In addition, these patients should have the thrill or palpable flow over the AV access area accessed and documented immediately preoperatively. Attention to positioning of the extremity and documentation of a persistent thrill or change in status should be done periodically during the perioperative period.

Patients scheduled for spine surgery under general anesthesia should be counseled about the risks of perioperative visual loss. An ASA Practice Advisory (50) defines high-risk patients as those who have spine surgery in the prone position that lasts more than an average of 6.5 hours, have blood loss in excess of half a blood volume, or both. Although expert and consensus opinion and the literature do not provide definitive guidelines or validated information, some data suggest that hypertension, glaucoma, carotid artery disease, smoking, obesity, and diabetes may be associated with perioperative visual loss. Preoperative anemia may play a role in addition to intraoperative anemia, but no lower limit of hemoglobin concentration has been shown to be associated with this complication. Preoperative consultation with neuro-ophthalmologists or other specialists is not recommended for the purposes of identifying patients at risk of perioperative visual loss given the absence of patient-specific predictive factors. The Advisory did not address other causes of visual loss such as cortical blindness, or visual loss occurring in the context of radical neck dissections or cardiac surgery. Although the incidence of perioperative visual loss secondary to anterior or posterior ischemia, optic neuropathy or central retinal artery occlusion is thought to be <0.2% of spine surgeries, it is a devastating complication. Patients scheduled for complex spine surgery under general anesthesia in a prone position should be counseled on a case-by-case basis.

Cases involving perioperative peripheral neuropathies have increased as a percentage of malpractice litigation. While the specific causes of these complications are not completely understood, a number of precautions may be taken. These include avoiding contact with hard surfaces that may put pressure on peripheral nerves, especially the radial nerve at the level of the midhumerus, the ulnar nerve at the elbow, and the peroneal nerve at the fibular head; judicious use of protective padding; and positioning the patient to avoid stretching of nerves and nerve plexuses. Preoperatively patients should be questioned about symptoms of extremity numbness or weakness, especially on awakening in the morning or associated with a particular position. The planned surgical position may also be simulated during the preoperative evaluation to determine the range of patient comfort and symptoms. The ASA has published a Practice Advisory for the Prevention of Peripheral Neuropathies in the absence of more rigorous evidence needed for a guideline or standard (51). This document may be helpful to review the basics and details of patient positioning. Patients may be counseled during a general discussion of perioperative risks that, although weakness and/or numbness of an extremity may occur postoperatively, this complication is uncommon and generally unpredictable.

Several circumstances preclude the use or provide possible indications for avoidance of nitrous oxide. Patients who have undergone sulfur hexafluoride gas installation to treat a detached retina should not receive nitrous oxide for several weeks. Patients who have undergone open craniotomy and have retained subdural air are at risk for expansion of these air pockets should they be exposed to nitrous oxide. The time period for this risk is not well defined, but one study showed persistence of air for several weeks postcraniotomy. Some patients with a history of middle ear disease or high risk for nausea and vomiting should probably not receive nitrous oxide as well.

REFERENCES

1. Warner M, Warner M, Weber J. Clinical significance of pulmonary aspiration during the perioperative period. *Anesthesiology*. 1993;78:56–62.
2. Olsson GL, Hallen B, Hambraeus-Jonzon K. Aspiration during anaesthesia: a computer aided study of 185,358 anaesthetics. *Acta Anaesthesiol Scand*. 1986;30:84–92.
3. Krantz ML, Edwards WL. The incidence of nonfatal aspiration in obstetrical patients. *Anesthesiology*. 1973;39:359.
4. Ezri T, Szmuk P, Stein A, et al. Peripartum general anaesthesia without tracheal intubation: incidence of aspiration pneumonia. *Anaesthesia*. 2000;55:421–426.
5. Harter RL, Kelly WB, Kramer MG, et al. A comparison of the volume and pH of gastric contents of obese and lean surgical patients. *Anesth Analg*. 1998;86:147–152.
6. Practice guidelines for preoperative fasting and the use of pharmacologic agents to reduce the risk of pulmonary aspiration: application to healthy patients undergoing elective procedures: a report by the American Society of Anesthesiologists Task Force on Preoperative Fasting. *Anesthesiology*. 1999;90:896–905.
7. Phillips S, Hutchinson S, Davidson T. Preoperative drinking does not affect gastric contents. *Br J Anaesth*. 1993;70:6–9.
8. Anderson FA, Wheeler HB. Venous thromboembolism. *Clin Chest Med*. 1995;16:235–251.
9. Silverstein MD, Heit JA, Mohr DN, et al. Trends in the incidence of deep vein thrombosis and pulmonary embolism—a 25 year population-based study. *Arch Int Med*. 1998;158:585–593.
10. Wilson W, Taubert K, Gewitz M, et al. Prevention of infective endocarditis. Guidelines from the American Heart Association. A

guideline from the American Heart Association Rheumatic Fever, Endocarditis, and Kawasaki Disease Committee, Council on Cardiovascular Disease in the Young, and the Council on Clinical Cardiology, Council on Cardiovascular Surgery and Anesthesia, and the Quality of Care and Outcomes Research Interdisciplinary Working Group. *Circulation*. Published online April 19, 2007. Available at http://circ.ahajournals.org.

11. Dajani AS, Taubert KA, Wilson W, et al. Prevention of bacterial endocarditis, recommendations by the American Heart Association. *JAMA*. 1997;277:1794–1801.

12. Smith SC Jr, Allen J, Blair SN, et al. AHA/ACC guidelines for secondary prevention for patients with coronary and other atherosclerotic vascular disease: 2006 update: endorsed by the National Heart, Lung, and Blood Institute. *Circulation*. 2006;113:2363–2372.

13. Comfere T, Sprung J, Kumar MM, et al. Angiotensin system inhibitors in a general surgical population. *Anesth Analg*. 2005;100:636–644.

14. Auerbach AD, Goldman L. β-blockers and reduction of cardiac events in noncardiac surgery. *JAMA*. 2002;287:1435–1444.

15. Poldermans D, Boersma E, Bax JJ, et al. The effect of bisoprolol on perioperative mortality and myocardial infarction in high-risk patients undergoing vascular surgery. *N Engl J Med*. 1999;341:1789–1794.

16. Fleisher LA, Beckman JA, Brown KA, et al. ACC/AHA 2006 guideline update on perioperative cardiovascular evaluation for noncardiac surgery: focused update on perioperative beta-blocker therapy: a report of the American College of Cardiology/American Heart Association Task Force on Practice Guidelines (writing committee to update the 2002 Guidelines on Perioperative Cardiovascular Evaluation for Noncardiac Surgery): developed in collaboration with the American Society of Echocardiography, American Society of Nuclear Cardiology, Heart Rhythm Society, Society of Cardiovascular Anesthesiologists, Society for Cardiovascular Angiography and Interventions, and Society for Vascular Medicine and Biology. *Circulation*. 2006;113:2662–2674.

17. Feringa HH, Bax JJ, Boersma E, et al. High-dose beta-blockers and tight heart rate control reduce myocardial ischemia and troponin T release in vascular surgery patients. *Circulation*. 2006;114(1 Suppl):I344–349.

18. Redelmeier D, Scales D, Kopp A. Beta blockers for elective surgery in elderly patients: population based, retrospective cohort study. *BMJ*. 2005;331:932.

19. Salpeter SS, Ormiston TM, Salpeter EE. Cardioselective (β-blockers in patients with reactive airway disease: a meta-analysis. *Ann Intern Med*. 2002;137:715–725.

20. London MJ, Itani KMF, Perrino AC, et al. Perioperative beta-blockade: a survey of physician attitudes in the department of Veteran Affairs. *J Cardiothorac Vasc Anesth*. 2004;18:14–24.

21. van de Pol MA, van Houdenhoven M, Hans EW, et al. Influence of cardiac risk factors and medication on length of hospitalization in patients undergoing major vascular surgery. *Am J Cardiol*. 2006;97:1423–1426.

22. Poldermans D, Bax JJ, Kertai MD, et al. Statins are associated with a reduced incidence of perioperative mortality in patients undergoing major noncardiac vascular surgery. *Circulation*. 2003;107:1848–1851.

23. Kapoor AS, Kanji H, Buckingham J, et al. Strength of evidence of preoperative use of statins to reduce cardiovascular risk: systemic review of controlled studies. *BMJ*. 2006: 333:1149–1155.

24. Durazzo AE, Machado FS, Ikeoka DT, et al. Reduction in cardiovascular events after vascular surgery with atorvastatin: a randomized trial. *J Vasc Surg*. 2004;39:967–975.

25. Schouten O, Kertai MD, Bax JJ, et al. Safety of perioperative statin use in high-risk patients undergoing major vascular surgery. *Am J Cardiol*. 2005;95:658–660.

26. Heeschen C, Hamm CW, Laufs U, et al. Withdrawal of statins increases event rates in patients with acute coronary syndromes. *Circulation*. 2002;105:1446–1452.

27. Aspirin for primary prevention of cardiovascular events—chemoprevention. U.S. Preventive Services Task Force. Available at: http://www.ahrq.gov/clinic/uspstf/uspsasmi.htm. Accessed June 30, 2007.

28. Burger W, Chemnitius JM, Kneissl GD, et al. Low-dose aspirin for secondary cardiovascular prevention—cardiovascular risks after its perioperative withdrawal versus bleeding risks with it continuation—review and meta-analysis. *J Intern Med*. 2005;257:399–414.

29. Lindblad B, Persson NH, Takolander R, et al. Does low-dose acetylsalicylic acid prevent stroke after carotid surgery? A double-blind, placebo-controlled randomized trial. *Stroke*. 1993;24:1125–1128.

30. Collet JP, Himbet F, Steg PG. Myocardial infarction after aspirin cessation in stable coronary artery disease patients. *Int J Cardiol*. 2000;76:257–258.

31. Senior K. Aspirin withdrawal increases risk of heart problems. *Lancet*. 2003;362:1558.

32. Albaladejo P, Geeraerts T, Francis F, et al. Aspirin withdrawal and acute lower limb ischemia. *Anesth Analg*. 2004;99:440–443.

33. Beving H, Zhao C, Albage, et al. Abnormally high platelet activity after discontinuation of acetylsalicylic acid treatment. *Blood Coagul Fibrinolysis*. 1996;7:80–84.

34. Horlocker TT, Wedel DJ, Offord KP. Does preoperative antiplatelet therapy increase the risk of hemorrhagic complications associated with regional anesthesia? *Anesth Analg*. 1990;70:631–634.

35. Horlocker TT, Wedel DJ, Schroeder DR, et al. Preoperative antiplatelet therapy does not increase the risk of spinal hematoma associated with regional anesthesia. *Anesth Analg*. 1995;80:303–309.

36. Horlocker TT, Wedel DJ, Benzon H, et al. Regional anesthesia in the anticoagulated patient: defining the risks (the Second ASRA Consensus Conference on Neuraxial Anesthesia and Anticoagulation). *Reg Anesth Pain Med*. 2003;28:172–197.

37. Clagett GP, Sobel M, Jackson MR, et al. Antithrombotic therapy in peripheral arterial occlusive disease: the Seventh ACCP

Conference on Antithrombotic and Thrombolytic Therapy. *Chest*. 2004;126(Suppl):609S–626S.

38. Harder S, Klinkhardt U, Alvarez JM. Avoidance of bleeding during surgery in patients receiving anticoagulant and/or antiplatelet therapy: pharmacokinetic and pharmacodynamic considerations. *Clin Pharmacokinet*. 2004;43:963–981.

39. Grines CL, Bonow RO, Casey DE, et al. Prevention of premature discontinuation of dual antiplatelet therapy in patients with coronary artery stents: a science advisory from the American Heart Association, American College of Cardiology, Society for Cardiovascular Angiography and Interventions, American College of Surgeons, and American Dental Association, with Representation from the American College of Physicians. *J Am Coll Cardiol*. 2007;49:734–739.

40. Schouten O, van Domburg RT, Bax JJ, et al. Noncardiac surgery after coronary stenting: early surgery and interruption of antiplatelet therapy are associated with an increase in major adverse cardiac events. *J Am Coll Cardiol*. 2007;49:122–124.

41. Kearon C, Hirsh J. Management of anticoagulation before and after elective surgery. *N Engl J Med*. 1997;336:1506–1511.

42. Likavec A, Moitra V, Greenberg J, et al. Comparison of preoperative blood glucose levels in patients receiving different insulin regimens. *Anesthesiology*. 2006;A567.

43. Salem M, Tainsh RE, Bromberg J, et al. Perioperative glucocorticoid coverage. A reassessment 42 years after emergence of a problem. *Ann Surg*. 1994;219:416–425.

44. Grady D, Wenger NK, Herrington D, et al. Postmenopausal hormone therapy increases risk for venous thromboembolic disease. The heart and estrogen/progestin replacement study. *Ann Intern Med*. 2000;132:689–696.

45. Qaseem A, Snow V, Fitterman N, et al. Risk assessment for and strategies to reduce perioperative pulmonary complications for patients undergoing noncardiothoracic surgery: a guideline from the American College of Physicians. *Ann Intern Med*. 2006;144:575–580.

46. Spell NO III. Stopping and restarting medications in the perioperative period. *Med Clin North Am*. 2001;85:1117–1128.

47. Del Savio GC, Zelicof SB, Wexler LM, et al. Preoperative nutritional status and outcome of elective total hip replacement. *Clin Orthop*. 1996;326:153–161.

48. The Veterans Affairs Total Parenteral Nutrition Cooperative Study Group. Perioperative total parenteral nutrition in surgical patients. *N Engl J Med*. 1991;325:525–532.

49. Detsky AS, Smalley PS, Chang J. Is this patient malnourished? *JAMA*. 1994;271:54–58.

50. Practice Advisory for Perioperative Visual Loss Associated with Spine Surgery. A report by the American Society of Anesthesiologists Task Force on Perioperative Blindness. *Anesthesiology*. 2006;104:1319–1328.

51. Practice Advisory for the Prevention of Perioperative Peripheral Neuropathies. A report by the American Society of Anesthesiologists Task Force on Prevention of Perioperative Peripheral Neuropathies. *Anesthesiology*. 2000;92:1168–1182.

Organizational Infrastructure of a Preoperative Evaluation Center

Angela M. Bader and Darin J. Correll

Hospitals are currently challenged to provide efficient, value-based, preoperative assessments leading to maximum operating room efficiency. A variety of organizational structures can successfully achieve these results. The structures must be capable of assessing patients who need high-acuity care and who are undergoing complex surgical procedures. Before decisions are made regarding organizational structure, an understanding of the goals of preoperative assessment is necessary. These goals are summarized in Table 18.1.

Although some institutions cite financial constraints as the reason for not establishing a coordinated process, they are still obligated to meet the goals of medical optimization and regulatory compliance. For cost containment, manpower resources must be maximized and unnecessary consultations, testing requirements, and redundant provider interviews must be eliminated. The absence of a preoperative system organized to achieve the goals in Table 18.1 may in fact result in a greater cost to the institution. Shifting patient assessment to the day of the procedure does not decrease the level of assessment; it merely shifts the assessment to a far more expensive time because of the risk of operating room (OR) cancellations or delays. A number of studies have demonstrated cost reductions from the establishment of a preoperative clinic, beginning with Fischer's article in 1996, which described the cost savings from fewer consultations and laboratory tests (1). More recently, Ferschl et al. compared patients who were assessed on the day of the procedure to a similar group who visited a preoperative clinic before the day of surgery (DOS). Patient visits to an anesthesiologist-directed clinic for preoperative evaluation reduced DOS case cancellations and case delays significantly (2).

A preoperative visit can reduce cancellations and delays because of the ability to identify and obtain information before surgery regarding comorbid conditions, their stability, and new problems first identified at the time of the preoperative visit. Correll et al. reported that a significant number of patients in the preoperative clinic had either known comorbidities that required retrieval of information from other institutions or new problems for which testing was needed before surgery (3). Leaving these issues unknown until the morning of surgery potentially results in case cancellation or delay. Other cancellations and delays due to inappropriate or inconsistent patient preoperative instructions can also be prevented with a preoperative visit during which standard instructions can be given.

Table 18.1.   Goals of a preoperative assessment system

1. Clinically excellent assessments of uniform quality (paper vs. electronic method options)
2. Medical optimization; intervention that could potentially reduce perioperative risk and improve outcome (e.g., institution of protocols such as those for perioperative beta blockade or reduction of surgical site infections)
3. Process standardization to ensure appropriate coding and billing
4. Minimization of operating room delays and cancellations due to missing paperwork or inadequate patient preparation (retrieval of information regarding known comorbidities needed to establish medical status; management of new problems identified at the preoperative visit)
5. Appropriate testing without redundancy
6. Patient education and preoperative instruction (e.g., appropriate preoperative patient instructions regarding fasting guidelines, bowel preparation, etc.)
7. Patient/family satisfaction
8. Systems checks/chart organization for the operating room
9. Efficient methods of collecting, recording, and transmitting data to the care teams
10. Compliance with regulatory requirements and patient safety initiatives (e.g., The Joint Commission, Centers for Medicare and Medicaid Services, Centers for Disease Control, National Surgical Quality Improvement Program)

Time of day influences the incidence of anesthetic events; patients anesthetized at the end of the workday had a higher incidence of anesthetic adverse events than those anesthetized at the beginning of the day, possibly because of factors such as case load, fatigue, and care transitions (4). Decreasing delays during the day in institutions with high OR utilization rates may result in fewer anesthetic adverse outcomes.

ESTABLISHMENT OF A PREOPERATIVE ASSESSMENT PROCESS

There is no one best preoperative process and a number of institutions have established a variety of ways to meet the goals outlined in Table 18.1. Institutions that do not have an organized process and that struggle with the issues of controllable OR cancellations and delays, unnecessary testing, and difficulty with regulatory requirements often have leaders who do not understand the need to invest in such a process. Without an organized process, overall accountability for the preoperative evaluation is absent and integration among multiple disciplines is difficult. "Who's in charge?" and "Who's going to pay for it?" become insurmountable barriers.

The anesthesiologist, with specific OR experience and knowledge of perioperative medicine, is the natural clinician to manage preoperative assessment processes. Anesthesiologists, however, may be reluctant to take on administrative roles in preoperative assessment. Until recently anesthesia residency programs have not emphasized preoperative assessment skills, patient interaction skills, and the roles of the anesthesiologist outside the OR. One survey of residency training in preoperative evaluation revealed that 32% of anesthesiologists were in programs that either did not have a preoperative clinic or had a clinic but did not rotate residents through it (5). Almost 33% of programs had 10%, or fewer, staff with expertise in this area. According to the new requirements of the Residency Review Committee (RRC) for anesthesiology programs, perioperative care must now include 1 month in a preoperative evaluation clinic, and any unit may not be <1 week. In addition to clinical skills, programs must now specifically focus on performance as a member of a health care team, effective communication, and good business practices. Once residency programs address these new areas of emphasis, anesthesiologists will be better equipped to take on the expanded role of preoperative evaluation.

FINANCIAL JUSTIFICATION FOR PREOPERATIVE ASSESSMENT SYSTEMS

An important part of the preoperative assessment process is financial justification:

- *Reduction in the cost of OR cancellations and delays.* With cancellations, dollars are wasted on unnecessary setups without billing for OR time. Revenues lost from cancellations range from $1,430 to $1,700 per hour plus variable costs in hospitals not on a fixed budget (6). Reducing delays can decrease staffing costs for ORs with high utilization rates by decreasing the need for overtime payments if staff are paid hourly instead of being salaried (2). With a standardized process, the OR chart can be organized before the DOS; the necessary paperwork and documents are ready, eliminating DOS delays while paperwork and consents are collected. Delays for collection of regulatory information are also eliminated. The elements of the nursing assessment required by The Joint Commission, formerly Joint Commission on Accreditation of Healthcare Organizations, which includes information not captured by the surgical or anesthesia assessments, can be collected and placed in the chart in advance, eliminating the need for nursing resources on the day of the procedure. The Joint Commission requirement of medicine reconciliation, which calls for a single medicine list for every admission to be reconciled throughout the hospitalization and at discharge, can be generated in the preoperative clinic and put in the OR chart for use at the time of the procedure.
- *Reduction in the cost of nonreimbursed laboratory tests.* How can an institution be sure that only appropriate tests are ordered for a patient? Designing guidelines for testing based on the literature is a much simpler feat if a standardized preoperative process is in place rather than implementing the guidelines among many different surgeons and anesthesiologists. Ordering appropriate testing only after a patient's comorbidities have been identified requires an organized process. When anesthesiologists order directed preoperative laboratory testing, significant cost savings can be achieved (1). The Centers for Medicare and Medicaid Services (CMS) are now denying reimbursement for

any "screening" preoperative laboratory tests. Institutions that order laboratory tests based on patient age, for example, are not reimbursed for the tests. Documentation of comorbidities in addition to the surgical diagnosis is required. Standardization of paperwork, coding, and test ordering in the preoperative process ensures reimbursement.

- *Reduction in the cost of unnecessary preoperative consultations.* Anesthesiologists and surgeons who are unfamiliar with preoperative evaluation and assessment may rely on consultations to provide "clearance" for patients before surgery. A standardized preoperative process implemented by clinicians who are familiar with preoperative assessment guidelines and algorithms reduces the need for outside consultation. The process provides alignment among clinicians. It is unlikely that cases evaluated preoperatively will be cancelled or delayed on the DOS because of differences in clinical judgment. Tsen et al. demonstrated that a standardized preoperative process with algorithms for consultation and educational programs in cardiac assessment and electrocardiogram (ECG) interpretation significantly decreased consultation requests (7). The consultations that were obtained after the programs were implemented showed improved efficacy in that patients were far more likely to receive testing and not just be deemed stable and ready for the procedure. Patients were also far less likely to be referred for consultation for unimportant ECG abnormalities.
- *Maximizing reimbursement by standardization and accuracy of documentation in the preoperative assessment.* In many institutions, nonclinical personnel review preoperative history and physical (H&P) assessments, from which comorbidities are coded for reimbursement for the surgical diagnosis and procedure. A variety of clinicians may be submitting preoperative H&P assessments in nonstandard ways, making coding difficult. Their assessments may focus on the surgical diagnosis without listing all existing comorbidities. If an institution does not have a standardized process for preoperative H&P recording, correct reimbursement may not be attained, losing revenue for the institution.
- *Maximizing revenue from pay for performance (P4P) measures.* Numerous strategies, including P4P measures, are being instituted across the country in attempts to improve quality and patient safety. While P4P programs attempt to be evidence based, there are presently little data that they actually affect changes in outcome (8). If P4P measures continue to increase, standardizing preoperative processes before the DOS will allow the development and implementation of protocols so the measures are met and documented. Presently this could include implementing some of the Surgical Care Improvement Project (SCIP) measures (e.g., appropriate venous thromboembolism prophylaxis in the perioperative period or appropriate perioperative beta blocker therapy). See Chapters 3, 7, and 17.
- *Maximizing reimbursement for the preoperative process.* Institutions will have to make individual decisions regarding billing for portions of the preoperative assessment. Patient preoperative assessment is considered part of anesthesia reimbursement for the case and cannot be billed separately if it is just routine

preoperative screening. If the surgeon refers the patient for a special anesthesia evaluation because of a specific issue not related to the surgical diagnosis, then the anesthesiologist can bill for a consultation. Billing a "facility fee" can only be done if the patient is being seen as a consultation, not if they are presenting for a routine preoperative evaluation. The cost of the surgical H&P is included in the global fee that the surgeon receives for the procedure. An internist or primary care physician cannot bill for a routine presurgical H&P unless they and the surgeon bill with a modifier that will result in the surgeon receiving a reduced fee. If the surgeon refers the patient to a specialist for a consultation because of a specific question regarding management of a comorbidity, not related to the indication for surgery, then the specialist can bill for the consultation. In order for any consultation to be billable, the requesting physician must document the medically necessary reason for the consultation (i.e., he or she must have the intention to use the information for the further care of the patient or to make the decision to proceed with surgery or not). Laboratory tests and ECGs cannot be ordered as "screening" or "preoperative" and be submitted for reimbursement to CMS. Billable tests are only those that are reasonable and necessary for the diagnosis or treatment of an illness.

- *Preoperative medical management that reduces potential complications can impact cost of admission and length of stay.* Because preoperative risk factors are effective predictors of hospital costs (9), preoperative intervention to reduce risk could lead to significant cost savings. There are several important examples of such interventions. Perioperative beta blockade has been recommended by the American Heart Association and American College of Cardiology (10) (see Chapters 3 and 17). Despite the evidence, a significant number of patients who are candidates for perioperative beta blockade are not receiving it at the time of the preoperative visit. The guidelines are applied inconsistently by surgeons and referring physicians, again because accountability for the preoperative assessment and process is not clearly defined. Standardization of the preoperative process means the appropriate protocols can be implemented before the DOS to decrease the cost of admission from perioperative cardiac complications. A second example is the reduction of surgical site infections. The Centers for Disease Control and Prevention (CDC) has reported that bacterial colony counts are significantly reduced for patients who have two preoperative antiseptic showers (11). The CDC recommends that patients shower or bathe with an antiseptic agent at least the night before the operative day (category IB recommendation). A standardized preoperative process provides a means for patients to be given the antiseptic agents at the time of the preoperative visit.

ESTABLISHING A STANDARDIZED PREOPERATIVE PROCESS

Once they understand the positive financial and medical impact of a standardized preoperative process, administrative and clinical leaders can begin to strategize for the best possible process in their institutions. The best process will vary widely depending on the needs of the institution; however, all must meet the basic requirements of The Joint Commission and CMS regulations outlined in Table 18.2. The following questions are useful during the development of a plan:

- What is the surgical volume and acuity of the patients' medical conditions?
- How will volume projections over time impact the current numbers?
- What space is available?
- Can all assessments be provided in the space available or will different portions of the assessment be performed in different places?
- What will be the impact on patient satisfaction of different locations for parts of the process?
- What percentages of patients have medical conditions of low acuity making them eligible for screening by telephone? Telephone screening requires the development of algorithms and education of office personnel.
- What will the organizational chart and accountability structure look like? Who is ultimately the clinician-leader responsible for the process?
- Where will clerical staff organize assessments into the chart for the OR?
- How will system checks be built into the process? For example, who is responsible for reviewing laboratory results that were not available at the time of the patient's preoperative visit? Who will be responsible for ECG interpretation and follow-up of significantly abnormal ECG?
- Who will bill for the preoperative process, laboratory tests, and ECGs? Financial justification can be calculated from projected decreases in controllable cancellations or unreimbursed testing.

Once the process has been defined by the questions above, an organizational chart can be drafted that includes staffing numbers and reporting lines for both clinical and nonclinical staff. Then the total budget for labor and nonlabor costs can be estimated.

Table 18.2.   Basic regulatory requirements for preoperative assessment

1. The Joint Commission requires that a surgical H&P be performed within 30 days of surgery. CMS requires that the surgical H&P be performed within 7 days of surgery (or updated within 7 days if it has been done within 30 days). The Joint Commission also requires a surgical reassessment to be documented within 24 hours of the time of surgery.
2. A nursing assessment containing all required elements specified by The Joint Commission must be completed.
3. An anesthesia assessment must be completed.
4. No specific testing is required by either The Joint Commission or CMS; all testing should be appropriate for the patient and based on surgical procedure and comorbidities.

CMS, Centers for Medicare and Medicaid Services; JCAHO, Joint Commission on Health Care Organizations.

Overall accountability and long-term planning for the unit necessitates the appointment of a medical/administrative director.

ORGANIZATIONAL EXAMPLES

When planning a preoperative evaluation process, the operational goals defined in Table 18.3 are important. Processes designed to address issues at a tertiary care center, seeing a large volume of patients with high-acuity medical conditions and who are scheduled for complex procedures, may not be transferable to other institutions with other types of patients (e.g., a small ambulatory surgicenter). Various options to consider include:

- Low-risk patients may initially be screened by phone and the anesthesia assessment completed on the day of the procedure provided the surgical H&P is done outside the process.
- The ideal clinic is a collaborative effort of the departments of nursing, anesthesia, surgery, and hospital administration.
- The clinic can exist as a separate cost center or be funded by a variety of means (e.g., departments of surgery, anesthesiology, or the hospital corporation).
- Anesthesia leadership should be responsible for the overall multidisciplinary process in conjunction with a practice manager responsible for day-to-day unit operations.
- The clinic should have a multidisciplinary approach, providing all assessments and testing necessary for the preoperative process on site.
- Insurance certification can be obtained as part of the process.
- When a surgery is booked, the same process can generate either an appointment for a preoperative clinic visit or screening via telephone, depending on algorithms used in the surgeons' offices.
- At the time of the visit in the surgeon's office, patients can receive information describing the surgical process.
- Before patients come to the clinic, the opportunity can exist for them to enter information at home via an Internet-based questionnaire that is then accessed by clinic providers.
- Having a single practitioner (e.g., a nurse practitioner) perform the three necessary assessments (surgical history and

Table 18.3. Goals in the design of a preoperative process

1. Provide all required assessments (surgical, nursing, anesthesia, testing) during one patient visit; eliminate redundant interviews and multiple waiting times.
2. Assume accountability for all aspects of the preoperative assessment process. The expectation of the surgeon, as well as the anesthesia team assigned to the case, is that all medical issues, test values, etc., will be evaluated and handled by the clinic staff in conjunction with the patient's primary care provider and specialists. The clinic will also assume responsibility for initiation of perioperative protocols, such as prescriptions for beta blockade.
3. Assemble a complete operating room chart (medical issues, regulatory compliance, and paperwork); this chart is generally sent to the operating room the afternoon before surgery.

physical, anesthesia, and nursing) on combined forms can eliminate redundant questioning and documentation.
- Having the surgeon's office note available at the time of the clinic visit is helpful, with all other documentation generated at the visit.
- All The Joint Commission requirements, including advance directives, specific patient education, and the initial medication list for medicine reconciliation, can be performed at this time.
- If an ECG and/or laboratory tests are required, they can be obtained in the same examination room where the other assessments take place to limit time spent by the patient moving from location to location.
- The surgeons' offices should be encouraged to schedule patients to allow for a preoperative visit at least 48 hours before the procedure so that there is time to review all results and resolve all issues.
- An anesthesia attending should always be present in the clinic so the practitioner evaluating each patient can discuss the case before the patient leaves.
- The anesthesia attending or the practitioner evaluating the patient can consult with the primary care physician or specialist if appropriate.
- The anesthesia attending should review the ECG and decide whether further testing or other perioperative protocols such as beta blockade should be initiated.
- A specific practitioner should be assigned each day to review laboratory results for all patients from the previous day's appointments. Issues identified can then be dealt with by the practitioner in consultation with the anesthesia attending.
- A clerical assistant can be assigned to retrieve medical information for patients from outside institutions for the anesthesia attending to review.
- Issues that may impact OR scheduling or equipment requirements (e.g., potential difficult intubation, need for fetal heart rate monitoring) should be transmitted to the assigned anesthesia and nursing teams before the DOS (e.g., via e-mail to a centralized scheduling office, which then forwards the information).

The above outlined processes can markedly decrease controllable OR cancellations and delays. The efficiency of the admitting nurses on the day of the procedure can be improved because minimal further assessment or paperwork is needed.

PATIENT SATISFACTION WITH THE PREOPERATIVE PROCESS

Consumerism and transparency in quality measures, with patient satisfaction being one of the quality measures, are becoming ever more important issues in health care. Measuring patient satisfaction with the various elements of the process is essential to evaluate success and plan improvement. The benefits of an effective preoperative process on efficiency have been well documented; however, there is limited information on the benefit of preoperative clinics to the patient experience. Patient satisfaction has been advocated as a unique clinical endpoint and as an indicator of the quality of health care provided. Fung and Cohen valued the insight from this outcome more than rare, major outcomes such as death or common, minor outcomes such as pain and nausea, which can be influenced by many other factors (12). In one study of anesthetic care, patient satisfaction was more meaningful than incidence of nausea, vomiting, or death because the latter are influenced by many institutional and patient factors. The overall perioperative experience showed improvement in provider scores and an overall high patient satisfaction rate with all clinical aspects of a preoperative clinic visit after implementation of the processes described above (13). (A copy of the questionnaire used is available in the reference.) The vast majority of patients said they were well prepared for their upcoming procedure.

USE OF DECISION SUPPORT SYSTEMS AND INFORMATION TECHNOLOGY IN PREOPERATIVE ASSESSMENT

Decision support algorithms can suggest clinical management and preoperative tests from factors documented in the patient's H&P. These algorithms can be generated by clinical leadership and distributed as part of the educational and orientation process for the preoperative clinic providers. Algorithms can be built into computer software. The ability to integrate these algorithms with patient data stored as part of the hospital's electronic medical record would be particularly valuable. At large institutions with extensive information technology support, these systems may be internally generated. Because institutions may store data in programs using different platforms, integrating multiple data storage programs within a single institution or integrating patient data with commercially available systems is difficult. When clinical and testing algorithms are used by clinicians, even in the absence of computer-based prompts, the cost of laboratory tests has decreased because unnecessary or unreimbursed testing and consultations are eliminated (1,7). A number of barriers to implementation of electronic preoperative systems are described in Table 18.4.

Table 18.4.   Barriers to computer/Internet-based preoperative systems

1. Lack of uniformity in coding of medical conditions; limitations of drop-down menus; coding inconsistent with physician thought processes
2. Inability to integrate across different interfaces both within institutions and with outside institutions and physician offices
3. Concern regarding confidentiality of transmitted information; federal regulation and privacy issues
4. Cost of systems; capital investment required to purchase commercially available systems whose longevity is not established; use of internal resources if "in-house" development is done
5. Change in workflow that utilization of such systems requires; interference with current work styles

The lack of uniformity in coding of medical conditions is one impediment to computer-based preoperative assessment systems. Coding these data is extremely complex in contrast to computer records of laboratory data. Most of the commercially available systems contain pull-down menus, which may or may not be consistent with physician thought processes. With pull-down menus, information may be recorded where it "best fits" and therefore may not be completely accurate. When free text is used, a plan cannot be generated from decision support and aggregate data cannot be used for reporting. Coding data should be used for individual patient billing as well as for reporting quality performance measures. It is difficult to demonstrate the impact of quality reporting programs on clinical outcomes until adequate coding of medical conditions through information technology can be achieved. Technology development both internally and commercially should be focused so that data from preoperative assessments can be recorded to demonstrate the impact on clinical outcomes of perioperative protocols and hospital quality improvement processes. Because focus is lacking in coding, regulatory quality reporting programs have influenced hospital improvement activities but have not been shown to have a positive impact on outcomes (14).

Integration of information depends on facts from a wide variety of sources that contain important preoperative information: Reports from the patient's specialists and primary care physicians, testing from outside institutions, and previous anesthesia and surgical records. An electronic preoperative assessment program must integrate information from all the sources. In fact, incompatibility in intrainstitutional interfaces may make retrieval of this data into an electronic preoperative assessment system impossible. It is, therefore, difficult to estimate a return on investment for any of the commercial systems if manual entry of all patient data is required. Issues of standardization and interoperability must be resolved before commercial systems can be adopted.

Confidentiality in protecting computer-based data from interception is of great concern. Like paper-based records, computer-stored data have the potential for security risks from unauthorized access to information. Proper policies and education of staff regarding privacy are essential. The Health Insurance Portability and Accountability Act (HIPAA) is legislation regarding the privacy of health care information and related transactions. HIPAA requirements are outlined in Table 18.5. Business partners of health care institutions must comply with these regulations.

Cost prevents some institutions from investment in commercially available systems whose longevity has not been established. If the focus of a system is on anesthesia assessment, as many currently are, the financial benefit to the institution for regulatory and billing information based on elements contained in the surgical H&P is absent. Most computerized anesthesia preoperative systems focus on the intraoperative period and include few preoperative predictors (15,16). There is no good literature demonstrating successful implementation, quality outcomes, and resource management using either commercial-based or internally developed systems that address all of the necessary elements.

Table 18.5.   Regulations of the Health Insurance Portability and Accountability Act

1. Providers and health plans must give patients a written explanation if their health information is used and disclosed.
2. Patients have access to their medical records. A history of nonroutine disclosures must be made available to patients.
3. Patient consent must be obtained before information is released for treatment, payment, and health care operations. Patients can request restrictions on the disclosure of their information.
4. Civil penalties have been established for violating patient rights to privacy.
5. Employers or financial institutions may not use health information covered by this rule for purposes not related to health care.
6. Covered entities must establish and train employees in these policies and procedures and ensure that they are followed.

From Department of Health and Human Services. 45 CFR Parts 160 and 164 Standards for Privacy of Individually Identifiable Health Information; Final Rule. Federal Register 2000;65:82461–82510. From www.hhs.gov/ocr/hipaa/finalreg.html. Accessed October 3, 2007.

Change in workflow raises concern that the efficiency of established workflow patterns would be diminished, especially if many elements of the H&P must be manually entered. The effect on the patient interview must also be considered. The quality of an interview may suffer if the clinician divides time between the computer terminal and the patient. The resource savings may not be demonstrated if merely typing information replaces writing it, again emphasizing the need for integration among platforms to achieve success.

DECISION ANALYSIS TOOLS FOR PREOPERATIVE ASSESSMENT

Even if an overall computer-based preoperative assessment tool is lacking, individual decision analysis tools may be useful. More and more institutions are developing computer-based physician order entry (CPOE) systems. Groups such as Leapfrog and the National Surgical Quality Improvement Program (NSQIP) encourage the development and use of such systems, although only a small percentage of hospitals have adopted them (17). No "off-the-shelf" products are available and no standards have been developed between vendors and institutions, thus requiring hospitals to develop expensive, customized programs (17). Regulatory groups promote the ability of such systems to decrease medication errors; however, physicians are concerned about cost and the impact on workflow. The use of such systems may actually increase physician workload; one study estimated that CPOE systems took up 5% of a resident's weekly work hours (18). The automatic integration of medications already known by the patient's primary care physician or specialist into such systems would vastly increase their appeal and efficiency. Eight commercially available programs for digital assistants were tested for sensitivity, specificity, and positive and negative predictive values for a number of well-documented drug–drug interactions within simulated patient profiles. Of the systems studied, Epocrates Rx and Epocrates Rx Pro most reliably detected the clinically relevant interactions without alerts for those of no clinical significance. These programs are regularly updated and easily accessible online (18).

INTERDISCIPLINARY AND INTERNATIONAL INTEREST IN PREOPERATIVE ASSESSMENT

Institutions both nationally and internationally face similar issues in attempting to provide evidence-based, efficient care. An international forum provides a basis for discussion, education, and benchmarking. The Society for Perioperative Assessment and Quality Improvement (SPAQI) was formed in 2006 to provide this forum (www.spaqi.org). SPAQI is an international society based in the United States with the goal of bringing together a variety of professionals in various disciplines to work together on all facets influencing optimal surgical outcomes. These elements include proper preoperative assessment and evaluation, optimization of presurgical status, appropriate and efficient resource use, proper planning for postoperative pain management, and appropriate use of alternative and complementary medicine techniques. The society is designed to share best practices, promote research, and provide a pathway for communication among members and the rest of the medical community.

SUMMARY

Successful preoperative assessment processes require multidisciplinary collaboration and an understanding of the particular demographic and operational issues of an institution. Analysis of clinical protocols, algorithms, and staff workflows is required. Regulatory requirements must be met and quality improvement processes must be maintained and continually evaluated. There are a number of barriers to successful implementation of electronic preoperative assessment; strong support for data storage methods that permit information to be drawn from multiple sources into the electronic preoperative assessment is essential for accuracy, optimal resource management, and clinician acceptance.

REFERENCES

1. Fischer SP. Development and effectiveness of an anesthesia preoperative evaluation clinic in a teaching hospital. *Anesthesiology*. 1996;85:190–206.
2. Ferschl MB, Tung A, Sweitzer BJ, et al. Preoperative visits reduce operating room cancellations and delays. *Anesthesiology*. 2005;103:855–859.
3. Correll DJ, Bader AM, Hull MW, et al. The value of preoperative clinic visits in identifying issues with potential impact on operating room efficiency. *Anesthesiology*. 2006;105:1254–1259.
4. Wright MC, Phillips-Bute B, Mark JB, et al. Time of day effects on the incidence of anesthetic adverse events. *Qual Saf Health Care*. 2006;15:258–263.
5. Tsen LC, Segal S, Pothier M, et al. Survey of residency training in preoperative evaluation. *Anesthesiology*. 2000;98:1134–1137.

6. Dexter F, Marcario E, Epstein RH, et al. Validation of statistical methods to compare cancellation rates on the day of surgery. *Anesth Analg*. 2005;101:465–473.

7. Tsen LC, Segal S, Pothier M, et al. The effect of alterations in a preoperative assessment clinic on reducing the number and improving the yield of cardiology consultations. *Anesth Analg*. 2002;95:1563–1568.

8. Birkmeyer NJO, Birkmeyer JD. Strategies for improving surgical quality — should payers reward excellence or effort? *N Engl J Med*. 2006;354:864–870.

9. Davenport DL, Henderson WG, Khuri SF, et al. Preoperative risk factors and surgical complexity are more predictive of costs than postoperative complications: a case study using the national surgical quality improvement program (NSQIP) database. *Ann Surg*. 2005;242:463–471.

10. Fleisher LA, Beckman JA, Brown KA, et al. ACC/AHA guidelines on perioperative cardiovascular evaluation and care for noncardiac surgery. *J Am Coll Cardiol*. 2007;20:3159–3241.

11. Mangram AJ, Horan TC, Pearson, ML, et al. Guideline for prevention of surgical site infection, 1999. *Infect Control Hosp Epidemiol*. 1999;20:247–278.

12. Fung D, Cohen M. Measuring patient satisfaction with anesthetic care: a review of current methodology. *Anesth Analg*. 1998;87:1089–1098.

13. Hepner DL, Bader AM, Hurwitz S, et al. Patient satisfaction with preoperative assessment in a preoperative testing clinic. *Anesth Analg*. 2004;98:1099–1105.

14. Pham HH, Coughlan J, O'Malley AS. The impact of quality-reporting programs on hospital operations. *Health Aff*. 2006;25:1412–1422.

15. Rose DK, Cohen MM, Wigglesworth DF, et al. Development of a computerized database for the study of anesthesia care. *Can J Anaesth*. 1992;39:716–723.

16. Chase CR, Merz BA, Mazuzan JE. Computer assisted patient evaluation (CAPE): a multipurpose computer system for an anesthesia service. *Anesth Analg*. 1983;62:198–206.

17. Berger RG, Kichak JP. Computerized physician order entry: helpful or harmful? *J Am Med Inform Assoc*. 2004;11:100–103.

18. Perkins NA, Murphy JE, Malone DC, et al. Performance of drug-drug interaction software for personal digital assistants. *Ann Pharmacother*. 2006;40:850–855.

Preoperative Assessment for Specific Procedures or Locations

Thomas W. Cutter

INTRODUCTION

The preoperative assessment and management of patients scheduled for anesthesia first requires determining what is appropriate for the particular setting. Procedures that once were exclusively inpatient are now performed on an outpatient basis and some patients with an American Society of Anesthesiologists (ASA) physical status (PS) score of 4 safely undergo select procedures in a nontraditional facility. Although guidelines and standards apply, the blanket application of strict protocols and restrictions eliminates certain patients from having anesthesia in the ambulatory setting.

Care given in a nonhospital setting must be equivalent to the care rendered in the traditional inpatient setting. The Joint Commission on Accreditation of Healthcare Organizations, the Center for Medicare and Medicaid Services, and other accrediting and regulating entities hold all anesthetics to equivalent standards. The preparation and evaluation of any patient should be of the same quality, although the quantity may change depending on the proposed anesthetic or procedure. There must be a carefully integrated assessment and management of the patient, the procedure, the personnel, and the facility.

FACILITIES

Anesthesia can be administered in a number of different facilities, ranging from a private office to a hospital, with the latter designating specific operating rooms for outpatients or using the same rooms for outpatients and inpatients. In between these two extremes are the freestanding facility and the separate on-campus facility. The location of and equipment in the facility will affect the procedures that can be performed outside of the traditional hospital setting.

In the traditional hospital setting, any patient can easily become an inpatient. The same is true for an on-campus facility, depending on the ease with which a patient may be transferred to the hospital proper. In freestanding surgicenters, imaging facilities, and office-based facilities, distance or transportation-related difficulties may preclude procedures that have a high risk of complications requiring patient admission afterwards.

Fleisher et al. (1) found that outpatients >85 years of age with a history of hospital admission within the previous 6 months had a higher risk of postoperative admission than those without a previous admission. He also found that patients anesthetized in on-campus facilities had a higher rate of hospital admission and death than patients in freestanding surgicenters or physicians' offices, but patient selection criteria may have been a confounding factor.

A facility must be capable of dealing with all anticipated pre-, post-, and intraoperative events. Anesthesia supplies must include medications and equipment to safely administer and monitor an anesthetic. If a life-threatening complication is possible, the facility must be prepared to diagnose and temporize the situation until the definitive intervention can be performed. For example, if a general anesthetic with volatile agents will be administered, a blood gas machine and malignant hyperthermia treatment must be nearby. If significant blood loss is anticipated, a means to measure hemoglobin is needed and blood should be readily available. The allowable complexity of the patient and the procedure is facility dependent.

PERSONNEL

The presence or absence of an anesthesiologist may affect the decision to accept a patient or procedure in a particular facility. Some patients may be better served by a senior anesthesiologist (2), rather than by a junior clinician or by a nurse supervised by the operating physician. Adequate nursing staff is needed during the procedure and in the preanesthesia and postanesthesia care units. Nurses with advanced training are required for those patients recovering from a general anesthetic versus those recovering from intravenous sedation and analgesia. With adequate numbers of adequately trained personnel, any procedure can be performed in a facility with the appropriate equipment.

PROCEDURES

Last century, the "ideal" ambulatory procedure was one that could be performed in <90 minutes, did not result in excessive blood loss or fluid shifts, did not require highly specialized operating equipment or postanesthesia care, and resulted only in nominal pain that could be managed at home, typically with oral medications (3).

Today, the only inviolate requirement of an ambulatory procedure is that the patient return home the same day as the surgery, with some advocating that all elective surgery should be on an ambulatory basis (4). Open heart procedures have not yet made the list, but laparoscopic cholecystectomies, total knee arthroplasties, and vaginal hysterectomies are examples of procedures that have transitioned to outpatient status. Same-day discharge may be prevented by the prolonged need for an endotracheal tube, the presence of pain requiring nursing or physician intervention, postoperative nausea and vomiting, excessive bleeding or fluid shifts, or the need for frequent patient monitoring by a health care professional.

A novel method for developing a list of acceptable ambulatory procedures is proposed by Dexter et al (5). A list of proposed procedures is generated (Fig. 19.1) using the International Classification of Diseases, Ninth Revision, Clinical Modification (ICD-9-CM); the American Medical Association's Current Procedural Terminology (CPT) codes; and the ASA Relative Value Guide (RVG). Procedures that have seven or fewer RVG basic

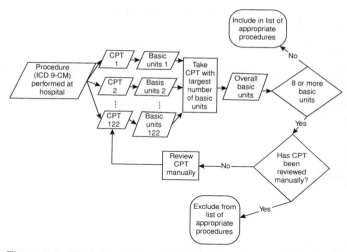

Figure 19.1.   Methodology to identify the maximum number of basic units for each procedure based on the International Classification of Diseases, Ninth Revision, Clinical Modification (ICD-9-CM). CPT, current procedural terminology. (Reprinted from Dexter F, Macario A, Penning, D, et al. Development of an appropriate list of surgical procedures of a specified maximum anesthetic complexity to be performed at a new ambulatory surgery facility. *Anesth Analg.* 2002;95:78–82.)

units are acceptable, while those with eight or more must be reviewed before inclusion by the staff.

Different procedures also incur different levels of risk and may be selected for a facility based on risk. Table 19.1 stratifies the cardiac risk of various procedures into three grades (6). High-risk procedures are probably not suitable for an ambulatory setting. Low-risk procedures are eminently appropriate, although the example of "Ambulatory surgery" should be excluded in the context of this chapter. Intermediate-risk procedures should be selected based on the available resources.

Safely performing any procedure in an ambulatory unit depends on the ability of the personnel to prevent significant morbid postoperative events and to safely and promptly mitigate them when they occur.

PATIENT

Once the facility, personnel, and procedure have been established, attention may be focused on the patient. Among the first considerations are the patient's psychological status and psychosocial support, including the caregivers after the patient is discharged. The patient and caregivers must understand and accept the responsibilities of care after the surgery. Any physical, cognitive, or emotional limitations of the patient or the caregivers must be identified and managed before the patient is scheduled for the procedure. The next step is to determine if the patient's unique

Table 19.1. Cardiac risk[a] stratification for noncardiac surgical procedures

Risk Stratification	Procedure Examples
Vascular (reported cardiac risk often more than 5%)	Aortic and other major vascular surgery
	Peripheral vascular surgery
Intermediate (reported cardiac risk generally 1% to 5%)	Intraperitoneal and intrathoracic surgery
	Carotid endarterectomy
	Head and neck surgery
	Orthopedic surgery
	Prostate surgery
Low[b] (reported cardiac risk generally less than 1%)	Endoscopic procedures
	Superficial procedure
	Cataract surgery
	Breast surgery
	Ambulatory surgery

[a]Combined incidence of cardiac death and nonfatal myocardial infarction.
[b]These procedures do not generally require further preoperative cardiac testing.
(From Fleisher LA, Beckman JA, Brown KA, et al. ACC/AHA 2007 Guidelines on perioperative cardiovascular evaluation and care for noncardiac surgery. A report of the American College of Cardiology/American Heart Association Task Force on Practice Guidelines. *J Am Coll Cardiol*, 2007;50:3159.

comorbidities and the planned procedure combine to yield an acceptable candidate.

Chung et al. (7) retrospectively considered the relationship between adverse events and pre-existing disease in 17,638 ambulatory patients. Tables 19.2 and 19.3 show the incidence of intraoperative or postoperative adverse events relative to the patient's medical condition. A history of congestive heart failure was most frequently associated with intraoperative cardiovascular events, followed by hypertension and previous cerebrovascular events. The events associated with hypertension are likely attributable more to its ubiquitous presence than to any predisposing feature unique to hypertension itself. Postoperatively, only respiratory adverse events were associated with a pre-existing condition, notably in those patients with a history of smoking, obesity, or asthma.

Ansell and Montgomery (8) retrospectively examined the outcomes for 28,921 patients, 896 (3.1%) of whom were ASA-PS 3 undergoing ambulatory surgery, and found no difference in postoperative complications or admission rates when compared to patients who were ASA-PS 1 or 2.

Fleisher et al. (9), retrospectively reviewing the outcomes of 783,483 outpatient procedures performed in the hospital setting, identified certain risk factors (Table 19.4) for either hospital admission or death immediately following the procedure.

The presence of two or more yielded the odds ratios shown in Table 19.5.

Chung et al. (10) considered the effect of age as an independent factor and found that patients >65 years of age had 1.4 times the risk for any event and two times the risk for a cardiovascular event. This risk did not constitute a contraindication, but rather

Table 19.2. Incidence of intraoperative adverse events by pre-existing medical condition

	Any Event [No. (%)]	Cardiovascular Event [No. (%)]	Respiratory Event [No. (%)]	Intubation-Related Event [No. (%)]
Hypertension	206 (8.4)	187 (7.7)	9 (0.4)	6 (0.3)
Angina pectoris	52 (6.9)	49 (6.5)	0 (0.0)	2 (0.3)
Myocardial infarction	30 (6.7)	29 (6.5)	0 (0.0)	1 (0.2)
Arrhythmia	29 (6.2)	28 (5.9)	1 (0.2)	0 (0.0)
Valvular disease	13 (4.3)	12 (4.0)	1 (0.3)	0 (0.0)
Congestive heart failure	16 (11.1)	16 (11.1)	0 (0.0)	0 (0.0)
Smoking	104 (4.2)	59 (2.4)	27 (1.1)	9 (0.4)
Asthma	40 (4.0)	23 (2.3)	7 (0.7)	4 (0.4)
COPD	28 (7.3)	23 (6.0)	2 (0.5)	0 (0.0)
URI	2 (2.1)	1 (1.1)	1 (1.1)	0 (0.0)
GERD	32 (5.0)	20 (3.1)	6 (0.9)	10 (1.6)
Renal disease	15 (7.4)	12 (5.9)	1 (0.5)	0 (0.0)
Diabetes mellitus	55 (6.0)	51 (5.5)	0 (0.0)	2 (0.2)
Thyroid disease	43 (5.4)	34 (4.3)	1 (0.1)	5 (0.6)
Obesity	137 (4.9)	89 (3.2)	29 (1.0)	15 (0.5)
Arthritis	86 (7.5)	69 (6.0)	5 (0.4)	7 (0.6)
CVA or TIA	19 (8.1)	18 (7.7)	0 (0.0)	0 (0.0)
Seizure	5 (4.2)	4 (3.4)	1 (0.9)	0 (0.0)

COPD, chronic obstructive pulmonary disease; CVA, cerebrovascular accident; GERD, gastroesophageal reflux disease; TIA, transient ischemic attack; URI, upper respiratory infection.
Adapted from: Chung F, Mezei G, Tong D. Pre-existing medical conditions as predictors of adverse events in day-case surgery. *Br J Anaesth*. 1999;83:262–270.

Table 19.3. Incidence of adverse events in the postanesthesia care unit by pre-existing medical condition

	Any Event [No. (%)]	Cardiovascular Event [No. (%)]	Respiratory Event [No. (%)]	Excessive Pain [No. (%)]	N/V [No. (%)]
Hypertension	121 (5.0)	36 (1.5)	12 (0.5)	52 (2.1)	20 (0.8)
Angina pectoris	35 (4.7)	11 (1.5)	7 (0.9)	12 (1.6)	6 (0.8)
Myocardial infarction	19 (4.2)	6 (1.3)	1 (0.2)	6 (1.3)	2 (0.5)
Arrhythmia	20 (4.3)	5 (1.1)	3 (0.6)	4 (0.9)	8 (1.7)
Valvular disease	36 (11.9)	1 (0.3)	0 (0.0)	22 (7.3)	9 (3.0)
Congestive heart failure	5 (3.5)	1 (0.7)	1 (0.7)	0 (0.0)	2 (1.4)
Smoking	295 (11.8)	16 (0.6)	16 (0.6)	185 (7.4)	62 (2.4)
Asthma	127 (12.7)	4 (0.4)	13 (1.3)	57 (5.7)	46 (4.6)
COPD	14 (3.7)	3 (0.8)	4 (1.0)	4 (1.0)	1 (0.3)
URI	11 (11.6)	1 (1.1)	0 (0.0)	6 (6.3)	3 (3.2)
GERD	51 (7.9)	4 (0.6)	5 (0.8)	26 (4.0)	15 (2.3)
Renal disease	14 (6.9)	2 (1.0)	1 (0.5)	8 (3.9)	0 (0.0)
Diabetes mellitus	28 (3.0)	10 (1.1)	5 (0.5)	12 (1.3)	2 (0.2)
Thyroid disease	53 (6.7)	9 (1.1)	5 (0.6)	21 (2.7)	17 (2.2)
Obesity	289 (10.3)	17 (0.6)	27 (1.0)	160 (5.7)	77 (2.8)
Arthritis	85 (7.4)	13 (1.1)	2 (0.2)	43 (3.8)	21 (1.8)
CVA or TIA	16 (6.8)	5 (2.1)	2 (0.9)	3 (1.3)	5 (2.1)
Seizure	21 (17.8)	1 (0.9)	0 (0.0)	16 (13.6)	4 (3.4)

COPD, chronic obstructive pulmonary disease; CVA, cerebrovascular accident; GERD, gastroesophageal reflux disease; N/V, nausea, vomiting; TIA, transient ischemic attack; URI, upper respiratory infection.

Adapted from: Chung F, Mezei G, Tong D. Pre-existing medical conditions as predictors of adverse events in day-case surgery. *Br J Anaesth.* 1999;83:262–270.

Table 19.4.   Risk factors for hospital admission or death after outpatient procedure in the hospital setting

- Operating room duration >60 min
- Cardiac disease
- Peripheral vascular disease
- Cerebrovascular disease
- Malignancy
- HIV positive
- General anesthesia
- Age >85

Adapted from: Fleisher LA, Pasternak R, Lyles A. A novel index of elevated risk for hospital admission or death immediately following outpatient surgery. *Anesthesiology.* 2002;96:A38.

indicated the need for careful intraoperative management. Aldwinkle and Montgomery (11) also concluded that age >70 years is not an exclusion criterion for ambulatory procedures.

Pregnancy is not an absolute contraindication for nonobstetric procedures, ambulatory or otherwise (12). The timing of surgery during pregnancy may be important (13), at least with regard to laparoscopic procedures. The second trimester may be preferrable to the first, since organogenesis is complete and spontaneous abortions are fewer. The second trimester has also been associated with fewer episodes of preterm labor than the third trimester.

Davies et al. (14) found that outpatient anesthesia for the morbidly obese patient (body mass index [BMI] >35) was not associated with increased unplanned admissions or postoperative complications. They concluded that morbid obesity should not be used as an exclusion criterion but cautioned that the equipment (e.g., tables and gurneys) must be able to accommodate the patient's weight.

Diabetes mellitus is typically not a significant concern in the ambulatory setting (15). An exception is a brittle diabetic patient presenting with an infection or some other disease state that exacerbates the already difficult glycemic control.

An excellent review of the controversies surrounding the management of ambulatory anesthesia (16,17) uses specific examples

Table 19.5.   Odds ratios for hospital admission or death after an outpatient procedure in the hospital setting[a]

Risk Factor	% of Population	Odds Ratio
0, 1	76	0.117
2	22	8.564
≥3	2	5.875

[a]A greater total score is associated with increased risk.
Adapted from: Fleisher LA, Pasternak R, Lyles A. A novel index of elevated risk for hospital admission or death immediately following outpatient surgery. *Anesthesiology.* 2002;96:A38.

Table 19.6.   Summary of patient issues for ambulatory anesthesia

Medical Condition	Further Workup	Concerns
Elderly (>65)	None	Hemodynamic variation
Reactive airway disease	None	Minor respiratory complications
Coronary artery disease	None if functional capacity is adequate	
Obstructive sleep apnea	None	Difficult airway; avoid narcotics; CPAP available
Diabetes mellitus	None	None
Morbid obesity	None	Minor respiratory complications
Ex-premature infant	Hct >30% >60 weeks postconceptual age	
Malignant hyperthermia	None	Treatment available

CPAP, continuous positive airway pressure; Hct, hematocrit.
Adapted from: Bryson GL, Chung F, Cox RG, et al. Patient selection in ambulatory anesthesia—evidence-based review: Part I. *Can J Anesth*. 2004;51:768–781, and Bryson GL, Chung F, Cox RG, et al. Patient selection in ambulatory anesthesia—evidence-based review: Part II. *Can J Anesth*. 2004;51:782–794.

of patients and associated comorbidities to make suggestions for proceeding and for what to expect. The review is based on available research and expert opinion and is summarized in Table 19.6.

Outcome studies in ambulatory surgery often do not consider the type of surgery or anesthetic. One of the first studies to consider the procedure was for cataract surgery by Schein et al. (18), with results later corroborated by Imasogie et al. (19). Both found that perioperative morbidity and mortality for cataract surgery were not reduced by routine perioperative laboratory testing.

The interrelationship of procedure and comorbidity is shown in the results of a survey of Canadian anesthesiologists (20), who were asked if they would administer general anesthesia to ambulatory patients with various comorbidities for procedures such as laparoscopic cholecystectomy, knee arthroscopy, or operative hysteroscopy. The results appear in Tables 19.7, 19.8, and 19.9.

While neither definitive nor scientific, the results demonstrate the willingness of certain anesthesiologists to proceed with an invasive procedure and a general anesthetic even in the face of significant comorbidities.

Once the decision to go forward has tentatively been made on the basis of an acceptable fit between the patient, the personnel, the facility, and the procedure, further patient evaluation is warranted. Evaluation can take place at any time before surgery,

Table 19.7. Ambulatory patient selection criteria—agreement or disagreement to proceed with surgery

Presented Condition	Yes (%, n = 1,337)	No (%, n = 1,337)
ASA 3	93.9	4.5
ASA 4	17.1	82.4
Angina pectoris[a] 2	96.4	2.7
Angina pectoris[a] 3	66.3	32.8
Angina pectoris[a] 4	4.0	95.3
Prior MI (1–6 mo)	15.9	83.1
Prior MI (>6 mo)	94.8	3.9
CHF 1	93.5	6.1
CHF 2	70.3	29.3
CHF 3	16.7	82.6
CHF 4	1.3	98.4
Asymptomatic valvular disease	93.4	5.3
Sleep apnea—monitored anesthesia care	91.5	7.2
Sleep apnea—RA without narcotics	97.0	2.7
Sleep apnea—RA with narcotics postop	35.3	64.0
Sleep apnea—GA without narcotics postop	63.4	36.0
Sleep apnea—GA with narcotics postop	14.7	84.2
Obesity (BMI = 35–44) without CV or respiratory comorbidity	91.0	9.0
Obesity (BMI = 35–44) with CV or respiratory comorbidity	18.1	81.7
Obesity (BMI = 45) without CV or respiratory comorbidity	49.5	50.1
Obesity (BMI = 45) without CV or respiratory comorbidity	4.7	95.2
Insulin-dependent diabetes mellitus	92.8	6.6
Malignant hyperthermia susceptible	82.0	17.6
Proven malignant hyperthermia	49.7	49.5
Substance abuse	69.0	29.8
Monoamine oxidase inhibitor treatment	69.5	29.6
Sickle cell anemia	53.2	45.5
Chronic renal failure	72.2	27.4
Age >90	59.6	39.8
No escort	11.2	88.1

Yes, agreement to proceed with surgery; no, disagreement.

[a] Canadian Cardiovascular Society Functional Classification; ASA, American Society of Anesthesiologists physical status; BMI, body mass index; CHF, congestive heart failure—New York Heart Association Classification; CV, cardiovascular; GA, general anesthesia; MI, myocardial infarction; RA, regional anesthesia.

Adapted from: Friedman Z, Chung F, Wong DT. Ambulatory surgery adult patient selection criteria—a survey of Canadian anesthesiologists. *Can J Anesth.* 2004;51:437–443.

Table 19.8. Ambulatory patient selection criteria with over 75% agreement to proceed with surgery

Presented Condition	% (n = 1,337)
ASA 3	93.9
Angina pectoris 2[a]	96.4
Prior MI (>6 mo)	94.8
CHF I	93.5
Asymptomatic valvular disease	93.4
Sleep apnea—monitored anesthesia care	91.5
Sleep apnea—RA without narcotics	97.0
Obesity (BMI = 35–44) without CV or respiratory complications	91.0
Insulin-dependent diabetes mellitus	92.8
Malignant hyperthermia susceptible	82.0

[a]Canadian Cardiovascular Society Functional Classification; ASA, American Society of Anesthesiologists physical status; BMI, body mass index; CHF = congestive heart failure—New York Heart Association Classification; CV, cardiovascular; MI, myocardial infarction; RA, regional anesthesia.
Adapted from: Friedman Z, Chung F, Wong DT. Ambulatory surgery adult patient selection criteria—a survey of Canadian anesthesiologists. *Can J Anesth.* 2004;51:437–443.

but cancellations and delays are reduced when the patient is assessed before the day of surgery (21–23). Determining which patients need a preoperative visit can be guided by prescreening inquiries via telephone or during the patient's visit with the surgeon. Written questionnaires and computerized programs are also available (24) (see Chapter 2). An example of comorbidities

Table 19.9. Ambulatory patient selection criteria with over 75% agreement NOT to proceed with surgery

Presented Condition	% (n = 1,337)
ASA 4	82.4
Angina pectoris 4[a]	95.3
Prior MI (1–6 mo)	83.1
CHF 3	82.6
CHF 4	98.4
Sleep apnea—GA with narcotics postop	84.2
Obesity (BMI = 35–44) with CV or respiratory complications	81.7
Obesity (BMI = 45) with CV or respiratory complications	95.2
No escort	88.1

[a]Canadian Cardiovascular Society Functional Classification; ASA, American Society of Anesthesiologists physical status; BMI, body mass index; CHF, congestive heart failure—New York Heart Association Classification; CV, cardiovascular; GA, general anesthesia; MI, myocardial infarction.
Adapted from: Friedman Z, Chung F, Wong DT. Ambulatory surgery adult patient selection criteria—a survey of Canadian anesthesiologists. *Can J Anesth.* 2004;51:437–443.

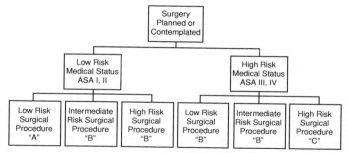

Figure 19.2. Illustrative algorithm for preanesthesia evaluation. High-risk procedure, significant perioperative and postoperative physiologic stress; low-risk procedure, poses minimal physiologic stress and risk to the patient independent of medical condition (e.g., office based, minor surgery); medium-risk procedure, moderate physiologic stress and risk with minimal blood loss, fluid shift, or postoperative change in normal physiology. "A": Preanesthesia assessment on day of surgery; "B": May require preanesthesia assessment prior to day of surgery; "C": Requires preanesthesia assessment prior to day of surgery. From: Pasternak LR. Preoperative screening for ambulatory patients. *Anesthesia Clin North Am.* 2003; 21: 229–242.

that may benefit from a preoperative evaluation prior to the procedure can be found in Table 2.8 in Chapter 2.

Figure 19.2 (25) illustrates an algorithm for determining the need for preanesthesia evaluation. Patients at low risk (on the left) are more likely to be evaluated by an anesthesiologist on the day of surgery; those at greater risk (on the right) would likely benefit from an evaluation before the day of surgery.

Preoperative testing may not involve the anesthesiologist, but when primary responsibility for preoperative testing is assigned to the anesthesiologist, efficiency and cost effectiveness are increased without an associated increase in untoward perioperative events (24–26). There are no laboratory tests that should be routinely ordered without a specific clinical indication for adults (25–28) or for children (29). Many anesthesiologists forgo preoperative testing for low-risk surgeries and patients in the ambulatory setting (20,21,29). A strategy for preoperative testing can be found in Chapter 2.

SPECIAL CONSIDERATIONS

Considerations for Patients

Some disease states may exclude a patient from having an ambulatory anesthetic. The American College of Cardiologists (ACC)/American Heart Association (AHA) Guideline Update for Perioperative Cardiovascular Evaluation for Noncardiac Surgery (6) states. In patients being considered for elective noncardiac surgery, the presence of unstable coronary disease, decompensated HF, H(eart) F(ailure), or severe arrhythima or valvular heart disease usually leads to cancellation or delay of surgery until the cardiac problem has been clarified and treated appropriately. Patients with these conditions should probably not be anesthetized in a freestanding ambulatory setting. On the other hand, patients with ASA PS 3 or 4, a history of sleep apnea, morbid obesity, chronic renal failure, or stable ischemic heart disease have safely undergone a procedure in an ambulatory setting. While there are few standards or guidelines, the following recommendations, based on research, clinical experience, and common sense, may provide some direction.

Hypertension

Most outpatients with a history of hypertension successfully and easily tolerate an ambulatory anesthetic without sequelae. Although significant hemodynamic changes are possible, it is not uncommon to proceed with elective surgery even in the presence of poorly controlled hypertension (30). Malignant hypertension is a contraindication (see Chapter 4.)

Ischemic Heart Disease

Many patients with ischemic heart disease live a virtually normal lifestyle and are able to ambulate into and out of a surgicenter. They are candidates for the ambulatory setting if their status has not changed as evident from history, physical examination, and supporting studies, if indicated (see Chapter 3.)

The patient with unstable angina is more problematic. If the procedure is relatively noninvasive and the anesthetic technique relatively benign (e.g., cataract surgery), then there are no absolute restrictions in the ambulatory setting, provided that immediate access to further aftercare is available and, if not, provisions should be made to perform the procedure elsewhere.

Valvular Heart Disease

Patients with valvular heart disease may have ambulatory surgery, although someone with severe disease, especially aortic stenosis, should likely undergo only the most minor of procedures (e.g., cataract surgery under monitored anesthesia care or finger surgery with a digital nerve block). If anything more complex is even remotely anticipated, additional resources for an immediate intervention must be available (see Chapter 4.)

Congestive Heart Failure/Cardiomyopathy

Cardiomyopathy by itself does not eliminate a patient from an ambulatory setting. Indeed, even a very low ejection fraction should not, in and of itself, preclude an ambulatory anesthetic. If the patient can walk in the door and the procedure and anesthetic technique are minor, then the patient is an acceptable candidate. Caveats include close monitoring and a procedure that entails only minimal fluid shifts.

Pacemaker/Internal Cardiac Defibrillator

Patients with pacemakers should present no significant difficulties in the ambulatory setting, assuming that their pacemakers have been recently evaluated and the reason for the pacemaker is well understood. A magnet should be available if difficulties arise.

An implantable cardioverter defibrillator (ICD) is problematic because it often indicates a more lethal underlying cardiac problem than one treated with a pacemaker. A patient with an ICD should be permitted in an ambulatory setting for only the most benign of procedures and anesthetics and only if personnel who can interrogate and program the device are immediately available (see Chapter 4.)

Obstructive Sleep Apnea

Patients with obstructive sleep apnea can be difficult to intubate and have a higher rate of significant postoperative adverse events (31). While no data firmly support a proscription against outpatient procedures for persons with sleep apnea, monitored anesthesia care or regional anesthesia is probably safest and narcotics should be avoided (see Chapter 13.)

Chronic Renal Failure

There are no absolute contraindications to the ambulatory setting for patients with chronic renal failure. Potassium levels measured preoperatively on the day of surgery should be obtained and arrangements should be made for possible postoperative hemodialysis (see Chapter 8.)

Need for Blood Transfusion

Procedures that require blood transfusion are best performed in an inpatient setting. Ambulatory facilities that perform certain procedures (e.g., hysterectomies, arteriovenous fistula thrombectomies, tonsillectomies) should make provisions for transfusion, maintaining at the very least a blood refrigerator with type O blood.

Anticipated Difficult Airway

Whether a patient with a difficult airway may have an ambulatory procedure depends on the skill of the providers and the equipment in the facility. Intubation is avoided by using an alternative anesthetic technique or is performed in a conservative fashion. The resources required to provide a surgical airway must be immediately available (see Chapter 16.)

Diabetes

Diabetes mellitus is typically not of significant concern in an ambulatory setting if blood sugar can be monitored. An exception is the brittle diabetic patient with an infection or some other disease state that exacerbates his or her already difficult control. If the patient's blood sugar cannot be managed with subcutaneous insulin postoperatively, the patient should not be accepted into an ambulatory unit (see Chapter 6.)

Extremes of Age

Virtually no one is too young or too old to be safely cared for in an ambulatory setting. The notable exception is an ex-premature baby who is <60 weeks postconceptual age. These children should never undergo anesthesia in an ambulatory setting unless arrangements are made for overnight observation to monitor for postanesthetic apnea (see Chapter 13.)

Advanced Pregnancy

A woman with an advanced pregnancy should have only the most nominal of procedures and anesthetics in an ambulatory setting where the fetus can be monitored and delivered if necessary (see Chapter 14.)

Reactive Airway Disease

Asthma and chronic obstructive airway disease can increase intraoperative and postoperative airway events. Smoking exacerbates these pre-existing conditions (7). Patients should be optimized and instructed to bring their inhalers to the facility (see Chapter 5.)

Psychiatric Disease

The depressed patient taking monoamine oxidase inhibitors poses no increased risk if the medications and the anesthetic are properly managed. Schizophrenia should be under control with medication so there is no risk to either the patient or others (see Chapter 12.)

Patients at Risk for Malignant Hyperthermia

All facilities that provide general anesthesia must have the means to treat someone with malignant hyperthermia. If a patient has either a personal or a family history of malignant hyperthermia, the anesthetic technique must avoid all triggering agents. In no case should succinylcholine or volatile anesthetics be used (see Chapter 16.)

Sickle Cell Disease

Patients with sickle cell disease must not be in "crisis" and their hematologist should have prepared them for the stresses and consequences of surgery and anesthesia. They must have an adequate hemoglobin (exchange transfusion if necessary) and no underlying infections or other undertreated diseases that would stress them (see Chapter 7.)

Neuromuscular Disease

Patients with Duchenne muscular dystrophy or myasthenia gravis should not undergo general anesthesia requiring muscle relaxation because of the potential need for postoperative ventilation.

PROCEDURE SPECIFIC PREOPERATIVE ASSESSMENT

For otherwise healthy patients undergoing minimally invasive procedures (e.g., cataract extraction with intraocular lens placement, diagnostic knee arthroscopy, breast biopsy, angiography) or moderately invasive procedures in which blood loss or hemodynamic changes are uncommon (e.g., laparoscopic cholecystectomy, ventral hernia repair), no routine laboratory tests are recommended. An exception is a baseline creatinine when a procedure includes the injection of contrast dye.

The type of anesthesia may dictate the need for further testing. Since the disruption to normal physiology is much less significant, patients expected to have monitored anesthesia care may require fewer preoperative tests than those scheduled for a regional or a general anesthetic. Anesthesia with major neuraxial blockade requires a normal coagulation status, so platelet count and relevant coagulation studies (e.g., prothrombin time, partial thromboplastin time) should be obtained if the patient bruises easily, has bleeding gums, or takes medications such as Warfarin.

For procedures that significantly disrupt normal physiology or require blood transfusions, or invasive monitoring, a complete blood count with platelets, electrolytes, a blood urea nitrogen, and creatinine should be obtained, regardless of the health of the patient. Other tests are warranted based on comorbid conditions. Figure 19.2 integrates patient and procedure with regard to the extent and timing of preoperative assessment before the day of surgery.

The current trend follows the adage "less is more," an example of which can be found in the evaluation for endovascular surgery, specifically an abdominal aortic aneurysm stent. Although many of these patients have significant comorbidities, including ischemic heart disease, renal failure, diabetes mellitus, chronic obstructive pulmonary disease, and hypertension, because the procedures are considered low risk, their preoperative assessment is less extensive than if they were having an open abdominal procedure.

CONCLUSION

The scope of anesthesia practice has gone far beyond the traditional operating room setting. Patient assessment and management in the nontraditional setting is evolving because procedures and anesthetic techniques continue to evolve. Definitions of high and low risk for both patients and procedures vary among practitioners, yielding even more diversity. Because the possible combinations of patient, place, and procedure are virtually unlimited, a unique and thoughtful approach is required for each patient.

REFERENCES

1. Fleisher LA, Pasternak LR, Herbert R, et al. Inpatient hospital admission and death after outpatient surgery in elderly patients: importance of patient and system characteristics and location of care. *Arch Surg.* 2004;139:67–72.

2. Ni KM, Watts JC. Day case surgery in an isolated unit may require more stringent selection of cases. *Anaesthesia.* 2001; 56:485–502.

3. White PF. *Ambulatory Anesthesia and Surgery.* Philadelphia: WB Saunders; 1997.

4. Baskerville P. A new vision for day surgery. *J Periop Pract.* 2006;16:327–332.

5. Dexter F, Macario A, Penning, D, et al. Development of an appropriate list of surgical procedures of a specified maximum anesthetic complexity to be performed at a new ambulatory surgery facility. *Anesth Analg.* 2002;95:78–82.

6. Fleisher LA, Beckman JA, Brown KA, et al. ACC/AHA guideline update for perioperative cardiovascular evaluation and care for noncardiac surgery. *J Am Coll Cardiol.* 2007;50:e159–241. Available at: http://www.acc.org. Accessed September 28, 2007.

7. Chung F, Mezei G, Tong D. Pre-existing medical conditions as predictors of adverse events in day-case surgery. *Br J Anaesth.* 1999;83:262–270.

8. Ansell GL, Montgomery JE. Outcome of ASA III patients undergoing day case surgery. *Br J Anaesth.* 2004;92:171–174.

9. Fleisher LA, Pasternak R, Lyles A. A novel index of elevated risk for hospital admission or death immediately following outpatient surgery. *Anesthesiology.* 2002;96:A38.

10. Chung F, Mexei G, Tong D. Adverse events in ambulatory surgery. A comparison between elderly and younger patients. *Can J Anesth.* 1999;46:309–321.

11. Aldwinckle RJ, Montgomery JR. Unplanned admission rates and post discharge complications in patients over the age of 70 following day case surgeries. *Anaesthesia.* 2004;59:57–59.

12. Melnick DM, Wahl WL, Dalton VK. Management of general surgery problems in the pregnant patient. *Am J Surg.* 2004;187:170–180.

13. O'Rourke N, Kodali, BS. Laparoscopic surgery during pregnancy. *Curr Opin Anaesthesiol.* 2006;19:254–259

14. Davies KE, Houghton K, Montgomery JE. Obesity and day care surgery. *Anaesthesia.* 2001;56:1090–1115.

15. Marks JB. Perioperative management of diabetes. *Am Fam Physician.* 2003;67:93–100.

16. Bryson GL, Chung F, Finegan BA, et al. Patient selection in ambulatory anesthesia—an evidence-based review: part I. *Can J Anesth.* 2004;51:768–781.

17. Bryson GL, Chung F, Cox RG, et al. Patient selection in ambulatory anesthesia—an evidence-based review: part II. *Can J Anesth.* 2004;51:782–794.

18. Schein OD, Katz J, Bass EB, et al. The value of routine preoperative medical testing before cataract surgery. *N Engl J Med.* 2000;342:168–175.

19. Imasogie N, Wong DT, Luk K, et al. Elimination of routine testing in patients undergoing cataract surgery allows substantial savings in laboratory costs. A brief report. *Can J Anesth.* 2003;50:246–248.

20. Friedman Z, Chung F, Wong DT. Ambulatory surgery adult patient selection criteria—a survey of Canadian anesthesiologists. *Can J Anesth.* 2004;51:437–443.

21. Parker BM, Tetzlaff JE, Litaker DL, et al. Redefining the preoperative evaluation process and the role of the anesthesiologist. *J Clin Anesth.* 2000;12:350–356.

22. Ferschl MB, Tung A, Sweitzer BJ, et al. Preoperative clinic visits reduce operating room cancellations and delays. *Anesthesiology.* 2005;103:855–859.

23. Pasternak LR. Preoperative screening for ambulatory patients. *Anesthesiol Clin North Am.* 2003;21:229–242.

24. Starsnic MA, Guarnieri DM, Norris MC. Efficacy and financial benefit of an anesthesiologist-directed university preadmission evaluation center. *J Clin Anesth.* 1997;9:299–305.

25. Allison JG, Bromley HR. Unnecessary preoperative investigations: evaluation and cost analysis. *Am Surg.* 1996;62:686–689.

26. Mancuso CA. Impact of new guidelines on physicians' ordering of preoperative tests. *J Gen Intern Med.* 1999;14:166–172.

27. Haug RH, Reifeis RL. A prospective evaluation of the value of

preoperative laboratory testing for office anesthesia and sedation. *J Oral Maxillofac Surg*. 1999;57:16–20.

28. Yuan H, Chung F, Wong D, et al. Current preoperative testing practices in ambulatory surgery are widely disparate: a survey of CAS members. *Can J Anesth*. 2005;52:675–679.

29. Meneghini L, Zadra N, Zanette G, et al. The usefulness of routine preoperative laboratory tests for one-day surgery in healthy children. *Paediatr Anaesth*. 1988;8:11–15.

30. Lermitte J, Chung F. Patient selection in ambulatory surgery. *Curr Opin Anaesthesiol*. 2005;18:598–602.

31. Gupta RM, Parvizi J, Hanssen AD, et al. Postoperative complications in patients with obstructive sleep apnea syndrome undergoing hip or knee replacement: a case-control study. *Mayo Clinic Proc*. 2001;76:897–905.

Case Studies in Preoperative Evaluation

Douglas C. Shook and BobbieJean Sweitzer

The preoperative evaluation is an important part of the patient's perioperative care. This unique evaluation combines primary care issues with those of the perioperative environment. The perioperative physician reviews the patient's history, current medical condition, and proposed surgery to determine how to optimize perioperative outcome. Often information needs to be obtained from the primary care physician and specialists to make informed decisions. Knowledge of the surgeon and the surgical procedure is imperative. The cases that follow illustrate how a complete history and physical examination with selected diagnostic studies facilitate perioperative patient care and patient satisfaction.

Case 1

A 57-year-old obese woman with a history of type 2 diabetes mellitus (DM) and elevated cholesterol comes to the preoperative clinic 2 days before a total abdominal hysterectomy and bilateral salpingo-oophorectomy (TAH-BSO) for cervical dysplasia and possible cervical cancer.

Medical History

Diabetes Mellitus (See Chapter 6)

Information regarding the duration of disease, glucose management and control, and symptoms or signs of diabetes-induced end-organ damage are sought in the patient's history.

The patient had not been evaluated by a physician for more than 10 years before a consultation a couple of months ago. At that time her type 2 DM was diagnosed. Her medications include Lantus 18 units subcutaneously in the evening and metformin 500 mg once a day. Her fasting blood glucose ranges from 140 to 200 mg/dL and her hemoglobin A_{1c} (Hgb A_{1c}) was 8.8 one month ago.

The duration of this patient's DM is unknown. She likely has had DM for a number of years during which she did not receive regular medical attention. Her Hgb A_{1c} is elevated, correlating with poor control. She is at risk for cardiovascular and peripheral vascular disease (PVD), neuropathies (autonomic and peripheral), renal insufficiency, increased rates of infection, and poor wound healing. The history focuses on eliciting end-organ dysfunction related to DM to optimize her perioperative care.

She has no history of myocardial infarction (MI), angina, or heart failure (HF). She denies a history of hypertension or tobacco use. She started atorvastatin for elevated cholesterol when the DM was diagnosed. She can ambulate slowly for 5 minutes before having to stop because of leg pain. She states that the leg pain is caused by osteoarthritis in her knees but admits to aching calves with pain that resolves with rest. Her family does most of her chores because of her restricted mobility. She denies a history of stroke. She has occasional heartburn and early satiety, but denies symptoms of reflux into her throat or a bitter taste in her mouth when lying flat. She has numbness in her hands and feet and complains of blurry night vision. Occasionally, she gets dizzy when standing up.

This patient does not have a history of coronary artery disease (CAD), but silent myocardial ischemia should be considered (1). Patients with DM are at least twice as likely to have CAD as nondiabetics. In addition, the risk of MI in diabetics is similar to the risk in nondiabetics who have a history of previous MI and the risk is considered a CAD equivalent (2,3). This patient also has poor functional capacity, possibly related to claudication. Her complaint of dizziness indicates possible autonomic dysfunction. She also has signs of peripheral neuropathy, retinopathy, and gastroparesis.

Obstructive Sleep Apnea (See Chapter 13)

She may have obstructive sleep apnea (OSA) because of her obesity.

She states that she does not snore. Her partner has not noticed apneic episodes at night, and she is able to lie flat without difficulty. She denies daytime somnolence.

Physical Examination

The examination focuses on delineating end-organ damage from type 2 DM, on physical findings of cardiovascular disease (e.g., heart murmur, irregular heart beat), and on autonomic or peripheral neuropathy. Vital signs, airway examination, and musculoskeletal abnormalities from osteoarthritis that may impact patient positioning in the operating room (OR) are evaluated.

The patient is 5 feet 2 inches tall and weighs 220 pounds. When she is sitting, her blood pressure (BP) is 140/82 mm Hg; heart rate (HR) is 94 beats per minute (bpm). When she stands, her BP is 112/58 mm Hg; HR is 108 bpm.

Funduscopic examination reveals small retinal hemorrhages. She is edentulous, with a Mallampati class 3 airway; the mouth opening is 3 cm; atlanto-occipital joint extension is limited with no pain or numbness on extension; and thyromental distance is 4 cm. Her neck is short, the neck circumference is 52 cm, and the trachea is midline. No carotid bruits are auscultated and no jugular venous distension (JVD) is noted.

Symmetric expansion is observed during quiet breathing. Breath sounds are equal bilaterally with no rhonchi or wheezes. The heart examination reveals a regular rate and rhythm with absence of HR variability during deep inspiration and expiration. No murmurs or gallops are heard. Pulses are diminished in her legs and absent below the ankles.

The abdomen is obese but otherwise unremarkable. Muscle strength is equal bilaterally with diminished sensation in her hands and feet. No edema is noted in her extremities.

Physical examination revealed retinopathy and neuropathy likely related to type 2 DM. No evidence of left or right heart failure was found, but she does have evidence of PVD. The airway examination indicates potential challenges. She is morbidly obese (BMI = 40), which is associated with both difficult mask ventilation and tracheal intubation (4).

Diagnostic Testing (See Chapter 2)

Electrolytes, blood urea nitrogen (BUN), creatinine, and glucose should be measured because of the history of DM. The creatinine is particularly important since this patient is taking metformin, which is cleared by the kidneys and is associated with perioperative lactic acidosis, especially in patients with renal insufficiency (5,6). An electrocardiogram (ECG) and hematocrit (Hct) determination are also necessary.

The electrolytes are normal; the glucose is 182 mg/dL; BUN is 18 mg/dL; creatinine is 1.2 mg/dL; and Hct is 33%. The ECG is significant for normal sinus rhythm, low-voltage QRS, and nonspecific ST- and T-wave changes.

The laboratory results reveal mild renal insufficiency likely related to the DM. The ECG changes are nonspecific but could be the result of underlying cardiac ischemia.

Assessment

This patient is an American Society of Anesthesiologists Physical Status (ASA-PS) class 3 patient for a not completely elective intermediate-risk procedure. She has type 2 DM with DM-related end-organ dysfunction and a potentially challenging airway. The history of DM, poor functional capacity, PVD, and abnormal ECG increases her risk for perioperative cardiac complications.

According to the 2007 American College of Cardiology/American Heart Association (ACC/AHA) Guidelines for Perioperative Cardiovascular Evaluation for Noncardiac Surgery, DM is a clinical risk factor for increased perioperative cardiovascular risk (7). Since TAH-BSO is considered an intermediate-risk surgery and she has DM, the ACC/AHA guidelines recommend noninvasive cardiac testing only if it will change management (7) (see Chapter 3). Because the patient may have cervical cancer, the consequences of delaying the operation for cardiac testing and possible intervention must be considered.

Noninvasive cardiac testing has excellent negative predictive value, but poor positive predictive value for determining patients at risk for perioperative MI (8) (see chapter 3). If testing shows ischemia and the patient undergoes coronary angiography, stenting, or bypass grafting, her surgery will likely be delayed for several weeks to months (9). On the other hand, patients with significant CAD diagnosed by coronary angiography did not benefit from preoperative revascularization before elective high-risk vascular surgery (10).

Several recent studies have advocated the use of perioperative beta blockade in patients with one or more clinical predictors. In this patient, the ACC/AHA would assign a class IIB recommendation for starting a perioperative beta blocker (7,8,11). There is good evidence to support this treatment and surgery can be performed given the possibility of underlying cancer.

This patient has a potentially difficult airway, which may be further complicated by DM. DM causes glycosylation of tissue proteins that can result in a stiff joint syndrome (12). Tissues throughout the body can be affected, but if the atlanto-occipital joint becomes less mobile, laryngoscopy and intubation will be difficult. Mask ventilation (MV) in this patient also may be difficult. Of the five independent criteria associated with difficult MV (age >55 years, BMI >26, beard, lack of teeth, and history of snoring), the presence of two indicates a likely difficult MV (13). This patient has three criteria for difficult MV: Age, BMI, and edentulous. To further complicate possible endotracheal tube placement, the patient likely has gastroparesis, given her history of early satiety and examination findings consistent with autonomic neuropathy (see Chapter 6).

The patient is taking metformin, which is rarely associated with lactic acidosis (14). Metformin should not be reinstituted perioperatively until the possibility of worsening renal or hepatic function is not an issue. According to the Cockcroft-Gault formula to estimate creatinine clearance and correcting for female muscle mass she already has mild renal insufficiency (creatinine clearance = 45 mL/min).

$$\text{Creatinine clearance} = \frac{(140 - \text{age}) \times \text{Lean body weight (kg)}}{(72 \times \text{Plasma creatinine})}$$
$$\times .85 \text{ (if female)}$$

Management

Whether, to postpone surgery and obtain noninvasive cardiac testing or proceed with HR control with beta blockers, should be made with the patient, with the surgeon, and possibly after consultation with a cardiologist. If the choice is to proceed with the surgery, then a cardioselective beta blocker is started as early as possible before surgery. The beta blocker can be prescribed in the preoperative clinic to modify perioperative cardiac risk. Oral metoprolol is commonly used with twice-a-day dosing, but twice-a-day dosing of atenolol, which has a longer half-life, may offer better 24-hour coverage. Medications started before surgery are more likely to be continued intra- and postoperatively. The patient should continue the statin perioperatively because HMG-CoA reductase inhibitors reduce perioperative cardiac complications, especially when combined with a beta blocker (15,16). She should be informed of the possible need for additional hemodynamic monitoring and lower red cell transfusion triggers. Postoperatively, additional cardiac monitoring and testing may be necessary.

The patient should take the full dose of her usual Lantus insulin the night before surgery. The day before surgery, the patient may take her usual dose of metformin, but not on the day of surgery. Her blood glucose must be checked on arrival to the preoperative area.

Epidural anesthesia, with or without general anesthesia (GA), should be discussed with the patient. Epidural analgesia provides optimal pain relief and may decrease the stress response of surgery, which may improve perioperative glucose management and decrease cardiac complications. Avoidance of GA also prevents problems with managing her airway. Possible awake fiberoptic intubation should be discussed with the patient. She is given the reasons for choosing this method of endotracheal tube placement and assured that her comfort will be maintained during the procedure. Metoclopramide, a histamine (H_2) blocker, and sodium citrate are indicated preoperatively because of her history of DM, obesity, heartburn, and probable gastroparesis.

Case 2

A 14-year-old female with recurrent pharyngotonsillitis comes to the preoperative clinic 7 days before an elective tonsillectomy. Her parents tell you that she has a cold. They also notify you that they are Jehovah's Witnesses. The patient has no previous surgical history.

Medical History

The important issues to be explored are the specifics of the patient's respiratory illness and medical history. Further questioning is needed about the family's wishes regarding blood and blood products.

Respiratory Tract Infection (See Chapter 15)

The decision to proceed with or delay an elective surgical procedure in a patient who has a current or recent respiratory tract infection is controversial. The etiology, length, and severity of the symptoms must be determined. Parents are an important source of information because of their knowledge of their child's day-to-day activities and general health (17).

The patient has had a sore throat, nasal congestion, and a dry cough for a couple of days. The sore throat is different than that experienced typically with tonsillitis. She denies shortness of breath (SOB), fevers, chest pain, or purulent nasal discharge. She has been attending school, but has had increased malaise in the past 24 hours. Many of her friends have had similar symptoms recently. She has no history of reactive airway disease, allergies, or allergic rhinitis.

Jehovah's Witness (See Chapters 13 and 15)

The beliefs of both the patient and the parents must be considered. If possible, the patient is interviewed without her parents, so that their presence does not influence her answers. All types of blood products should be discussed (e.g., red blood cells, plasma, platelets, albumin, clotting factors, erythropoietin, autologous donation) and methods of blood salvaging (e.g., cell saver, hemodilution). Even though the patient is a minor, her autonomy and wishes should be respected.

The parents are adamant that under no circumstances should their daughter be given any type of blood products. They also refuse all blood salvaging techniques. The patient is very articulate and mature. She is well versed in her family's faith and reaffirms that she will not accept blood products or blood salvaging even if it means that she will die without the treatment.

Pregnancy (See Chapters 2 and 15)

A menstrual/pregnancy history must be obtained from the patient. Ideally this should be done confidentially because of the effect parents can have on answers given by an adolescent patient (18). In addition, a history of abnormal bleeding should be sought.

A conversation with the parents and patient regarding the possibility of pregnancy is uneasy. The patient denies any sexual contact, but the answers do not appear reliable. The parents are unwilling to leave the room. The patient has no history of excessive bleeding from dental work, menses, or prolonged epistaxis.

Given the unreliable pregnancy history, the question of doing a pregnancy test becomes important.

Physical Examination

The physical examination focuses on determining the nature and significance of the patient's acute illness and evaluation of the airway, given her history of recurrent pharyngotonsillitis.

The patient appears comfortable, in no distress, and occasionally blows her nose. Her temperature is 37.5°C, respiratory rate is 14/minute, HR is 77, BP is 100/70 mm Hg, and oxygen saturation on room air is 99%.

Her nasal congestion is clear. She has a Mallampati class 1 airway with bilateral large tonsils, and her throat is inflamed with no purulence. There is no lymphadenopathy of the neck.

She is breathing comfortably without using accessory muscles. Her lungs are clear bilaterally and the cardiovascular examination is normal.

Diagnostic Testing (See Chapter 2)

The patient is postmenarchal and scheduled to undergo a procedure with possible blood loss, so a hematocrit (Hct) is indicated. Pregnancy testing is controversial (19). Anesthesia and surgery may be associated with an increased incidence of miscarriage. Additionally, certain medications may be teratogenic. This information should be shared with the patient and her parents so that they understand the reasons for the previous questions and the possible need for pregnancy testing. The reason for the testing is that virtually all patients will postpone elective surgery if they find out they are unexpectedly pregnant.

Assessment

In this 14-year-old girl with a respiratory tract infection who is scheduled for elective tonsillectomy, the initial decision is determining whether the infection is upper respiratory or lower respiratory. Elective procedures should be postponed in patients with fever or symptoms suggestive of a lower respiratory tract infection such as pneumonia or severe bronchitis. This patient's history is most consistent with symptoms of a mild, uncomplicated upper respiratory tract infection (URI) (17) (see Chapter 15).

In a study of 1,087 children ranging in age from 1 month to 18 years, no differences were found between children with active URIs, children with recent URIs (within 4 weeks), and asymptomatic children with respect to the incidences of laryngospasm and bronchospasm (20). Incidence of overall respiratory events was greater in the active and recent URI groups, but none of the patients had increased long-term morbidity. Adverse event rates were similar in children with recent URIs or with acute URIs. Given the similar incidence of perioperative respiratory events in children with active and recent URIs, a procedure in a child with a URI must be delayed for at least 6 weeks after the URI has resolved to significantly change the incidence of adverse respiratory events (21).

The Jehovah's Witness Society is the most rapidly growing religious organization in the Western world (22). In 1945, after discussion in the *Watch Tower*, it was determined that accepting blood transfusions violates God's law based on three Biblical passages forbidding transfusion (23). The punishment for accepting blood products is loss of eternal life and excommunication on earth (24).

In any religious society, not everyone has exactly the same beliefs. In this case, both the patient and her parents refuse to allow blood products for lifesaving measures. However, this patient is a minor. The U.S. judicial system has been pretty clear regarding unemancipated minors still under parental authority: A child of Jehovah's Witness parents cannot be allowed to die because of the parents' refusal to consent to the administration of blood products (23,24). Legal decisions have given courts the responsibility of *parens patriae,* the right and duty to protect a child's welfare. This protection includes justifying medical treatment (e.g., transfusion) to avoid physical harm (24).

Traditionally, U.S. minors have no legal rights. Therefore, physicians can transfuse blood products if indicated (24). Some states have a "mature minor" doctrine that allows minors to consent to or refuse medical treatment without parental consent (24). Under this doctrine, a judge must determine if a minor is mature enough to make health care choices.

Finally, should this patient be tested for possible pregnancy? The ASA Task Force on Preanesthesia Evaluation concluded that pregnancy testing may be considered for all female patients of childbearing age (25). Malviya et al. found that a detailed preoperative sexual history obtained from adolescent patients was consistently in agreement with pregnancy test results (26). The study suggested obtaining a "detailed history regarding the last menstrual period, contraception, sexual activity, and the possibility of pregnancy" and ordering a pregnancy test only if indicated by history. Anesthesia groups should develop guidelines in accordance with state statutes regarding pregnancy testing to help guide testing decisions.

Management

Should the surgery be delayed until the URI resolves and airway hyperreactivity is back to baseline (requiring at least 6 weeks)? The surgeon should be involved in this decision. One consideration is that coughing postoperatively may increase the risk of postoperative hemorrhage. The family also must be told about the risks of proceeding. They must have the ability to monitor the child closely postdischarge and have ready access to care.

If it is decided to proceed with the surgery and the patient's symptoms become more severe over the next week, then the decision may need to be reassessed.

The likelihood of the need for a lifesaving transfusion is low, given the patient's overall good health and the relatively low rate of hemorrhage after tonsillectomy (approximately 3.5%) (27). The preoperative clinic is the ideal place to discuss with the family the possible transfusion and the different blood products available. The decision-making options for avoiding transfusion should be discussed (28). The family should understand that unless the child is recognized as a "mature minor," blood products will be given if deemed necessary. A court order should be sought if necessary. This conversation should be documented in the chart and if the family decides to proceed with surgery, no written consent is needed for the transfusion.

The pregnancy test should be performed in the preoperative clinic if there is any question that the patient is pregnant. It may be helpful to enlist the help of the patient's pediatrician or the hospital's social services if further explanation is necessary.

Case 3

A 68-year-old obese male arrives in the ambulatory surgical center for elective cataract surgery. He has a history of ischemic cardiomyopathy and a pacemaker. There were no recent diagnostic tests ordered for the surgery. He is scheduled to go to the OR in the next couple of hours, and his son took the day off from work to be with him.

Medical History

Ischemic Cardiovascular Disease (See Chapter 3)

The history focuses on determining prior MI, HF, arrhythmias, and current and past cardiovascular (CV) symptoms. The frequency and intensity of anginal symptoms and precipitating factors that produce the angina are noted. Symptoms such as dyspnea, orthopnea, paroxysmal nocturnal dyspnea (PND), exercise capacity, and extremity edema may suggest possible left or right heart dysfunction. Recent hospital admissions, interventions, diagnostic tests, and specialist care can be informative, especially in patients who are poor historians. The patient's medications and any recent changes in his regimen or dosages are ascertained

The patient had coronary artery bypass grafting (CABG) 8 years ago after an MI. His last stress test was more than 5 years ago and he does not know the results. He has not had a cardiac catheterization since his surgery. He has occasional angina, usually at the end of his daily walks (one to two miles) or after climbing several flights of stairs. He has not had chest pain during the past month. He was last admitted to the hospital 2 years ago for HF. Since that admission he gets dyspneic "when he overexerts himself" (e.g., walking several flights of stairs). He denies orthopnea or PND when lying supine.

He takes lisinopril 5 mg, atenolol 50 mg, and atorvastatin 40 mg once a day. The dosages have been unchanged for several months. He took his atorvastatin last night and the atenolol and lisinopril this morning.

Obesity (See Chapter 13)

The preoperative history in obese patients focuses on the pulmonary system, the cardiovascular system, and related diseases such as OSA.

The patient denies a history of asthma, bronchitis, or pneumonia. He quit smoking 16 years ago but he has an 18 pack-year history (number of packs × number of years). His son says that his father snores, and in fact was diagnosed with OSA, but never used continuous positive airway pressure (CPAP). He has lost 40 pounds in the past year as recommend by his physician.

Because this case is scheduled for sedation with topical anesthesia, the ability of the patient to lie flat is important, especially given his history of HF and OSA.

The patient states that he sleeps on his side with two pillows under his head. His snoring is worse when he tries to lie flat. He had an esophagogastroduodenoscopy (EGD) a year ago without complications at an outpatient facility. He does not recall being intubated for the procedure.

Pacemaker (See Chapter 4)

The type, indication, dependency, and date of pacemaker placement must be determined. Most patients have a manufacturer's identification card with important information. The most recent interrogation and current programming are ascertained. Implantable cardioverter defibrillators (ICDs) must be differentiated from pacemakers, both commonly referred to as cardiac rhythm management devices (CRMDs) (29). Manufacturers can be contacted for information and perioperative recommendations.

The patient explains that the pacemaker was placed after his heart surgery because "his heart was not beating fast enough." His identification card shows that he has a dual-chamber pacemaker with ICD function. A note in the chart indicates that it was last interrogated 3 months ago and found to be functioning well, and the ICD has never discharged. The current programming for the device is not in the note.

Physical Examination

The physical examination focuses on the CV system, the pulmonary system, and the airway. The location of the CRMD should be determined.

The patient is 5 feet 10 inches tall and weighs 250 pounds. His HR is 70 bpm, respiratory rate is 18/minute, BP is 118/72 mm Hg, and oxygen saturation on room air is 98%. There are no orthostatic changes when the patient moves from lying to standing. The patient is able to lie flat on the examination table for 5 minutes with his head elevated 30 degrees.

He has a Mallampati class 2 airway with intact teeth. His mouth opening is 7 cm and thyromental distance is 8 cm with moderately limited flexion and extension of his neck. His neck circumference is 64 cm. No carotid bruits or JVD is noted.

Examination of his lungs and heart reveal no abnormalities. Pulses are equal in all extremities and no peripheral edema is noted. The CRMD is palpated over the left chest with no evidence of infection. The rest of the examination is unremarkable.

The physical examination confirms the history. The patient's BMI is 36, which is consistent with extreme obesity (see Chapter 13). He has no evidence of left heart failure (e.g., left heart gallop, crackles) or pulmonary hypertension with right heart failure (e.g., loud closure of P_2, gallop, murmur of tricuspid insufficiency, peripheral edema, JVD). Pulmonary hypertension is difficult to diagnose by physical examination unless it is severe. Most patients will have no physical findings and only mild symptoms. The range of motion of his cervical spine is limited, which is common in obese patients. His obesity and large neck are associated with OSA.

Diagnostic Testing

Diagnostic test results from 6 months ago are in the chart.

His complete blood count, electrolytes, BUN, and creatinine are normal and his ECG is consistent with ventricular pacing. Transthoracic echocardiogram (TTE) from 2 years ago shows a dilated left ventricle (LV), global hypokinesis, and an ejection fraction (EF) of 35%. The right ventricle (RV) was mildly dilated with normal function. There was mild mitral regurgitation (MR) and mild tricuspid regurgitation (TR). Doppler interrogation of the TR jet is consistent with a pulmonary artery systolic pressure of 26 mm Hg plus right atrial pressure. The inferior vena cava (IVC) has normal respiratory variation in size consistent with right atrial pressures <10 mm Hg.

Assessment

The patient has a history of MI with chronic stable angina (Canadian class II) and compensated ischemic cardiomyopathy. His daily activities are consistent with moderate functional capacity of at least 4 metabolic equivalents (METs). According to the ACC/AHA Guidelines for Preoperative Cardiac Evaluation for Noncardiac Surgery, previous MI, compensated HF, and mild angina are stable clinical risk factors of increased perioperative CV risk (7). He is scheduled for a low-risk surgical procedure. Patients who undergo low-risk noncardiac procedures (e.g., endoscopic, breast, cataract, superficial procedures) do not need further preoperative cardiac testing unless active cardiac conditions are present (4) (see Chapter 3).

The patient took his statin last night and atenolol this morning. As discussed in the first case, beta blockers and HMG-CoA reductase inhibitors likely reduce perioperative cardiac risk and taking them perioperatively is recommended (11,16). Taking his morning dose of lisinopril, an angiotensin-converting enzyme inhibitor (ACEI), is more controversial. Taking angiotensin receptor blockers (ARBs), such as losartan, on the day of surgery is also controversial (30,31). These drugs have beneficial effects on the heart and regional organ perfusion. But in patients who are chronically treated, these classes of drugs can cause intraoperative hypotension, especially during induction of anesthesia (32). The incidence and severity of hypotension with anesthesia may be associated with the patient's severity of hypertension, number of antihypertensive medications taken, dose and timing of the ACEI/ARB, and LV diastolic dysfunction. Patients taking an

ACEI are more dependent on intravascular volume for maintenance of BP than patients not taking an ACEI (30). Most hypotensive episodes can be treated with fluid, ephedrine, and/or phenylephrine. In rare instances, vasopressin may be necessary (30).

The patient's obesity and OSA are a concern. He may have restrictive lung disease with decreased lung compliance, which increases the work of breathing (4) (see Chapters 5 and 13). He may not be able to maintain adequate oxygenation with sedation or induction of anesthesia. Mask ventilation and endotracheal tube placement may be more difficult (33). Since the patient does not use CPAP and his OSA is untreated, he is at risk for obesity hypoventilation syndrome or, in severe cases, pulmonary hypertension with right heart failure (4).

The weight loss over the last year likely improved his OSA and respiratory compliance. The TTE from 2 years ago shows normal pulmonary artery pressure (PAP) and normal RV function. The patient was able to recline on the table during the physical examination, and he tolerated sedation for a previous EGD. However, EGDs are usually performed with the patient in the lateral position and may not reflect his tolerance of sedation when lying supine.

A preanesthetic interrogation of the CRMD should be performed (7,29). Placing a magnet on the device does not guarantee that the pacemaker will revert to an asynchronous mode nor disable the ICD. Various devices have different responses to magnet placement. The best way to clarify the effect of magnet placement is to call the manufacturer. Many patients have pacemakers with rate-adaptive functions that must be disabled perioperatively. There are multiple reports of abnormal rate-responsive pacing at the upper activity rate in response to electrocautery, mechanical ventilation, and monitoring devices (34). There are numerous reports of rate-responsive tachycardia in patients attached to monitors that use bioelectric impedance to measure respiratory rate through the ECG leads (35).

The ACC/AHA recommend interrogating pacemakers before and after surgery, disabling ICDs before surgery, and turning them on before a patient is discharged from the postanesthesia care unit (PACU). An external defibrillator must be available while the ICD is turned off. During preoperative interrogation of pacemakers in one study, 15.7% required intervention before an elective procedure (36). If the pacemaker has a rate-adaptive function, unexpected tachycardia in a patient with depressed ventricular function and/or CAD can be harmful. Likewise, an unexpected discharge from an ICD during an eye case could be disastrous.

No other preoperative laboratory testing is needed for this procedure. Laboratory testing solely because of surgery is rarely necessary for most low-risk procedures (see Chapter 2). If the history and physical examination indicate acute changes in the patient's health status, then laboratory tests may be needed. Routine medical testing before cataract surgery with sedation did not improve outcomes in a study that excluded patients who received general anesthesia or had an MI in the preceding 3 months (37). All patients had first seen a primary care physician who could order tests if deemed necessary regardless of the surgery.

Management

Given the low risk of this procedure, the patient's stable condition, and current medical therapy, no further preoperative medical evaluation is necessary (7). Interrogation of the CRMD is performed in the preoperative holding area.

Interrogation reveals that the patient is pacemaker dependent. The pacemaker is appropriately capturing and pacing and is programmed for rate-adaptive pacing. The ICD is programmed on and will respond to magnet placement. It has never discharged.

The ICD is disabled for the surgery and the rate-adaptive pacemaker function is suspended. Since the patient is pacemaker dependent, the CRMD is reprogrammed to an asynchronous mode based on a conversation with the manufacturer and cardiologist. Bipolar cautery should be used if cautery is necessary. Temporary pacing and an external cardioverter-defibrillator must be immediately available during the procedure. After surgery, the patient's CRMD must be reprogrammed and the pacing/ICD functions returned to their original settings before the patient leaves a monitored setting.

Because the patient took his lisinopril this morning, vasopressin should be readily available in the rare chance that hypotension develops and does not resolve with sympathetic agonists and/or fluids. He is likely to tolerate sedation without significant hypotension, and the procedure poses minimal risk for significant hemodynamic challenges. Because of his OSA and obesity, minimal sedation should be planned with comfort provided by topical or peribulbar anesthesia. Preparations should be made for the possibility of advanced airway management if the patient does not tolerate sedation or lying flat.

Extreme obesity alone is not an exclusion criterion for day-surgery cases. The proposed surgery and the patient's medical conditions are more important considerations (38). Caring for this patient in an ambulatory surgery environment should be safe if the above management conditions can be met (see Chapter 19.)

REFERENCES

1. McAnulty GR, Robertshaw HJ, Hall GM. Anaesthetic management of patients with diabetes mellitus. *Br J Anaesth.* 2000;85:80–90.
2. Haffner SM, Lehto S, Ronnemaa T, et al. Mortality from coronary heart disease in subjects with type 2 diabetes and in nondiabetic subjects with and without prior myocardial infarction. *N Engl J Med.* 1998;339:229–234.
3. Fox CS, Coady S, Sorlie PD, et al. Trends in cardiovascular complications of diabetes. *JAMA.* 2004;292:2495–2499.
4. Adams JP, Murphy PG. Obesity in anaesthesia and intensive care. *Br J Anaesth.* 2000;85:91–108.
5. American Diabetes Association. Standards of medical care in diabetes—2006. *Diabetes Care.* 2006;29(Suppl 1):S4–42.
6. Misbin RI, Green L, Stadel BV, et al. Lactic acidosis in patients with diabetes treated with metformin. *N Engl J Med.* 1998;338:265–266.
7. Fleisher LA, Beckman JA, Brown KA, et al. ACC/AHA guidelines for perioperative cardiovascular evaluation and care for

noncardiac surgery. *J Am Coll Cardiol*. 2007;50:e159–241. Available at: http://www.acc.org. Accessed September 28, 2007.

8. Grayburn PA, Hillis LD. Cardiac events in patients undergoing noncardiac surgery: shifting the paradigm from noninvasive risk stratification to therapy. *Ann Intern Med*. 2003;138:506–511.

9. Wilson SH, Fasseas P, Orford JL, et al. Clinical outcome of patients undergoing non-cardiac surgery in the two months following coronary stenting. *J Am Coll Cardiol*. 2003;42:234–240.

10. McFalls EO, Ward HB, Moritz TE, et al. Coronary-artery revascularization before elective major vascular surgery. *N Engl J Med*. 2004;351:2795–2804.

11. Fleisher LA, Beckman JA, Brown KA, et al. ACC/AHA 2006 guideline update on perioperative cardiovascular evaluation for noncardiac surgery: focused update on perioperative beta-blocker therapy: a report of the American College of Cardiology/American Heart Association Task Force on Practice Guidelines (writing committee to update the 2002 Guidelines on Perioperative Cardiovascular Evaluation for Noncardiac Surgery). *J Am Coll Cardiol*. 2006;47:2343–2355.

12. Warner ME, Contreras MG, Warner MA, et al. Diabetes mellitus and difficult laryngoscopy in renal and pancreatic transplant patients. *Anesth Analg*. 1998;86:516–519.

13. Langeron O, Masso E, Huraux C, et al. Prediction of difficult mask ventilation. *Anesthesiology*. 2000;92:1229–1236.

14. Mercker SK, Maier C, Neumann G, et al. Lactic acidosis as a serious perioperative complication of antidiabetic biguanide medication with metformin. *Anesthesiology*. 1997;87:1003–1005.

15. Lindenauer PK, Pekow P, Wang K, et al. Lipid-lowering therapy and in-hospital mortality following major noncardiac surgery. *JAMA*. 2004;291:2092–2099.

16. Kertai MD, Boersma E, Westerhout CM, et al. A combination of statins and beta-blockers is independently associated with a reduction in the incidence of perioperative mortality and nonfatal myocardial infarction in patients undergoing abdominal aortic aneurysm surgery. *Eur J Vasc Endovasc Surg*. 2004;28:343–352.

17. Tait AR, Malviya S. Anesthesia for the child with an upper respiratory tract infection: still a dilemma? *Anesth Analg*. 2005;100:59–65.

18. Orr RJ, Ramamoorthy C. Controversies in pediatric ambulatory anesthesia. *Anesthesiol Clin North Am*. 1996;14:767–780.

19. Maxwell LG. Age-associated issues in preoperative evaluation, testing, and planning: pediatrics. *Anesthesiol Clin North Am*. 2004;22:27–43.

20. Tait AR, Malviya S, Voepel-Lewis T, et al. Risk factors for perioperative adverse respiratory events in children with upper respiratory tract infections. *Anesthesiology*. 2001;95:299–306.

21. Cote CJ. The upper respiratory tract infection (URI) dilemma: fear of a complication or litigation? *Anesthesiology*. 2001;95:283–285.

22. Stark R, Iannaconne LR. Why the Jehovah's Witnesses grow so rapidly: a theoretical application. *Contemporary Religion*. 1997;12:133–157.

23. Benson KT. The Jehovah's Witness patient: considerations for the anesthesiologist. *Anesth Analg*. 1989;69:647–656.

24. Woolley S. Children of Jehovah's Witnesses and adolescent Jehovah's Witnesses: what are their rights? *Arch Dis Child.* 2005;90:715–719.
25. Practice advisory for preanesthesia evaluation: a report by the American Society of Anesthesiologists Task Force on Preanesthesia Evaluation. *Anesthesiology.* 2002;96:485–496.
26. Malviya S, D'Errico C, Reynolds P, et al. Should pregnancy testing be routine in adolescent patients prior to surgery? *Anesth Analg.* 1996;83:854–858.
27. Liu JH, Anderson KE, Willging JP, et al. Posttonsillectomy hemorrhage: what is it and what should be recorded? *Arch Otolaryngol Head Neck Surg.* 2001;127:1271–1275.
28. Goodnough LT, Shander A, Spence R. Bloodless medicine: clinical care without allogeneic blood transfusion. *Transfusion.* 2003;43:668–676.
29. Practice advisory for the perioperative management of patients with cardiac rhythm management devices: pacemakers and implantable cardioverter-defibrillators: a report by the American Society of Anesthesiologists Task Force on Perioperative Management of Patients with Cardiac Rhythm Management Devices. *Anesthesiology.* 2005;103:186–198.
30. Colson P, Ryckwaert F, Coriat P. Renin angiotensin system antagonists and anesthesia. *Anesth Analg.* 1999;89:1143–1155.
31. Groban L, Butterworth J. Perioperative management of chronic heart failure. *Anesth Analg.* 2006;103:557–575.
32. Comfere T, Sprung J, Kumar MM, et al. Angiotensin system inhibitors in a general surgical population. *Anesth Analg.* 2005;100:636–644.
33. Hiremath AS, Hillman DR, James AL, et al. Relationship between difficult tracheal intubation and obstructive sleep apnoea. *Br J Anaesth.* 1998;80:606–611.
34. Rozner MA, Nishman RJ. Electrocautery-induced pacemaker tachycardia: why does this error continue? *Anesthesiology.* 2002;96:773–774.
35. Hartman S, Rinia M, Kalkman C. Monitor-induced tachycardia in a patient with a rate responsive pacemaker. *Anaesthesia.* 2006;61:399–401.
36. Rozner MA, Roberson J, Nguyen AD. Unexpected high incidence of serious pacemaker problems detected by pre- and postoperative interrogations: a two-year experience. [Abstract]. *J Am Coll Cardiol.* 2004;43:113A.
37. Schein OD, Katz J, Bass EB, et al. The value of routine preoperative medical testing before cataract surgery. Study of Medical Testing for Cataract Surgery. *N Engl J Med.* 2000;342:168–175.
38. Davies KE, Houghton K, Montgomery JE. Obesity and day-case surgery. *Anaesthesia.* 2001;56:1112–1115.

Index

Page numbers followed by *f* indicate figure; those followed by *t* indicate table.